DRUG TARIFF

NATIONAL HEALTH SERVICE
ENGLAND AND WALES

MARCH 2007

**Compiled on behalf of the Department of Health
by the NHS Business Services Authority,
Prescription Pricing Division**

Available on the NHS Business Services Authority website at
www.nhsbsa.nhs.uk
or
www.ppa.org.uk

TSO: London

D0280137

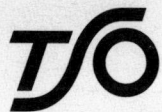

Published by TSO (The Stationery Office) and available from:

Online
www.tsoshop.co.uk

Mail, Telephone, Fax & E-mail
TSO
PO Box 29, Norwich, NR3 1GN
Telephone orders/General enquiries: 0870 600 5522
Fax orders: 0870 600 5533
E-mail: customer.services@tso.co.uk
Textphone: 0870 240 3701

TSO Shops
123 Kingsway, London, WC2B 6PQ
020 7242 6393 Fax 020 7242 6394
16 Arthur Street, Belfast BT1 4GD
028 9023 8451 Fax 028 9023 5401
71 Lothian Road, Edinburgh EH3 9AZ
0870 606 5566 Fax 0870 606 5588

TSO@Blackwell and other Accredited Agents

Technical Specifications are available singly from:
NHS Business Services Authority
Prescription Pricing Division
Bridge House
152 Pilgrim Street
Newcastle upon Tyne
NE1 6SN

ISBN 978-0-11-783162-9

ISSN 0962 3582

TO: General Medical Practitioners, Pharmacy Contractors, Appliance Contractors

PREFACE

AMENDMENTS TO THE DRUG TARIFF

March 2007

1. In accordance with regulation 56(1) of the National Health Service (Pharmaceutical Services) Regulations 2005, the Secretary of State for Health as respects England and in accordance with regulation 18(1) of the National Health Service (Pharmaceutical Services) Regulations 1992, the National Assembly for Wales have amended the Drug Tariff and as a consequence of article 4 of the National Health Service (Pre-Consolidation Amendments) Order 2006, determinations made in respect of the amendments to the Drug Tariff shall have effect from 1 March 2007.

    Before the Secretary of State and the National Assembly for Wales make further determinations they will consult with such organisations as appear to be representative of persons to whose remuneration the determination would relate and such other persons as they consider appropriate in respect of determinations which relate to persons providing pharmaceutical services, or a category of such services in accordance with section 165 of the National Health Service Act 2006 and section 89 of the National Health Service (Wales) Act 2006, regulations made under those sections and under section 164 of the National Health Service Act 2006 and section 88 of the National Health Service (Wales) Act 2006.

2. Please note that you are now being supplied each month with the Drug Tariff which incorporates all amendments to date. All entries showing a change in price are not specifically included in this preface but are indicated in the Drug Tariff by $\triangledown$ for price reduction and $\triangle$ for price increase; changes to the text relating to code, product description, or the inclusion of a new product are indicated by a vertical line in the margin.

3. While every effort is made to ensure that each monthly publication of the Drug Tariff includes all amendments made by the Secretary of State and the National Assembly for Wales to the price applicable to the relevant period, the need to observe printing deadlines sometimes defeats those efforts. Any omitted amendments will be effective from the date on which they came into force, even if publication of the details is unavoidably delayed.

4. **ADVANCE NOTICE**

4.1 **ADDITIONS TO APRIL 2007 DRUG TARIFF**

4.1.1 **ADDITIONS TO PART VIII EFFECTIVE FROM 1 APRIL 2007**

♦ **Calendar Pack**
■ **Special Container**

Bisoprolol 3.75mg tablets	♦	28	Category C *Cardicor*
Bisoprolol 7.5mg tablets	♦	28	Category C *Cardicor*
Cinchocaine 1mg/Prednisolone hexonate 1.3mg suppositories		12	Category C *Scheriproct*
Dimeticone 22%/Benzalkonium chloride 0.1% cream	■	100g	Category C *Conotrane*
		500g	Category C *Conotrane*
Doxepin 25mg capsules		28	Category C *Sinepin*
Doxepin 50mg capsules		28	Category C *Sinepin*
Hydrocortisone acetate 25mg/1ml suspension for injection ampoules		10	Category C *Hydrocortistab*
Hyoscine butylbromide 20mg/1ml solution for injection ampoules		10	Category C *Buscopan*
Ivabradine 5mg tablets	♦	56	Category C *Procoralan*
Ivabradine 7.5mg tablets	♦	56	Category C *Procoralan*

Olmesartan medoxomil 20mg/Hydrochlorothiazide 12.5mg tablets	28	Category C *Olmetec Plus*
Olmesartan medoxomil 20mg/Hydrochlorothiazide 25mg tablets	28	Category C *Olmetec Plus*
Propantheline bromide 15mg tablets	112	Category C *Pro-Banthine*
Ropinirole 250microgram tablets	12	Category C *Adartrel*
Ropinirole 500microgram tablets	12	Category C *Adartrel*
Salicylic acid 11%/Lactic acid 4% gel	■ 5g	Category C *Cuplex*
Salicylic acid 2% solution	■ 177ml	Category C *Acnisal*
Sulpiride 200mg/5ml oral solution sugar free	150ml	Category C *Sulpor*
Tramadol 50mg soluble tablets sugar free	20	Category C *Zydol*
	100	Category C *Zydol*
Trandolapril 1mg capsules	♦ 28	Category C *Gopten*

4.2   DELETIONS FROM APRIL 2007 DRUG TARIFF

4.2.1   DELETIONS FROM PART VIII EFFECTIVE FROM 1 APRIL 2007

*   **This pack only (others still available)**

Benzoyl peroxide 5% gel	40g	Category C
Clotrimazole 1%/Hydrocortisone 1% cream	30g	Category C
* Danazol 100mg capsules	100	Category M
Estradiol 150micrograms/dose nasal spray	60 dose	Category C
Macrogol 4000 10g oral powder sachets sugar free	20	Category C
* Naproxen 250mg tablets	250	Category M
Prochlorperazine 5mg suppositories	10	Category C
Triamcinolone 0.1% oromucosal paste	10g	Category C

4.2.2   DELETIONS FROM PART IX EFFECTIVE FROM 1 APRIL 2007

See Pages: 160, 182, 183, 185, 194, 220

4.3   OTHER CHANGES TO APRIL 2007 DRUG TARIFF

4.3.1   OTHER CHANGES TO PART VIII EFFECTIVE FROM 1 APRIL 2007

Aceclofenac 100mg tablets	60	Category C *Preservex* will be:
	60	Category A
Ammonia solution aromatic	500ml	Category A will be:
	500ml	Category C *Loveridge*
Betamethasone valerate 0.1% cream	100g	Category C *Betnovate* will be:
	100g	Category A
Betamethasone valerate 0.1% ointment	100g	Category C *Betnovate* will be:
	100g	Category A

---

5.   PART VIA - PAYMENT FOR ESSENTIAL SERVICES (PHARMACY CONTRACTORS)

Contractors should note a change to **paragraph 6.4**.

6.   PART IXA - APPLIANCES

Contractors should note changes to the layout of **Blom-Singer** Tracheostomy Breathing Aids.

PREFACE

---

7.   **PART IXB - INCONTINENCE APPLIANCES**

Contractors should note that certain **Incontinence Sheaths** which moved to be listed under **Rochester Medical Ltd** in February 2007 have been moved back to be listed under **Jade-Euro-Med**. The product names have also been changed back to their original names. Please also note new **additions** under **Rochester Medical Ltd**.

8.   **PART IXB - INCONTINENCE APPLIANCES AND PART IXC - STOMA APPLIANCES**

Contractors should note several products listed under **Coloplast Ltd** and **Mentor Medical Ltd** can now be found under **Jade-Euro-Med Ltd**.

9.   <u>**CHANGES TO MARCH 2007 DRUG TARIFF**</u>

9.1   **ADDITIONS TO MARCH 2007 DRUG TARIFF**

9.1.1 **PART II - REQUIREMENTS ENABLING PAYMENTS TO BE MADE FOR THE SUPPLY OF DRUGS, APPLIANCES AND CHEMICAL REAGENTS**

PAGE 12 - DRUGS FOR WHICH DISCOUNT IS NOT DEDUCTED
Enbrel 25mg/0.5ml solution for injection pre-filled syringes
Enbrel 50mg/1ml solution for injection pre-filled syringes
Enbrel Paediatric 25mg powder and solvent for solution for injection vials

PAGE 18 -
PKU cooler 10 liquid
PKU cooler 20 liquid
Presinex 10micrograms/dose nasal spray

9.1.2 **PART VIII - BASIC PRICES OF DRUGS**

■   **Special Container**
*   **This pack only (others already available)**

PAGE 90 -

Dipyridamole 50mg/5ml oral suspension sugar free		150	ml	3525	A

PAGE 99 -

Griseofulvin 125mg tablets		100		3380	A
Griseofulvin 500mg tablets		100		8760	A

PAGE 101 -

Indometacin 100mg suppositories		10		1091	A

PAGE 109 -

* Miconazole 2% / Hydrocortisone 1% cream	■	15	g	273	C	*Daktacort Hydrocortisone*

PAGE 131 -

Varenicline 1mg tablets	28		2730	C	*Champix*
Varenicline 500microgram tablets	56		5460	C	*Champix*

9.1.3 PART IXA - APPLIANCES

PAGE 137 - ATOMIZERS, HAND OPERATED
(b) Devices for use with Pressurised Aerosols
Spacer/Holding Chamber Devices
NebuChamber with child mask   856

PAGE 154 - CATHETERS, URINARY, URETHRAL
(C)(ii)(a)Foley Catheter - 2 Way For Long Term Use - Adult pack of 1
Coloplast Ltd
Folysil X-tra silicone   100% silicone with pre-filled syringe
          (Male)   (AA8112-AA8120)   10   12-20   597
          (Female)   (AA8512-AA8518)   10   12-18   597

PAGE 157 -
(C)(ii)(b) Foley Catheter - 2 Way For Long Term Use - Paediatric pack of 1
Coloplast Ltd
Folysil X-tra silicone   100% silicone with pre-filled syringe
          (Paediatric)   (AP8106-AP8110)   1.5   6-10   597

PAGE 161 - DRESSINGS
Absorbent Dressing Pads, Sterile
Xupad Dressing Pad   10cm x 20cm   17
                                                              20cm x 20cm   28
                                                              20cm x 40cm   40

PAGE 181 -
Wound Management Dressings
Polyurethane Foam Film Dressing - Sterile - With Adhesive BorderModerate to heavily exuding wounds
PolyMem
Square   15cm x 15cm   (wound contact pad 9cm x 9cm + border 3cm)   272
Rectangular   10cm x 13cm   (wound contact pad 5cm x 8cm + border 2.5cm)   202
Oval   5cm x 7.6cm   (wound contact pad 2.5cm x 5cm + irregular border)   107
              8.8cm x 12.7cm   (wound contact pad 5cm x 7.6cm + irregular border)   190
              16.5cm x 20.9cm (wound contact pad 10.1cm x 14.6cm + irregular border) 625
Sacral   18.4cm x 20cm   (wound contact pad 11.4cm x 12cm + border 3.5-4cm)   420

PAGE 182 -
Wound Management Dressings
Polyurethane Foam Film Dressing - Sterile - Without Adhesive Border Moderate to heavily exuding wounds
Kerraboot   Boot Shaped   Extra Small (Clear)   1427
                                                 Extra Small (White)   1427
                                                 Extra Large (Clear)   1427
                                                 Extra Large (White)   1427

PolyMem   Square   8cm x 8cm   147
                                                 10cm x 10cm   229
                                                 13cm x 13cm   382
                                Rectangular   17cm x 19cm   564
                                Roll   10cm x 61cm   1215

PAGE 183 -
PolyMem Max   Square   11cm x 11cm   275

PAGE 185 -
Wound Management Dressings
Soft Polymer Wound Contact Dressing
Urgotul   11cm x 11cm   292
                                                 16cm x 21cm   826

Soft Polymer Wound Contact Dressing Impregnated with Silver
Urgotul SSD   11cm x 11cm   289
                                                 16cm x 21cm   819

PREFACE

PAGE 187 -
Wound Management Dressings
Wound Drainage Pouch
Indications: Suitable for wounds with a high volume of exudate
Oakmed Option Wound Manager pack of 10

Extra Small (wounds upto 90mm x 180mm)	(WWM-XS)	10700
Large (wounds upto 160mm x 260mm)	(WWM-L)	14500
Extra Small with Access Port (wounds upto 90mm x 180mm)	(WWM-XSA)	11700
Large with Access Port (wounds upto 160mm x 260mm)	(WWM-LA)	15500

PAGE 194 - HYPODERMIC EQUIPMENT
F. Lancets - Sterile, Single-Use each

Unistik 3 Comfort	1.8mm/28 gauge	100	624
(Owen Mumford Ltd)		200	1220
Unistik 3 Normal	1.8mm/23 gauge	100	624
(Owen Mumford Ltd)		200	1220
Unistik 3 Extra	2.0mm/21 gauge	100	624
(Owen Mumford Ltd)		200	1220

G. Accessories

Sharpsafe	1 litre	85

PAGE 197 - LYMPHOEDEMA GARMENTS
Jobst Bellavar - Sahara

Style	Lengths	Sizes	
Class 2 (23-32mmHg)			Price per pair
Knee High, Open Toe	Short, Long	I, II, III, IV, V, VI	2550
Thigh High, Open Toe, With Knitted Band	Standard	I, II, III, IV, V, VI	4900
Thigh High, Open Toe, With Silicone Band	Standard	I, II, III, IV, V, VI	4900
Class 3 (34-46mmHg)			Price per pair
Knee High, Open Toe	Short, Long	I, II, III, IV, V, VI	2800

PAGE 199 -
Jobst Opaque

Style	Colour	Lengths	Sizes	
Class 1 (18-21mmHg)				Price per pair
Knee High Closed Toe	Black, Sand	Short, Long	I, II, III, IV, V, VI	2550
Knee High Open Toe	Black, Sand	Short, Long	I, II, III, IV, V, VI	2550
Thigh High Open Toe with Silicone Band Standard Width	Black, Sand	Short, Long	I, II, III, IV, V, VI	4900
Thigh High Open Toe with Silicone Band Wide Width	Black, Sand	Short, Long	I, II, III, IV, V, VI	4900
Class 2 (23-32mmHg)				Price per pair
Knee High Closed Toe	Black, Sand	Short, Long	I, II, III, IV, V, VI	2550
Knee High Open Toe	Black, Sand	Short, Long	I, II, III, IV, V, VI	2550
Thigh High Open Toe with Silicone Band Standard Width	Black, Sand	Short, Long	I, II, III, IV, V, VI	4900
Thigh High Open Toe with Silicone Band Wide Width	Black, Sand	Short, Long	I, II, III, IV, V, VI	4900

9.1.4 PART IXB - INCONTINENCE APPLIANCES

⊗ **Non-adhesive sheath without liner**
⊙ **Sheath with self-adhesive liner**
S **These leg bags are supplied sterile**

PAGE 224 - INCONTINENCE SHEATHS

Rochester Medical Ltd (formerly Coloplast Ltd, Mentor Medical Ltd & Rochester Medical Corporation)	⊙	Clear Advantage with Aloe silicone sheath, style 1 Standard			
		24mm	1243	30	4722
		28mm	1283	30	4722
		32mm	1323	30	4722
		36mm	1363	30	4722
		40mm	1403	30	4722
	⊙	Clear Advantage with Aloe silicone sheath, style 2 Pop-On			
		24mm	2243	30	4722
		28mm	2283	30	4722
		32mm	2323	30	4722
		36mm	2363	30	4722
		40mm	2403	30	4722
	⊙	Clear Advantage with Aloe silicone sheath, style 3 Wideband			
		24mm	3243	30	4722
		28mm	3283	30	4722
		32mm	3323	30	4722
		36mm	3363	30	4722
		40mm	3403	30	4722

PAGE 225 -

	⊗	Natural Clear Non-Adhesive Sheath			
		25mm (small)	38301	30	4471
		29mm (medium)	38302	30	4471
		32mm (intermediate)	38303	30	4471
		36mm (large)	38304	30	4471
	⊙	UltraFlex Clear Sheath (Self-adhesive)			
		small	33101	30	4471
		medium	33102	30	4471
		intermediate	33103	30	4471
		large	33104	30	4471
		ex-large	33105	30	4471

PAGE 232 - LEG BAGS

Manfred Sauer UK Ltd (formerly Manfred Sauer GmbH)

S	Smartflow Children's leg bag				
	210ml, direct inlet	CBDirectS	10	2748	
	210ml, 30cm adjustable inlet	CB30S	10	2748	

PAGE 241 - URINAL SYSTEMS

C S Bullen Ltd
Acti-Brief Uri-Drain System with 10 pouches
Sizes S, M, L, XL

Flange size	27.5mm	AB/18/27.5	1	2375
	32.5mm	AB/18/32.5	1	2375

Uri-Drain System with 10 pouches

Flange Size	27.5mm	LU/18/27.5	1	2375
	32.5mm	LU/18/32.5	1	2375

9.1.5 PART IXC - STOMA APPLIANCES

PAGE 390 - TWO PIECE OSTOMY SYSTEMS

Peak Medical   Combimate Colocap 2-piece stoma cap with high capacity filter

38mm flange	CCB238	30	3347
45mm flange	CCB245	30	3347
57mm flange	CCB257	30	3347

Combimate Softflex 2-piece Flange

38mm flange			
starter hole 13mm	FFB3813	5	1800
pre-cut 22mm	FFB3822	5	1800
pre-cut 25mm	FFB3825	5	1800
pre-cut 28mm	FFB3828	5	1800
45mm flange			
starter hole 13mm	FFB4513	5	1800
pre-cut 22mm	FFB4522	5	1800
pre-cut 25mm	FFB4525	5	1800
pre-cut 28mm	FFB4528	5	1800
pre-cut 32mm	FFB4532	5	1800
pre-cut 35mm	FFB4535	5	1800
57mm flange			
starter hole 13mm	FFB5713	5	1800
pre-cut 32mm	FFB5732	5	1800
pre-cut 35mm	FFB5735	5	1800
pre-cut 38mm	FFB5738	5	1800
70mm flange			
starter hole 13mm	FFB7013	5	1800

9.1.6 PART IXR - CHEMICAL REAGENTS

PAGE 412 - DETECTION STRIPS, BLOOD FOR GLUCOSE
Biosensor Strips - to be read only with the appropriate meter

* 2.2.10 Microdot		50	1296

* The manufacturer of this product does not provide additional free patient support services

9.1.7 PART XV - BORDERLINE SUBSTANCES

PAGE 442 - LIST A

Frebini Original Fibre Protein
    See: Frebini Original Fibre

PAGE 445 -
Gluten-Free Products (Not necessarily low-protein, lactose or sucrose free).
Innovative Solutions brown rice flour
Innovative Solutions potato flour
Innovative Solutions tapioca flour
Innovative Solutions white rice flour

PAGE 448 -
Innovative Solutions Products
    See: Gluten-Free Products

PAGE 456 -
Pku Express Cooler
    See: Pku Cooler 15

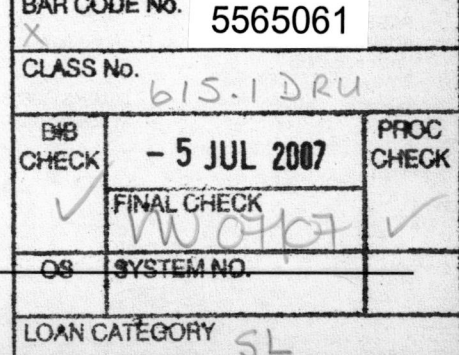

PAGE 458 -

Resource Energy Dessert
See: Resource Dessert Energy

9.2 DELETIONS FROM MARCH 2007 DRUG TARIFF

9.2.1 PART II - REQUIREMENTS ENABLING PAYMENTS TO BE MADE FOR THE SUPPLY OF DRUGS, APPLIANCES AND CHEMICAL REAGENTS

PAGE 15 - DRUGS FOR WHICH DISCOUNT IS NOT DEDUCTED
Ketek 400mg tablets

PAGE 20 -
Sustiva 50mg capsules

9.2.2 PART VIII - BASIC PRICES OF DRUGS

♦ **Calendar Pack**
● **Item Requiring Reconstitution**
* **This pack only (others still available)**

PAGE 80 -

* Carbamazepine 400mg tablets		28		735	M

PAGE 81 -

Cefaclor 250mg/5ml oral suspension	●	100	ml	990	A

PAGE 87 -

* Danazol 200mg capsules		100		7813	M

PAGE 121 -

Ranitidine bismuth citrate 400mg tablets	♦	14		1209	C	*Pylorid*

9.2.3 PART IXA - APPLIANCES

PAGE 156 - CATHETERS, URINARY, URETHRAL
(C)(ii)(a)Foley Catheter - 2 Way For Long Term Use - Adult
Tyco Healthcare (formerly The Kendall Company (UK) Ltd)

Ultramer	(Male) (1622-1M)	5	22	625
	(1420-1M)	30	20	625
	(Female) (1222-1F)	30	22	625

PAGE 157 -
(C)(ii)(b) Foley Catheter - 2 Way For Long Term Use - Paediatric
Unomedical Ltd
2 Way Foley All Silicone

(Paediatric)	(MMS43150605-MMS43151005)	1.5-3	6-10	560

9.2.4 PART IXB - INCONTINENCE APPLIANCES

PAGE 240 - TUBING AND ACCESSORIES

Mentor Medical Ltd	Plastic connector with tube	WS152-25-C	1	352

PAGE 245 - URINAL SYSTEMS

Jade-Euro-Med Ltd	Inner sheath	I/S	5	1430

9.2.5 PART IXC - STOMA APPLIANCES

♦ **Cloth Fabric**

PAGE 263 - BAG COVERS

Jade Euro Med Ltd	♦ Bag Cover	KM51	1	486

PAGE 331 - ILEOSTOMY (DRAINABLE) BAGS
Marlen USA
UltraLite Ileostomy Bag (formerly UltraLite Small Bag)

	Transparent starter hole	561312	15	3396

9.2.6 PART IXR - CHEMICAL REAGENTS

● **Please refer to manufacturer for availability**

PAGE 412 - DETECTION STRIPS, BLOOD FOR GLUCOSE
Biosensor Strips - to be read only with the appropriate meter

●	2.2.13	SeNova	50	1525

9.2.7 PART XVIIA - DENTAL PRESCRIBING

PAGE 507 -

Amphotericin Oral Suspension BP 100mg/ml

9.3   OTHER CHANGES TO MARCH 2007 DRUG TARIFF

PAGE 2 - DEFINITIONS

(j)   The term pharmacy means any premises where drugs are provided by a pharmacist as part of pharmaceutical services under section 41 (arrangements for pharmaceutical services) of the Act.

Now Reads

(j)   The term pharmacy means any premises where drugs are provided by a pharmacist as part of pharmaceutical services under section 126 (arrangements for pharmaceutical services) of the National Health Service Act 2006.

9.3.1 PART II - REQUIREMENTS ENABLING PAYMENTS TO BE MADE FOR THE SUPPLY OF DRUGS, APPLIANCES AND CHEMICAL REAGENTS

PAGE 11 - DRUGS FOR WHICH DISCOUNT IS NOT DEDUCTED
Doxorubicin Cytosafe 10mg/5ml solution for injection vials
Doxorubicin Cytosafe 50mg/25ml solution for injection vials
Now Reads

Doxorubicin 10mg/5ml solution for injection Cytosafe vials
Doxorubicin 50mg/25ml solution for injection Cytosafe vials

PREFACE

PAGE 13 -
Frebini Fibre liquid
Now Reads

Frebini Original Fibre liquid

Frebini liquid
Now Reads

Frebini Original liquid

PAGE 18 -
PKU express cooler liquid
Now Reads

PKU cooler 15 liquid

PAGE 24 - PRODUCTS INCLUDED IN CLAUSE 10B(III)
Liquid preparations for external use:

(a)	Oilatum Junior Bath Formula	(150ml and 300ml)
(a)	Oilatum Junior Emollient (Bath Oil) (Fragrance Free)	(250ml, 500ml and 1 litre)

Now Reads

(a)	Oilatum Junior Emollient Bath Additive	(150ml, 250ml, 300ml, 500ml and 1 litre)

9.3.2 PART VIII - BASIC PRICES OF DRUGS

■   **Special Container**

PAGE 97 -

Furosemide 20mg/5ml oral solution sugar free		150	ml	1207	C	*Frusol*

Now Reads

Furosemide 20mg/5ml oral solution sugar free		150	ml	1207	A	

PAGE 123 -

Sevelamer 800mg tablets	■	180	12276	C	*Renagel*

Now Reads

Sevelamer 800mg tablets		180	12276	C	*Renagel*

9.3.3 PART XIV - REWARD SCHEME - FRAUDULENT PRESCRIPTION FORMS

PAGE 432 - PHARMACISTS WHO ARE ELIGIBLE TO CLAIM A REWARD UNDER THE SCHEME SHOULD CONTACT:

England
Alan Harrison
NHSBSA, Counter Fraud
and Security Management Division
3rd Floor Sandyford House Archbold Terrace
Jesmond
Newcastle Upon Tyne
NE2 1DB
Freephone: 0800-068-6161
Tel: 0191-203-5738
Now Reads

England
Patient Fraud Support Unit
NHSBSA, CFSMS
2nd Floor Sandyford House
Archbold Terrace
Jesmond
Newcastle Upon Tyne
NE2 1DB
Freephone: 0800-068-6161
Tel: 0191-2046300

9.3.4 PART XV - BORDERLINE SUBSTANCES

PAGE 436 - LIST A

A.S. Saliva Orthana
    Patients suffering from a dry mouth as a result of having or having undergone radiotherapy or sicca syndrome/Xerostomia.
Now Reads

A.S. Saliva Orthana
    Patients suffering from xerostomia (dry mouth) as a result of having or having undergone radiotherapy or sicca syndrome.

PAGE 437 -

Biotene Oralbalance Dry Mouth Saliva Replacement Gel
    Patients suffering from a dry mouth as a result of having or having undergone radiotherapy or sicca syndrome/Xerostomia.
Now Reads

Biotene Oralbalance Dry Mouth Saliva Replacement Gel
    Patients suffering from xerostomia (dry mouth) as a result of having or having undergone radiotherapy or sicca syndrome.

PAGE 437 -

Bioxtra Gel Mouthspray
Bioxtra Moisturing Gel
    Patients suffering from a dry mouth as a result of having or having undergone radiotherapy or sicca syndrome/Xerostomia.
Now Reads

Bioxtra Gel Mouthspray
Bioxtra Moisturing Gel
    Patients suffering from xerostomia (dry mouth) as a result of having or having undergone radiotherapy or sicca syndrome.

PAGE 442 -

Frebini Original Fibre Protein
    As a sole source of nutrition, or as a nutritional supplement for children aged 1-6 years with disease-related malnutrition and/or growth failure, proven inflammatory bowel disease, following total gastrectomy, short bowel syndrome, intractable malabsorption, dysphagia, bowel fistulae, and for the pre-operative preparation of patients who are malnourished. Not to be prescribed for any child under one year.
Now Reads

Frebini Original Fibre (Formerly Frebini Original Fibre Protein)
    As a sole source of nutrition, or as a nutritional supplement for children aged 1-6 years with disease-related malnutrition and/or growth failure, proven inflammatory bowel disease, following total gastrectomy, short bowel syndrome, intractable malabsorption, dysphagia, bowel fistulae, and for the pre-operative preparation of patients who are malnourished. Not to be prescribed for any child under one year.

PAGE 443 -

Glandosane
    Patients suffering from a dry mouth as a result of having or having undergone radiotherapy or sicca syndrome/Xerostomia.
Now Reads

Glandosane
    Patients suffering from xerostomia (dry mouth) as a result of having or having undergone radiotherapy or sicca syndrome.

PAGE 450 -

Low-protein Products
Promin low-protein imitation rice pudding
Now Reads

Promin low-protein imitation rice pudding (apple, banana, strawberry and original flavours)

PAGE 451 -

Luborant Saliva Replacement
    Patients suffering from a dry mouth as a result of having or having undergone radiotherapy or sicca syndrome/Xerostomia.
Now Reads

Luborant Saliva Replacement
    Patients suffering from xerostomia (dry mouth) as a result of having or having undergone radiotherapy or sicca syndrome.

PAGE 452 -

Neocate
    Proven whole protein intolerance, short bowel syndrome, intractable malabsorption, and other gastrointestinal disorders where an elemental diet is specifically indicated.
Neocate Advance (Unflavoured, Banana Vanilla Flavour And Strawberry Vanilla Flavour)
    Proven whole protein intolerance, short bowel syndrome, intractable malabsorption, and other gastrointestinal disorders where an elemental diet is specifically indicated.
Now Reads

Neocate

Neocate Active (Unflavoured And Blackcurrant Flavour)

Neocate Advance (Unflavoured, Banana Vanilla Flavour And Strawberry Vanilla Flavour)
    Proven whole protein intolerance, short bowel syndrome, intractable malabsorption, and other gastrointestinal disorders where an elemental diet is specifically indicated.

PREFACE

Nepro
> Patients with chronic renal failure who are on haemodialysis or complete ambulatory peritoneal dialysis (CAPD), or patients with cirrhosis or other conditions requiring a high energy, low fluid, low electrolyte diet.

Now Reads

Nepro (Can, Ready To Hang And Tetrapak)
> Patients with chronic renal failure who are on haemodialysis or complete ambulatory peritoneal dialysis (CAPD), or patients with cirrhosis or other conditions requiring a high energy, low fluid, low electrolyte diet.

PAGE 456 -

Pku Express Cooler
> For use in the dietary management of phenylketonuria.

Now Reads

Pku Cooler 15 (Formerly Pku Express Cooler)
> For use in the dietary management of phenylketonuria.

PAGE 458 -

Resource Energy Dessert
> As a necessary nutritional supplement prescribed on medical grounds for:
> Short bowel syndrome, intractable malasorption, pre-operative preparation of patients who are undernourished, patients with proven inflammatory bowel disease, following total gastrectomy, dysphagia, bowel fistulae, disease-related malnutrition, continuous ambulatory peritoneal dialysis (CAPD) and haemodialysis. Not to be prescribed for any child under one year; use with caution for young children up to five years of age.

Now Reads

Resource Dessert Energy (Formerly Resource Energy Dessert)
> As a necessary nutritional supplement prescribed on medical grounds for:
> Short bowel syndrome, intractable malasorption, pre-operative preparation of patients who are undernourished, patients with proven inflammatory bowel disease, following total gastrectomy, dysphagia, bowel fistulae, disease-related malnutrition, continuous ambulatory peritoneal dialysis (CAPD) and haemodialysis. Not to be prescribed for any child under one year; use with caution for young children up to five years of age.

PAGE 458 -

Saliveze
Salivix Pastilles
> Patients suffering from a dry mouth as a result of having or having undergone radiotherapy or sicca syndrome/Xerostomia.

Now Reads

Saliveze
Salivix Pastilles
> Patients suffering from xerostomia (dry mouth) as a result of having or having undergone radiotherapy or sicca syndrome.

9.3.5   PART XVIIB(I) - NURSE PRESCRIBING

Page 510 - Medicinal Preparations
Emollient Bath Additives as listed below:
Oilatum Fragrance Free Junior
Now Reads

Oilatum Junior Emollient Bath Additive

This Page is Intentionally Blank

CONTENTS

DEFINITIONS

(a) Except where the context otherwise requires, the terms to which a meaning is assigned by the Regulations or the Terms of Service have the same meaning in this Tariff.

(b) The term contractor has the same meaning as chemist as defined in the Regulations.

(c)   A pharmacy contractor is a person with whom the Primary Care Trust (PCT) for England and Local Health Board (LHB) for Wales has made arrangements for the provision of pharmaceutical services in respect of the supply of drugs, appliances and chemical reagents.

(d) An appliance contractor is a person with whom the PCT for England and LHB for Wales has made arrangements for the provision of pharmaceutical services so far as it relates to the supply of appliances included within Part IXA/B/C of this Tariff.

(e) The term persons includes a body of persons corporate or unincorporate.

(f) The term Pricing Authority means, as the case may require, the NHS Business Services Authority (NHSBSA) or the Health Solutions Wales.

(g) The term appliances as used in this Tariff includes dressings.

(h) The term prescription refers to an item on a prescription form or dispensed in accordance with a repeatable prescription.

(i) The term prescription form includes, where appropriate, a repeatable prescription.

(j) The term pharmacy means any premises where drugs are provided by a pharmacist as part of pharmaceutical services under section 126 (arrangements for pharmaceutical services) of the National Health Service Act 2006.

In the preparation of this Tariff the Secretary of State for Health and the National Assembly for Wales have consulted the Pharmaceutical Services Negotiating Committee.

REQUIREMENTS FOR THE SUPPLY OF DRUGS, APPLIANCES AND CHEMICAL REAGENTS

CLAUSE 1   DRUGS
Any drug included in this Tariff or in the British National Formulary including the Nurse Prescribers' Formulary, Dental Practitioner's Formulary, European Pharmacopoeia, British Pharmacopoeia or the British Pharmaceutical Codex, supplied as part of pharmaceutical services, must comply with the standard or formula specified therein unless the prescriber has indicated to the contrary. Any drug supplied which is not so included must be of a grade or quality not lower than that ordinarily used for medicinal purposes.

CLAUSE 2   APPLIANCES
The only appliances which may be supplied as part of the pharmaceutical services are those listed in Part IXA/B/C, and Part X (see Clause 4 below), of the Tariff and which comply with the specifications therein. The items within Part IXA which are **not** prescribable on Forms FP10(CN) and FP10(PN) are annotated ⊗

CLAUSE 3   CHEMICAL REAGENTS
The only chemical reagents which may be supplied as part of the pharmaceutical services are those listed in Part IXR of the Tariff. The items within Part IXR which are **not** prescribable on forms FP10(CN) and FP10(PN) are annotated ⊗

CLAUSE 4   DOMICILIARY OXYGEN THERAPY SERVICE
The requirements for the supply of domiciliary oxygen and its associated appliances together with the arrangements for reimbursement of those contractors included on the PCT's for England and LHB's for Wales lists of contractors authorised to provide this service, are set out in Part X of the Tariff.

CLAUSE 5   CLAIMS FOR PAYMENT
Contractors shall endorse prescription forms as required in Clause 9 (Endorsement Requirements) of this Tariff. Contractors shall sort and despatch forms in such a manner as the PCT for England and LHB for Wales may direct. Contractors shall despatch the forms together with the appropriate claim form not later than the fifth day of the month following that in which the supply was made.

CLAUSE 5A   CLAIMS FOR PAYMENT - REPEAT DISPENSING SERVICES

A   Contractors shall endorse batch issues (rather than repeatable prescriptions) as required in Clause 9 (Endorsement Requirements) of this Tariff. In addition, a batch issue relating to drugs, appliances or chemical reagents which have been dispensed shall be stamped with the contractor's stamp and dated with the date on which the items were dispensed.

B   Contractors shall sort and despatch batch issues and repeatable prescriptions in such a manner as the Primary Care Trust may direct.

   (i)   Contractors shall despatch batch issues relating to drugs, appliances or chemical reagents which have been dispensed, together with the appropriate claim form, not later than the fifth day of the month following that in which the supply was made.

   (ii)   Contractors shall retain repeatable prescriptions until they have expired or are no longer required, and shall then despatch them (separately from the batch issues) in the month following that in which they expired or the contractor became aware that they were no longer required.

   (iii)   Contractors shall destroy any batch issues relating to drugs, appliances or chemical reagents which are not required, or which should not be dispensed, because the contractor has been notified to that effect by the doctor who issued them or because the relevant repeatable prescription has expired.

This Page is Intentionally Blank

REQUIREMENTS ENABLING PAYMENTS TO BE MADE FOR THE SUPPLY OF DRUGS, APPLIANCES AND CHEMICAL REAGENTS

CLAUSE 6   ****CALCULATION OF PAYMENTS**

A   Pharmacy Contractors

Payment for services provided by pharmacy contractors in respect of the supply of drugs, appliances and chemical reagents supplied against prescriptions at each separate place of business shall comprise:-

(i)   (a) The total of the prices of the drugs, appliances and chemical reagents so supplied calculated in accordance with the requirements of this Tariff.

LESS

*(b) An amount, based on the total of the prices at (i)(a) above, calculated from the table at Part V ("Deduction Scale").

AND

(ii)   The appropriate professional fee as set out in Part IIIA

AND

(iii)   The allowance for containers and specified measuring devices as set out in Part IV.

*NOTE 1

No deduction will be made in respect of prescriptions for items listed on page 9 to page 22 for which the contractor has not been able to obtain a discount:

**NOTE 2

(Wales only) Payments in respect of October 1999 to March 2000.

Contractors in agreement with LHBs in Wales who have notified the LHB that they accept the revised basis of calculation of payments for the period 1 October 1999 to 31 March 2000 set out in the National Assembly's offer letters on 20 November 2000 and 3 April 2001 shall be paid in accordance with the provisions of these letters.

B   Appliance Contractors

Payment for services provided by appliance contractors in respect of the supply of appliances so supplied against prescriptions at each separate place of business, shall comprise:-

(i)   The total of the prices of the appliances, calculated in accordance with Part IXA/B/C

PLUS

(ii)   An amount based on the number of prescriptions against which supply is made each month, calculated from the Table at Part VIB ("Oncost Allowance" scale) and applied to the total of the prices at (i) above.

PROVIDED THAT

(a)   Where prescription forms are received by the Pricing Authority from two or more contractors whose names are separately entered on the pharmaceutical list for the supply of appliances only in respect of the provision of services at the same place of business, all such prescription forms shall be aggregated for the purpose of the calculation as at (ii) above and the rate so calculated shall be applied to the total of the prices calculated in accordance with (i) above in respect of the prescriptions received from each of those persons.

(b)   A contractor's name shall not be entered on the Pharmaceutical List separately for the same place of business in respect of (1) the supply of appliances, (2) the supply of drugs and appliances, or (3) the supply of drugs, except in the case of a contractor for whom separate entries on the Pharmaceutical List relating to the same place of business were allowed prior to the first day of November 1961.

REQUIREMENTS ENABLING PAYMENTS TO BE MADE FOR THE SUPPLY OF DRUGS, APPLIANCES AND CHEMICAL REAGENTS

(c)   Where a contractor's name is entered on the Pharmaceutical List in respect of the provision of services at more than one place of business, the calculation as at (ii) above shall be made separately in relation to the total of the prices calculated in accordance with (i) above in respect of prescriptions received in respect of the services provided at each place of business.

AND

(iii)   The appropriate fees as set out in Part IIIB

CLAUSE 7   PAYMENTS FOR DRUGS, APPLIANCES AND CHEMICAL REAGENTS

A   The price on which payment is based for a quantity of a drug, appliance or chemical reagent supplied is calculated proportionately from the basic price (see Clause 8 - Basic Price).

B   Subject to the provisions of Clause 10 (Quantity to be supplied) payment will be calculated on the basis that the exact quantity ordered by the prescriber has been supplied.

C   Where a prescription form has been returned to the contractor for endorsement or elucidation and it is returned to the Pricing Authority unendorsed, or incompletely endorsed, or without further explanation, then the price for the drug, appliance or chemical reagent which it orders shall be determined by the Secretary of State for Health and the National Assembly for Wales.

D   If a contractor's overall supply of a product appears to justify payment being based on the cost of a larger size than that normally required pursuant to orders on prescription forms and notice has been given to that effect to the contractor, the basic price will be the price of that larger size, the prescription form being deemed to have been endorsed.

CLAUSE 8   BASIC PRICE

A   The basic price for those drugs, appliances and chemical reagents ordered by a name, or a synonym of that name, included in Parts VIII or IX shall be the price listed in the Drug Tariff.

B   In exceptional circumstances, where, in the opinion of the Secretary of State for Health and the National Assembly of Wales (NAW), there is no product available to contractors, at the price in Part VIII, claims for reimbursement for a product with a higher price than that listed may be accepted. Such claims shall be made by endorsement as set out in Clause 9C but only in the circumstances described in that Clause. If the Secretary of State for Health and the NAW are satisfied that the contractor was not able reasonably to obtain the product at a lower price, the basic price shall be the list price, for supplying to contractors, of the product and pack size so used, or such other price as the Secretary of State for Health and the NAW shall determine.
The Secretary of State for Health and the NAW will publish details of any preparations to which this applies and the month(s) in which it applies. The Secretary of State for Health and the NAW may in addition specify the products for which endorsement will be accepted.

C   The basic price for a drug which is not listed in Part VIII of the Tariff shall be the list price, for supplying to contractors, of the pack size to be used for a prescription for that quantity, published by the manufacturer, wholesaler or supplier. In default of any such list price, the price shall be determined by the Secretary of State for Health and the NAW.

REQUIREMENTS ENABLING PAYMENTS TO BE MADE FOR THE SUPPLY OF DRUGS, APPLIANCES AND CHEMICAL REAGENTS

CLAUSE 9   ENDORSEMENT REQUIREMENTS

A   Contractors shall endorse prescription forms for drugs, appliances and chemical reagents listed in this Tariff as required by this Clause and when so required by the provisions of Part II Clauses 10 (Quantity to be Supplied) and 11 (Broken Bulk), Part III (Fees) and Note 2 to Part IXA/B/C (Appliances).

B   Prescriptions for drugs not listed in Part VIII of the Tariff shall be endorsed by the contractor with the pack size from which the order was supplied and, if the order is in pharmacopoeial or 'generic' form, with the brand name or the name of the manufacturer or wholesaler from whom the supply was purchased. Where the preparation is in Part VIII of the Tariff and more than one pack size is listed, contractors shall endorse the pack size from which the order was supplied. Where the preparation is in Part VIII of the Tariff and only one pack size is listed, no endorsement of pack size is necessary. Where additional specific endorsement is necessary contractors shall endorse prescription forms when so required by the provisions of Part II Clauses 10 (Quantity to be Supplied) and 11 (Broken Bulk), Part III (Fees).

C   Where the preparation is in Part VIII of the Tariff and, as described in Clause 8B, in the opinion of the Secretary of State for Health and the NAW there is no product available to contractors at the appropriate price, endorsements of brand name or of manufacturer or wholesaler of the product and pack size so used may be accepted. Contractors shall not so endorse unless they have made all reasonable efforts to obtain the product at the appropriate price but have not succeeded. The endorsement shall be initialled and dated by or on behalf of the contractor, and shall be further endorsed "no cheaper stock obtainable" or "NCSO" to indicate that the contractor has taken all such responsible steps.

D   Where insufficient information is available to enable the Pricing Authority to process the prescription, the form shall be returned to the contractor who shall endorse the prescription form with the information requested.

E   Where a contractor supplies a quantity at variance with that ordered, ie under the provisions set out in Clause 10 (Quantity to be Supplied), the prescription shall be endorsed with the quantity supplied. An exception to this requirement is where a drug is supplied in a Calendar Pack and the quantity ordered differs from that pack. In such cases and in the absence of an endorsement to the contrary, the contractor will be deemed to have supplied the quantity available in the nearest number of packs or sub-packs to that ordered.

CLAUSE 10   QUANTITY TO BE SUPPLIED

A   Subject to the requirements of the Weights and Measures (Equivalents for Dealing with Drugs) Regulation, 1970, with regard to the supply in metric quantities of orders expressed in imperial quantities, payment will normally be calculated on the basis that the exact quantity ordered by the prescriber has been supplied, except only of those preparations referred to in B and C below:

B   **Drugs and Chemical Reagents in Special Containers.**

Where the quantity ordered by the prescriber does not coincide with that of an original pack and the drug or chemical reagent is:

(i)   Sterile

(ii)   Effervescent or hygroscopic, or

(iii)   (a) Liquid preparations for addition to bath water

(b) Coal Tar preparations

(c) Viscous external preparations

(iv)   Packed in a castor, collapsible tube, drop-bottle, pressurised aerosol, puffer pack, roll-on-bottle, sachet, shaker, spray, squeeze pack, container with an integral means of application, or any other container from which it is not practicable to dispense the exact quantity:

the contractor shall supply in the special container or containers the quantity nearest to that ordered and endorse the prescription form with the number and size of those containers. Although payment will normally be based on the quantity nearest to that ordered, some items are available in a larger size pack or container than that normally required pursuant to orders on prescription forms. Where the amount ordered on a prescription form, or the frequency of supply, justifies supply from such larger size pack or container, payment will be based on the cost of that larger size in the absence of endorsement.

REQUIREMENTS ENABLING PAYMENTS TO BE MADE FOR THE SUPPLY OF DRUGS, APPLIANCES AND CHEMICAL REAGENTS

C   **Manufacturers' Calendar Packs (including Oral Contraceptives)**

(i)   A manufacturer's calendar pack is a blister or strip pack showing the days of the week or month against each of the several units in the pack. Although payment is normally based on the number of packs or sub-packs nearest to the quantity ordered (see Clause 9E (Endorsement Requirements)) there may be occasions when, in the pharmacist's professional opinion, the prescriber's intention is that an exact quantity should be supplied. In such cases the contractor should supply accordingly and endorse the prescription form with the quantity supplied. Payment will then be based on the quantity shown by the endorsement.

(ii)   Payment for a Manufacturer's Calendar Pack or Original Pack will be based on the smallest pack size available when one or a number of such packs are ordered. Some original packs contain more than one monthly cycle and prescriptions ordering three or more such packs will be returned to the contractor for clarification.

* Products included in Clause 10B(iii) are listed on page 23 and 24.

CLAUSE 11   BROKEN BULK

A   This clause applies to drugs, incontinence and stoma appliances in Part IXB and IXC and chemical reagents other than items supplied in special containers covered by Clause 10B.

B   When the quantity ordered on a prescription form is other than the minimum quantity the manufacturer, wholesaler or supplier is prepared to supply and the contractor, having purchased such minimum quantity as may be necessary to supply the quantity ordered cannot readily dispose of the remainder, payment will be made for the whole of the quantity purchased. Subsequent prescriptions, received during the next six months, will be deemed to have been supplied from the remainder and no further payment will be made to drug costs other than fees and container allowances until that remainder has been used up. Thereafter contractors must endorse prescription forms to indicate when a claim for payment is being made.

CLAUSE 12   OUT OF POCKET EXPENSES

Where, in exceptional circumstances, out-of-pocket expenses have been incurred in obtaining a drug, appliance or chemical reagent other than those priced in Part VIII Category A and M, Part IXA and Part IXR of the Tariff and not required to be frequently supplied by the contractor, or where out-of-pocket expenses have been incurred in obtaining oxygen from a manufacturer, wholesaler or supplier specially for supply against a prescription, payment of the amount by which such expenses on any occasion exceed 10p may be made where the contractor sends a claim giving full particulars to the Pricing Authority with the appropriate prescription form.

CLAUSE 13   DRUG PREPARATIONS REQUIRING RECONSTITUTION FROM GRANULES OR POWDER

A   This clause applies to a drug preparation requiring reconstitution from granules or powder by the contractor and resulting in a liquid of limited stability.

B   When the quantity reconstituted from an original pack or packs is unavoidably greater than the quantity ordered, and it has not been possible for the contractor to use the remainder for or towards supplying against another prescription (See "CLAUSE 11 BROKEN BULK" on page 8.) payment, which attracts the standard professional fee (but see also Part IIIA, 2D), will be calculated from the Basic Price of the preparation and will be based on the nearest pack or number of packs necessary to cover the quantity ordered.

REQUIREMENTS ENABLING PAYMENTS TO BE MADE FOR THE SUPPLY OF DRUGS, APPLIANCES AND CHEMICAL REAGENTS

Drugs for which discount is not deducted

Contractors who have not received discount in respect of the following products need not endorse the prescription. The prescription price reimbursement will have no discount deduction applied.
However, there is an exception for specials.

For specials and other unlicensed medicines sourced from within the UK on a named-patient basis, other than those containing Controlled Drugs in schedules 1, 2 and 3 of the Misuse of Drugs Regulations 2001, where discount has not been obtained from the supplier, contractors need to endorse 'DNG' for 'discount not given' to avoid discount being removed.

If discount was obtained by the contractor no endorsement should be made.

"Specials"
Specials are unlicensed relevant medicinal products for human use which have been specially prepared to meet a prescription ordered for individual patients without the need for the manufacturer to hold a marketing authorisation for the medicinal product concerned.

Items sourced from outside the UK
All specials and other unlicensed medicines sourced from outside the UK for supply on a named-patient basis should be endorsed 'DNG' if discount has not been obtained, irrespective of whether they contain Controlled Drugs.

Acetic acid 33% liquid
Acetic acid dilute 420microlitres/5ml oral solution sugar free
Acetic acid glacial
Aciclovir 400mg/5ml oral suspension sugar free
Actinac lotion
Additrace solution for injection 10ml ampoules
Ainsworth special solution for injection 1ml ampoule
Alprostadil 40microgram powder and solvent for solution for injection vials
Ametop 4% gel
Ametop 4% gel dispensing pack
Aminogran Food Supplement powder
Aminogran PKU 1g tablets
Ammonaps 500mg tablets
Ammonaps 940mg/g granules
Ammonia solution strong
Ammonium chloride powder
Anapen Junior 150micrograms/0.3ml (1 in 2,000) solution for injection auto-injectors
Andropatch 5mg/24hours patches
Anectine 100mg/2ml solution for injection ampoules
Anise water concentrated
APO-go 20mg/2ml solution for injection ampoules
APO-go 50mg/5ml solution for injection ampoules
APO-go PEN 30mg/3ml solution for injection
APO-go PFS 50mg/10ml solution for infusion pre-filled syringes
Aptivus 250mg capsules
Aquasol A 100,000units/2ml solution for injection ampoules
Aranesp 100micrograms/0.5ml solution for injection pre-filled syringes
Aranesp 10micrograms/0.4ml solution for injection pre-filled syringes
Aranesp 150micrograms/0.3ml solution for injection pre-filled syringes
Aranesp 15micrograms/0.375ml solution for injection pre-filled syringes
Aranesp 20micrograms/0.5ml solution for injection pre-filled syringes
Aranesp 300micrograms/0.6ml solution for injection pre-filled syringes
Aranesp 30micrograms/0.3ml solution for injection pre-filled syringes
Aranesp 40micrograms/0.4ml solution for injection pre-filled syringes
Aranesp 500micrograms/1ml solution for injection pre-filled syringes
Aranesp 50micrograms/0.5ml solution for injection pre-filled syringes
Aranesp 60micrograms/0.3ml solution for injection pre-filled syringes
Aranesp 80micrograms/0.4ml solution for injection pre-filled syringes

REQUIREMENTS ENABLING PAYMENTS TO BE MADE FOR THE SUPPLY OF DRUGS, APPLIANCES AND CHEMICAL REAGENTS

Drugs for which discount is not deducted

Aranesp SureClick 100micrograms/0.5ml solution for injection pre-filled disposable devices
Aranesp SureClick 150micrograms/0.3ml solution for injection pre-filled disposable devices
Aranesp SureClick 20micrograms/0.5ml solution for injection pre-filled disposable devices
Aranesp SureClick 300micrograms/0.6ml solution for injection pre-filled disposable devices
Aranesp SureClick 40micrograms/0.4ml solution for injection pre-filled disposable devices
Aranesp SureClick 500micrograms/1ml solution for injection pre-filled disposable devices
Aranesp SureClick 60micrograms/0.3ml solution for injection pre-filled disposable devices
Aranesp SureClick 80micrograms/0.4ml solution for injection pre-filled disposable devices
Arixtra 10mg/0.8ml solution for injection pre-filled syringes
Arixtra 2.5mg/0.5ml solution for injection pre-filled syringes
Arixtra 5mg/0.4ml solution for injection pre-filled syringes
Arixtra 7.5mg/0.6ml solution for injection pre-filled syringes
Arnica tincture
Atimos Modulite 12micrograms/dose inhaler
Ativan 4mg/1ml solution for injection ampoules
Atracurium besilate 250mg/25ml solution for injection vials
Atracurium besilate 25mg/2.5ml solution for injection ampoules
Atracurium besilate 50mg/5ml solution for injection ampoules
Avandamet 4mg/1000mg tablets
Avonex 30microgram powder and solvent for solution for injection vials
Avonex 30micrograms/0.5ml solution for injection pre-filled syringes
Baraclude 0.5mg tablets
Baraclude 1mg tablets
Becodisks 400microgram & Diskhaler
Becodisks 400microgram refill pack
BeneFIX 1,000unit powder and solvent for solution for injection vials
BeneFIX 250unit powder and solvent for solution for injection vials
BeneFIX 500unit powder and solvent for solution for injection vials
Benzocaine powder
Benzoic acid powder
Benzoin compound tincture
Benzoin tincture
Benzoyl peroxide 5% / Clindamycin 1% gel
Benzyl benzoate 25% application
Benzyl benzoate crystals
Betaferon 300microgram powder and solvent for solution for injection vials
Bisacodyl 10mg/37ml rectal tube
Bismuth subnitrate and Iodoform paste
Bismuth subnitrate and Iodoform paste 30g sachets
Bismuth subnitrate powder
Bondronat 6mg/6ml concentrate for solution for infusion vials
Botox 100unit powder for solution for injection vials
Brochlor 0.5% eye drops
Caffeine citrate powder
Calamine and coal tar ointment
Calcitonin (salmon) 200 units/dose nasal spray
Calcium carbonate 250mg dispersible tablets
Calcium folinate 50mg/5ml solution for injection ampoules
Camphor racemic powder
Camphor water concentrated
Cancidas 50mg powder for solution for injection vials
Cancidas 70mg powder for solution for injection vials
Caprilon powder
Capsicum tincture
Cardamom compound tincture
Catapres TTS 1 patches
Catapres TTS 2 patches
Caverject 40microgram powder and solvent for solution for injection vials
Cerezyme 200unit powder for solution for injection vials
Cerezyme 400unit powder for solution for injection vials
Cetrimide powder

REQUIREMENTS ENABLING PAYMENTS TO BE MADE FOR THE SUPPLY OF DRUGS, APPLIANCES AND CHEMICAL REAGENTS

Drugs for which discount is not deducted

Chloral hydrate crystals
Chloramphenicol 0.5% eye drops
Chloramphenicol 10% ear drops
Chloramphenicol 5% ear drops
Chlorhexidine gluconate 0.5% solution
Chlorhexidine gluconate 4% solution
Chlorocresol powder
Chloroform liquid
Chloroform and morphine tincture
Chloroform spirit
Chloroform water concentrated
Chloromycetin Redidrops 0.5%
Citric acid monohydrate powder
Citronella oil liquid
Clexane 100mg/1ml solution for injection pre-filled syringes
Clexane 20mg/0.2ml solution for injection pre-filled syringes
Clexane 40mg/0.4ml solution for injection pre-filled syringes
Clexane 60mg/0.6ml solution for injection pre-filled syringes
Clexane 80mg/0.8ml solution for injection pre-filled syringes
Clexane Forte 120mg/0.8ml solution for injection pre-filled syringes
Clexane Forte 150mg/1ml solution for injection pre-filled syringes
Clomethiazole 250mg/5ml oral solution sugar free
Clove oil liquid
Clozaril 100mg tablets
Coal tar solution
Coal tar solution strong
Combivir tablets
Comminuted chicken meat
Controlled Drugs in schedules 1, 2 and 3 of the Misuse of Drugs Regulations 2001
Copaxone 20mg powder and solvent for solution for injection vials
Copaxone 20mg/1ml solution for injection pre-filled syringes
Copper sulphate pentahydrate powder
Crystal violet powder BP 1980
Cubicin 350mg powder for concentrate for solution for infusion vials
Cyclopentolate 0.5% eye drops
Cyclopentolate 1% eye drops
Cystagon 150mg capsules
Cystagon 50mg capsules
Cytotoxic or Cytostatic items
Daktacort cream
DDAVP 100micrograms/ml intranasal solution
DDAVP 4micrograms/1ml solution for injection ampoules
Decapeptyl SR 11.25mg powder and solvent for suspension for injection vials
Decapeptyl SR 3mg powder and solvent for suspension for injection vials
Denzapine 100mg tablets
Desferal 500mg powder for solution for injection vials
Desmopressin 100micrograms/ml intranasal solution
Dialamine powder
Diethylstilbestrol 5mg tablets
Digibind 38mg powder for solution for injection vials
Dithranol powder
Doxorubicin 10mg/5ml solution for injection Cytosafe vials
Doxorubicin 50mg/25ml solution for injection Cytosafe vials
Duac Once Daily gel
Duodupa intestinal gel 100ml cassette
Dysport 500unit powder for solution for injection vials
Easiphen liquid
Eldoquin 4% cream
Elemental 028 Extra liquid
Elemental 028 Extra powder
Elemental 028 powder

REQUIREMENTS ENABLING PAYMENTS TO BE MADE FOR THE SUPPLY OF DRUGS, APPLIANCES AND CHEMICAL REAGENTS

Drugs for which discount is not deducted

Elmiron 100mg capsules
Emsogen powder
Emtriva 10mg/ml oral solution
| Enbrel 25mg/0.5ml solution for injection pre-filled syringes
Enbrel 25mg powder and solvent for solution for injection vials
| Enbrel 50mg/1ml solution for injection pre-filled syringes
Enbrel 50mg powder and solvent for solution for injection vials
| Enbrel Paediatric 25mg powder and solvent for solution for injection vials
Energivit powder
Enoxaparin sodium 100mg/ml solution for injection pre-filled syringes
Enoxaparin sodium 120mg/0.8ml solution for injection pre-filled syringes
Enoxaparin sodium 150mg/1ml solution for injection pre-filled syringes
Enoxaparin sodium 20mg/0.2ml solution for injection pre-filled syringes
Enoxaparin sodium 40mg/0.4ml solution for injection pre-filled syringes
Enoxaparin sodium 60mg/0.6ml solution for injection pre-filled syringes
Enoxaparin sodium 80mg/0.8ml solution for injection pre-filled syringes
Enrich liquid
Enrich Plus liquid
EpiPen Jr. 150micrograms/0.3ml (1 in 2,000) solution for injection auto-injectors
Epivir 150mg tablets
Epivir 300mg tablets
Eprex 1,000units/0.5ml solution for injection pre-filled syringes
Eprex 10,000units/1ml solution for injection pre-filled syringes
Eprex 2,000units/0.5ml solution for injection pre-filled syringes
Eprex 3,000units/0.3ml solution for injection pre-filled syringes
Eprex 4,000units/0.4ml solution for injection pre-filled syringes
Eprex 40,000units/1ml solution for injection vials
Eprex 5,000units/0.5ml solution for injection pre-filled syringes
Eprex 6,000units/0.6ml solution for injection pre-filled syringes
Eprex 8,000units/0.8ml solution for injection pre-filled syringes
Ergometrine 500micrograms/1ml solution for injection ampoules
Esmeron 100mg/10ml solution for injection vials
Esmeron 50mg/5ml solution for injection vials
Estracyt 140mg capsules
Ethanol 70% duty paid
Ethanol 90% including duty
Ethanol Absolute Duty Paid
Ether solvent
Etopophos 100mg powder for solution for injection vials
Eucalyptus oil liquid
Evotrox 100micrograms/5ml oral solution
Evotrox 25micrograms/5ml oral solution
Evotrox 50micrograms/5ml oral solution
Fabrazyme 5mg powder for solution for injection vials
Fabrazyme 35mg powder for solution for injection vials
Fanhdi 1,000unit powder and solvent for solution for injection vials
Fanhdi 500unit powder and solvent for solution for injection vials
Faslodex 250mg/5ml solution for injection pre-filled syringes
Fasturtec 1.5mg powder and solvent for solution for injection vials
Fasturtec 7.5mg powder and solvent for solution for injection vials
Ferric chloride solution
Ferrous sulphate heptahydrate powder
Fibrogammin P 250unit powder and solvent for solution for injection vials
Flexible collodion methylated
Floxapen 1g powder for solution for injection vials
Fluticasone 500micrograms/dose/Salmeterol 50micrograms/dose dry powder inhaler
Formaldehyde solution
Forsteo 20micrograms/80microlitres solution for injection 3ml pre-filled disposable devices
Fortini liquid
Fortini Multifibre liquid
Fortisip Multi Fibre liquid

REQUIREMENTS ENABLING PAYMENTS TO BE MADE FOR THE SUPPLY OF DRUGS, APPLIANCES AND CHEMICAL REAGENTS

Drugs for which discount is not deducted

Fortum 1g powder for solution for injection vials
Fortum 250mg powder for solution for injection vials
Fortum 2g powder for solution for injection vials
Fortum 3g powder for solution for injection vials
Fortum 500mg powder for solution for injection vials
Fortum Monovial 2g powder for solution for injection vials
Fostimon 150unit powder and solvent for solution for injection vials
Fostimon 75unit powder and solvent for solution for injection vials
Fragmin 12,500units/0.5ml solution for injection pre-filled syringes
Frebini Energy Drink
Frebini Energy Fibre liquid
Frebini Energy Fibre liquid neutral
Frebini Energy liquid
Frebini Original Fibre liquid
Frebini Original liquid
Fresubin 1000 Complete liquid
Fresubin 1200 Complete liquid
Fresubin Energy Fibre liquid
Fresubin Energy liquid
Fresubin HP Energy liquid
Fresubin Original Fibre liquid
Fresubin Original liquid
Fungizone Intravenous 50mg powder for solution for injection vials
Galactomin 17 powder
Galactomin 19 powder
Generaid Plus powder
Genotropin 12mg powder and solvent for solution for injection cartridges
Genotropin 5.3mg powder and solvent for solution for injection cartridges
Genotropin MiniQuick 1.2mg powder and solvent for solution for injection pre-filled disposable devices
Genotropin MiniQuick 1.4mg powder and solvent for solution for injection pre-filled disposable devices
Genotropin MiniQuick 1.6mg powder and solvent for solution for injection pre-filled disposable devices
Genotropin MiniQuick 1.8mg powder and solvent for solution for injection pre-filled disposable devices
Genotropin MiniQuick 1mg powder and solvent for solution for injection pre-filled disposable devices
Genotropin MiniQuick 200microgram powder and solvent for solution for injection pre-filled disposable devices
Genotropin MiniQuick 2mg powder and solvent for solution for injection pre-filled disposable devices
Genotropin MiniQuick 400microgram powder and solvent for solution for injection pre-filled disposable devices
Genotropin MiniQuick 600microgram powder and solvent for solution for injection pre-filled disposable devices
Genotropin MiniQuick 800microgram powder and solvent for solution for injection pre-filled disposable devices
Ginger tincture strong
Glivec 100mg capsules
Glivec 100mg tablets
Glivec 400mg tablets
GlucaGen Hypokit 1mg powder and solvent for solution for injection
Gonal-f 1050unit powder and solvent for solution for injection vials
Gonal-f 300units/0.5ml solution for injection pre-filled syringes
Gonal-f 450unit powder and solvent for solution for injection vials
Gonal-f 450units/0.75ml solution for injection pre-filled syringes
Gonal-f 75unit powder and solvent for solution for injection ampoules
Gonal-f 75unit powder and solvent for solution for injection vials
Gonal-f 900units/1.5ml solution for injection pre-filled syringes
Gonapeptyl Depot 3.75mg powder and solvent for suspension for injection pre-filled disposable devices
Granocyte-13 powder and solvent for solution for injection vials
Granocyte-34 powder and solvent for solution for injection vials
Guaifenesin powder
Gutron 2.5mg tablets
Haemate P 1,000unit powder and solvent for solution for injection vials
Haemate P 500unit powder and solvent for solution for injection vials
HCU gel oral powder 20g sachets
Helixate NexGen 1,000unit powder and solvent for solution for injection vials
Helixate NexGen 250unit powder and solvent for solution for injection vials
Helixate NexGen 500unit powder and solvent for solution for injection vials

REQUIREMENTS ENABLING PAYMENTS TO BE MADE FOR THE SUPPLY OF DRUGS, APPLIANCES AND CHEMICAL REAGENTS

Drugs for which discount is not deducted

Hemabate 250micrograms/1ml solution for injection ampoules
Heminevrin 250mg/5ml syrup
Hepsera 10mg tablets
Humatrope 1.3mg powder and solvent for solution for injection vials
Humatrope 12mg powder and solvent for solution for injection cartridges
Humatrope 24mg powder and solvent for solution for injection cartridges
Humatrope 5.3mg powder and solvent for solution for injection vials
Humatrope 6mg powder and solvent for solution for injection cartridges
Humira 40mg/0.8ml solution for injection pre-filled syringes
Hydrocortisone powder
Hydrogen peroxide 6% solution
Hydrogen peroxide 9% solution
Hydrogen peroxide 35% solution

Ichthammol liquid
Imigran Radis 100mg tablets
Imigran Subject 6mg/0.5ml solution for injection pre-filled syringes
Imigran Subject 6mg/0.5ml solution for injection syringe refill pack
ImmuCyst 81mg powder for reconstitution for instillation vials
Immukin 100micrograms/0.5ml solution for injection vials
Immunoglobulins
Industrial methylated spirit 70%
Industrial methylated spirit 95%
Industrial methylated spirit 99%
Infatrini liquid
Innohep 10,000units/0.5ml solution for injection pre-filled syringes
Innohep 14,000units/0.7ml solution for injection pre-filled syringes
Innohep 18,000units/0.9ml solution for injection pre-filled syringes
Innohep 20,000units/2ml solution for injection vials
Innohep 4,500units/0.45ml solution for injection pre-filled syringes
Innohep 40,000units/2ml solution for injection vials
Insulins for Injection
Integrilin 20mg/10ml solution for injection vials
Integrilin 75mg/100ml solution for injection vials
IntronA 10million unit powder and solvent for solution for injection vials
IntronA 18million units/1.2ml solution for injection multidose pens
IntronA 25million units/2.5ml solution for injection multidose vials
IntronA 30million units/1.2ml solution for injection multidose pens
IntronA 3million unit powder and solvent for solution for injection vials
IntronA 60million units/1.2ml solution for injection multidose pens
Invicorp 1 solution for injection
Invicorp 2 solution for injection
Iodine alcoholic solution
Iodine aqueous oral solution
Iodine solution strong
Iodoform powder BPC 1954
Iodoform compound paint BPC 1954
Ipecacuanha liquid extract
Iscador 1ml solution for injection ampoules
Iscador oral drops
Iscador M solution for injection ampoules
Isoleucine Amino Acid supplement oral powder 4g sachets
Isopropyl alcohol 70% / Triclosan 0.5% topical solution
Isopropyl alcohol liquid
Isosource Energy Fibre liquid
Isosource Energy liquid
Isosource Fibre liquid
Isosource Junior liquid
Isosource Standard liquid
Jevity 1.5kcal liquid
Jevity liquid
Jevity Plus liquid

REQUIREMENTS ENABLING PAYMENTS TO BE MADE FOR THE SUPPLY OF DRUGS, APPLIANCES AND CHEMICAL REAGENTS

Drugs for which discount is not deducted

Kaletra 133.3mg/33.3mg capsules
Kaletra 80mg/20mg/1ml oral solution
Ketalar 1g/10ml solution for injection vials
Ketalar 200mg/20ml solution for injection vials
Ketalar 500mg/10ml solution for injection vials
KetoCal powder
Ketovite liquid
Ketovite tablets
Kindergen powder
Kineret 100mg/0.67ml solution for injection pre-filled syringes
Kivexa 600mg/300mg tablets
Kogenate Bayer 1,000unit powder and solvent for solution for injection vials
Kogenate Bayer 250unit powder and solvent for solution for injection vials
Kogenate Bayer 500unit powder and solvent for solution for injection vials

Lactic acid liquid
Lamictal 100mg dispersible tablets
Lamictal 100mg tablets
Lamictal 200mg tablets
Lamotrigine 100mg dispersible tablets
Lamotrigine 100mg tablets
Lamotrigine 200mg tablets
Lanvis 40mg tablets
LarvE
Latanoprost 50micrograms/ml eye drops
Lavender oil liquid
Lederfolin 350mg/35ml solution for injection vials
Lemon spirit
Levothyroxine Sodium 100mcg/5ml oral solution sugar free
Levothyroxine Sodium 25mcg/5ml oral solution sugar free
Levothyroxine Sodium 50mcg/5ml oral solution sugar free
Liquigen emulsion
Locasol powder
MabCampath 30mg/1ml concentrate for solution for infusion vials
MabThera 100mg/10ml concentrate for solution for infusion vials
MabThera 500mg/50ml concentrate for solution for infusion vials
Macugen 300micrograms/0.09ml solution for injection pre-filled syringes
Magenta powder
Magnesiocard tablets
Malarone tablets
Mapleflex oral powder 29g sachets
Mastic compound paste
MCT Pepdite powder
Mefenamic acid 50mg/5ml oral suspension
Melatonin 2.5mg capsules
Melatonin 2mg capsules
Melatonin 3mg capsules
Melatonin 5mg capsules
Menopur 75unit powder and solvent for solution for injection vials
Menthol crystals
Merional 150unit powder and solvent for solution for injection vials
Merional 75unit powder and solvent for solution for injection vials
Meronem 1g powder for solution for injection vials
Meronem 500mg powder for solution for injection vials
Mestinon retard 180mg tablets
Metformin 1g/Rosiglitazone 4mg tablets
Methyl salicylate 25% liniment
Methyl salicylate 50% ointment
Metvix 16% cream
Miacalcic 100units/1ml solution for injection ampoules
Miacalcic 200units/dose nasal spray
Miacalcic 400units/2ml multidose solution for injection vials

REQUIREMENTS ENABLING PAYMENTS TO BE MADE FOR THE SUPPLY OF DRUGS, APPLIANCES AND CHEMICAL REAGENTS

Drugs for which discount is not deducted

Miacalcic 50units/1ml solution for injection ampoules
Miconazole 2% / Hydrocortisone 1% cream
Midodrine 5mg tablets
Midon 2.5mg tablets
Milupa PKU 2 granules
Milupa PKU 3 granules
Milupa Prejomin granules
Mimpara 30mg tablets
Mimpara 60mg tablets
Mimpara 90mg tablets
Minaphlex powder
Mineralised methylated spirit
Minijet amiodarone 300mg/10ml solution for injection pre-filled syringes
Minijet sodium bicarbonate 4.2% solution for injection 10ml pre-filled syringes
Minijet sodium bicarbonate 8.4% solution for injection 10ml pre-filled syringes
Minims chloramphenicol 0.5% eye drops 0.5ml unit dose
Minims proxymetacaine 0.5% eye drops 0.5ml unit dose
Minims proxymetacaine 5% / Fluorescein 0.25% eye drops 0.5ml unit dose
Modulen IBD powder
Monoclate-P 1,000unit powder and solvent for solution for injection vials
Monogen powder
Mononine 1,000unit powder and solvent for solution for injection vials
Mononine 500unit powder and solvent for solution for injection vials
MSUD Aid 111 powder
MSUD Analog powder
MSUD express oral powder 25g sachets
MSUD Maxamaid powder
MSUD Maxamum powder
Muse 1000microgram urethral sticks
Muse 125microgram urethral sticks
Muse 250microgram urethral sticks
Muse 500microgram urethral sticks
Mydrilate 0.5% solution
Mydrilate 1% solution

Nabilone 1mg capsules
Nardil 15mg tablets
Neocate Advance powder
Neocate powder
NeoRecormon 1,000units/0.3ml solution for injection pre-filled syringes
NeoRecormon 10,000unit powder and solvent for solution for injection pre-filled disposable devices
NeoRecormon 10,000units/0.6ml solution for injection pre-filled syringes
NeoRecormon 100,000unit powder and solvent for solution for injection vials
NeoRecormon 2,000units/0.3ml solution for injection pre-filled syringes
NeoRecormon 20,000unit powder and solvent for solution for injection pre-filled disposable devices
NeoRecormon 20,000units/0.6ml solution for injection pre-filled syringes
NeoRecormon 3,000units/0.3ml solution for injection pre-filled syringes
NeoRecormon 30,000units/0.6ml solution for injection pre-filled syringes
NeoRecormon 4,000units/0.3ml solution for injection pre-filled syringes
NeoRecormon 5,000units/0.3ml solution for injection pre-filled syringes
NeoRecormon 50,000unit powder and solvent for solution for injection vials
NeoRecormon 500units/0.3ml solution for injection pre-filled syringes
NeoRecormon 6,000units/0.3ml solution for injection pre-filled syringes
NeoRecormon 60,000unit powder and solvent for solution for injection pre-filled disposable devices
Nepro liquid
Neulasta 6mg/0.6ml solution for injection pre-filled syringes
Neulasta SureClick 6mg/0.6ml solution for injection pre-filled disposable devices
Neupogen 30million units/1ml solution for injection vials
Neupogen 48million units/1.6ml solution for injection vials
Neupogen Singleject 30million units/0.5ml solution for injection pre-filled syringes
Neupogen Singleject 48million units/0.5ml solution for injection pre-filled syringes
Nimbex 10mg/5ml solution for injection ampoules

REQUIREMENTS ENABLING PAYMENTS TO BE MADE FOR THE SUPPLY OF DRUGS, APPLIANCES AND CHEMICAL REAGENTS

Drugs for which discount is not deducted

II

Nimbex 20mg/10ml solution for injection ampoules
Nimbex 5mg/2.5ml solution for injection ampoules
Nimbex Forte 150mg/30ml solution for injection vials
Norditropin SimpleXx 10mg/1.5ml solution for injection cartridges
Norditropin SimpleXx 15mg/1.5ml solution for injection cartridges
Norditropin SimpleXx 5mg/1.5ml solution for injection cartridges
Norvir 100mg capsules
Novasource Forte liquid
NovoSeven 120,000unit powder and solvent for solution for injection vials
NovoSeven 240,000unit powder and solvent for solution for injection vials
NovoSeven 60,000unit powder and solvent for solution for injection vials
Noxafil 40mg/ml oral suspension
Nutrini Energy liquid
Nutrini Energy Multifibre liquid
Nutrini liquid
Nutrini Low Energy Multifibre liquid
Nutrini Multifibre liquid
Nutriprem 2 liquid
Nutrison 1200 Complete Multi Fibre liquid
Nutrison Energy liquid
Nutrison Energy Multi Fibre liquid
Nutrison MCT liquid
Nutrison Multi Fibre liquid
Nutrison Protein Plus liquid
Nutrison Protein Plus Multifibre liquid
Nutrison Soya liquid
Nutrison Standard liquid
NutropinAq 10mg/2ml solution for injection cartridges
Octim 150micrograms/dose nasal spray
Octim 15micrograms/1ml solution for injection ampoules
OncoTICE 12.5mg powder for reconstitution for instillation vials
One-Alpha 1micrograms/0.5ml solution for injection ampoules
One-Alpha 2micrograms/1ml solution for injection ampoules
One-Alpha 2micrograms/ml drops
Optivate 500unit powder and solvent for solution for injection vials
Optrex Infected Eyes 0.5% eye drops
Orange tincture BP 2001
Orfadin 10mg capsules
Orgalutran 250micrograms/0.5ml solution for injection pre-filled syringes
Osmolite liquid
Osmolite Plus liquid
Otosporin ear drops
Ovitrelle 250micrograms/0.5ml solution for injection pre-filled syringes
OxBipp paste
Pabal 100micrograms/1ml solution for injection ampoules
Pabrinex Intramuscular High Potency solution for injection 5ml and 2ml ampoules
Paediasure liquid
Paediasure Plus liquid
Paediasure Plus with fibre liquid
Paediasure with fibre liquid
Pancrex gastro-resistant granules
Pancrex V 125mg capsules
Pancrex V capsules
Pancrex V Forte gastro-resistant tablets
Pancrex V gastro-resistant tablets
Pancrex V oral powder
Pancuronium bromide 4mg/2ml solution for injection ampoules
Pegasys 135micrograms/0.5ml solution for injection pre-filled syringes
Pegasys 180micrograms/0.5ml solution for injection pre-filled syringes
PegIntron 100microgram powder and solvent for solution for injection vials
PegIntron 120microgram powder and solvent for solution for injection vials

REQUIREMENTS ENABLING PAYMENTS TO BE MADE FOR THE SUPPLY OF DRUGS, APPLIANCES AND CHEMICAL REAGENTS

Drugs for which discount is not deducted

PegIntron 150microgram powder and solvent for solution for injection vials
PegIntron 50microgram powder and solvent for solution for injection vials
PegIntron 80microgram powder and solvent for solution for injection vials
Pentagastrin 500micrograms/2ml solution for injection ampoules
Pepdite 1+ powder
Pepdite 1+ powder banana
Pepdite powder
Peppermint water concentrated
Peptamen liquid
Peptamen liquid unflavoured
Peptisorb liquid
Perative liquid
Phenelzine 15mg tablets
Phenol crystals
Phenol liquefied
Phenoxyethanol BP
Phenylephrine 10% eye drops
Phlexy-10 bar
Phlexy-10 500mg capsules
Phlexy-10 drink mix
Phlexy-10 tablets
Phlexy-Vits powder
PK Aid 4 powder
PKU cooler 10 liquid
PKU cooler 15 liquid
PKU cooler 20 liquid
PKU express powder
PKU gel powder
Podophyllum resin powder
Potassium permanganate powder
Pregnyl 1,500unit powder and solvent for solution for injection ampoules
Pregnyl 5,000unit powder and solvent for solution for injection ampoules
Presinex 10micrograms/dose nasal spray
Proctosedyl suppositories
Pro-Epanutin 750mg/10ml solution for injection vials
Proflavine hemisulphate powder
Prograf 1mg capsules
Prograf 500microgram capsules
Prograf 5mg capsules
Proleukin 18million unit powder for solution for injection vials
Prostin E2 1mg vaginal gel
Prostin E2 2mg vaginal gel
Prostin E2 3mg vaginal tablets
Prostin E2 5mg/0.5ml solution for injection ampoules
Prostin E2 750micrograms/0.75ml solution for injection ampoules
Prostin VR 500micrograms/1ml solution for injection ampoules
ProSure liquid
Provide Xtra liquid
Pulmozyme 2.5mg nebuliser liquid 2.5ml ampoules
Puregon 100units/0.5ml solution for injection vials
Puregon 150units/0.5ml solution for injection vials
Puregon 200units/0.5ml solution for injection vials
Puregon 50units/0.5ml solution for injection vials
Puregon 600units/0.72ml solution for injection cartridges
Puregon 900units/1.08ml solution for injection cartridges
Puri-Nethol 10mg tablets
Rapamune 1mg/ml oral solution
Raptiva 125mg powder and solvent for solution for injection vials
Rebif 22micrograms/0.5ml solution for injection pre-filled syringes
Rebif 44micrograms/0.5ml solution for injection pre-filled syringes
ReFacto 1,000unit powder and solvent for solution for injection vials

REQUIREMENTS ENABLING PAYMENTS TO BE MADE FOR THE SUPPLY OF DRUGS, APPLIANCES AND CHEMICAL REAGENTS

Drugs for which discount is not deducted

II

ReFacto 2,000unit powder and solvent for solution for injection vials
ReFacto 250unit powder and solvent for solution for injection vials
ReFacto 500unit powder and solvent for solution for injection vials
Regranex 0.01% gel
Remicade 100mg powder for solution for injection vials
Renapro powder
ReoPro 10mg/5ml solution for injection vials
Replagal 1mg/1ml solution for injection vials
Replagal 3.5mg/3.5ml solution for injection vials
Replenate 1,000unit powder and solvent for solution for injection vials
Replenate 500unit powder and solvent for solution for injection vials
Replenine-VF 1,000unit powder and solvent for solution for injection vials
Replenine-VF 500unit powder and solvent for solution for injection vials
ReQuip 1mg tablets
ReQuip 2mg tablets
ReQuip 5mg tablets
ReQuip tablets follow on pack
Resource Junior complete sip feed
Restandol 40mg capsules
Retrovir 250mg capsules
Reyataz 100mg capsules
Reyataz 150mg capsules
Reyataz 200mg capsules
Rilutek 50mg tablets
Riluzole 50mg tablets
Risperdal Consta 25mg powder and solvent for suspension for injection vials
Risperdal Consta 37.5mg powder and solvent for suspension for injection vials
Risperdal Consta 50mg powder and solvent for suspension for injection vials
Rivotril 2.5mg/1ml drops
Roaccutane 20mg capsules
Robinul 1mg tablets
Robinul forte 2mg tablets
Robinul powder
Roferon-A 18million units/0.6ml solution for injection cartridges
Roferon-A 18million units/1ml solution for injection vials
Roferon-A 3million units/0.5ml solution for injection pre-filled syringes
Roferon-A 4.5million units/0.5ml solution for injection pre-filled syringes
Roferon-A 6million units/0.5ml solution for injection pre-filled syringes
Roferon-A 9million units/0.5ml solution for injection pre-filled syringes
Rogitine 10mg/1ml solution for injection ampoules
Ropinirole 1mg tablets
Ropinirole 2mg tablets
Ropinirole 5mg tablets

Saizen 1.33mg powder and solvent for solution for injection vials
Saizen 3.33mg powder and solvent for solution for injection vials
Saizen 8mg click.easy powder and solvent for solution for injection vials
Salazopyrin 500mg suppositories
Salicylic acid 12% collodion
Salicylic acid powder
Sandimmun 100mg capsules
Sandimmun 100mg/ml oral solution
Sandimmun 25mg capsules
Sandimmun 50mg capsules
Sandimmun 50mg/1ml solution for injection ampoules
Sandostatin 100micrograms/1ml solution for injection ampoules
Sandostatin 1mg/5ml solution for injection vials
Sandostatin 500micrograms/1ml solution for injection ampoules
Sandostatin 50micrograms/1ml solution for injection ampoules
Sandostatin LAR 10mg powder and solvent for suspension for injection vials
Sandostatin LAR 20mg powder and solvent for suspension for injection vials
Sandostatin LAR 30mg powder and solvent for suspension for injection vials

REQUIREMENTS ENABLING PAYMENTS TO BE MADE FOR THE SUPPLY OF DRUGS, APPLIANCES AND CHEMICAL REAGENTS

Drugs for which discount is not deducted

Seretide 500 Accuhaler
Silver nitrate powder
Simulect 10mg powder and solvent for solution for injection vials
Simulect 20mg powder and solvent for solution for injection vials
SMA High Energy milk
Sodium bicarbonate 1.4% solution for injection 250ml bottles
Sodium bicarbonate 8.4% solution for injection 100ml bottles
Sodium bicarbonate 8.4% solution for injection 10ml ampoules
Sodium bicarbonate 8.4% solution for injection 300ml bottles
Sodium bicarbonate 8.4% solution for injection 500ml bottles
Sodium salicylate powder
Solgar CoQ-10 100mg capsules
Somatuline Autogel 120mg/0.5ml solution for injection pre-filled syringes
Somatuline Autogel 60mg/0.3ml solution for injection pre-filled syringes
Somatuline Autogel 90mg/0.3ml solution for injection pre-filled syringes
Somatuline LA 30mg powder and solvent for suspension for injection vials
Somavert 10mg powder and solvent for solution for injection vials
Somavert 15mg powder and solvent for solution for injection vials
Somavert 20mg powder and solvent for solution for injection vials
Squill liquid extract
Streptomycin 1g powder for solution for injection vials
Sumatriptan 6mg/0.5ml solution for injection pre-filled syringes
Sumatriptan 6mg/0.5ml solution for injection syringe refill
Suplena liquid
Surgical spirit
Survimed OPD liquid
Sustiva 100mg capsules
Sustiva 200mg capsules
Sustiva 30mg/ml oral solution
Sustiva 600mg tablets
Suxamethonium chloride 100mg/2ml solution for injection ampoules
Synacthen 250micrograms/1ml solution for injection ampoules
Synacthen Depot 1mg/1ml suspension for injection ampoules
Synagis 100mg powder and solvent for solution for injection vials
Synagis 50mg powder and solvent for solution for injection vials
Synercid powder for solution for injection vials
Syntocinon 10units/1ml solution for injection ampoules
Syntocinon 5units/1ml solution for injection ampoules
Syntometrine 500micrograms/1ml solution for injection ampoules
Syprol 10mg/5ml oral solution
Tacrolimus 1mg capsules
Tacrolimus 500microgram capsules
Tacrolimus 5mg capsules
Tarceva 100mg tablets
Tarceva 150mg tablets
Tentrini Energy liquid
Tentrini Energy Multifibre liquid
Tentrini liquid
Tentrini Multifibre liquid
Testosterone 40mg capsules
Testosterone 5mg/24hours patches
Thalidomide 50mg capsules
Thyrogen 900microgram powder for solution for injection vials
Timodine cream
Timolol 5mg/ml/Latanoprost 50mcg/ml eye drops
Tobi 300mg/5ml nebuliser solution 5ml ampoules
Tracleer 125mg tablets
Tracleer 62.5mg tablets
Tracrium 250mg/25ml solution for injection vials
Tracrium 25mg/2.5ml solution for injection ampoules
Tracrium 50mg/5ml solution for injection ampoules

REQUIREMENTS ENABLING PAYMENTS TO BE MADE FOR THE SUPPLY OF DRUGS, APPLIANCES AND CHEMICAL REAGENTS

Drugs for which discount is not deducted

Tractocile 37.5mg/5ml solution for injection vials
Tractocile 6.75mg/0.9ml solution for injection vials
Trientine dihydrochloride 300mg capsules
Trizivir tablets
Truvada tablets
Turpentine oil liquid
Tygacil 50mg powder for solution for injection vials
TYR gel oral powder 20g sachets

Vaccines and Antisera
Valine Amino Acid supplement oral powder 4g sachets
Valtrex 250mg tablets
Vancomycin 125mg capsules
Vancomycin 250mg capsules
Varidase Topical 125,000unit powder vials and diluent
Ventolin 5mg/5ml solution for injection ampoules
VFEND 40mg/ml oral suspension
Videx 200mg chewable dispersible tablets
Videx 25mg chewable dispersible tablets
Videx EC 200mg capsules
Videx EC 250mg capsules
Videx EC 400mg capsules
Vinblastine 10mg/10ml solution for injection vials
Viraferon 18million units/1.2ml solution for injection multidose pens
Viraferon 18million units/3ml solution for injection multidose vials
ViraferonPeg 100microgram powder and solvent for solution for injection pre-filled disposable devices
ViraferonPeg 100microgram powder and solvent for solution for injection vials
ViraferonPeg 120microgram powder and solvent for solution for injection pre-filled disposable devices
ViraferonPeg 120microgram powder and solvent for solution for injection vials
ViraferonPeg 150microgram powder and solvent for solution for injection pre-filled disposable devices
ViraferonPeg 150microgram powder and solvent for solution for injection vials
ViraferonPeg 50microgram powder and solvent for solution for injection pre-filled disposable devices
ViraferonPeg 50microgram powder and solvent for solution for injection vials
ViraferonPeg 80microgram powder and solvent for solution for injection pre-filled disposable devices
ViraferonPeg 80microgram powder and solvent for solution for injection vials
Viramune 200mg tablets
Viread 245mg tablets
Vitamins B and C high potency intramuscular solution for injection 5ml and 2ml ampoules
Vitlipid N Adult emulsion for injection 10ml ampoules
Vitlipid N Infant emulsion for injection 10ml ampoules
Wellvone 750mg/5ml oral suspension
White liniment
Xalacom eye drops
Xalatan 50micrograms/ml eye drops
Xigris 5mg powder for solution for injection vials
XLEU Analog powder
XLYS Analog powder
XLYS Maxamaid powder
XLYS TRY Maxamaid powder
XMET Analog powder
XMET Maxamaid powder
XMET Maxamum powder
XMTVI Analog powder
XMTVI Maxamaid powder
XMTVI Maxamum powder
Xolair 150mg powder and solvent for solution for injection vials
XP Analog powder
XP Analog LCP powder
XP Maxamaid Concentrate powder
XP Maxamaid powder
XP Maxamum powder
XPHEN TYR Analog powder

REQUIREMENTS ENABLING PAYMENTS TO BE MADE FOR THE SUPPLY OF DRUGS, APPLIANCES AND CHEMICAL REAGENTS

Drugs for which discount is not deducted

XPHEN TYR Maxamaid powder
XPTM Analog powder
Xylocaine 1% with Adrenaline 100micrograms/20ml (1 in 200,000) solution for injection vials
Xylocaine 2% with Adrenaline 100micrograms/20ml (1 in 200,000) solution for injection vials
Xyloproct ointment
Zeffix 100mg tablets
Zenalb 20% solution for injection 50ml bottles
Zenalb 4.5% solution for injection 100ml bottles
Zenapax 25mg/5ml solution for injection vials
Zerit 15mg capsules
Zerit 20mg capsules
Zerit 30mg capsules
Zerit 40mg capsules
Ziagen 20mg/ml oral solution
Ziagen 300mg tablets
Zofran 16mg suppositories
Zofran 4mg tablets
Zofran 4mg/5ml syrup
Zofran 8mg tablets
Zofran Flexi-amp 4mg/2ml solution for injection
Zofran Flexi-amp 8mg/4ml solution for injection
Zofran Melt 4mg oral lyophilisates
Zofran Melt 8mg oral lyophilisates
Zomacton 4mg powder and solvent for solution for injection vials
Zonegran 100mg capsules
Zonegran 50mg capsules
Zovirax 400mg dispersible tablets
Zovirax Shingles Treatment Pack 800mg dispersible tablets
Zyvox 600mg tablets

REQUIREMENTS ENABLING PAYMENTS TO BE MADE FOR THE SUPPLY OF DRUGS, APPLIANCES AND CHEMICAL REAGENTS

PRODUCTS INCLUDED IN CLAUSE 10B(iii)

Products included in Clause 10B(iii) are listed below.
Liquid preparations for external use:

SubPara	Name	Pack(s)
(c)	Alcoderm Lotion	(200ml)
(a)	Alpha Keri Bath Oil	(240ml and 480ml)
(b)	Alphosyl Lotion	(250ml)
(c)	Alphosyl Shampoo 2 in 1	(125ml and 250ml)
(c)	Ascabiol Emulsion	(100ml)
(a)	Aveeno Bath Oil	(250ml)
(c)	Aveeno Lotion	(400ml pump pack)
(a)	Balneum Bath Oil	(200ml, 500ml and 1000ml)
(a)	Balneum Plus Bath Oil 82.95%/15%	(500ml)
(c)	Betadine Shampoo	(250ml)
(b)	Capasal Therapeutic Shampoo	(250ml)
(c)	Ceanel Concentrate	(50ml, 150ml and 500ml)
(a)	Cetraben Bath Oil	(500ml)
(c)	Dentinox Cradle Cap Shampoo	(125ml)
(a)	Dermalo Bath Emollient	(500ml)
(c)	Dermol 200 Shower Emollient	(200ml)
(c)	Dermol 500 Lotion	(500ml pump)
(c)	Dermol 600 Bath Emollient	(600ml)
(a)	Diprobath Emollient	(500ml)
(a)	E45 Bath Oil	(250ml and 500ml)
(c)	E45 Lotion	(250ml and 500ml pump)
(c)	E45 Shower Creme Emollient	(200ml)
(c)	E45 Wash	(250ml)
(a)	Eurax Dermatological Bath Oil	(200ml)
(a)	Emmolate Bath Oil	(200ml)
(a)	Emulsiderm Emollient	(300ml and 1 litre)
(b)	Exorex Lotion	(100ml and 250ml)
(b)	Gelcosal Gel	(50g)
(b)	Gelcotar Gel	(50g and 500g)
(b)	Gelcotar Liquid	(150ml and 350ml)
(a)	Hydromol Emollient	(150ml, 350ml, 500ml and 1 litre)
(c)	Keri Therapeutic Lotion	(190ml and 380ml pump packs)
(a)	Imuderm Therapeutic Oil	(250ml)
(a)	Infaderm Therapeutic Oil	(250ml)
(c)	Lacticare Lotion	(150ml)
(c)	Meted Shampoo	(120ml)

REQUIREMENTS ENABLING PAYMENTS TO BE MADE FOR THE SUPPLY OF DRUGS, APPLIANCES AND CHEMICAL REAGENTS

Products included in Clause 10B(iii) are listed below.
Liquid preparations for external use:

SubPara	Name	Pack(s)
(a)	Oilatum Bath Formula	(150ml and 300ml)
(c)	Oilatum Cream	(1050ml)
(a)	Oilatum Emollient	(250ml and 500ml)
(a)	Oilatum Emollient, Fragrance Free	(500ml)
(c)	Oilatum Junior Cream	(1050ml)
(a)	Oilatum Junior Emollient Bath Additive	(150ml, 250ml, 300ml, 500ml and 1 litre)
(a)	Oilatum Junior Flare-Up Bath Treatment	(150ml)
(a)	Oilatum Plus Emollient	(500ml and 1 litre)
(a)	Pinetarsol Bath Oil	(200ml and 500ml)
(a)	Pinetarsol Solution	(200ml and 500ml)
(a)	Pinetarsol Gel	(100g)
(b)	Pentrax Shampoo	(120ml)
(b)	Polytar AF Liquid	(150ml and 250ml)
(b)	Polytar Emollient	(350ml and 500ml)
(b)	Polytar Liquid	(150ml, 250ml and 500ml)
(b)	Polytar Plus (Scalp Cleanser)	(350ml and 500ml)
(b)	Pragmatar Cream	(25g and 100g)
(b)	Psorin Ointment	(50g and 100g)
(b)	Psoriderm Bath Emulsion	(200ml)
(b)	Psoriderm Cream	(225ml)
(b)	Psoriderm Scalp Lotion Shampoo	(250ml)
(c)	Quellada-M Cream Shampoo	(40g)
(a)	Quellada-M Liquid (Aqueous)	(50ml and 200ml)
(c)	Quinoderm Lotio-Gel 5%	(30ml)
(c)	Selsun Suspension	(50ml, 100ml and 150ml)
(a)	Ster-Zac Bath Concentrate	(28.5ml)
(b)	T-Gel Shampoo	(125ml and 250ml)
(b)	T-Gel Shampoo Anti-Dandruff	(125ml and 250ml)

PROFESSIONAL FEES (PHARMACY CONTRACTORS)

See Part II, Clause 6A (ii) (page 5)

	*Fee per prescription p	Endorsements required by contractors

* Endorsements under this heading apply only to claims for the appropriate professional fee. The endorsement codes to be used are:
ED=Extemporaneously Dispensed
MF= Measured and Fitted
Further endorsement may be necessary for other purposes eg Part II "CLAUSE 8 BASIC PRICE, "CLAUSE 9 ENDORSEMENT REQUIREMENTS and Notes to Part VIII (page 69)

1. **ALL PRESCRIPTIONS** attract a Professional Fee with a value of: 90   NIL

2. **ADDITIONAL FEES:**

   A.   PREPARATIONS WHEN EXTEMPORANEOUSLY DISPENSED *AND* ENDORSED

   (a)   Liquids being 'special formula preparations' e.g. mixtures, lotions, nasal drops (not including dilutions)   155   ED

   (b)   Liquid preparations prepared by straightforward dilution (not including reconstitution)   85   ED

   (c)   Ointments, creams, pastes being 'special formula preparations' (not including dilutions)   310   ED

   (d)   Ointments, creams, pastes prepared by dilution or admixture of standard or proprietary ointments, creams and pastes   155   ED

   B.   APPLIANCES

   (a)   Elastic Hosiery (Compression Hosiery) requiring measurement and endorsed "measured and fitted"   128   MF

   (b)   Trusses requiring measurement and endorsed "measured and fitted"   197   MF

   C.   Where liquid preparations extemporaneously dispensed are ordered by the prescriber to be supplied in more than one container, each extra quantity ordered   128   NIL

   D.   Where a preparation which requires the addition of a vehicle/diluent by the pharmacy contractor results in a liquid of stability of less than 14 days, and for pharmaceutical reasons necessitates supply in more than one container and the prescription form is endorsed with the number of extra quantities supplied, for each extra supply   155   Number of extra containers supplied

PROFESSIONAL FEES (PHARMACY CONTRACTORS)

	*Fee per prescription p	Endorsements required by contractors
E. Where the prescription is for a Controlled Drug in Schedule 2 or 3 of the Misuse of Drugs Regulations 2001		
Schedule 2 drug	128	NIL
Schedule 3 drug	43	NIL

F.   Expensive Prescription Fee

A fee equivalent to 2% of the net ingredient cost will be payable on all prescriptions over £100.

Note - Expensive Prescription Fee is not included in calculation of ESPS payments

SCALE OF FEES (APPLIANCE CONTRACTORS)

See Part II, Clause 6B(iii) (page 6)

		Fee per prescription p
1. APPLIANCES		
ELASTIC HOSIERY (Compression Hosiery)		
Anklets, Kneecaps, Leggings		13
Below-knee, Above-knee and Thigh Stockings		18
TRUSSES		
Spring	Single	50
	Double	78
Elastic Band	Single	23
	Double	30
Repairs		5
2. OTHER APPLIANCES		2

IIIB

SCALE OF FEES (APPLIANCE CONTRACTORS)

This Page is Intentionally Blank

CONTAINERS

See Part II Clause 6A (iii)

---

1. A Pharmacy Contractor shall supply in a *suitable container* any drug which he is required to supply under Part II of Schedule 2 to the Regulations.

    Capsules, tablets, pills, pulvules etc shall be supplied in airtight containers of glass, aluminium or rigid plastics; card containers may be used only for foil/strip packed tablets etc.
    For ointments, creams, pastes, card containers shall not be used

    Eye, ear and nasal drops shall be supplied in dropper bottles, or with a separate dropper where appropriate.

2. *Payment for containers* is at the average rate of **3.24p** per prescription for every prescription (except an oxygen prescription) supplied by contractors whether or not a container is supplied.

    This payment includes provision for supply of a *5ml plastic measuring spoon* which shall comply with BS 3221:Part 6:1987 and shall be made with every oral liquid medicine except where the manufacturer's pack includes one. However, when the prescribed dose is not 5ml or whole multiples of 5ml, and the pack does not already contain a suitable measuring device, a 5ml plastics oral syringe measure, wrapped together with a bottle adaptor and instruction leaflet, shall be supplied. This shall comply with BS 3221: Part 7: 1995, or an equivalent European Standard.

    In very exceptional circumstances, or where specifically requested by the prescriber dilution may still take place. The prescription should be endorsed accordingly.

3. Payment for containers is payable to pharmacy contractors only.

CONTAINERS

This Page is Intentionally Blank

DEDUCTION SCALE (PHARMACY CONTRACTORS)

(Revised with effect from 1st September 2006)
See Part II Clause 6A(i) (b) (page 5)

Monthly Total of Prices £		Deduction Rate %	Monthly Total of Prices £		Deduction Rate %	Monthly Total of Prices £		Deduction Rate %
From	To		From	To		From	To	
1	125	5.63	5626	5750	6.42	11251	11375	7.20
126	250	5.65	5751	5875	6.43	11376	11500	7.22
251	375	5.66	5876	6000	6.45	11501	11625	7.24
376	500	5.68	6001	6125	6.47	11626	11750	7.26
501	625	5.70	6126	6250	6.49	11751	11875	7.27
626	750	5.72	6251	6375	6.50	11876	12000	7.29
751	875	5.73	6376	6500	6.52	12001	12125	7.31
876	1000	5.75	6501	6625	6.54	12126	12250	7.33
1001	1125	5.77	6626	6750	6.56	12251	12375	7.34
1126	1250	5.79	6751	6875	6.57	12376	12500	7.36
1251	1375	5.80	6876	7000	6.59	12501	12625	7.38
1376	1500	5.82	7001	7125	6.61	12626	12750	7.40
1501	1625	5.84	7126	7250	6.63	12751	12875	7.41
1626	1750	5.86	7251	7375	6.64	12876	13000	7.43
1751	1875	5.87	7376	7500	6.66	13001	13125	7.45
1876	2000	5.89	7501	7625	6.68	13126	13250	7.47
2001	2125	5.91	7626	7750	6.70	13251	13375	7.48
2126	2250	5.93	7751	7875	6.71	13376	13500	7.50
2251	2375	5.94	7876	8000	6.73	13501	13625	7.52
2376	2500	5.96	8001	8125	6.75	13626	13750	7.54
2501	2625	5.98	8126	8250	6.77	13751	13875	7.55
2626	2750	6.00	8251	8375	6.78	13876	14000	7.57
2751	2875	6.01	8376	8500	6.80	14001	14125	7.59
2876	3000	6.03	8501	8625	6.82	14126	14250	7.61
3001	3125	6.05	8626	8750	6.84	14251	14375	7.62
3126	3250	6.07	8751	8875	6.85	14376	14500	7.64
3251	3375	6.08	8876	9000	6.87	14501	14625	7.66
3376	3500	6.10	9001	9125	6.89	14626	14750	7.68
3501	3625	6.12	9126	9250	6.91	14751	14875	7.69
3626	3750	6.14	9251	9375	6.92	14876	15000	7.71
3751	3875	6.15	9376	9500	6.94	15001	15125	7.73
3876	4000	6.17	9501	9625	6.96	15126	15250	7.75
4001	4125	6.19	9626	9750	6.98	15251	15375	7.76
4126	4250	6.21	9751	9875	6.99	15376	15500	7.78
4251	4375	6.22	9876	10000	7.01	15501	15625	7.80
4376	4500	6.24	10001	10125	7.03	15626	15750	7.82
4501	4625	6.26	10126	10250	7.05	15751	15875	7.83
4626	4750	6.28	10251	10375	7.06	15876	16000	7.85
4751	4875	6.29	10376	10500	7.08	16001	16125	7.87
4876	5000	6.31	10501	10625	7.10	16126	16250	7.89
5001	5125	6.33	10626	10750	7.12	16251	16375	7.90
5126	5250	6.35	10751	10875	7.13	16376	16500	7.92
5251	5375	6.36	10876	11000	7.15	16501	16625	7.94
5376	5500	6.38	11001	11125	7.17	16626	16750	7.96
5501	5625	6.40	11126	11250	7.19	16751	16875	7.97

DEDUCTION SCALE (PHARMACY CONTRACTORS)

Monthly Total of Prices £		Deduction Rate %	Monthly Total of Prices £		Deduction Rate %	Monthly Total of Prices £		Deduction Rate %
From	To		From	To		From	To	
16876	17000	7.99	23001	23125	8.85	40501	41000	9.61
17001	17125	8.01	23126	23375	8.88	41001	41750	9.62
17126	17250	8.03	23376	23625	8.92	41751	42250	9.63
17251	17375	8.04	23626	24000	8.97	42251	43000	9.64
17376	17500	8.06	24001	24250	9.01	43001	43750	9.65
17501	17625	8.08	24251	24625	9.06	43751	44250	9.66
17626	17750	8.10	24626	24875	9.09	44251	45000	9.67
17751	17875	8.11	24876	25250	9.15	45001	45500	9.68
17876	18000	8.13	25251	25500	9.18	45501	46250	9.69
18001	18125	8.15	25501	25875	9.23	46251	46750	9.70
18126	18250	8.17	25876	26125	9.27	46751	47500	9.71
18251	18375	8.18	26126	26375	9.30	47501	48250	9.72
18376	18500	8.20	26376	26750	9.36	48251	48750	9.73
18501	18625	8.22	26751	27000	9.39	48751	49500	9.74
18626	18750	8.24	27001	27375	9.40	49501	50000	9.75
18751	18875	8.25	27376	27625	9.41	50001	50750	9.76
18876	19000	8.27	27626	28000	9.41	50751	51250	9.77
19001	19125	8.29	28001	28250	9.41	51251	52000	9.78
19126	19250	8.31	28251	28625	9.42	52001	52750	9.79
19251	19375	8.32	28626	28875	9.42	52751	53250	9.80
19376	19500	8.34	28876	29250	9.43	53251	54000	9.81
19501	19625	8.36	29251	29500	9.43	54001	54500	9.81
19626	19750	8.38	29501	29875	9.44	54501	55250	9.83
19751	19875	8.39	29876	30125	9.44	55251	55750	9.83
19876	20000	8.41	30126	30500	9.45	55751	56500	9.85
20001	20125	8.43	30501	30750	9.45	56501	57250	9.86
20126	20250	8.45	30751	31125	9.46	57251	57750	9.86
20251	20375	8.46	31126	31375	9.46	57751	58500	9.88
20376	20500	8.48	31376	31750	9.47	58501	59000	9.88
20501	20625	8.50	31751	32000	9.47	59001	59750	9.89
20626	20750	8.52	32001	32375	9.48	59751	60250	9.90
20751	20875	8.53	32376	32625	9.48	60251	61000	9.91
20876	21000	8.55	32626	32875	9.49	61001	61750	9.93
21001	21125	8.57	32876	33250	9.49	61751	62250	9.93
21126	21250	8.59	33251	33500	9.49	62251	63000	9.94
21251	21375	8.60	33501	33875	9.50	63001	63500	9.95
21376	21500	8.62	33876	34125	9.50	63501	64250	9.96
21501	21625	8.64	34126	34500	9.51	64251	64750	9.97
21626	21750	8.66	34501	34750	9.51	64751	65500	9.98
21751	21875	8.67	34751	35125	9.52	65501	66250	9.99
21876	22000	8.69	35126	35375	9.52	66251	66750	10.00
22001	22125	8.71	35376	36000	9.53	66751	67500	10.01
22126	22250	8.73	36001	36500	9.54	67501	68000	10.02
22251	22375	8.74	36501	37250	9.55	68001	68750	10.03
22376	22500	8.76	37251	37750	9.56	68751	69250	10.04
22501	22625	8.78	37751	38500	9.57	69251	70000	10.05
22626	22750	8.80	38501	39250	9.58	70001	70750	10.06
22751	22875	8.81	39251	39750	9.59	70751	71250	10.07
22876	23000	8.83	39751	40500	9.60	71251	72000	10.08

DEDUCTION SCALE (PHARMACY CONTRACTORS)

Monthly Total of Prices £		Deduction Rate %	Monthly Total of Prices £		Deduction Rate %	Monthly Total of Prices £		Deduction Rate %
From	To		From	To		From	To	
72001	72500	10.09	101501	102000	10.54	127001	127500	10.93
72501	73250	10.10	102001	102750	10.55	127501	128000	10.93
73251	73750	10.11	102751	103250	10.56	128001	128500	10.94
73751	74500	10.12	103251	103750	10.57	128501	129000	10.95
74501	75250	10.13	103751	104250	10.57	129001	129500	10.96
75251	75750	10.14	104251	104750	10.58	129501	130000	10.97
75751	76500	10.15	104751	105250	10.59	130001	130500	10.97
76501	77000	10.16	105251	105750	10.60	130501	131000	10.98
77001	77750	10.17	105751	106250	10.60	131001	131500	10.99
77751	78250	10.18	106251	106750	10.61	131501	132000	11.00
78251	79000	10.19	106751	107250	10.62	132001	132500	11.00
79001	79750	10.20	107251	107750	10.63	132501	133000	11.01
79751	80250	10.21	107751	108250	10.63	133001	133500	11.02
80251	81000	10.22	108251	108750	10.64	133501	134000	11.03
81001	81500	10.23	108751	109250	10.65	134001	134750	11.04
81501	82250	10.24	109251	109750	10.66	134751	135250	11.05
82251	82750	10.25	109751	110500	10.67	135251	135750	11.05
82751	83500	10.26	110501	111000	10.68	135751	136250	11.06
83501	84250	10.27	111001	111500	10.68	136251	136750	11.07
84251	84750	10.28	111501	112000	10.69	136751	137250	11.08
84751	85500	10.29	112001	112500	10.70	137251	137750	11.08
85501	86000	10.29	112501	113000	10.71	137751	138250	11.09
86001	86750	10.31	113001	113500	10.71	138251	138750	11.10
86751	87250	10.31	113501	114000	10.72	138751	139250	11.11
87251	88000	10.33	114001	114500	10.73	139251	139750	11.11
88001	88750	10.34	114501	115000	10.74	139751	140250	11.12
88751	89250	10.34	115001	115500	10.74	140251	140750	11.13
89251	90000	10.36	115501	116000	10.75	140751	141250	11.14
90001	90500	10.36	116001	116500	10.76	141251	141750	11.14
90501	91250	10.37	116501	117000	10.77	141751	142500	11.16
91251	91750	10.38	117001	117500	10.77	142501	143000	11.16
91751	92500	10.39	117501	118000	10.78	143001	143500	11.17
92501	93250	10.41	118001	118750	10.79	143501	144000	11.18
93251	93750	10.41	118751	119250	10.80	144001	144500	11.19
93751	94500	10.42	119251	119750	10.81	144501	145000	11.19
94501	95000	10.43	119751	120250	10.82	145001	145500	11.20
95001	95500	10.44	120251	120750	10.82	145501	146000	11.21
95501	96000	10.45	120751	121250	10.83	146001	146500	11.22
96001	96500	10.45	121251	121750	10.84	146501	147000	11.22
96501	97000	10.46	121751	122250	10.85	147001	147500	11.23
97001	97500	10.47	122251	122750	10.85	147501	148000	11.24
97501	98000	10.48	122751	123250	10.86	148001	149000	11.25
98001	98500	10.49	123251	123750	10.87	149001	150000	11.27
98501	99000	10.49	123751	124250	10.88	150001	160000	11.42
99001	99500	10.50	124251	124750	10.89	160001	& above	11.50
99501	100000	10.51	124751	125250	10.89			
100001	100500	10.52	125251	125750	10.90			
100501	101000	10.52	125751	126500	10.91			
101001	101500	10.53	126501	127000	10.92			

DEDUCTION SCALE (PHARMACY CONTRACTORS)

This Page is Intentionally Blank

PAYMENT FOR ESSENTIAL SERVICES (PHARMACY CONTRACTORS)

1.   Establishment Payments

1.1   Pharmacy contractors who dispense the stated number of prescription items or more in any month will receive an Establishment Payment from 1 April 2005.

1.2   From 1 April 2005 to 30 September 2006 pharmacy contractors who dispense 2,000 prescription items or more in any month will receive an Establishment Payment. The Establishment Payments for the six month period from 1 April 2006 to 30 September 2006 are set out in the table below:

Number of items per month	Establishment Payment for the six months 1 April 2006 to 30 September 2006 £
2,000 - 2,249	£10,000
2,250 - 2, 499	£10,456
2,500+	£10,911

VIA

1.3   From 1 October 2006, pharmacy contractors who dispense 2,060 prescription items or more in any month will receive an Establishment Payment. The Establishment Payments for the six month period from 1 October 2006 to 31 March 2007 are set out in the table below:

Number of items per month	Establishment Payment for the six months 1 October 2006 to 31 March 2007 £
2,060 - 2,319	£11,639
2,320 - 2, 574	£12,095
2,575+	£12,550

1.4   The Establishment Payment will be paid monthly, calculated as 1/6th of the payment, on the basis of the number of prescription items submitted, and reimbursed by the Pricing Authority, in the relevant month.

1.5   Where total monthly payments in relation to prescriptions passed for pricing between 1 April and 31 March in any year are less than the amount which would have been paid had the payment been calculated on an annual or six monthly* basis, pharmacy contractors may make a claim for a top up payment to their PCT for England and LHB for Wales. This should take account of any Protected Professional Allowance Payment made, such that pharmacy contractors do not receive both an Establishment Payment and a Protected Professional Allowance Payment for the same month. They should submit, by the following 30 November, copies of FP/WP34 statements for the relevant period (April to March) as evidence of the total number of prescription items passed for pricing during this period.

*For 2006-07, this should be applied on a six monthly basis taking into account the Establishment Payment due for April to September and for October to March.

PAYMENT FOR ESSENTIAL SERVICES (PHARMACY CONTRACTORS)

2.   **Practice Payments**

2.1   All pharmacy contractors will receive a Practice Payment from 1 April 2005.

2.2   Practice Payments from 1 April 2006 to 30 September 2006, which includes a contribution for provision of auxiliary aids for people eligible under the Disability Discrimination Act 1995 (DDA), are set out in the table below:

Number of items per month	Practice Payment for the six months 1 April 2006 to 30 September 2006	Contribution in Practice Payment for DDA for the six months 1 April 2006 to 30 September 2006
Up to 1,099	£250	£250
1,100 - 1,599	£1,500	£500
1,600 - 1,999	£2,125	£625
2,000+	29.7p per item	5.5p per item

2.3   Practice Payments for the six month period from 1 October 2006 to 31 March 2007 are set out in the table below:

Number of items per month	Practice Payment for the six months 1 October 2006 to 31 March 2007	Contribution in Practice Payment for DDA for the six months 1 October 2006 to 31 March 2007
Up to 1,099	£300	£300
1,100 - 1,599	£1,800	£600
1,600 - 2,059	£2,550	£750
2,060+	35.6p per item	6.6p per item

2.4   Practice Payments will be paid monthly, calculated, subject to 2.5 to 2.7 below, as 1/6th of the payment, on the basis of the number of prescription items submitted, and reimbursed by the Pricing Authority, in the relevant month.

2.5   From 1 October 2005, in order to receive the full Practice Payment pharmacy contractors must have, and must have declared to the Pricing Authority on the appropriate claim form for the relevant month minimum dispensing staff levels as set out in the table below:

Number of items per month	Minimum dispensing staff level (Hours per week)*
2,000 - 3,499	40 hours
3,500 - 4,999	56 hours
5,000 - 6,499	75 hours
6,500 - 7,999	94 hours
8,000 - 9,499	112 hours
9,500 - 10,999	131 hours
11,000**	150 hours

* Dispensing staff include: a pharmacist; a non-practising pharmacist working as a dispenser; a pre-registration trainee (only half of the pre-registration trainees hours should be counted for this purpose) or an assistant trained to undertake the functions being performed. Where a staff member has multiple roles, only the number of hours spent supporting the dispensing process may be counted in the staffing declaration.

In determining the dispensing staff level to declare on the appropriate claim form the number of hours should be rounded as follows:
0.5 or less round down to the nearest whole number of hours
Above 0.5 round up to the nearest whole number of hours.

**Pharmacy Contractors will be required to employ a staff member for an extra 19 hours per week for each additional 1,500 items the pharmacy contractor dispensed per month above 11,000 items.

PAYMENT FOR ESSENTIAL SERVICES (PHARMACY CONTRACTORS)

2.6   From 1 October 2005, where for any month a pharmacy contractor has declared to the Pricing Authority dispensing staff levels lower than those set out in the table in 2.5 above, the Practice Payment for the relevant month will be paid at the level that would be paid if the pharmacy only dispensed the number of items at the lowest level in the band that corresponds in the above table to its declared dispensing staff levels.   (Example: A pharmacy contractor dispensing 7,000 prescription items a month who employs dispensing staff for only 75 hours per week, including a pharmacist, would receive the Practice Payment for 5,000 prescriptions items per month, ie 5,000 x 29.7p = £1,485 or 5,000 x 35.6p = £1,780, whichever is applicable).

2.7   From 1 October 2005, where for any month a pharmacy contractor has not declared dispensing staff levels to the Pricing Authority, the Practice Payment for the relevant month will be paid at the minimum level (i.e. 1/6th of £250 or 1/6th of £300, whichever is applicable).

2.8   Subject to 2.8.1 and 2.8.2, where total monthly payments in relation to prescriptions passed for pricing between 1 April and 31 March in any year are less than the amount which would have been paid had the payment been calculated on an annual or six monthly* basis, pharmacy contractors may make a claim for a top up payment to their PCT for England and LHB for Wales.   They should submit, by the following 30 November, copies of FP/WP34 statements for the relevant period (April to March) as evidence of the total number of prescription items passed for pricing during this period.

2.8.1   Where, in any month, Practice Payments were paid at a lower level because minimum dispensing staff levels were not met, those months shall be disregarded (in terms of both the number of items passed for pricing and the payments received) when calculating the amount of any top up payment which may be payable.

2.8.2   Where, in any month, Practice Payments were paid at a lower level because a pharmacy contractor did not declare dispensing staff levels, those months shall be disregarded (in terms of both the number of items passed for pricing and the payments received) when calculating the amount of any top up payment which may be payable, unless the pharmacy contractor can satisfy their PCT for England and LHB for Wales that their dispensing staff levels were sufficient in respect of the table in 2.5 for the relevant month.

* For 2006-07, this should be applied on a six monthly basis taking into account the Practice Payment due for April to September and for October to March.

3.   **Protected Professional Allowance Payments**

3.1   From 1 April 2005, where in any month a pharmacy:

3.1.1   is providing as a minimum Schedule 1 (Terms of Service) of the NHS (Pharmaceutical Services) Regulations 2005 (subject to transitional arrangements in respect of their terms of service Part 6 Regulation 74) and the National Health Service (Pharmaceutical Services)(Amendment)(Wales) Regulations 2005;

3.1.2   received, at any time during the year ending 31 March 2005, the "Payment for Additional Professional Services" as set out in the Drug Tariff Part VIA at that time; and

3.1.3   from 1 April 2005 to 30 September 2006 dispenses at least 1,100, but less than 2,000 prescription items, and from 1 October 2006 dispenses at least 1,100, but less than 2,060 prescription items;

        the pharmacy contractor will, subject to 3.2 below, be entitled to be paid a Protected Professional Allowance calculated in accordance with paragraph 3.3

3.2   Such pharmacy contractors will only be entitled to continue to receive this payment until 31 March 2008 or such time as the pharmacy ceases to provide services, whichever is the earlier.

3.3   The basis of calculation for the Protected Professional Allowance payment is as follows:

        Pharmacy contractors who have had passed for payment by the Pricing Authority between 1,100 and 1,600 prescriptions in the relevant month will receive a payment of £775 (at 1,100 prescriptions) rising to £1,500 (at 1,600 or more prescriptions).

PAYMENT FOR ESSENTIAL SERVICES (PHARMACY CONTRACTORS)

4.   **Repeat Dispensing**

   4.1   All pharmacy contractors will receive a repeat dispensing annual payment of £1,500 from 1 April 2005. The payment will be paid monthly calculated as 1/12th of the annual payment (£125 per month).

   4.2   Pharmacists undertaking repeat dispensing should undertake appropriate training. Appropriate training for these purposes includes successful completion of the Centre for Pharmacy Postgraduate Education's (CPPE) open learning programme 'From pathfinder to practice'. For pharmacists in Wales, suitable training would be 'Repeat Dispensing', a programme available from the Welsh Centre for Postgraduate Pharmaceutical Education.

5.   **Transitional Payment**

   5.1   All pharmacy contractors will receive Transitional Payments from 1 April 2005. Transitional Payments will be paid monthly on the basis of the number of prescription items submitted and reimbursed by the Pricing Authority, in the relevant month.

   5.2   Transitional Payments from 1 April 2005 to 30 September 2006 are set out in the table below:

Number of items per month	Payment
1 - 500	£38.50
501 - 1,000	£77.00
1,001 - 1,500	£115.50
Rising in bands of 500	Increased by £38.50 each band

   5.3   Transitional Payments for the six month period from 1 October 2006 to 31 March 2007 are set out in the table below:

Number of items per month	Payment
1 - 500	£54.06
501 - 1,000	£108.12
1,001 - 1,500	£162.18
Rising in bands of 500	Increased by £54.06 each band

PAYMENT FOR ESSENTIAL SERVICES (PHARMACY CONTRACTORS)

6.   **Electronic Transmission of Prescriptions Allowances**

6.1   The Electronic Prescription Service will be deployed in phases with two releases (Release 1 and Release 2) of ETP Compliant pharmacy systems. Further details of service implementation and deployment can be found at www.cfh.nhs.uk.

6.2   In order to be able to use the Electronic Prescription Service pharmacy contractors will need to have

●an ETP compliant pharmacy system accredited as such by NHS Connecting for Health (either Release 1 or Release 2)

●appropriate network connectivity to be able to operate the Electronic Prescription Service (details of connectivity arrangements for community pharmacies will be made available by NHS Connecting for Health)

●staff operating the service who are registered users and have been issued with smart cards and PIN numbers by their PCT's Registration Authority.

6.3   All pharmacy contractors will be paid two allowances of £1,300 (ie a total of £2,600 with one payment of £1,300 in December 2005 *and* one in February 2006). These allowances are linked to a pharmacy deploying Release 1 of the Electronic Prescription Service. If the pharmacy has not deployed Release 1 of the service (by a date as yet to be determined of which three months notice will be given), the PCT will be able to reclaim these allowances from the pharmacy contractor through a deduction via the monthly schedule of payments.

6.4   A further allowance of £1,000 will be paid linked to the pharmacy deploying Release 2 of the Electronic Prescription Service. If the pharmacy has not deployed Release 2 of the service (by a date as yet to be determined of which three months notice will be given), the PCT will be able to reclaim this allowance from the pharmacy contractor through a deduction via the monthly schedule of payments.

6.5   When the Pharmacy Contractor is able to operate the Electronic Prescription Service if an appropriate prescription is presented or requested, the pharmacy can claim £200/month from the PCT. This will need to be done via form PPAETP1 (available at www.nhsbsa.nhs.uk) (Gateway reference PPA-05-007). If at a later date the pharmacy contractor becomes unable to operate the Electronic Prescription Service, they must inform the PCT in writing immediately so that payment of this ongoing allowance is stopped.

VIA

PAYMENT FOR ESSENTIAL SERVICES (PHARMACY CONTRACTORS)

7.   **Electronic Transfer of Prescriptions (Wales)**

Community Pharmacy IM & T Programme

IM&T Allowances for Community Pharmacy Contractors (Wales)

7.1   This guidance replaces the Welsh 'IM & T Allowances for Community Pharmacy Contractors' statement, issued in November 2005 and published in the Drug Tariff, part VIA.

7.2   There are parallel strategic developments within England and Wales in relation to the technical architecture that underpins the 'NHS Care Records Service' (England) and the 'Individual Health Record' (Wales). At present, some components of the Pharmacy IM & T solutions accredited for England may not be applicable to Wales and may have to be modified or disabled until such time that Wales, via its national IM & T Programme Board, has determined appropriate and comparable solutions.

7.3   The delivery of the IM & T component of the Pharmacy contract will be a pragmatic, phased approach ensuring alignment to the overall strategic direction for Wales and is described below:

•   Phase 1 - 'IT Infrastructure', (hardware, software and secure network connectivity)

•   Phase 2 -

• Release 1 - 2D Barcoded Prescription forms

• Release 2 - Transmission of Pharmacy claims

7.4   The following updated guidance is intended to advise on how previously advised IT allowances should be used by Community Pharmacy Contractors and also provide an indication of when future payments can be expected.

Phase 1 - £2,600 allowances (previously allocated 2005/06)

7.5   All existing Pharmacy Contractors received two allowances of £1,300 in 2005/06 (i.e. a total of £2,600, with one payment of £1,300 in December 2005 and one in February 2006).

7.6   These allowances are linked to investment in IT infrastucture, to support the Programme's key objectives associated with Phase 1.

7.7   Specifically, Phase 1 funding must be targeted to ensure any investment in IT is "fit for purpose" and **capable** of running the latest version of the Pharmacy Contractors' PMR system, as well as supporting secure/managed connectivity, enabling access to the NHS Wales network, including its web-based applications, such as web eMail and HOWIS (Health of Wales Information Services) resources.

7.8   Community Pharmacy Contractors are therefore advised that any investment in IT facilities must be provided or approved by their Pharmacy System Supplier who will ensure that the IT facilities and services are appropriately configured to support the latest version of their respective Patient Medication Records (PMRs), together with the security requirements for secure access to the NHS Wales network.

7.9   As a minimum, all Community Pharmacy Contractors are required to initiate discussions with their respective Pharmacy System Supplier to arrange for an 'approved' connectivity package described below.

PAYMENT FOR ESSENTIAL SERVICES (PHARMACY CONTRACTORS)

7.10   A choice of two 'approved' methods of connectivity have been identified, namely:

- An indirect 'managed' broadband connection with an **N3-accredited** broadband network provider (known as an 'Aggregator'), arranged through your Pharmacy System Supplier.

    [recommended for 'independents' and small chains]

    In this option, the Pharmacy System Supplier may have a 'package' of services available to its clients, which could also include managed service support and maintenance, as well as providing connectivity access to an N3-accredited Aggregator.

- A direct connection to N3, using an accredited 3rd party Gateway.

    [recommended for 'multiples' and corporates]

    This option is more suitable for the larger chains and corporate retailers ('multiples'), who may already have a direct connection to N3 for its English outlets. In the same way as above, their direct connections to N3 can then 'route' their Welsh branches onto the NHS Wales network.

7.11   In both cases, only Welsh Community Pharmacy Contractors will be able to access the NHS Wales network and its associated resources.

7.12   Failure to place an order for an 'approved' connectivity package by 31st March 2007 will mean that the LHB will seek to reclaim these allowances.

7.13   Community Pharmacy Contractors should be mindful of future developments relating to Phase 2 of the Programme, when making investment in IT infrastructure.

Phase 1 - £200 per month recurring funding

7.14   The trigger for £200 per month payment by the LHB to a Community Pharmacy Contractor will be on receipt of confirmation that an 'approved' connection has been installed, live and active.

7.15   If at a later date the Community Pharmacy Contractor cancels their connectivity or breaches the Acceptable Use Policy (AUP) for access to the NHS Wales network, recurring payments for connectivity will be withdrawn.

Phase 2 - £1,000 allowance (2007/08)

7.16   Subject to successful testing and evaluation, Phase 2 is expected to be delivered through 2 Releases. In Release 1, 2D Barcoded prescription forms will be provisionally implemented across Community Pharmacy in Wales. Release 2 will provide a mechanism for electronically transmitting pharmacy claims to the payment authority in Wales. It is anticipated that testing of Phase 2 will commence during 2007/8.

7.17   A further one-off allowance of £1,000 will be paid to Community Pharmacy Contractors during 2007/08 to support the implementation requirements of Phase 2, Releases 1 and 2.

7.18   Further details on Release 1 and 2 developments and requirements will be provided to key stakeholders, specifically Community Pharmacies and their respective Pharmacy System Suppliers, in due course.

7.19   This funding was included in the LHBs' 2006-07 Pharmacy Contract allocation. LHBs should therefore ensure that they are able to re-provide for the Phase 2 payment in 2007-08.

7.20   If at a later date the Community Pharmacy Contractor fails to implement Phase 2 their LHB will be entitled to reclaim this additional allowance.

Further Information

7.21   These allowances and guidelines will be published in Part VIA of the Drug Tariff.

7.22   Further supplementary guidance will follow to provide clarification on the procedures to support the payment mechanisms and implementation of Phases 1 and 2.

PAYMENT FOR ESSENTIAL SERVICES (PHARMACY CONTRACTORS)

This Page is Intentionally Blank

SCALE OF ON-COST ALLOWANCES (APPLIANCE CONTRACTORS)

See Part II Clause 6B(ii) (page 5)

Number of prescriptions dispensed during month		On-cost %	Number of prescriptions dispensed during month		On-cost %
From	To		From	To	
1	505	25.0	1036	1048	20.3
506	515	24.9	1049	1062	20.2
516	526	24.8	1063	1076	20.1
527	537	24.7	1077	1090	20.0
538	549	24.6	1091	1105	19.9
550	561	24.5	1106	1120	19.8
562	574	24.4	1121	1136	19.7
575	588	24.3	1137	1152	19.6
589	602	24.2	1153	1169	19.5
603	617	24.1	1170	1186	19.4
618	632	24.0	1187	1203	19.3
633	649	23.9	1204	1221	19.2
650	666	23.8	1222	1240	19.1
667	684	23.7	1241	1259	19.0
685	704	23.6	1260	1279	18.9
705	724	23.5	1280	1300	18.8
725	746	23.4	1301	1321	18.7
747	756	23.3	1322	1342	18.6
757	762	23.2	1343	1365	18.5
763	770	23.1	1366	1388	18.4
771	777	23.0	1389	1413	18.3
778	785	22.9	1414	1438	18.2
786	792	22.8	1439	1463	18.1
793	800	22.7	1464	1490	18.0
801	808	22.6	1491	1518	17.9
809	816	22.5	1519	1547	17.8
817	824	22.4	1548	1577	17.7
825	833	22.3	1578	1608	17.6
834	841	22.2	1609	1641	17.5
842	850	22.1	1642	1675	17.4
851	859	22.0	1676	1710	17.3
860	868	21.9	1711	1747	17.2
869	878	21.8	1748	1785	17.1
879	887	21.7	1786	1825	17.0
888	897	21.6	1826	1867	16.9
898	907	21.5	1868	1911	16.8
908	918	21.4	1912	1957	16.7
919	928	21.3	1958	2006	16.6
929	939	21.2	2007	2056	16.5
940	950	21.1	2057	2110	16.4
951	961	21.0	2111	2166	16.3
962	973	20.9	2167	2226	16.2
974	984	20.8	2227	2288	16.1
985	996	20.7	2289	2355	16.0
997	1009	20.6	2356	2425	15.9
1010	1022	20.5	2426	2500	15.8
1023	1035	20.4			

VIB

SCALE OF ON-COST ALLOWANCES (APPLIANCE CONTRACTORS)

This Page is Intentionally Blank

ADVANCED SERVICES (PHARMACY CONTRACTORS)

MEDICINES USE REVIEW AND PRESCRIPTION INTERVENTION SERVICE

1. The Medicines Use Review and Prescription Intervention Service forms part of the Advanced Services within the community pharmacy contractual framework. A fee per Medicines Use Review (MUR) is payable with effect from 1 April 2005 to all pharmacy contractors meeting the requirements for this service. These are set out below in the principal Directions to PCTs (as amended by the Amendment Directions of 8 March 2006) in England and the principal Directions to LHBs (as amended by the Amendment Directions of 16 December 2006) in Wales.

2. From 1 April 2005 to 30 September 2006, a fee of £23 per Medicines Use Review (MUR) is payable. From 1 October 2006, a fee per MUR of £25 is payable.

3. In England and Wales, for the year April 2006 to March 2007, payment will be made up to a maximum of 400 MURs per pharmacy, with the exception of pharmacies who have not made arrangements before 1 October 2006, in which case payment will be made up to a maximum of 200 MURs per pharmacy (see Amendment Directions dated 15 September 2006 (England) and 16 December 2006 (Wales) below).

4. Contractors will be paid monthly, via the Pricing Authority or appropriate body, on the basis of the number of MURs declared by the pharmacy to the Pricing Authority or appropriate body on the appropriate claim form in the relevant month.

VIC

DIRECTIONS

THE NATIONAL HEALTH SERVICE ACT 1977

The Pharmaceutical Services (Advanced and Enhanced Services) (England) Directions 2005

The Secretary of State for Health, in exercise of the powers conferred upon him by sections 17, 41A, 41B and 126(4) of the National Health Service Act 1977(1), and of all other powers enabling him in that behalf, hereby gives the following Directions:

Citation, commencement and application

1.—(1) These Directions may be cited as the Pharmaceutical Services (Advanced and Enhanced Services) (England) Directions 2005 and shall come into force on 1st April 2005.

---

(1) 1977 c.49. Section 17 of the 1977 Act is as substituted by the Health Act 1999 (c.8) ("the 1999 Act"), section 12(1), and thereafter amended by the Health and Social Care Act 2001 (c.15) ("the 2001 Act"), Schedule 5, paragraph 5(3), and the National Health Service Reform and Health Care Professions Act 2002 (c.17) ("the 2002 Act"), Schedule 1, paragraph 7. Section 41A of the 1977 Act was inserted into the 1977 Act by the National Health Service (Primary Care) Act 1997 (c. 46) ("the 1997 Act"), section 27(1); and has been amended by the 2001 Act, section 43(1) and the 2002 Act, Schedule 2, Part 1, paragraphs 1 and 14. Section 41B was inserted into the 1977 Act by the 1997 Act, section 28(1) ans has been amended by the 2002 Act, Schedule 2, Part 1, paragraphs 1 and 15. Section 126(4) of the 1977 Act was amended by the National Health Service and Community Care Act 1990 (c.19), section 65(2). As regards Wales, the functions of the Secretary of State under the 1977 Act were transferred to the National Assembly for Wales by virtue of article 2 of, and Schedule 1 to, the National Assembly for Wales (Transfer of Functions) Order 1999 (S.I. 1999/672), as amended by section 66(5) of the 1999 Act and as read with section 40(1) of the 2002 Act.

ADVANCED SERVICES (PHARMACY CONTRACTORS)

(2) These Directions are given to Primary Care Trusts in England and apply in relation to England only.

Interpretation

2. In these Directions—

"the Act" means the National Health Service Act 1977;

"clinical management plan" has the same meaning as in the POM Order;

"drug misuser" means a person who is misusing drugs by self-injection;

"drugs" includes medicines;

"Drug Tariff" means the Drug Tariff published under regulation 56 (standards of, and payments for, drugs and appliances) of the Pharmaceutical Services Regulations;

"gluten free foods" means only those gluten free foods that are listed in Part XV (borderline substances) of the Drug Tariff;

"GMS contract essential services" has the meaning given to it in regulation 2(1) of the National Health Service (General Medical Services Contracts) Regulations 2004(**2**);

"health care professional" means a person who is a member of a profession regulated by a body mentioned in section 25(3) (the Council for the Regulation of Health Care Professionals) of the National Health Service Reform and Health Care Professions Act 2002(**3**);

"independent prescriber" means a doctor or dentist who is a party to a clinical management plan with a supplementary prescriber;

"MUR certificate" means a statement of satisfactory performance certificate awarded or endorsed by a higher education institute being evidence that he has satisfactorily completed an assessment relating to the competency framework for pharmacists providing MUR services approved by the Secretary of State(**4**);

"out of hours period" means, in relation to a pharmacy, the days and times at which the pharmacy is not obliged to remain open by virtue of paragraph 22(1) (pharmacy opening hours: general) of Schedule 1 (terms of service of pharmacists) to the Pharmaceutical Services Regulations;

"patient's care record" means the patient records kept by the person or body who is providing the patient with GMS contract essential services or their equivalent;

"pharmaceutical essential services" has the same meaning as that given to essential services in the Pharmaceutical Services Regulations;

"pharmaceutical list" means a list referred to in regulation 4(1)(a) (preparation of lists) of the Pharmaceutical Services Regulations;

"Pharmaceutical Services Regulations" means the National Health Service (Pharmaceutical Services) Regulations 2005(**5**);

"pharmacist" means, except where the context otherwise requires—

(a) a registered pharmacist; or

(b) a person lawfully conducting a retail pharmacy business in accordance with section 69 (general provisions) of the Medicines Act 1968,

whose name is included in the pharmaceutical list of a Primary Care Trust (including a pharmacist who is suspended from such a list), but does not include a supplier of appliances only;

"pharmacy" has the meaning given to it in the Pharmaceutical Services Regulations;

(**2**) S.I. 2004/291. There are no relevant amendments.
(**3**) 2002 c.17.
(**4**) This document "Competency Framework for the Assessment of Pharmacists Providing the Medicines Use Review (MUR) and Prescription Intervention Service" dated 23rd December 2004 is published by the Department of Health on its website www.dh.gov.uk/mpi.
(**5**) S.I. 2005/641.

ADVANCED SERVICES (PHARMACY CONTRACTORS)

"the POM Order" means the Prescription Only Medicines (Human Use) Order 1997(**6**); and "supplementary prescriber" has the meaning given to it in the Pharmaceutical Services Regulations.

Advanced Services: Medicines Use Review and Prescription Intervention Service

3.—(1) Each Primary Care Trust shall make arrangements for the provision of medicines use review and prescription intervention services ("MUR services") for persons within or outside its area with any pharmacist on its pharmaceutical list who—

    (a) meets the conditions set out in paragraphs (3), (4) and (5); and

    (b) wishes to enter into such arrangements or is required to do so by virtue of regulation 13(3) or 14 of the Pharmaceutical Services Regulations.

(2) The underlying purpose of MUR services is, with the patient's agreement, to improve his knowledge and use of drugs by in particular—

    (a) establishing the patient's actual use, understanding and experience of taking drugs;

    (b) identifying, discussing and assisting in the resolution of poor or ineffective use of drugs by the patient;

    (c) identifying side effects and drug interactions that may affect the patient's compliance with instructions given to him by a health care professional for the taking of drugs; and

    (d) improving the clinical and cost effectiveness of drugs prescribed to patients thereby reducing the wastage of such drugs.

(3) The first condition is—

    (a) if the pharmacist is a registered pharmacist, that he has an MUR certificate;

    (b) if the pharmacist is a registered pharmacist, but he intends to employ or engage a registered pharmacist to provide MUR services, that that registered pharmacist has an MUR certificate; or

    (c) if the pharmacist is not a natural person, that any registered pharmacist that it intends to employ or engage to provide MUR services has an MUR certificate,

and the pharmacist has supplied a copy of such certificates to the Primary Care Trust prior to entering into an arrangement to provide MUR services.

(4) The second condition is that the pharmacy meets the following requirements, namely that it has a consultation area which—

    (a) must be a clearly designated area for confidential consultations which is distinct from the general public areas of the pharmacy; and

    (b) must be an area where both the person receiving MUR services and the registered pharmacist providing MUR services can sit down together and talk at normal speaking volumes without being overheard by other visitors to the pharmacy or by any other person, including pharmacy staff.

(5) Subject to direction 6(2), the third condition is that the pharmacist is satisfactorily complying with his obligation under Schedule 1 to the Pharmaceutical Services Regulations to provide pharmaceutical essential services and has an acceptable system of clinical governance.

(6) The Primary Care Trust shall ensure that the arrangements made pursuant to paragraph (1) provide that—

    (a) only a registered pharmacist who has an MUR certificate may perform MUR services;

    (b) MUR services that are provided in a pharmacy may only be provided from a consultation area that meets the requirements set out in paragraph (4) unless the pharmacy is closed to other members of the public in which case the consultation may take place in another part of the pharmacy provided the condition in paragraph (4)(b) is met;

(**6**) S.I. 1997/1830; relevant amending instruments are S.I. 2000/1917 and 2003/2915.

ADVANCED SERVICES (PHARMACY CONTRACTORS)

(c) MUR services may be provided outside the pharmacy or exceptionally by telephone only where the Primary Care Trust consents;

(d) no more than 200 MUR services consultations may be carried out in each pharmacy (or outside it in accordance with subparagraph (c)) in any one period of twelve months under the arrangements;

(e) an MUR service consultation shall not be offered to a patient unless the patient has been receiving pharmaceutical services from the pharmacy for a period of at least three consecutive months;

(f) a patient may not have more than one MUR service consultation in any one period of twelve months unless in the reasonable opinion of the registered pharmacist the patient's circumstances have changed sufficiently to justify one or more further consultations during this period;

(g) where the Primary Care Trust has notified pharmacists in its area of the categories of patients who would benefit from the provision of MUR services, the pharmacist shall have regard to the notification in determining who to offer an MUR service consultation to;

(h) the pharmacist shall ensure that a written record of each MUR service consultation held with a patient is prepared by the registered pharmacist carrying out the consultation on a form approved for this purpose by the Secretary of State(7);

(i) the pharmacist shall be required to provide a copy of the record prepared pursuant to sub-paragraph (h) to the patient and to a person with whom the patient is registered for the provision of GMS contract essential services or their equivalent;

(j) the pharmacist shall keep a copy of the record prepared pursuant to sub-paragraph (h) for such period as the Primary Care Trust may reasonably require; and

(k) the arrangements shall be terminated where after 1st October 2005 the pharmacist is not satisfactorily complying with his obligation under Schedule 1 to the Pharmaceutical Services Regulations to provide pharmaceutical essential services and to have an acceptable system of clinical governance.

(7) The record referred to in paragraph (6)(h) may be in the form of an electronic record and may be sent or stored electronically.

Enhanced services

4.—(1) Each Primary Care Trust is authorised to arrange for the provision of the following additional pharmaceutical services to persons within or outside its area with pharmacists included in its pharmaceutical list or in the pharmaceutical list of a neighbouring Primary Care Trust—

(a) an Anticoagulant Monitoring Service, the underlying purpose of which is for the pharmacist to test the patient's blood clotting time, review the results and adjust (or recommend the adjustment to) the anticoagulant dose accordingly;

(b) a Care Home Service, the underlying purpose of which is for the pharmacist to provide advice and support to residents and staff in a care home relating to—

    (i) the proper and effective ordering of drugs and appliances for the benefit of residents in the care home,

    (ii) the clinical and cost effective use of drugs,

    (iii) the proper and effective administration of drugs and appliances in the care home,

    (iv) the safe and appropriate storage and handling of drugs and appliances, and

    (v) the recording of drugs and appliances ordered, handled, administered, stored or disposed of;

(c) a Disease Specific Medicines Management Service, the underlying purpose of which is for the pharmacist to advise on, support and monitor the treatment of patients with

---

(7) A copy of the form is published by the Department of Health on its website at www.dh.gov.uk/mpi.

specified conditions, and where appropriate to refer the patient to another health care professional;

(d)   a Gluten Free Food Supply Service, the underlying purpose of which is for the pharmacist to supply gluten free foods to patients;

(e)   a Home Delivery Service, the underlying purpose of which is for the pharmacist to deliver drugs and appliances to patients at their home;

(f)   a Language Access Service, the underlying purpose of which is for the pharmacist to provide, either orally or in writing, advice and support to patients in a language understood by them relating to—

    (i)   drugs which they are using,

    (ii)   their health, and

    (iii)   general health matters relevant to them,

and where appropriate referral to another health care professional;

(g)   a Medication Review Service, the underlying purpose of which is for the pharmacist to—

    (i)   conduct a review of the drugs used by a patient, including on the basis of information and test results included in the patient's care record, with the objective of considering the continued appropriateness and effectiveness of the drugs for the patient,

    (ii)   advise and support a patient regarding his use of drugs including encouraging the active participation of the patient in decision making relating to his use of drugs, and

    (iii)   where appropriate, refer the patient to another health care professional;

(h)   a Medicines Assessment and Compliance Support Service, the underlying purpose of which is for the pharmacist to—

    (i)   assess the knowledge of, compliance with and use of, drugs by vulnerable patients and patients with special needs, and

    (ii)   offer advice, support and assistance to vulnerable patients and patients with special needs regarding the use of drugs with a view to improving the patient's knowledge of, compliance with and use of, such drugs;

(i)   a Minor Ailment Scheme, the underlying purpose of which is for the pharmacist to provide advice and support to eligible patients complaining of a minor ailment, and where appropriate to supply drugs to them for the treatment of the minor ailment;

(j)   a Needle and Syringe Exchange Service, the underlying purpose of which is for the pharmacist to—

    (i)   provide sterile needles, syringes and associated materials to drug misusers,

    (ii)   receive from drug misusers used needles, syringes and associated materials, and

    (iii)   offer advice to drug misusers and where appropriate referral to another health care professional or a specialist drug treatment centre;

(k)   an On Demand Availability of Specialist Drugs Service, the underlying purpose of which is for the pharmacist to ensure that patients or health care professionals have prompt access to specialist drugs;

(l)   Out of Hours Services, the underlying purpose of which is for the pharmacist to dispense drugs and appliances in the out of hours period (whether or not for the whole of the out of hours period);

(m)   a Patient Group Direction Service, the underlying purpose of which is for the pharmacist to supply a prescription only medicine to a patient under a Patient Group Direction;

(n)   a Prescriber Support Service, the underlying purpose of which is for the pharmacist to support health care professionals who prescribe drugs, and in particular to offer advice on—

    (i)   the clinical and cost effective use of drugs,

    (ii) prescribing policies and guidelines, and

    (iii) repeat prescribing;

(o) a Schools Service, the underlying purpose of which is for the pharmacist to provide advice and support to children and staff in schools relating to—

    (i) the clinical and cost effective use of drugs in the school,

    (ii) the proper and effective administration and use of drugs and appliances in the school,

    (iii) the safe and appropriate storage and handling of drugs and appliances, and

    (iv) the recording of drugs and appliances ordered, handled, administered, stored or disposed of;

(p) a Screening Service, the underlying purpose of which is for the pharmacist to—

    (i) identify patients at risk of developing a specified disease or condition,

    (ii) offer advice regarding testing for a specified disease or condition,

    (iii) carry out such a test with the patient's consent, and

    (iv) offer advice following a test and referral to another health care professional where appropriate;

(q) a Stop Smoking Service, the underlying purpose of which is for the pharmacist to—

    (i) advise and support patients wishing to give up smoking, and

    (ii) where appropriate, to supply appropriate drugs and aids;

(r) a Supervised Administration Service, the underlying purpose of which is for the pharmacist to supervise the administration of prescribed medicines in the pharmacy; and

(s) a Supplementary Prescribing Service, the underlying purpose of which is for the pharmacist who is a supplementary prescriber to implement with an independent prescriber a clinical management plan for a patient with that patient's agreement.

(2) The Primary Care Trust shall ensure that the arrangements for the services referred to in paragraph (1) make provision for those services to be provided—

(a) only by appropriately trained and qualified persons;

(b) in accordance with relevant national guidelines or standards;

(c) from premises that are suitable for the purpose; and

(d) using the appropriate or necessary equipment.

Revocation

5. The Directions to Health Authorities concerning arrangements for providing additional pharmaceutical services which came into force on 1st April 1999 are hereby revoked.

Transitional provisions

6.—(1) Any arrangements pursuant to the Directions referred to in direction 5 shall continue in effect for a period of twelve months beginning with the date of the coming into force of these Directions unless—

(a) the pharmacist notifies the Primary Care Trust in writing that the arrangements should terminate before the end of this period, in which case the arrangements shall terminate on—

    (i) the date specified by the pharmacist in his notice,

    (ii) the date agreed with the Primary Care Trust, or

    (iii) if no date is specified or agreed, on the last day of the calendar month following the giving of the notice;

ADVANCED SERVICES (PHARMACY CONTRACTORS)

(b) the Primary Care Trust requests the pharmacist to enter into arrangements for a Care Home Service or Out of Hours Services pursuant to direction 4 and the pharmacist refuses such a request, in which case the arrangements shall terminate on the last day of the third calendar month following the date of the Primary Care Trust's request; or

(c) the arrangements would otherwise come to an end before this date, for example, because the pharmacist ceases to be included in the Primary Care Trust's pharmaceutical list.

(2) Direction 3(5) shall not apply to any arrangement entered into before 1st October 2005.

Signed by authority of the Secretary of State for Health

Jeannette Howe   Department of Health

31 March 2005   A member of the Senior Civil Service

DIRECTIONS

THE NATIONAL HEALTH SERVICE ACT 1977

The Pharmaceutical Services (Advanced and Enhanced Services) (England) Amendment Directions 2006

The Secretary of State for Health gives the following directions in exercise of the powers conferred upon her by sections 17, 41A, 41B and 126(4) of the National Health Service Act 1977(1).

Citation, commencement and application

1.—(1) These Directions may be cited as the Pharmaceutical Services (Advanced and Enhanced Services) (England) Amendment Directions 2006 and shall come into force on 1st October 2006.

(2) These Directions are given to Primary Care Trusts in England and apply in relation to England only.

Amendment of the Pharmaceutical Services (Advanced and Enhanced Services) (England) Directions 2005

2.—(1) The Pharmaceutical Services (Advanced and Enhanced Services) (England) Directions 2005(2) are amended as follows.

(2) In direction 3 (advanced services: Medicines Use Review and Prescription Intervention Service)—

(a) in paragraph (6)(d)(3), for "250" substitute "400"; and

(b) after paragraph (6), insert the following sub-paragraph(4)—

"(6A) Paragraph (6)(d) shall apply as if for "400" there were substituted "200" as regards the first financial year of any arrangements made pursuant to paragraph (1), if the arrangements made pursuant to paragraph (1) only took effect on or after 1st October of that financial year, but for these purposes, arrangements with a pharmacist to provide MUR services at an acceptable location to which paragraph (4)(a) applies are to be treated as taking effect once the pharmacist has—

---

(1) 1977 c.49. Section 17 is as substituted by the Health Act 1999 (c.8) ("the 1999 Act"), section 12(1), and thereafter amended by the Health and Social Care Act 2001 (c.15) ("the 2001 Act"), Schedule 5, paragraph 5(3), and the National Health Service Reform and Health Care Professions Act 2002 (c.17) ("the 2002 Act"), Schedule 1, paragraph 7. Section 41A was inserted into the 1977 Act by the National Health Service (Primary Care) Act 1997 (c. 46) ("the 1997 Act"), section 27(1); and has been amended by the 2001 Act, section 43(1), and the 2002 Act, Schedule 2, Part 1, paragraphs 1 and 14. Section 41B was inserted into the 1977 Act by the 1997 Act, section 28(1), and has been amended by the 2002 Act, Schedule 2, Part 1, paragraphs 1 and 15. Section 126(4) of the 1977 Act was amended by the National Health Service and Community Care Act 1990 (c.19), section 65(2). As regards Wales, the functions of the Secretary of State under the 1977 Act were transferred to the National Assembly for Wales by virtue of article 2 of, and Schedule 1 to, the National Assembly for Wales (Transfer of Functions) Order 1999 (S.I. 1999/672), as amended by section 66(5) of the 1999 Act and as read with section 40(1) of the 2002 Act.

(2) Signed on 31st March 2005 and available on www.dh.gov.uk. These Directions were amended by the Pharmaceutical Services (Advanced and Enhanced Services) (England) (Amendment) Directions 2005, signed on 6th December and available on www.dh.gov.uk, and by the National Health Service (Miscellaneous Amendments Relating to Prescribing, Pharmaceutical Services and Local Pharmaceutical Services etc.) (England) Directions 2006, signed on 8th March 2006 and available on www.dh.gov.uk.

(3) Sub-paragraph (d) of paragraph (6) was substituted by the National Health Service (Miscellaneous Amendments Relating to Prescribing, Pharmaceutical Services and Local Pharmaceutical Services etc.) (England) Directions 2006, direction 3(3)(b).

(4) The paragraph (6A) that was inserted by the Pharmaceutical Services (Advanced and Enhanced Services) (England) (Amendment) Directions 2005 was revoked by the National Health Service (Miscellaneous Amendments Relating to Prescribing, Pharmaceutical Services and Local Pharmaceutical Services etc.) (England) Directions 2006.

Amendment of the Pharmaceutical Services (Advanced and Enhanced Services) (England) Directions 2005

3.—(1) The Pharmaceutical Services (Advanced and Enhanced Services) (England) Directions 2005(**a**) are amended in accordance with this direction.

(2) In direction 2 (interpretation)—

  (a) insert the following definition at the appropriate place in the alphabetical order—

     ""financial year" means the period of twelve months ending on 31st March in any year; "; and

  (b) insert the following definition at the appropriate place in the alphabetical order—

     ""pharmacist independent prescriber" has the meaning given in regulation 2(1) of the Pharmaceutical Services Regulations;";

(3) In direction 3 (advanced services: Medicines Use Review and Prescription Intervention Service)—

  (a) for paragraph (4) substitute the following paragraphs—

     "(4) Subject to paragraph (4A), the second condition is that the MUR services are provided at an acceptable location, and for these purposes, an "acceptable location" means—

       (a) an area for confidential consultations within the pharmacist's pharmacy, which is—

         (i) clearly designated as an area for confidential consultations,

         (ii) distinct from the general public areas of the pharmacy, and

         (iii) an area where both the person receiving MUR services and the pharmacist providing those services are able to sit down together and talk at normal speaking volumes without being overheard by any other person (including pharmacy staff),

       except that paragraphs (i) and (ii) shall not apply in circumstances where the pharmacy is closed to other members of the public;

       (b) an area for confidential consultations which is not at the pharmacist's pharmacy but which—

         (i) is clearly designated as an area for confidential consultations—

         (ii) is distinct from the general public areas of the premises in which it is situated, and

         (iii) is an area where both the person receiving MUR services and the pharmacist providing those services are able to sit down together and talk at normal speaking volumes without being overheard by any other person,

       and the Primary Care Trust has approved the premises where the area is situated as being premises at which MUR services may be provided (and that approval has not been withdrawn); or

       (c) premises to which neither sub-paragraph (a) or (b) applies, but which are —

         (i) premises as regards which the pharmacist has obtained the approval of the Primary Care Trust to provide MUR services to a particular patient on a particular occasion, or

         (ii) premises or a category of premises as regards which the pharmacist has obtained the approval of the Primary Care Trust (which has not been withdrawn) to provide MUR services to a particular category of patients, in such circumstances and subject to such conditions as the Primary Care Trust may have specified (which the Primary Care Trust may vary without withdrawing its approval).

(**a**) Signed on 31st March 2005 and available on www.dh.gov.uk. These Directions were amended by the NHS Pharmaceutical Services (Advanced and Enhanced Services) (England) (Amendment) Directions 2005, signed on 6th December and available on www.dh.gov.uk.

(4A) A pharmacist may provide MUR services other than at an acceptable location, if he does so—

    (a) by telephone to a particular patient on a particular occasion;

    (b) in circumstances where the telephone conversation cannot be overheard (except by someone whom the patient wants to hear the conversation, for example a carer); and

    (c) having obtained the approval of the Primary Care Trust to do so on that occasion.";

  (b) for sub-paragraphs (b) to (d) of paragraph (6) substitute the following sub-paragraphs—

    "(b) MUR services are only provided—

        (i) at an acceptable location, except in the circumstances set out in paragraph (4A), and

        (ii) at a location for which the PCT's approval is required by virtue of paragraph (4)(b) or (c) for the location to be considered acceptable, if the necessary approval has been given by the PCT and has not been withdrawn;

    (c) where MUR services are provided other than at an acceptable location, they are only provided by telephone, and with its approval, to a particular patient on a particular occasion;

    (d) no more than 250 MUR services consultations may be carried out under the arrangements with a pharmacist to provide those services, whether at an acceptable location or in the circumstances set out in paragraph (4A), in any financial year;";

  (c) in sub-paragraph (e) of paragraph (6), after "an MUR service consultation" insert "which is not triggered by concerns over patient concordance"; and

  (d) omit paragraph (6A)(**a**).

(4) In direction 4 (enhanced services)—

  (a) after paragraph (1), insert the following paragraph—

    "(1A) Each Primary Care Trust is authorised to arrange for the provision of an Independent Prescribing Service, the underlying purpose of which is to provide a framework within which pharmacist independent prescribers may act as such under arrangements to provide an additional pharmaceutical service between the Primary Care Trust and a person included in the Primary Care Trust's pharmaceutical list or in a pharmaceutical list of a neighbouring Primary Care Trust."; and

  (b) in paragraph (2), for "paragraph (1)" substitute "paragraphs (1) and (1A)".

[...]

Revocation of the Pharmaceutical Services (Advanced and Enhanced Services) (England) (Amendment) Directions 2005

7. The Pharmaceutical Services (Advanced and Enhanced Services) (England) (Amendment) Directions 2005(**b**) are revoked.

Signed by authority of the Secretary of State for Health

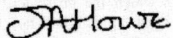

J.A. Howe
A member of the Senior Civil Service
Department of Health

8 March 2006

(**a**) Inserted by the NHS Pharmaceutical Services (Advanced and Enhanced Services) (England) (Amendment) Directions 2005, signed on 6th December and available on www.dh.gov.uk.

(**b**) Signed on 6th December 2005 and available at www.dh.gov.uk.

DIRECTIONS

THE NATIONAL HEALTH SERVICE ACT 1977

The Pharmaceutical Services (Advanced and Enhanced Services) (England) Amendment Directions 2006

The Secretary of State for Health gives the following directions in exercise of the powers conferred upon her by sections 17, 41A, 41B and 126(4) of the National Health Service Act 1977**(1)**.

Citation, commencement and application

1.—(1) These Directions may be cited as the Pharmaceutical Services (Advanced and Enhanced Services) (England) Amendment Directions 2006 and shall come into force on 1st October 2006.

(2) These Directions are given to Primary Care Trusts in England and apply in relation to England only.

Amendment of the Pharmaceutical Services (Advanced and Enhanced Services) (England) Directions 2005

2.—(1) The Pharmaceutical Services (Advanced and Enhanced Services) (England) Directions 2005**(2)** are amended as follows.

(2) In direction 3 (advanced services: Medicines Use Review and Prescription Intervention Service)—

    (a) in paragraph (6)(d)**(3)**, for "250" substitute "400"; and

    (b) after paragraph (6), insert the following sub-paragraph**(4)**—

        "(6A) Paragraph (6)(d) shall apply as if for "400" there were substituted "200" as regards the first financial year of any arrangements made pursuant to paragraph (1), if the arrangements made pursuant to paragraph (1) only took effect on or after 1st October of that financial year, but for these purposes, arrangements with a pharmacist to provide MUR services at an acceptable location to which paragraph (4)(a) applies are to be treated as taking effect once the pharmacist has—

---

(1) 1977 c.49. Section 17 is as substituted by the Health Act 1999 (c.8) ("the 1999 Act"), section 12(1), and thereafter amended by the Health and Social Care Act 2001 (c.15) ("the 2001 Act"), Schedule 5, paragraph 5(3), and the National Health Service Reform and Health Care Professions Act 2002 (c.17) ("the 2002 Act"), Schedule 1, paragraph 7. Section 41A was inserted into the 1977 Act by the National Health Service (Primary Care) Act 1997 (c. 46) ("the 1997 Act"), section 27(1); and has been amended by the 2001 Act, section 43(1), and the 2002 Act, Schedule 2, Part 1, paragraphs 1 and 14. Section 41B was inserted into the 1977 Act by the 1997 Act, section 28(1), and has been amended by the 2002 Act, Schedule 2, Part 1, paragraphs 1 and 15. Section 126(4) of the 1977 Act was amended by the National Health Service and Community Care Act 1990 (c.19), section 65(2). As regards Wales, the functions of the Secretary of State under the 1977 Act were transferred to the National Assembly for Wales by virtue of article 2 of, and Schedule 1 to, the National Assembly for Wales (Transfer of Functions) Order 1999 (S.I. 1999/672), as amended by section 66(5) of the 1999 Act and as read with section 40(1) of the 2002 Act.

(2) Signed on 31st March 2005 and available on www.dh.gov.uk. These Directions were amended by the Pharmaceutical Services (Advanced and Enhanced Services) (England) (Amendment) Directions 2005, signed on 6th December and available on www.dh.gov.uk, and by the National Health Service (Miscellaneous Amendments Relating to Prescribing, Pharmaceutical Services and Local Pharmaceutical Services etc.) (England) Directions 2006, signed on 8th March 2006 and available on www.dh.gov.uk.

(3) Sub-paragraph (d) of paragraph (6) was substituted by the National Health Service (Miscellaneous Amendments Relating to Prescribing, Pharmaceutical Services and Local Pharmaceutical Services etc.) (England) Directions 2006, direction 3(3)(b).

(4) The paragraph (6A) that was inserted by the Pharmaceutical Services (Advanced and Enhanced Services) (England) (Amendment) Directions 2005 was revoked by the National Health Service (Miscellaneous Amendments Relating to Prescribing, Pharmaceutical Services and Local Pharmaceutical Services etc.) (England) Directions 2006.

ADVANCED SERVICES (PHARMACY CONTRACTORS)

    (a) declared in writing to the Primary Care Trust, in terms, that he has an acceptable location that meets the requirements of paragraph (4)(a); and

    (b) supplied the Primary Care Trust with a copy of the MUR certificate that he has to supply in order to meet the first condition."

Signed by authority of the Secretary of State for Health

Jeannette Howe   Department of Health

15th September 2006   A member of the Senior Civil Service

NATIONAL ASSEMBLY FOR WALES

DIRECTIONS

NATIONAL HEALTH SERVICE, WALES

The Pharmaceutical Services (Advanced and Enhanced Services) (Wales) Directions 2005

The National Assembly for Wales in exercise of the powers conferred by sections 16BB(4), 41A, 41B and 126(4) of the National Health Service Act 1977(**1**) hereby gives the following Directions:

Title, commencement and application

1.—(1) The title of these Directions is the Pharmaceutical Services (Advanced and Enhanced Services) (Wales) Directions 2005 and will come into force on 5 May 2005.

(2) These Directions are given to Local Health Boards and apply in relation to Wales.

2. In these Directions—

"the Act" means the National Health Service Act 1977;

"clinical management plan" has the same meaning as in the POM Order;

"drug misuser" means a person who is misusing drugs by self-injection;

"drugs" includes medicines;

"Drug Tariff" means the Drug Tariff published under regulation 18 of the Pharmaceutical Services Regulations;

"gluten free foods" means only those gluten free foods that are listed in Part XV (borderline substances) of the Drug Tariff;

(**1**)   1977 c.49 ("the 1977 Act"); section 16BB(4) was inserted by the National Health Service Reform and Health Care Professions Act 2002 (c.17)("the 2002 Act"), section 6(1).   Date in force 10.10.02;   see SI 2002/2532 and was amended by section 184 of and paragraphs 7 and 10 of Schedule 11 to the Health and Social Care (Community Health and Standards Act 2003 (c.43) ("the 2003 Act").

Section 41A was inserted into the 1977 by the National Health Service (Primary Care) Act 1997 (c.46) ("the 1997 Act"), section 27(1); and has been amended by the Health and Social Care Act 2001 (c.15) ("the 2001 Act), section 43(1)(b) and the 2002 Act, section 2(5) and Schedule 2, Part I, paragraphs 1 and 14.

Section 41B was inserted into the 1977 Act by the 1997 Act, section 28(1) and has been amended by the 2002 Act, section 2(5) and Schedule 2, Part 1, paragraphs 1 and 15.

Section 126(4) was amended by the National Health Service and Community Care Act 1990 (c.19), section 65(2); and by the 2001 Act, section 67(1) and Schedule 5, Part 1, paragraphs 5(1) and 13(b), by the 2002 Act, section 6(3)(c) and by the Health and Social Care (Community Health and Standards) Act 2003 (c.43) ("the 2003 Act"), section 184 and Schedule 11, paragraphs 7 and 38.

The functions of the Secretary of State under sections 41A, 41B and 126(4) of the 1977 Act were transferred to the National Assembly for Wales by the National Assembly for Wales (Transfer of Functions) Order 1999, SI 1999/672, article 2 and Schedule 1, as amended by the 1999 Act, section 66(5), the 2001 Act, section 68(1), the 2002 Act, section 40(1) and by the 2003 Act, section 197(1).

"GMS contract essential services" has the meaning given to it in regulation 2(1) of the National Health Service (General Medical Services Contracts) (Wales) Regulations 2004(**1**);

"health care professional" means a person who is a member of a profession regulated by a body mentioned in section 25(3) (the Council for the Regulation of Health Care Professionals) of the National Health Service Reform and Health Care Professions Act 2002(**2**);

"independent prescriber" means a doctor or dentist who is a party to a clinical management plan with a supplementary prescriber;

"MUR certificate" means a statement of satisfactory performance awarded or endorsed by a higher education institute being evidence that a person has satisfactorily completed an assessment relating to the competency framework for chemists providing MUR services approved by the National Assembly for Wales;(**3**)

"out of hours period" means, in relation to a pharmacy, the days and times at which the pharmacy is not obliged to remain open by virtue of paragraph 21(1) (pharmacy opening hours: general) of Schedule 2 to the Pharmaceutical Services Regulations;

"patient's care record" means the patient records kept by the person or body who is providing the patient with GMS contract essential services or their equivalent;

"pharmaceutical essential services" has the same meaning as that given to essential services in the Pharmaceutical Services Regulations;

"Pharmaceutical Services Regulations" means the National Health Service (Pharmaceutical Services) Regulations 1992(**4**);

"chemist" means, except where the context otherwise required—

(a) a registered pharmacist; or

(b) a person lawfully conducting a retail pharmacy business in accordance with section 69 (general provisions) of the Medicines Act 1968(**5**),

whose name is included in the pharmaceutical list of a Local Health Board (including a chemist who is suspended from such a list), but does not include a supplier of appliances only;

"pharmacy" has the meaning given to it in the Pharmaceutical Services Regulations;

"the POM Order" means the Prescription Only Medicines (Human Use) Order 1997(**6**); and

"supplementary prescriber" has the meaning given to it in the Pharmaceutical Services Regulations.

Advanced Services: Medicines Use Review and Prescription Intervention Service

3.—(1) Each Local Health Board must make arrangements for the provision of medicines use review and prescription intervention services ("MUR services") for persons within or outside its area with any pharmacist on its pharmaceutical list who—

(a) meets the conditions set out in paragraphs (3), (4) and (5); and

(b) wishes to enter into such arrangements.

(2) The underlying purpose of MUR services is, with the patient's agreement, to improve his or her knowledge and use of drugs by, in particular—

(a) establishing the patient's actual use, understanding and experience of taking drugs;

(b) identifying, discussing and assisting in the resolution of poor or ineffective use of drugs by the patient;

---

(1)   SI 2004/478 (W.48) to which there are no relevant amendments.
(2)   2002 c.17
(3)   A copy of the document "Competency Framework for the Assessment of Pharmacists Providing the Medicines Use
        Review (MUR) and prescription intervention service" dated 19th April 2005 is available on the NHS Wales website
        – www.wales.nhs.uk
(4)   SI 1992/662; for relevant amendments see SI 2005/1013 (W.67)
(5)   1968 c.67
(6)   SI 1997/1839; relevant amending instruments are SI 2000/1917 and 2003/2915.

ADVANCED SERVICES (PHARMACY CONTRACTORS)

(c) identifying side effects and drug interactions that may affect the patient's compliance with instructions given to him or her by a health care professional for the taking of drugs; and

(d) improving the clinical and cost effectiveness of drugs prescribed to patients thereby reducing the wastage of such drugs.

(3) The first condition is—

(a) if the chemist is a registered pharmacist, that he or she has an MUR certificate;

(b) if the chemist is a registered pharmacist, but he or she intends to employ or engage a registered pharmacist to provide MUR services, that that registered pharmacist has an MUR certificate;

(c) if the chemist is not a natural person, that any registered pharmacist that it intends to employ or engage to provide MUR services has an MUR certificate,

and the chemist has supplied a copy of the relevant certificates to the Local Health Board prior to entering into an arrangement to provide MUR services.

(4) The second condition is that the pharmacy meets the following requirements, namely that it has a consultation area which—

(a) must be a clearly designated area for confidential consultations which is distinct from the general public areas of the pharmacy; and

(b) must be an area where both the person receiving MUR services and the registered pharmacist providing MUR services can sit down together and talk at normal speaking volumes without being overheard by other visitors to the pharmacy or by any other person, including pharmacy staff.

(5) Subject to direction 6(2), the third condition is that the chemist is satisfactorily complying with his or her obligation under Schedule 2 to the Pharmaceutical Services Regulations to provide pharmaceutical essential services and has a system of clinical governance that is acceptable.

(6) The Local Health Board must ensure that the arrangements made pursuant to paragraph (1) provide—

(a) only a registered pharmacist who has an MUR certificate may perform MUR services;

(b) MUR services that are provided in a pharmacy may only be provided from a consultation area that meets the requirements set out in paragraph (4) unless the pharmacy is closed to other members of the public in which case the consultation may take place in another part of the pharmacy provided that the condition in paragraph (4)(b) is met;

(c) MUR services may be provided outside the pharmacy or exceptionally by telephone only where the Local Health Board consents;

(d) no more than 200 MUR services consultations may be carried out in each pharmacy (or outside it in accordance with sub-paragraph (c)) in any one period of twelve months under the arrangements;

(e) an MUR service consultation must not be offered to a patient unless the patient has been receiving pharmaceutical services from the pharmacy for a period of at least three consecutive months;

(f) a patient may not have more than one MUR service consultation in any one period of twelve months unless in the reasonable opinion of the registered pharmacist the patient's circumstances have changed sufficiently to justify one or more further consultations during this period;

(g) where the Local Health Board has notified chemists in its area of the categories of patients who would benefit from the provision of MUR services, the chemist must have regard to the notification in determining to whom to offer a MUR service consultation;

(h) the chemist must ensure that a written record of each MUR service consultation held with a patient is prepared by the registered pharmacist carrying out the consultation on a form approved by the National Assembly for Wales(1);

(i) the chemist must provide a copy of the record prepared pursuant to sub-paragraph (h) to the patient and to a person with whom the patient is registered for the provision of GMS contract essential services or their equivalent;

(j) the chemist must keep a copy of the record prepared pursuant to sub-paragraph (h) for such period as the Local Health Board may reasonable require; and

(k) the arrangements will be terminated where after 1 October 2005 the chemist is not satisfactorily complying with his or her obligation under Schedule 2 to the Pharmaceutical Services Regulations to provide pharmaceutical essential services and to have an acceptable system of clinical governance.

Enhanced services

4.—(1) Each Local Health Board is authorised to arrange for the provision of the following additional pharmaceutical services to persons within or outside its area with chemists included in its pharmaceutical list or in the pharmaceutical list of a neighbouring Local Health Board—

(a) an Anticoagulant Monitoring Service, the underlying purpose of which is for the chemist to test the patient's blood clotting time, review the results and adjust (or recommend an adjustment to) the anticoagulant dose accordingly;

(b) a Care Home Service, the underlying purpose of which is for the chemist to provide advice and support to residents and staff in a care home relating to—

   (i) the proper and effective ordering of drugs and appliances for the benefit of residents in the care home,

   (ii) the clinical and cost effective use of drugs,

   (iii) the proper and effective administration of drugs and appliances in the care home,

   (iv) the safe and appropriate storage and handling of drugs and appliances, and

   (v) the recording of drugs and appliances ordered, handled, administered, stored or disposed of;

(c) a Disease Specific Management Service, the underlying purpose of which is for the chemist to advise on, support and monitor the treatment of patients with specified conditions, and where appropriate, to refer the patient to another health care professional;

(d) a Gluten Free Food Supply service, the underlying purpose of which is for the chemist to supply gluten free foods to patients;

(e) a Home Delivery Service, the underlying purpose of which is for the chemist to deliver drugs and appliances to patients at their home;

(f) a Language Access Service, the underlying purpose of which is for the chemist to provide, either orally or in writing, advice and support to patients in a language understood by them relation to—

   (i) drugs which they are using,

   (ii) their health, and

   (iii) general health matters relevant to them,

   and where appropriate referral to another health care professional;

(g) a Medication Review Service, the underlying purpose of which is for the chemist to—

   (i) conduct a review of the drugs used by a patient on the basis of information and test results included in the patient's care record, with the objective of considering the continued appropriateness and effectiveness of the drugs for the patient,

---

(1) Details for obtaining copies of this form will be made available shortly.

ADVANCED SERVICES (PHARMACY CONTRACTORS)

    (ii) advise and support a patient regarding the use of his or her drugs including encouraging the active participation of the patient in decision making relating to his or her use of drugs, and

    (iii) where appropriate, refer the patient to another health care professional;

(h) a Medicines Assessment and Compliance Support Service, the underlying purpose of which is for the chemist to—

    (i) assess the knowledge of, compliance with and use of, drugs by vulnerable patients and patients with special needs, and

    (ii) offer advice, support and assistance to vulnerable patients and patients with special needs regarding the use of drugs with a view to improving the patient's knowledge of, compliance with and use of, such drugs;

(i) a Minor Ailment Scheme, the underlying purpose of which is for the chemist to provide advice and support to eligible patients complaining of a minor ailment, and where appropriate, to supply drugs to them for the treatment of the minor ailment;

(j) a Needle and Syringe Exchange Scheme, the underlying purpose of which is for the chemist to—

    (i) to provide sterile needles, syringes and associated materials to drug misusers,

    (ii) receive from drug misusers used needles, syringes and associated materials, and

    (iii) offer advice to drug misusers and where appropriate referral to another health care professional or a specialist drug treatment centre;

(k) an On Demand Availability of Specialist Drugs Service, the underlying purpose of which is for the chemist to ensure that patients or health care professionals have prompt access to specialist drugs;

(l) Out of Hours Services, the underlying purpose of which is for the chemist to dispense drugs and appliances in the out of hours period (whether or not for the whole of the out of hours period);

(m) a Patient Group Direction Service, the underlying purpose of which is for the chemist to supply a prescription only medicine to a patient under a Patient Group Direction;

(n) a Prescriber Support Service, the underlying purpose of which is for the chemist to support health care professionals who prescribe drugs, and in particular to offer advice on—

    (i) the clinical and cost effective use of drugs,

    (ii) prescribing policies and guidelines, and

    (iii) repeat prescribing;

(o) a Schools Service, the underlying purpose of which is for the chemist to provide advice and support to children and staff in schools relating to—

    (i) the clinical and cost effective use of drugs in the school,

    (ii) the proper and effective administration and use of drugs and appliances in the school,

    (iii) the safe and appropriate storage and handling of drugs and appliances, and

    (iv) the recording of drugs and appliances ordered, handled, administered, stored or disposed of;

(p) a Screening Service, the underlying purpose of which is for the chemist to—

    (i) identify patients at risk of developing a specified disease or condition,

    (ii) offer advice regarding testing for a specified disease or condition,

    (iii) carry out such a test with the patient's consent, and

    (iv) offer advice following a test and referral to another health care professional where appropriate;

(q) a Stop Smoking Service, the underlying purpose of which is for the chemist to—

ADVANCED SERVICES (PHARMACY CONTRACTORS)

> (i) advise and support patients wishing to give up smoking, and
>
> (ii) where appropriate, to supply appropriate drugs and aids;

(r) a Supervised Administration Service, the underlying purpose of which is for the chemist to supervise the administration of prescribed medicines in the pharmacy; and

(s) a Supplementary Prescribing Service, the underlying purpose of which is for the chemist who is a supplementary prescriber to implement with an independent prescriber a clinical management plan for a patient with that patient's agreement.

(2) The Local Health Board must ensure that the arrangements for the services referred to in paragraph (1) make provision for those services to be provided—

(a) only by appropriately trained and qualified persons

(b) in accordance with relevant national guidelines or standards;

(c) from premises that are suitable for the purpose; and

(d) using the appropriate or necessary equipment.

Signed by authority of the National Assembly for Wales

D. Ellis-Thomas

04-05-2005   Presiding Officer of the National Assembly

NATIONAL ASSEMBLY FOR WALES

SUBORDINATE LEGISLATION

NATIONAL HEALTH SERVICE, WALES

VIC

The Pharmaceutical Services (Advanced and Enhanced Services) (Wales) Amendment Directions 2006

Made   December 2006
Coming into force   11ᵗʰ December 2006

The National Assembly for Wales, in exercise of the powers conferred by sections 16BB(4), 41A, 41B and 126(4) of the National Health Service Act 1977(1) hereby gives the following directions.

Title, commencement, application and interpretation

1.—(1) The title of these directions is the Pharmaceutical Services (Advanced and Enhanced Services) (Wales) Amendment Directions 2006.

(2) These Directions come into force on 11ᵗʰ December 2006

(3) These Directions are given to Local Health Boards and apply in relation to Wales.

(4) In these Directions "the Principal Directions" means the Pharmaceutical Service (Advanced and Enhanced Services) (Wales) Directions 2005.

(**1**) 1977 c.49 ("the 1977 Act"); section 16BB(4) was inserted by the National Health Service Reform and Health Care Professions Act 2002 (c.17)("the 2002 Act") section 6(1). Date in force 10.10.02; see S.I. 2002/2532 and was amended by section 184 of and paragraphs 7 and 10 of Schedule 11 to the Health and Social Care (Community Health and Standards Act 2003 9 (c.43) ("the 2003 Act").

Section 41A was inserted into the 1977 Act by the National Heath Service (Primary Care)Act 1997 (c.46) ("the 1997 Act"), section 27(1) ; and has been amended by the Health and Social Care Act 2001 (c.15) ("the 2001 Act"), section 43(1)(b) and the 2002 Act, section 2(5) and Schedule 2, Part I, paragraphs 1and 14.

Section 41B was inserted into the 1977 Act, section 28(1) and has been amended by the 2002 Act, section 2(5) and Schedule 2, Part I paragraphs 1 and 15.

Section 126(4) was amended by the National Health Service and Community Care Act 1990 (c.19), section 65(2); and by the 2001 Act, section 67(1) and Schedule 5, Part I, paragraphs 5(1) and 13(b), by the 2002 Act, section 6(3)(c) and by the Health and Social Care (Community Health and Standards) Act 2003 (c.43) ("the 2003 Act"), section 184 and Schedule 11, paragraphs 7 and 38.

The functions of the Secretary of State under sections 41A, 41B and 126(4) of the 1977 Act were transferred to the National Assembly for Wales by the National Assembly for Wales (Transfer of Functions) Order 1999, S.I. 1999/672, article 2 and Schedule 1, as amended by the 1999 Act, section 66(5), the 2001 Act, section 68(1), the 2002 Act, section 40(1) and by the 2003 Act, section 197(1).

ADVANCED SERVICES (PHARMACY CONTRACTORS)

Amendment of the Direction 3 of the Principal Directions

2.—(1) Direction 3 of the Principal Directions (Advanced Services: Medicines Use Review and Prescription Intervention Service) is amended as follows.

(2) In subparagraph (6)(d)—

    (i) insert the words "subject to subparagraph (6)(dd)" at the beginning;

    (ii) delete the figure "200" and replace it with the figure "400".

(3) After subparagraph (6)(d), insert the following subparagraph

    "(dd) where arrangements made under paragraph (1) between an LHB and a pharmacist only take effect after 1st October of the financial year in question then the maximum number of MUR services consultations that can be carried out in that year is 200;".

(4) Delete subparagraph (6)(e).

Signed   Dr Brian Gibbons

Dated 11th December 2006

Minister for Health and Social Services

ENHANCED SERVICES (PHARMACY CONTRACTORS)

Directions have been issued to PCTs in England and LHBs in Wales authorising them to make arrangements for enhanced services. The directions are reproduced in Part VIC.

For enhanced services, PCTs and LHBs are the determining authority for the payment arrangements. PCTs and LHBs can commission enhanced services from pharmacies within neighbouring PCTs or LHBs. Determinations to allow for this on an England/Wales basis are detailed below.

Determination of payments for enhanced services

In accordance with Regulation 56(2) of the National Health Service (Pharmaceutical Services) Regulations 2005, each Primary Care Trust is the determining authority for the purposes of making a determination for the fees and allowances for the provision of the enhanced services referred to in direction 4 of the Pharmaceutical Services (Advanced and Enhanced Services) (England) Directions 2005, by pharmacists included in its pharmaceutical list or in the list of a neighbouring Primary Care Trust.

In Wales, in accordance with Regulation 18(1)(a) of the National Health Service (Pharmaceutical Services) Regulations 1992, each Local Health Board is the determining authority for the purposes of making a determination for the fees and allowances for the provision of the enhanced services referred to in direction 4 of the Pharmaceutical Services (Advanced and Enhanced Services) (Wales) Directions 2005, by pharmacists included in its pharmaceutical list or in the list of a neighbouring Local Health Board.

VID

ENHANCED SERVICES (PHARMACY CONTRACTORS)

This Page is Intentionally Blank

DRUGS WITH COMMON PACK

LIST OF DRUGS WITH A COMMONLY USED PACK SIZE
See Part II, Clause 7D (page 6)

If a drug specified in this list is supplied but the relative prescription form is not endorsed payment will be calculated on the basis of the price for the pack size listed

Drug	Common Pack	
Anusol suppositories	24	
Azathioprine 50mg tablets	100	
Benadryl Allergy Relief 8mg capsules	24	
Brufen 400mg tablets	250	
Capoten 25mg tablets	56	
Ceporex 250mg capsules	100	
Ceporex 500mg capsules	100	
Ceporex 250mg tablets	100	
Ceporex 500mg tablets	100	
Deltacortril Enteric 2.5mg tablets	100	
Deltacortril Enteric 5mg tablets	100	
Dexamethasone 2mg tablets	500	
Dexomon 75mg SR tablets	56	
Diclofenac sodium 50mg gastro-resistant tablets	84	
Diclovol 75mg SR tablets	28	
Dipyridamole 25mg tablets	100	
Elantan 10 tablets	84	
Elantan 20 tablets	84	
Galpseud 60mg tablets	100	
Gaviscon, Liquid aniseed	600	ml
Gaviscon, Liquid peppermint	600	ml
Imodium 2mg capsules	250	
Keflex 250mg capsules	100	
Keflex 500mg capsules	100	
Keflex 250mg tablets	100	
Keflex 500mg tablets	100	
Kolanticon gel	500	ml
Lasix 40mg tablets	28	
Metformin 850mg tablets	300	
Natrilix 2.5mg tablets	60	
Nicef 250mg capsules	100	
Nicef 500mg capsules	100	
Nicorette Microtab 2mg sublingual tablets	105	
Nicotinell Classic, Fruit, Liquorice, Mint 2mg gum	96	
Nicotinell Classic, Fruit, Liquorice, Mint 4mg gum	96	
Nicotinell 1mg lozenges	96	
Nicotinell 2mg lozenges	96	

DRUGS WITH COMMON PACK

Drug	Common Pack	
Nicotinell TTS 30 patches	21	
NiQuitin CQ 21mg patches	14	
NiQuitin CQ Clear 21mg patches	14	
NovoNorm 500microgram tablets	90	
NovoNorm 1mg tablets	90	
Nurofen for Children 100mg/5ml suspension	150	ml
Praxilene capsules	500	
Prednisolone 2.5mg gastro-resistant tablets	30	
Prednisolone 5mg gastro-resistant tablets	30	
Proflavine 0.1% cream	500	ml
Prothiaden 25mg capsules	100	
Provera 100mg tablets	100	
Stugeron 15mg tablets	100	
Sudafed, Non-Drowsy 60mg tablets	100	
Trandate 100mg tablets	250	
Trandate 200mg tablets	250	
Velosef 250mg capsules	100	
Velosef 500mg capsules	100	

BASIC PRICES OF DRUGS

BASIC PRICE OF DRUGS
COVERED BY PART II CLAUSE 8A

The price listed in respect of a drug specified in the following list is
the basic price (see Part II, Clause 8) on which payment will be calculated
pursuant to Part II Clause 6A for the dispensing of that drug

1. All drugs listed in this Part have a pack size and price which has been determined by the Secretary of State for Health as respects England and the National Assembly for Wales as respects Wales.

2. Categories A, B, C, E and M of the drugs (appearing in Col.4) are as under:

    2.1 Category A - Drugs which are readily available. Endorsement of pack size is required if more than one pack size is listed. Broken Bulk may be claimed if necessary.

    2.2 Category B - Drugs whose usage has declined over time. No endorsement is required other than a claim for Broken Bulk if necessary.

    2.3 Category C - Priced on the basis of a particular brand or particular manufacturer. Endorsement of pack size is required if more than one pack is listed. Broken Bulk may be claimed if necessary.

    2.4 Category E - Extemporaneously prepared items for which the fee listed under Part IIIA 2A (page 25) will be claimed. No endorsement is required. Broken Bulk is not allowed, but may be paid on the ingredients.

    2.5 Category M - Drugs which are readily available, where the Department of Health calculate the reimbursement price based on information submitted by manufacturers. Endorsement of pack size is required if more than one pack size is listed. Broken Bulk may be claimed if necessary.

3. Recommended International Non-proprietary Names

    With effect from 1 December 2003 drugs will be listed in this Part by their recommended International Non-proprietary Name (rINN), with the exception of Adrenaline and Noradrenaline (which will be listed by their BAN). Where such products are ordered by the former BAN, reimbursement will be made whether the manufacturer of those products is using the former BAN or the rINN to name them. Where prices are calculated for Category A products such prices will be included in the calculation whether they are listed by suppliers as a former BAN or as a rINN.

4. NHS dictionary of medicines and devices (NHS dm+d)

    The drugs listed in this Part will reflect the naming convention used in the NHS dictionary of medicines and devices. Where such products are ordered by another naming convention, reimbursement will be made using the Part VIII dm+d naming convention. Where prices are calculated for Category A products such prices will be included in the calculation whether they are listed by suppliers using the NHS dm+d naming convention or as other naming conventions.Products are displayed as Name, strength, modification (when present), presentation and 'freeness' (when present e.g. sugar free, gluten free).

    E.g. Aciclovir 400mg/5ml oral suspension sugar free.

    A salt will only be displayed if more than one clinically significant salt exists in that presentation.

    E.g. Calcium carbonate and Calcium gluconate.

    Please note that the NHS dm&d uses the Pharmeuropa List of Standard Terms 2002 e.g. gastro-resistant is used to describe enteric coated.

5. Symbols

    The following symbols are used in Part VIII

    - ♦   Calendar Pack
    - ■   Special Container
    - ●   Item requiring reconstitution
    - ★   Common pack
    - §   Selected List Scheme (SLS)

BASIC PRICES OF DRUGS

6.   Methylated Spirit

        Industrial Methylated Spirit should be supplied or used and payment will be calculated accordingly, where:

        6.1   "Methylated Spirit", "Spirit", "Spt. Vini. Meth.", "SVM", "IMS", is ordered alone or as an ingredient of a preparation for external use, or

        6.2   A liniment, lotion, etc., in the preparatioin of which Methylated Spirit is permitted, is ordered and the prescriber has not indicated to the contrary.

7.   Rectified Spirit

        7.1   Where Alcohol (96%), or Rectified Spirit (Ethanol 90%), or any other of the dilute Ethanols is prescribed alone or as an ingredient in a medicament for external application, payment will be made for supply of Industrial Methylated Spirit unless the prescriber has indicated that no alternative may be used.

        7.2   Where Alcohol (96%), or Rectified Spirit (Ethanol 90%), or any other of the dilute Ethanols is prescribed as an ingredient of a medicine for internal use, the price of the duty paid to Customs and Excise will be allowed, unless the contractor endorses the prescription form "rebate claimed".

8.   Purified Water
        (Exclusive of ordinary potable water)

        Payment for Purified Water will be made:

        8.1   where it is ordered:

        8.2   where the water is included in any preparation intended for application to the eye;

        8.3   where, in the opinion of the pharmacist the use of ordinary potable water in a particular preparation would result in an undesirable change in the medicament prescribed and he endorses the prescription form accordingly;

        8.4   where the PCT for England and LHB for Wales, after consultation with the Local Medical Committee and Local Pharmaceutical Committee, has decided with the approval of the Secretary of State for Health as respects England and the National Assembly for Wales as respects Wales that the water ordinarily available is unsuitable for dispensing purposes, and has notified the contractor accordingly.

        When Purified Water is used instead of potable water, it should be freshly boiled and cooled.

9.   A "Bulk" prescription is an order for two or more patients, bearing the name of a school or institution in which at least 20 persons normally reside, for the treatment of at least 10 of whom a particular doctor is responsible. Such a prescription must be an order for a drug which is prescribable under the NHS and which is not designated a "Prescription Only Medicine" (POM) under Section 58(1) of the Medicines Act 1968, or for a prescribable dressing which does not contain a product which is designated POM.

BASIC PRICES OF DRUGS

Drug		Quantity		Basic Price		Category	
Acacia spray dried powder		250	g	925		C	Loveridge
Acamprosate 333mg gastro-resistant tablets		168		2892		C	Campral EC
Acarbose 100mg tablets		90		1251		C	Glucobay 100
Acarbose 50mg tablets		90		660		C	Glucobay 50
Acebutolol 100mg capsules		84		1497		A	
Acebutolol 200mg capsules		56		1918		A	
Acebutolol 400mg tablets		28		1862		A	
Aceclofenac 100mg tablets		60		963		C	Preservex
Acemetacin 60mg capsules		90		2820		C	Emflex
Acenocoumarol 1mg tablets		100		462		C	Sinthrome
Acetazolamide 250mg modified-release capsules	♦	28		1155		C	Diamox SR
Acetazolamide 250mg tablets		112		1268		A	
Acetic acid 33% liquid		500	ml	230		C	Unichem
Acetone liquid		500	ml	251	△	A	
Acetylcysteine 5% eye drops	■	10	ml	463		C	Ilube
Aciclovir 200mg dispersible tablets		25		356		M	
Aciclovir 200mg tablets		25		401		A	
Aciclovir 200mg/5ml oral suspension sugar free		125	ml	2956		C	Zovirax
Aciclovir 3% eye ointment	■	4.5	g	992		C	Zovirax
Aciclovir 400mg dispersible tablets	♦	56		945		M	
Aciclovir 400mg tablets		56		731		A	
Aciclovir 400mg/5ml oral suspension sugar free		100	ml	3302		C	Zovirax Chickenpox Treatment
Aciclovir 5% cream	■	2	g	193		M	
	■	10	g	369		M	
Aciclovir 800mg dispersible tablets		35		1112		M	
Aciclovir 800mg tablets		35		921		A	
Acipimox 250mg capsules		90		4633		C	Olbetam
Adapalene 0.1% cream	■	45	g	1140		C	Differin
Adapalene 0.1% gel	■	45	g	1140		C	Differin
Adrenaline acid tartrate 1mg/1ml (1 in 1,000) solution for injection ampoules		10		462	▽	A	
Adrenaline acid tartrate 500micrograms/0.5ml (1 in 1,000) solution for injection ampoules		10		499	△	A	
Alclometasone 0.05% cream	■	50	g	268		C	Modrasone
Alclometasone 0.05% ointment	■	50	g	268		C	Modrasone
Alendronic acid 10mg tablets	♦	28		2627		M	
Alendronic acid 5mg tablets	♦	28		2543		C	Fosamax
Alendronic acid 70mg / Colecalciferol 70microgram tablets	■	4		2280		C	Fosavance
Alendronic acid 70mg tablets	■	4		722		M	
Alfacalcidol 1microgram capsules	■	30		2381		M	

VIII

BASIC PRICES OF DRUGS

Drug		Quantity		Basic Price		Category
Alfacalcidol 250nanogram capsules	■	30		865	M	
Alfacalcidol 500nanogram capsules	■	30		1063	M	
Alfuzosin 10mg modified-release tablets		30		1328	C	*Xatral XL*
Alfuzosin 2.5mg tablets		60		2120	C	*Xatral*
Alimemazine 10mg tablets		28		389	C	*Vallergan*
Alimemazine 30mg/5ml oral solution		100	ml	686	C	*Vallergan Forte Syrup*
Alimemazine 7.5mg/5ml oral solution		100	ml	444	C	*Vallergan Syrup*
Allopurinol 100mg tablets		28		143	M	
Allopurinol 300mg tablets		28		165	M	
Almond oil liquid		500	ml	612	△ A	
Almotriptan 12.5mg tablets		3		907	C	*Almogran*
		6		1814	C	*Almogran*
		9		2720	C	*Almogran*
§ Alprostadil 10microgram powder and solvent for solution for injection vials	■	1		924	C	*Caverject*
§ Alprostadil 20microgram powder and solvent for solution for injection vials	■	1		1194	C	*Caverject*
§ Alprostadil 40microgram powder and solvent for solution for injection vials	■	1		2158	C	*Caverject*
§ Alprostadil 5microgram powder and solvent for solution for injection vials	■	1		773	C	*Caverject*
Alum powder		500	g	230	C	*Unichem*
Aluminium hydroxide 475mg capsules		120		375	C	*Alu-Cap*
Alverine 120mg capsules		60		1380	C	*Spasmonal Forte*
Alverine 60mg capsules		100		1195	C	*Spasmonal*
Amantadine 100mg capsules		56		1688	C	*Symmetrel*
Amantadine 50mg/5ml oral solution	■	150	ml	555	C	*Symmetrel Syrup*
Amiloride 2.5mg / Cyclopenthiazide 250microgram tablets	♦	28		225	C	*Navispare*
Amiloride 5mg / Bumetanide 1mg tablets	♦	28		263	C	*Burinex A*
Amiloride 5mg tablets		28		142	M	
Aminophylline 250mg/10ml solution for injection ampoules		10		712	A	
Amiodarone 100mg tablets	♦	28		238	M	
Amiodarone 200mg tablets	♦	28		267	M	
Amisulpride 100mg tablets		60		3672	C	*Solian 100*
Amisulpride 200mg tablets		60		6138	C	*Solian 200*
Amisulpride 400mg tablets		60		12276	C	*Solian 400*
Amisulpride 500mg/5ml oral solution sugar free	■	60	ml	3069	C	*Solian*
Amisulpride 50mg tablets		60		3198	M	
Amitriptyline 10mg tablets		28		144	M	
Amitriptyline 25mg tablets		28		145	M	

BASIC PRICES OF DRUGS

Drug		Quantity		Basic Price	Category	
Amitriptyline 25mg/5ml oral solution sugar free		150	ml	1240	A	
Amitriptyline 50mg tablets		28		157	M	
Amitriptyline 50mg/5ml oral solution sugar free		150	ml	1350	A	
Amlodipine 10mg tablets	♦	28		288	M	
Amlodipine 5mg tablets	♦	28		238	M	
Ammonia and Ipecacuanha mixture		500	ml	184	A	
Ammonia solution aromatic		500	ml	400	A	
Ammonium acetate solution strong		500	ml	366	C	AAH
Ammonium bicarbonate powder		500	g	280	C	Loveridge
Ammonium chloride mixture		200	ml	44 △	E	
Ammonium chloride powder		500	g	395	C	Loveridge
Amobarbital 50mg / Secobarbital sodium 50mg capsules		100		1940	C	Tuinal Pulvule
Amorolfine 0.25% cream	■	20	g	483	C	Loceryl
Amorolfine 5% paint	■	5	ml	2143	C	Loceryl Lacquer
Amoxicillin 125mg/1.25ml oral suspension paediatric	●	20	ml	338	C	Amoxil
Amoxicillin 125mg/5ml oral suspension	●	100	ml	221	M	
Amoxicillin 125mg/5ml oral suspension sugar free	●	100	ml	225	M	
Amoxicillin 1g powder for solution for injection vials		10		1164	C	Amoxil
Amoxicillin 250mg capsules		21		165	M	
Amoxicillin 250mg/5ml oral suspension	●	100	ml	208	M	
Amoxicillin 250mg/5ml oral suspension sugar free	●	100	ml	263	M	
Amoxicillin 3g oral powder sachets sugar free		2		585	M	
Amoxicillin 500mg capsules		21		201	M	
		100		530	M	
Amoxicillin 500mg powder for solution for injection vials		10		582	C	Amoxil
Amphotericin 100mg tablets		56		774	C	Fungilin
Amphotericin 10mg lozenges		60		367	C	Fungilin
Ampicillin 125mg/5ml oral suspension	●	100	ml	378	M	
Ampicillin 250mg capsules		28		551	M	
Ampicillin 250mg/5ml oral suspension	●	100	ml	739	M	
Ampicillin 500mg capsules		28		798	M	
Anastrozole 1mg tablets	♦	28		6856	C	Arimidex
Anise oil liquid		100	ml	630	C	Loveridge
Anise water concentrated		100	ml	851 △	A	
Antazoline 0.5% / Xylometazoline 0.05% eye drops	■	10	ml	235	C	Otrivine-Antistin
Apraclonidine 0.5% eye drops	■	5	ml	1145	C	Iopidine
Aqueous calamine cream		100	ml	69	A	
Aqueous cream		500	g	263	M	

VIII

BASIC PRICES OF DRUGS

Drug		Quantity		Basic Price		Category	
Arachis oil 130ml enema	■	130	ml	96		C	Fletchers
Arachis oil liquid		200	ml	182	△ A		
Aripiprazole 10mg tablets		28		10163		C	Abilify
Aripiprazole 15mg tablets		28		10163		C	Abilify
Aripiprazole 30mg tablets		28		20326		C	Abilify
Aripiprazole 5mg tablets		28		10163		C	Abilify
Ascorbic acid 100mg tablets		28		123		A	
		100		90		A	
Ascorbic acid 200mg tablets		28		126		A	
		100		112		A	
Ascorbic acid 500mg tablets		28		266		M	
Ascorbic acid 50mg tablets		28		118		A	
Ascorbic acid powder		100	g	400	△ A		
Aspirin 300mg dispersible tablets		100		397		M	
Aspirin 300mg gastro-resistant tablets		100		482	▽ A		
Aspirin 300mg tablets		32		31		A	
Aspirin 75mg dispersible tablets		28		137		M	
		100		166		M	
Aspirin 75mg gastro-resistant tablets		28		167		M	
		56		202		M	
Aspirin 75mg tablets		28		87		C	Angettes 75
Aspirin 900mg / Metoclopramide 10mg oral powder sachets sugar free		6		700		C	Migramax
		20		2333		C	Migramax
Aspirin powder		250	g	640		C	Loveridge
Atenolol 100mg tablets	♦	28		145		M	
Atenolol 25mg tablets	♦	28		136		M	
Atenolol 25mg/5ml oral solution sugar free		300	ml	855		C	Tenormin Syrup
Atenolol 50mg tablets	♦	28		139		M	
Atomoxetine 10mg capsules		28		6006		C	Strattera
Atomoxetine 18mg capsules		28		6006		C	Strattera
Atomoxetine 25mg capsules		28		6006		C	Strattera
Atomoxetine 40mg capsules		28		6006		C	Strattera
Atomoxetine 60mg capsules		28		6006		C	Strattera
Atorvastatin 10mg tablets	♦	28		1803		C	Lipitor
Atorvastatin 20mg tablets	♦	28		2464		C	Lipitor
Atorvastatin 40mg tablets	♦	28		2821		C	Lipitor
Atorvastatin 80mg tablets	♦	28		2821		C	Lipitor
Atropine 1% eye drops	■	10	ml	90		A	
Atropine 1% eye ointment	■	3	g	297		A	
Atropine 600microgram tablets		28		902	△ A		
Atropine 600micrograms/1ml solution for injection ampoules		10		496		A	
Auranofin 3mg tablets		60		2520		C	Ridaura
Azathioprine 25mg tablets		28		499		M	
		100		1791		M	

BASIC PRICES OF DRUGS

Drug		Quantity		Basic Price	Category	
Azathioprine 50mg tablets		56		1047	M	
	★	100		1665	M	
Azelaic acid 20% cream	■	30	g	374	C	Skinoren
Azelastine 140micrograms/ actuation nasal spray	■	22	ml	1109	C	Rhinolast
Azithromycin 200mg/5ml oral suspension	●	15	ml	508	C	Zithromax
	●	22.5	ml	762	C	Zithromax
	●	30	ml	1380	C	Zithromax
Azithromycin 250mg capsules		4		895	C	Zithromax
		6		1343	C	Zithromax
Baclofen 10mg tablets		84		292	M	
Baclofen 5mg/5ml oral solution sugar free		300	ml	895	A	
Balsalazide 750mg capsules		130		3900	C	Colazide
Bambuterol 10mg tablets		28		1205	C	Bambec
Bambuterol 20mg tablets		28		1314	C	Bambec
Beclometasone 100microgram inhalation powder capsules		120		1599	C	Beclometasone 100 Cyclocaps
Beclometasone 100micrograms/ dose breath actuated inhaler	■	200	dose	1030	C	Beclazone 100 Easi-Breathe
Beclometasone 100micrograms/ dose breath actuated inhaler CFC free	■	200	dose	1721	C	Qvar Autohaler
Beclometasone 100micrograms/ dose inhaler	■	200	dose	605	M	
Beclometasone 200microgram inhalation powder capsules		120		2500	C	Beclometasone 200 Cyclocaps
Beclometasone 200micrograms/ dose inhaler	■	200	dose	814	C	Becotide 200
Beclometasone 250micrograms/ dose breath actuated inhaler	■	200	dose	2025	C	Beclazone 250 Easi-Breathe
Beclometasone 250micrograms/ dose inhaler	■	200	dose	1359	M	
Beclometasone 400microgram inhalation powder capsules		120		3225	C	Beclometasone 400 Cyclocaps
Beclometasone 50micrograms/dose breath actuated inhaler	■	200	dose	434	C	Beclazone 50 Easi-Breathe
Beclometasone 50micrograms/dose breath actuated inhaler CFC free	■	200	dose	787	C	Qvar Autohaler
Beclometasone 50micrograms/dose inhaler	■	200	dose	444	M	
Beclometasone 50micrograms/dose nasal spray	■	200	dose	514	M	
Beeswax white solid		500	g	820	C	Loveridge
Beeswax yellow solid		500	g	1210	C	Loveridge

VIII

BASIC PRICES OF DRUGS

Drug		Quantity		Basic Price	Category	
Bendroflumethiazide 2.5mg / Potassium chloride 630mg (potassium 8.4mmol) modified-release tablets		100		795	C	Neo-Naclex-K
Bendroflumethiazide 2.5mg tablets		28		128	M	
Bendroflumethiazide 5mg tablets		28		134	M	
Benperidol 250microgram tablets		112		10400	C	Anquil
Benzoic acid compound ointment		500	g	340	A	
Benzoin compound tincture		500	ml	540	C	Loveridge
Benzoin tincture		500	ml	560	C	Loveridge
Benzoyl peroxide 10% gel	■	40	g	207	C	Panoxyl Aquagel 10
Benzoyl peroxide 2.5% gel	■	40	g	176	C	Panoxyl Aquagel 2.5
Benzoyl peroxide 4% cream	■	40	g	330	C	Brevoxyl
Benzoyl peroxide 5% / Clindamycin 1% gel	■	25	g	995	C	Duac
	■	50	g	1990	C	Duac
Benzoyl peroxide 5% / Erythromycin 3% gel	■	46.6	g	1562	C	Benzamycin
Benzoyl peroxide 5% gel	■	40	g	192	C	Panoxyl Aquagel 5
Benzydamine 0.15% mouthwash	■	300	ml	401	C	Difflam
Benzydamine 0.15% oromucosal spray	■	30	ml	317	C	Difflam
Benzydamine 3% cream	■	35	g	263	C	Difflam
	■	100	g	684	C	Difflam
Benzyl benzoate 25% application		500	ml	250	C	Thornton & Ross
Benzyl benzoate crystals		500	g	480	C	Loveridge
Benzylpenicillin 1.2g powder for solution for injection vials		25		2164	C	Crystapen
Benzylpenicillin 600mg powder for solution for injection vials		25		1082	C	Crystapen
Betahistine 16mg tablets	♦	84		446	M	
Betahistine 8mg tablets		84		525	M	
		120		301	M	
Betamethasone 0.1% ear/eye/nose drops	■	10	ml	232	C	Betnesol
Betamethasone 0.1% eye ointment	■	3	g	141	C	Betnesol
Betamethasone 0.1% foam	■	100	g	975	C	Bettamousse
Betamethasone 500microgram soluble tablets sugar free		100		517	C	Betnesol
Betamethasone dipropionate 0.05% / Calcipotriol 0.005% ointment	■	60	g	3500	C	Dovobet
	■	120	g	6500	C	Dovobet
Betamethasone dipropionate 0.05% cream	■	30	g	224	C	Diprosone
	■	100	g	636	C	Diprosone
Betamethasone dipropionate 0.05% ointment	■	30	g	224	C	Diprosone
	■	100	g	636	C	Diprosone
Betamethasone dipropionate 0.05% scalp lotion	■	30	ml	283	C	Diprosone
	■	100	ml	810	C	Diprosone

BASIC PRICES OF DRUGS

Drug		Quantity		Basic Price	Category	
Betamethasone valerate 0.025% cream	■	100	g	334	C	*Betnovate-RD*
Betamethasone valerate 0.025% ointment	■	100	g	334	C	*Betnovate-RD*
Betamethasone valerate 0.1% cream	■	30	g	141	A	
	■	100	g	405	C	
Betamethasone valerate 0.1% lotion	■	100	ml	486	C	*Betnovate*
Betamethasone valerate 0.1% ointment	■	30	g	168	A	
	■	100	g	405	C	
Betamethasone valerate 0.1% scalp application	■	100	ml	392	C	*Betacap*
Betaxolol 0.25% eye drops	■	5	ml	280	C	*Betoptic Susp*
Betaxolol 0.5% eye drops	■	5	ml	200	C	*Betoptic Ophthalmic Solution*
Bezafibrate 200mg tablets		100		1147	M	
Bezafibrate 400mg modified-release tablets		30		809	C	*Bezalip-Mono*
Bicalutamide 150mg tablets	♦	28		24000	C	*Casodex*
Bicalutamide 50mg tablets	♦	28		12800	C	*Casodex*
Bimatoprost 300micrograms/ml eye drops	■	3	ml	1146	C	*Lumigan*
Bisacodyl 10mg suppositories		12		77	A	
Bisacodyl 5mg gastro-resistant tablets		1000		2575	M	
Bisacodyl 5mg suppositories		5		94	C	*Dulcolax*
Bismuth subcarbonate powder		250	g	1580	C	*Loveridge*
Bisoprolol 1.25mg tablets	♦	28		856	C	
Bisoprolol 10mg tablets		28		202	M	
Bisoprolol 2.5mg tablets	♦	28		490	C	*Cardicor*
Bisoprolol 5mg tablets		28		185	M	
Black currant syrup		500	ml	780	C	*Loveridge*
Boric acid powder		500	g	310	C	*Loveridge*
Brimonidine 0.2% eye drops	■	5	ml	685	C	*Alphagan*
Brinzolamide 10mg/ml eye drops	■	5	ml	690	C	*Azopt*
Bromocriptine 10mg capsules		100		6950	C	*Parlodel*
Bromocriptine 1mg tablets		100		990	C	*Parlodel*
Bromocriptine 2.5mg tablets		30		923	M	
Bromocriptine 5mg capsules		100		3757	C	*Parlodel*
Budesonide 100micrograms/dose / Formoterol 6micrograms/dose dry powder inhaler	■	120	dose	3300	C	*Symbicort 100/6*
Budesonide 100micrograms/dose dry powder inhaler	■	200	dose	1850	C	*Pulmicort Turbohaler 100*
Budesonide 200micrograms/dose / Formoterol 6micrograms/dose dry powder inhaler	■	120	dose	3800	C	*Symbicort 200/6*
Budesonide 200micrograms/dose dry powder inhaler	■	100	dose	1850	C	*Pulmicort Turbohaler 200*

VIII

BASIC PRICES OF DRUGS

Drug		Quantity		Basic Price	Category	
Budesonide 200micrograms/dose inhaler	■	200	dose	2090	C	Pulmicort
Budesonide 3mg gastro-resistant capsules		100		7670	C	Budenofalk
Budesonide 3mg gastro-resistant modified-release capsules	■	100		9900	C	Entocort CR
Budesonide 400micrograms/dose / Formoterol 12micrograms/ dose dry powder inhaler	■	60	dose	3800	C	Symbicort 400/12
Budesonide 400micrograms/dose dry powder inhaler	■	50	dose	1850	C	Pulmicort Turbohaler 400
Budesonide 50micrograms/dose inhaler	■	200	dose	733	C	Pulmicort LS
Budesonide 64micrograms/dose nasal spray	■	120	dose	449	C	Rhinocort Aqua 64
Bumetanide 1mg tablets	♦	28		199	M	
Bumetanide 1mg/5ml oral solution sugar free		150	ml	1522	A	
Bumetanide 500microgram / Potassium chloride 573mg (potassium 7.7mmol) modified-release tablets		28		112	C	Burinex K
Bumetanide 5mg tablets	♦	28		338	M	
Buprenorphine 10micrograms/hour patches		4		3272	C	BuTrans
Buprenorphine 200microgram sublingual tablets sugar free		50		533	C	Temgesic
Buprenorphine 20micrograms/hour patches		4		5959	C	BuTrans
Buprenorphine 2mg sublingual tablets sugar free		7		672	C	Subutex
Buprenorphine 35micrograms/hour patches		4		3090	C	Transtec
Buprenorphine 400microgram sublingual tablets sugar free		7		160	C	Subutex
		50		1066	C	Temgesic
Buprenorphine 52.5micrograms/ hour patches		4		4636	C	Transtec
Buprenorphine 5micrograms/hour patches		2		900	C	BuTrans
Buprenorphine 70micrograms/hour patches		4		6180	C	Transtec
Buprenorphine 8mg sublingual tablets sugar free		7		2016	C	Subutex
Bupropion 150mg modified-release tablets		60		3985	C	Zyban
Buspirone 10mg tablets		30		2428	M	
Buspirone 5mg tablets		30		1878	M	
Butobarbital 100mg tablets		56		1065	C	Soneryl
Cabergoline 1mg tablets	■	20		8300	C	Cabaser

BASIC PRICES OF DRUGS

Drug		Quantity		Basic Price	Category	
Cabergoline 2mg tablets	■	20		8300	C	*Cabaser*
Cabergoline 4mg tablets	■	16		7584	C	*Cabaser*
Cabergoline 500microgram tablets	■	8		3004	C	*Dostinex*
Cade oil liquid		100	ml	660	C	*Unichem*
Caffeine 100mg / Ergotamine 1mg tablets		30		502	C	*Cafergot*
Calamine lotion		2	litre	626	A	
Calamine powder		500	g	340	C	*Loveridge*
Calcipotriol 50micrograms/g cream	■	60	g	1202	C	*Dovonex*
	■	120	g	2404	C	*Dovonex*
Calcipotriol 50micrograms/g ointment	■	60	g	1202	C	*Dovonex*
	■	120	g	2404	C	*Dovonex*
Calcipotriol 50micrograms/ml scalp solution	■	60	ml	1304	C	*Dovonex*
Calcitonin (salmon) 200units/dose nasal spray	■	14	dose	2099	C	*Miacalcic*
Calcitriol 3micrograms/g ointment	■	100	g	1634	C	*Silkis*
Calcium acetate 1g tablets		180		1979	C	*Phosex*
Calcium and Ergocalciferol tablets		28		232	M	
Calcium carbonate 1.25g / Colecalciferol 200unit chewable tablets		100		1502	C	*Calcichew D3*
Calcium carbonate 1.25g / Colecalciferol 400unit chewable tablets		60		450	C	*Calcichew D3 Forte*
		100		750	C	*Calcichew D3 Forte*
Calcium carbonate 1.25g / Colecalciferol 440unit effervescent granules sachets		30		575	C	*Cacit D3*
Calcium carbonate 1.25g chewable tablets		100		933	C	*Calcichew*
Calcium carbonate 1.5g / Colecalciferol 400unit chewable tablets		56		406	C	*Adcal-D3*
		100		725	C	*Adcal-D3*
		112		799	C	*Adcal-D3*
Calcium carbonate 1.5g chewable tablets		100		725	C	*Adcal*
Calcium carbonate 2.5g chewable tablets		60		1316	C	*Calcichew Forte*
Calcium carbonate powder		500	g	245	C	*Loveridge*
Calcium gluconate 1g effervescent tablets	■	28		462	A	
Calcium lactate 300mg tablets		84		422	M	
Calcium phosphate 3.1g / Colecalciferol 800unit oral powder sachets		30		432	C	*Calfovit D3*
Camphor racemic powder		100	g	380	C	*Loveridge*
Camphor water concentrated		100	ml	285	C	*Unichem*
Candesartan 16mg tablets	♦	28		1272	C	*Amias*
Candesartan 2mg tablets	♦	7		299	C	*Amias*

VIII

BASIC PRICES OF DRUGS

Drug		Quantity		Basic Price		Category	
Candesartan 32mg tablets	♦	28		1613		C	Amias
Candesartan 4mg tablets	♦	7		324		C	Amias
	♦	28		815		C	Amias
Candesartan 8mg tablets	♦	28		989		C	Amias
Capsaicin 0.025% cream	■	45	g	1504		C	Zacin
Capsaicin 0.075% cream	■	45	g	1215		C	Axsain
Capsicum tincture		500	ml	397	△	A	
Captopril 12.5mg tablets		56		173		M	
Captopril 25mg tablets	♦	56		196		M	
Captopril 50mg tablets	♦	56		240		M	
Carbamazepine 100mg chewable tablets sugar free		56		354		C	Tegretol Chewtab
Carbamazepine 100mg tablets		28		375		M	
		84		243		C	Tegretol
Carbamazepine 100mg/5ml oral suspension sugar free		300	ml	686		C	Tegretol Liquid
Carbamazepine 200mg chewable tablets sugar free		56		659		C	Tegretol Chewtab
Carbamazepine 200mg modified-release tablets		56		526		C	Tegretol Retard
Carbamazepine 200mg tablets		28		350		M	
		84		450		C	Tegretol
Carbamazepine 400mg modified-release tablets		56		1034		C	Tegretol Retard
Carbamazepine 400mg tablets		56		590		C	Tegretol
Carbaryl 0.5% alcoholic lotion	■	50	ml	228		C	Carylderm
Carbaryl 1% aqueous liquid	■	50	ml	228		C	Carylderm
Carbimazole 20mg tablets		100		1912		C	Neo-Mercazole 20
Carbimazole 5mg tablets		100		515		C	Neo-Mercazole 5
Carbocisteine 125mg/5ml oral solution		300	ml	457		C	Mucodyne Syrup
Carbocisteine 250mg/5ml oral solution		300	ml	584		C	Mucodyne Syrup
Carbocisteine 375mg capsules		120		1668		C	Mucodyne
Carbomer 980 0.2% eye drops	■	10	g	280		C	GelTears Ophthalmic Gel
Carmellose 1% eye drops 0.4ml unit dose preservative free		30		575		C	Celluvisc
Carteolol 1% eye drops	■	5	ml	460		C	Teoptic
Carteolol 2% eye drops	■	5	ml	540		C	Teoptic
Carvedilol 12.5mg tablets	♦	28		291		M	
Carvedilol 25mg tablets	♦	28		356		M	
Carvedilol 3.125mg tablets	♦	28		580	▽	A	
Carvedilol 6.25mg tablets	♦	28		607	▽	A	
Castor oil liquid		500	ml	500		C	Loveridge
Cefaclor 125mg/5ml oral suspension	●	100	ml	836	△	A	
Cefaclor 125mg/5ml oral suspension sugar free	●	100	ml	836		M	
Cefaclor 250mg capsules		21		867		M	

BASIC PRICES OF DRUGS

Drug		Quantity		Basic Price	Category	
Cefaclor 250mg/5ml oral suspension sugar free	●	100	ml	990	M	
Cefaclor 375mg modified-release tablets		14		693	C	*Distaclor MR*
Cefaclor 500mg capsules		50		4466	M	
Cefadroxil 125mg/5ml oral suspension	●	60	ml	163	C	*Baxan*
Cefadroxil 250mg/5ml oral suspension	●	60	ml	324	C	*Baxan*
Cefadroxil 500mg capsules		20		525	C	*Baxan*
Cefadroxil 500mg/5ml oral suspension	●	60	ml	485	C	*Baxan*
Cefalexin 125mg/5ml oral suspension	●	100	ml	356	M	
Cefalexin 250mg capsules		28		341	M	
		100		705	M	
Cefalexin 250mg tablets		28		370	M	
		100		546	M	
Cefalexin 250mg/5ml oral suspension	●	100	ml	459	M	
Cefalexin 500mg capsules		21		419	M	
		100		794	M	
Cefalexin 500mg tablets		21		455	M	
		100		1236	M	
Cefalexin 500mg/5ml oral suspension	●	100	ml	557	C	*Ceporex Syrup*
Cefixime 100mg/5ml oral suspension	■	50	ml	1053	C	*Suprax*
	■	100	ml	1891	C	*Suprax*
Cefixime 200mg tablets		7		1323	C	*Suprax*
Cefotaxime 1g powder for solution for injection vials		10		4308	C	*Claforan*
Cefotaxime 2g powder for solution for injection vials		10		8573	C	*Claforan*
Cefotaxime 500mg powder for solution for injection vials		10		2143	C	*Claforan*
Cefpodoxime 100mg tablets		10		1018	C	*Orelox*
Cefradine 250mg capsules		20		647	M	
		100		2186	M	
Cefradine 250mg/5ml oral solution	●	100	ml	392	C	*Velosef Syrup*
Cefradine 500mg capsules		20		1234	M	
		100		4720	M	
Ceftriaxone 1g powder for solution for injection vials	■	1		1017	C	*Rocephin*
Ceftriaxone 250mg powder for solution for injection vials	■	1		255	C	*Rocephin*
Ceftriaxone 2g powder for solution for injection vials	■	1		2036	C	*Rocephin*
Cefuroxime 125mg tablets		14		484	C	*Zinnat*
Cefuroxime 250mg tablets		14		916	△ A	
Celecoxib 100mg capsules		60		2155	C	*Celebrex*
Celecoxib 200mg capsules		30		2155	C	*Celebrex*

BASIC PRICES OF DRUGS

Drug		Quantity		Basic Price		Category	
Celiprolol 200mg tablets	♦	28		1006		M	
Celiprolol 400mg tablets	♦	28		4370		M	
Cetirizine 10mg tablets		30		163		M	
Cetirizine 1mg/ml oral solution sugar free		200	ml	510		M	
Cetomacrogol cream (Formula A)		500	g	255		A	
Chalk powder		1	kg	280		C	Loveridge
Chloral hydrate crystals		100	g	515		C	Loveridge
Chloramphenicol 0.5% eye drops	■	10	ml	272		M	
Chloramphenicol 1% eye ointment	■	4	g	282		M	
Chloramphenicol 5% ear drops	■	10	ml	141		A	
Chlordiazepoxide 10mg capsules		100		547	▽	A	
		500		3044		M	
Chlordiazepoxide 10mg tablets		100		1487		M	
Chlordiazepoxide 5mg capsules		100		376	▽	A	
		500		2632		M	
Chlordiazepoxide 5mg tablets		100		1436		M	
Chlorhexidine 0.2% oral spray	■	60	ml	410		C	Corsodyl
Chlorhexidine 1% dental gel	■	50	g	121		C	Corsodyl
Chlorhexidine gluconate 0.2% mouthwash		300	ml	194		A	
Chloroform and Morphine tincture		500	ml	705	△	A	
Chloroform spirit		500	ml	248		C	Unichem
Chloroquine phosphate 250mg tablets		20		122		C	Avloclor
Chlorphenamine 10mg/1ml solution for injection ampoules		5		810		A	
Chlorphenamine 2mg/5ml oral solution		150	ml	228		C	Piriton Syrup
Chlorphenamine 2mg/5ml oral solution sugar free		150	ml	219		A	
Chlorphenamine 4mg tablets		28		181		M	
Chlorpromazine 100mg tablets		28		428		M	
Chlorpromazine 25mg tablets		28		346		M	
Chlorpromazine 25mg/5ml oral solution		150	ml	135		A	
Chlorpromazine 50mg tablets		28		369		M	
Chlortalidone 50mg tablets		28		164		C	Hygroton
Choline salicylate 8.7% oromucosal gel sugar free	■	15	g	179		C	Bonjela
Ciclesonide 160micrograms/dose inhaler CFC free	■	60	dose	1680		C	Alvesco 160
	■	120	dose	3360		C	Alvesco 160
Ciclesonide 80micrograms/dose inhaler CFC free	■	120	dose	2856		C	Alvesco 80
Ciclosporin 100mg capsules		30		5513		C	Neoral
Ciclosporin 100mg/ml oral solution sugar free	■	50	ml	9020		C	Neoral
Ciclosporin 25mg capsules		30		1320		C	Neoral
Ciclosporin 50mg capsules		30		2922		C	Neoral
Cilazapril 1mg tablets	♦	28		601		C	Vascace

BASIC PRICES OF DRUGS

Drug		Quantity		Basic Price	Category	
Cilazapril 2.5mg tablets	♦	28		764	C	*Vascace*
Cilazapril 500microgram tablets	♦	28		365	C	*Vascace*
Cilazapril 5mg tablets	♦	28		1328	C	*Vascace*
Cilostazol 100mg tablets		56		3531	C	*Pletal*
Cimetidine 200mg tablets		60		244	M	
Cimetidine 200mg/5ml oral solution		600	ml	2849	C	*Tagamet Syrup*
Cimetidine 200mg/5ml oral solution sugar free		300	ml	1424	A	
Cimetidine 400mg tablets		60		283	M	
Cimetidine 800mg tablets	♦	30		317	M	
Cinnarizine 15mg tablets		84		728	M	
Ciprofibrate 100mg tablets		28		1766	C	*Modalim*
Ciprofloxacin 0.3% eye drops	■	5	ml	494	C	*Ciloxan*
Ciprofloxacin 100mg tablets		6		173	M	
Ciprofloxacin 250mg tablets		10		176	M	
		20		210	M	
Ciprofloxacin 250mg/5ml oral suspension	●	100	ml	1650	C	*Ciproxin*
Ciprofloxacin 500mg tablets		10		191	M	
		20		228	M	
Ciprofloxacin 750mg tablets		10		323	M	
Citalopram 10mg tablets	♦	28		257	M	
Citalopram 20mg tablets	♦	28		326	M	
Citalopram 40mg tablets	♦	28		406	M	
Citalopram 40mg/ml oral solution sugar free	■	15	ml	2016	C	*Cipramil*
Citric acid monohydrate powder		500	g	290	C	*Thornton & Ross*
Clarithromycin 125mg/5ml oral suspension	●	70	ml	558	A	
	●	100	ml	960	A	
Clarithromycin 250mg tablets	♦	14		562	M	
Clarithromycin 250mg/5ml oral suspension	●	70	ml	1116	A	
Clarithromycin 500mg modified-release tablets	♦	7		800	C	*Klaricid XL*
	♦	14		1600	C	*Klaricid XL*
Clarithromycin 500mg tablets	♦	14		1005	M	
	♦	20		1714	C	*Klaricid 500*
Clemastine 1mg tablets		60		235	C	*Tavegil*
Clindamycin 1% alcoholic solution	■	30	ml	434	C	*Dalacin T Topical*
Clindamycin 1% aqueous lotion	■	30	ml	508	C	*Dalacin T Topical*
	■	50	ml	847	C	*Dalacin T Topical*
Clindamycin 1% gel	■	30	g	866	C	*Zindaclin*
Clindamycin 150mg capsules		24		2052	M	
Clindamycin 2% vaginal cream	■	40	g	1086	C	*Dalacin*
Clindamycin 75mg capsules		24		745	C	*Dalacin C*
Clioquinol 1% / Flumetasone 0.02% ear drops	■	7.5	ml	147	C	*Locorten Vioform*
Clioquinol 3% / Betamethasone valerate 0.1% cream	■	30	g	176	C	*Betnovate-C*

BASIC PRICES OF DRUGS

Drug		Quantity		Basic Price		Category	
Clioquinol 3% / Betamethasone valerate 0.1% ointment	■	30	g	176	C	Betnovate-C	
Clioquinol 3% / Hydrocortisone 1% cream	■	30	g	146	C	Vioform-Hydrocortisone	
Clioquinol 3% / Hydrocortisone 1% ointment	■	30	g	146	C	Vioform-Hydrocortisone	
§ Clobazam 10mg tablets		30		974	C	Frisium	
Clobetasol 0.05% cream	■	30	g	286	C	Dermovate	
	■	100	g	839	C	Dermovate	
Clobetasol 0.05% ointment	■	30	g	286	C	Dermovate	
	■	100	g	839	C	Dermovate	
Clobetasol 0.05% scalp application	■	30	ml	326	C	Dermovate	
	■	100	ml	1106	C	Dermovate	
Clobetasone 0.05% cream	■	30	g	197	C	Eumovate	
	■	100	g	577	C	Eumovate	
Clobetasone 0.05% ointment	■	30	g	197	C	Eumovate	
	■	100	g	577	C	Eumovate	
Clomethiazole 192mg capsules		60		478	C	Heminevrin	
Clomethiazole 250mg/5ml oral solution sugar free		300	ml	400	C	Heminevrin Syrup	
Clomifene 50mg tablets		30		1120	A		
Clomipramine 10mg capsules	♦	28		273	M		
Clomipramine 25mg capsules	♦	28		345	M		
		100		647	M		
Clomipramine 50mg capsules	♦	28		500	M		
Clomipramine 75mg modified-release tablets		28		883	C	Anafranil SR	
Clonazepam 2mg tablets		100		523	C	Rivotril	
Clonazepam 500microgram tablets		100		392	C	Rivotril	
Clonidine 100microgram tablets		100		560	C	Catapres	
Clonidine 25microgram tablets		112		1492	M		
Clonidine 300microgram tablets		100		1304	C	Catapres	
Clopidogrel 75mg tablets	♦	28		3531	C	Plavix	
Cloral betaine 707mg tablets		30		790	C	Welldorm	
Clotrimazole 1% / Betamethasone dipropionate 0.064% cream	■	30	g	634	C	Lotriderm	
Clotrimazole 1% / Hydrocortisone 1% cream	■	30	g	242	△ C	Canesten HC	
Clotrimazole 1% cream	■	20	g	264	M		
	■	50	g	380	A		
Clotrimazole 1% powder	■	30	g	152	C	Canesten Dermatological	
Clotrimazole 1% solution	■	20	ml	243	C	Canesten	
Clotrimazole 10% vaginal cream	■	5	g	450	C	Canesten VC	
Clotrimazole 100mg pessaries	■	6		363	△ C	Canesten	
Clotrimazole 2% cream	■	20	g	370	C	Canesten Thrush	
Clotrimazole 200mg pessaries	■	3		363	△ C	Canesten	
Clotrimazole 500mg pessaries	■	1		460	M		
Clotrimazole 500mg pessary and Clotrimazole 2% cream	■	1		521	△ C	Canesten Combi	
Clove oil liquid		50	ml	220	A		

BASIC PRICES OF DRUGS

Drug		Quantity		Basic Price		Category	
Coal tar prepared 1% lotion	■	100	ml	811		C	*Exorex*
	■	250	ml	1624		C	*Exorex*
Coal tar solution		500	ml	665	△	A	
Coal tar solution strong		500	ml	767	△	A	
Co-amilofruse 10mg/80mg tablets	♦	28		743		A	
Co-amilofruse 2.5mg/20mg tablets	♦	28		201		M	
	♦	56		239		M	
Co-amilofruse 5mg/40mg tablets	♦	28		246		M	
	♦	56		276		M	
Co-amilozide 2.5mg/25mg tablets	♦	28		188	△	A	
Co-amilozide 5mg/50mg tablets		28		176		M	
Co-amoxiclav 125mg/31mg/5ml oral suspension sugar free	●	100	ml	532		M	
Co-amoxiclav 250mg/125mg dispersible tablets		21		1022		C	*Augmentin Dispersible*
Co-amoxiclav 250mg/125mg tablets		21		628		M	
		100		1239		M	
Co-amoxiclav 250mg/62mg/5ml oral suspension sugar free	●	100	ml	594		M	
Co-amoxiclav 400mg/57mg/5ml oral suspension sugar free	●	35	ml	438		C	*Augmentin Duo 400/ 57*
	●	70	ml	615		C	*Augmentin Duo 400/ 57*
Co-amoxiclav 500mg/125mg tablets		21		1222		M	
Co-beneldopa 12.5mg/50mg capsules		100		620		C	*Madopar*
Co-beneldopa 12.5mg/50mg dispersible tablets		100		737		C	*Madopar*
Co-beneldopa 25mg/100mg capsules		100		864		C	*Madopar*
Co-beneldopa 25mg/100mg dispersible tablets		100		1306		C	*Madopar*
Co-beneldopa 50mg/200mg capsules		100		1473		C	*Madopar*
Cocaine hydrochloride powder		5	g	6149	▽	A	
Co-careldopa 10mg/100mg tablets		100		1637		M	
Co-careldopa 12.5mg/50mg tablets		90		654		C	*Sinemet 62.5*
Co-careldopa 25mg/100mg tablets		100		2369		M	
Co-careldopa 25mg/250mg tablets		100		3703		M	
Co-codamol 15mg/500mg tablets		100		750		C	*Codipar*
Co-codamol 30mg/500mg capsules		100		873		M	
Co-codamol 30mg/500mg effervescent tablets		100		1755		M	
Co-codamol 30mg/500mg tablets		100		609		M	
Co-codamol 8mg/500mg effervescent tablets		60		627		M	
		100		781		M	
Co-codamol 8mg/500mg tablets		30		202		M	
		32		210		M	
		100		294		M	

VIII

BASIC PRICES OF DRUGS

Drug	Quantity		Basic Price	Category	
Co-codaprin 8mg/400mg dispersible tablets	100		1112	M	
Coconut oil	500	g	283	C	Unichem
Co-cyprindiol 2000microgram/ 35microgram tablets ♦	63		557	M	
Co-danthramer 25mg/200mg capsules	60		1286	A	
Co-danthramer 25mg/200mg/5ml oral suspension sugar free	300	ml	1127	A	
Co-danthramer 37.5mg/500mg capsules	60		1555	A	
Co-danthramer 75mg/1000mg/5ml oral suspension sugar free	300	ml	3013	A	
Co-danthrusate 50mg/60mg capsules	63		1346	A	
Co-danthrusate 50mg/60mg/5ml oral suspension sugar free	200	ml	875	C	Normax
Codeine 15mg tablets	28		189	M	
	30		148	△ A	
Codeine 15mg/5ml linctus	200	ml	115	C	Thornton & Ross
Codeine 15mg/5ml linctus sugar free	2	litre	610	A	
Codeine 25mg/5ml oral solution	500	ml	449	A	
Codeine 30mg tablets	28		201	M	
Codeine 3mg/5ml linctus paediatric sugar free	2	litre	352	C	Galcodine
Codeine 60mg tablets	28		343	M	
	30		311	△ A	
Codeine phosphate powder	25	g	3910	C	Martindale
Co-dydramol 10mg/500mg tablets	30		209	M	
	100		310	M	
Co-fluampicil 125mg/125mg/5ml oral suspension ●	100	ml	499	C	Magnapen Syrup
Co-fluampicil 250mg/250mg capsules	28		540	M	
	100		1341	M	
Co-flumactone 25mg/25mg tablets	100		2023	C	Aldactide 25
Co-flumactone 50mg/50mg tablets	100		3823	C	Aldactide 50
Colchicine 500microgram tablets	100		1980	△ A	
Colestyramine 4g oral powder sachets	50		1632	C	Questran
Colestyramine 4g oral powder sachets sugar free	50		1653	△ A	
Conjugated oestrogens 1.25mg tablets ♦	84		1319	C	Premarin
Conjugated oestrogens 625microgram tablets ♦	84		972	C	Premarin
Co-phenotrope 2.5mg/0.025mg tablets	100		814	C	Lomotil
Copper sulphate pentahydrate powder	500	g	260	A	

BASIC PRICES OF DRUGS

Drug		Quantity		Basic Price	Category	
Co-prenozide 160mg/0.25mg modified-release tablets	♦	28		888	C	*Trasidrex*
Co-proxamol 32.5mg/325mg tablets		100		337	M	
Cortisone 25mg tablets		56		1092	A	
Co-simalcite 125mg/500mg/5ml oral suspension sugar free		500	ml	196	C	*Altacite Plus*
Co-tenidone 100mg/25mg tablets	♦	28		225	M	
Co-tenidone 50mg/12.5mg tablets	♦	28		203	M	
Co-triamterzide 50mg/25mg tablets	♦	30		95	C	*Dyazide*
Co-trimoxazole 160mg/800mg tablets		100		2346	C	*Septrin Forte*
Co-trimoxazole 80mg/400mg tablets		28		1031	M	
Crotamiton 10% cream	■	30	g	227	C	*Eurax*
	■	100	g	395	C	*Eurax*
Crotamiton 10% lotion		100	ml	299	C	*Eurax*
Cyanocobalamin 1mg/1ml solution for injection ampoules		5		833	C	*Cytamen*
§ Cyanocobalamin 50microgram tablets		50		377	C	*Cytacon*
Cyclizine 30mg / Dipipanone 10mg tablets		50		870	C	*Diconal*
Cyclizine 50mg tablets		100		741	C	*Valoid*
Cyclizine 50mg/1ml solution for injection ampoules		5		271	C	*Valoid*
Cyclopenthiazide 500microgram tablets		28		127	C	*Navidrex*
Cyclopentolate 0.5% eye drops	■	5	ml	97	C	*Mydrilate*
Cyclopentolate 1% eye drops	■	5	ml	119	C	*Mydrilate*
Cyclophosphamide 50mg tablets		100		1058	A	
Cyproheptadine 4mg tablets		30		86	C	*Periactin*
Cyproterone 100mg tablets		84		7768	C	*Cyprostat*
Cyproterone 50mg tablets		168		7768	C	*Cyprostat*
Danazol 100mg capsules	♦	28		1466	M	
		60		1704	C	*Danol*
		100		4547	M	
Danazol 200mg capsules		56		4969	M	
Dantrolene 100mg capsules		100		4307	C	*Dantrium*
Dantrolene 25mg capsules		100		1232	C	*Dantrium*
Dapsone 100mg tablets		28		1256	M	
Dapsone 50mg tablets		28		894	M	
Demeclocycline 150mg capsules		28		694	C	*Ledermycin*
Desloratadine 2.5mg/5ml oral solution		100	ml	704	C	*Neoclarityn*
Desloratadine 5mg tablets		30		704	C	*Neoclarityn*
Desmopressin 100micrograms/ml intranasal solution	■	2.5	ml	972	C	*DDAVP Nasal Solution*

BASIC PRICES OF DRUGS

Drug		Quantity		Basic Price		Category	
Desmopressin 10micrograms/dose nasal spray	■	50	dose	1969		C	Nocutil
	■	60	dose	2291	▽	A	
Desogestrel 75microgram tablets	♦	84		885		C	Cerazette
Dexamethasone 0.1% / Hypromellose 0.5% eye drops	■	5	ml	149		C	Maxidex
	■	10	ml	295		C	Maxidex
Dexamethasone 2mg tablets		50		660		A	
		100		1205		A	
	★	500		4333		A	
Dexamethasone 2mg/5ml oral solution sugar free		150	ml	4230		C	Dexsol
Dexamethasone 500microgram tablets		50		176		A	
		100		352		A	
		500		1753		A	
Dexamfetamine 5mg tablets		28		300		C	Dexedrine
Dexibuprofen 300mg tablets		60		947		C	Seractil
Dexibuprofen 400mg tablets		60		997		C	Seractil
Dexketoprofen 25mg tablets		20		367		C	Keral
		50		918		C	Keral
Diamorphine 100mg powder for solution for injection ampoules		5		2812		A	
Diamorphine 10mg powder for solution for injection ampoules		5		1445		A	
Diamorphine 10mg tablets		100		1230		A	
Diamorphine 30mg powder for solution for injection ampoules		5		1534		A	
Diamorphine 500mg powder for solution for injection ampoules		5		15513		A	
Diamorphine 5mg powder for solution for injection ampoules		5		887		A	
Diamorphine hydrochloride powder		2	g	1340		A	
Diazepam 10mg tablets		28		143		M	
Diazepam 10mg/2ml solution for injection ampoules		10		259		A	
Diazepam 2mg tablets		28		136		M	
Diazepam 2mg/5ml oral solution		100	ml	575	△	C	Sandoz Diazepam Syrup
Diazepam 2mg/ml rectal solution 2.5ml tube		5		636		A	
Diazepam 4mg/ml rectal solution 2.5ml tube		5		920		M	
Diazepam 5mg tablets		28		141		M	
Diclofenac 1% gel	■	100	g	700		C	Voltarol Emulgel
Diclofenac 100mg suppositories		10		304		A	
Diclofenac 12.5mg suppositories		10		71		C	Voltarol
Diclofenac 16mg/ml topical solution	■	60	ml	1600		C	Pennsaid
Diclofenac 25mg suppositories		10		126		C	Voltarol
Diclofenac 50mg dispersible tablets		21		619		C	Voltarol Dispersible
Diclofenac 50mg suppositories		10		207		C	Voltarol

BASIC PRICES OF DRUGS

Drug		Quantity		Basic Price		Category	
Diclofenac 75mg/3ml solution for injection ampoules		10		826		C	Voltarol I/M
Diclofenac potassium 25mg tablets		28		404		C	Voltarol Rapid
Diclofenac potassium 50mg tablets		28		773		C	Voltarol Rapid
Diclofenac sodium 100mg modified-release capsules	♦	28		871		C	
Diclofenac sodium 25mg gastro-resistant tablets		84		278		M	
Diclofenac sodium 3% gel	■	25	g	1665		C	Solaraze
Diclofenac sodium 50mg gastro-resistant / Misoprostol 200microgram tablets		60		1331		C	Arthrotec 50
Diclofenac sodium 50mg gastro-resistant tablets	★	84		484		M	
		100		570	△	A	
Diclofenac sodium 75mg gastro-resistant / Misoprostol 200microgram tablets		60		1759		C	Arthrotec 75
Diclofenac sodium 75mg gastro-resistant modified-release capsules		56		800		C	Motifene 75mg
Diclofenac sodium 75mg modified-release capsules	♦	56		1210		C	Diclomax SR
Dicycloverine 10mg tablets		100		504		C	Merbentyl
Dicycloverine 10mg/5ml oral solution		120	ml	184		C	Merbentyl Syrup
Dicycloverine 20mg tablets		84		847		C	Merbentyl 20
Diethylamine salicylate 10% cream	■	50	g	121		C	Algesal
Diethylstilbestrol 1mg tablets		28		3606	△	A	
Diethylstilbestrol 5mg tablets		28		25691		M	
Diflucortolone 0.1% oily cream	■	30	g	256		C	Nerisone Oily
Diflucortolone 0.3% oily cream	■	15	g	209		C	Nerisone Forte
Digitoxin 100microgram tablets		28		411		A	
Digoxin 125microgram tablets		28		266		M	
Digoxin 250microgram tablets		28		273		M	
Digoxin 50micrograms/ml oral solution	■	60	ml	535		C	Lanoxin PG Elixir
Digoxin 62.5microgram tablets		28		266		M	
Dihydrocodeine 10mg/5ml oral solution		150	ml	320		A	
Dihydrocodeine 120mg modified-release tablets		56		1157		C	DHC Continus
Dihydrocodeine 30mg tablets		28		318		M	
		30		329		M	
		100		515		M	
Dihydrocodeine 40mg tablets		100		1151		C	DF 118 Forte
Dihydrocodeine 50mg/1ml solution for injection ampoules		10		2294		A	
Dihydrocodeine 60mg modified-release tablets		56		550		C	DHC Continus
Dihydrocodeine 90mg modified-release tablets		56		866		C	DHC Continus

BASIC PRICES OF DRUGS

Drug		Quantity		Basic Price	Category	
Diltiazem 200mg modified-release capsules	♦	28		666	C	Tildiem LA 200
Diltiazem 60mg modified-release capsules		56		640	C	Dilzem SR 60
Diltiazem 60mg modified-release tablets		84		401	M	
		100		560	M	
Dimeticone 4% lotion	■	50	ml	298	C	Hedrin
	■	150	ml	683	C	Hedrin
Dipivefrine 0.1% eye drops	■	5	ml	381	C	Propine
	■	10	ml	477	C	Propine
Dipyridamole 100mg tablets		84		575	M	
Dipyridamole 200mg modified-release capsules	■	60		838	C	Persantin Retard
Dipyridamole 25mg tablets		84		460	M	
	★	100		322	M	
Dipyridamole 50mg/5ml oral suspension sugar free		150	ml	3525	A	
Disodium etidronate 200mg tablets		60		3730	A	
Disopyramide 100mg capsules		84		3637	M	
Disopyramide 150mg capsules		84		4882	M	
Disopyramide 250mg modified-release tablets		56		2885	C	Rythmodan Retard
Disulfiram 200mg tablets		50		2628	C	Antabuse
Docusate 100mg capsules		30		240	C	Dioctyl
		100		800	C	Dioctyl
Docusate 12.5mg/5ml oral solution sugar free		300	ml	163	C	Docusol
Docusate 50mg/5ml oral solution sugar free		300	ml	248	C	Docusol
Docusate sodium 0.5% ear drops	■	10	ml	126	C	Waxsol
Domperidone 10mg tablets		30		209	M	
		100		435	M	
Domperidone 30mg suppositories		10		318	C	Motilium
Domperidone 5mg/5ml oral suspension sugar free		200	ml	216	C	Motilium
Donepezil 10mg tablets	♦	28		8906	C	Aricept
Donepezil 5mg tablets	♦	28		6354	C	Aricept
Dorzolamide 2% / Timolol 0.5% eye drops	■	5	ml	1005	C	Cosopt
Dorzolamide 2% eye drops	■	5	ml	633	C	Trusopt Ophthalmic Solution
Dosulepin 25mg capsules		28		170	M	
		100		203	M	
Dosulepin 75mg tablets	♦	28		214	M	
Doxazosin 1mg tablets	♦	28		171	M	
Doxazosin 2mg tablets	♦	28		276	M	
Doxazosin 4mg modified-release tablets	♦	28		633	C	
Doxazosin 4mg tablets	♦	28		443	M	

BASIC PRICES OF DRUGS

Drug		Quantity		Basic Price	Category	
Doxazosin 8mg modified-release tablets	♦	28		1267	C	*Cardura XL*
Doxycycline 100mg capsules		8		211	M	
		50		782	M	
Doxycycline 100mg dispersible tablets sugar free		8		491	C	*Vibramycin-D*
Doxycycline 20mg tablets		56		1650	C	*Periostat*
Doxycycline 50mg capsules	♦	28		427	M	
Duloxetine 30mg gastro-resistant capsules		28		2240	C	*Cymbalta*
Duloxetine 60mg gastro-resistant capsules		28		2772	C	*Cymbalta*
Dutasteride 500microgram capsules		30		2481	C	*Avodart*
Dydrogesterone 10mg tablets		60		404	C	*Duphaston*

Drug		Quantity		Basic Price		Category	
Econazole 1% / Hydrocortisone 1% cream	■	30	g	209		C	*Econacort*
Eflornithine 11.5% cream	■	30	g	2604		C	*Vaniqua*
Eletriptan 20mg tablets		6		2250		C	*Relpax*
Eletriptan 40mg tablets		6		2250		C	*Relpax*
Emedastine 0.05% eye drops	■	5	ml	769		C	*Emadine*
Emulsifying ointment		500	g	354		M	
Emulsifying wax		500	g	510		A	
Enalapril 10mg tablets	♦	28		181		M	
Enalapril 2.5mg tablets	♦	28		159		M	
Enalapril 20mg / Hydrochlorothiazide 12.5mg tablets		28		1297	△	A	
Enalapril 20mg tablets	♦	28		199		M	
Enalapril 5mg tablets	♦	28		164		M	
Enoxaparin sodium 100mg/1ml solution for injection pre-filled syringes		10		6687		C	*Clexane*
Enoxaparin sodium 120mg/0.8ml solution for injection pre-filled syringes		10		9770		C	*Clexane Forte*
Enoxaparin sodium 150mg/1ml solution for injection pre-filled syringes		10		11101		C	*Clexane Forte*
Enoxaparin sodium 20mg/0.2ml solution for injection pre-filled syringes		10		3152		C	*Clexane*
Enoxaparin sodium 40mg/0.4ml solution for injection pre-filled syringes		10		4200		C	*Clexane*
Enoxaparin sodium 60mg/0.6ml solution for injection pre-filled syringes		10		4750		C	*Clexane*
Enoxaparin sodium 80mg/0.8ml solution for injection pre-filled syringes		10		5399		C	*Clexane*

BASIC PRICES OF DRUGS

Drug		Quantity		Basic Price		Category	
Entacapone 200mg tablets		30		1800		C	Comtess
		100		6000		C	Comtess
Ephedrine 0.5% nasal drops	■	10	ml	124	▽	A	
Ephedrine 1% nasal drops	■	10	ml	130	▽	A	
Ephedrine hydrochloride 15mg tablets		28		345	△	A	
Ephedrine hydrochloride 30mg tablets		28		450	△	A	
Epinastine 500micrograms/ml eye drops	■	5	ml	990		C	Relestat
Eplerenone 25mg tablets		28		4272		C	Inspra
Eplerenone 50mg tablets		28		4272		C	Inspra
Eprosartan 300mg tablets	♦	28		1163		C	Teveten
Eprosartan 400mg tablets	♦	56		1577		C	Teveten
Eprosartan 600mg tablets	♦	28		1431		C	Teveten
Ergocalciferol 1.25mg tablets		100		3027	△	A	
Ergocalciferol 250microgram tablets		100		2194	△	A	
Ergocalciferol 300,000units/1ml solution for injection ampoules		10		5924		A	
Ergocalciferol 600,000units/2ml solution for injection ampoules		10		7070		A	
Erythromycin 2% / Isotretinoin 0.05% gel	■	30	g	778		C	Isotrexin
Erythromycin 2% solution	■	50	ml	800		C	Stiemycin
Erythromycin 250mg gastro-resistant capsules		28		595		C	Erymax
		30		672		M	
Erythromycin 250mg gastro-resistant tablets		28		259		M	
		500		3041		M	
Erythromycin 4% gel	■	30	g	497		C	Eryacne 4
Erythromycin 40mg/ml / Zinc acetate 12mg/ml lotion	■	30	ml	771		C	Zineryt
	■	90	ml	2224		C	Zineryt
Erythromycin ethyl succinate 125mg/5ml oral suspension	●	100	ml	270		M	
Erythromycin ethyl succinate 125mg/5ml oral suspension sugar free	●	100	ml	280		M	
Erythromycin ethyl succinate 250mg/5ml oral suspension	●	100	ml	382		M	
Erythromycin ethyl succinate 250mg/5ml oral suspension sugar free	●	100	ml	365		M	
Erythromycin ethyl succinate 500mg tablets	♦	28		1078		C	Erythroped A
Erythromycin ethyl succinate 500mg/5ml oral suspension	●	100	ml	588		M	
Erythromycin ethyl succinate 500mg/5ml oral suspension sugar free	●	100	ml	577		M	

BASIC PRICES OF DRUGS

Drug		Quantity		Basic Price		Category	
Erythromycin stearate 250mg tablets		100		1820		C	Erythrocin
Erythromycin stearate 500mg tablets		100		3640		C	Erythrocin 500
Escitalopram 10mg tablets		28		1491		C	Cipralex
Escitalopram 20mg tablets		28		2520		C	Cipralex
Escitalopram 5mg tablets		28		897		C	Cipralex
Esomeprazole 20mg gastro-resistant tablets		28		1850		C	Nexium
Esomeprazole 40mg gastro-resistant tablets	♦	28		2519		C	Nexium
Estradiol 150micrograms/dose nasal spray	■	60	dose	741		C	Aerodiol
Estradiol 1mg gel sachets		28		608		C	Sandrena
		91		1826		C	Sandrena
Estradiol 25mg implant	■	1		1295		A	
Estradiol 25microgram vaginal tablets		15		880		C	Vagifem
Estradiol 500microgram gel sachets		28		528		C	Sandrena
Estradiol 50mg implant	■	1		2108		A	
Estriol 500microgram pessaries		15		492		C	Ortho-Gynest
Estropipate 1.5mg tablets		28		377		C	Harmogen
Etamsylate 500mg tablets		100		878		C	Dicynene
Ethambutol 100mg tablets		56		1177 ▽		A	
Ethambutol 400mg tablets		56		4327 ▽		A	
Ethanol 90% including duty		100	ml	697		A	
Ethanolamine oleate 5% solution for injection 2ml ampoules		10		2620		C	Martindale
Ethanolamine oleate 5% solution for injection 5ml ampoules		10		2297		A	
Ether solvent		500	ml	880		A	
Ethinylestradiol 10microgram tablets		21		1299 △		A	
Ethinylestradiol 1mg tablets		28		2885		A	
Ethinylestradiol 50microgram tablets		21		1547 △		A	
Ethosuximide 250mg capsules		56		3823		C	Emeside
Ethosuximide 250mg/5ml oral solution		200	ml	448		C	Zarontin
Etodolac 300mg capsules		60		814		C	Eccoxolac
Etodolac 600mg modified-release tablets		30		1550		C	
Etoricoxib 120mg tablets		7		603		C	Arcoxia
		28		2411		C	Arcoxia
Etoricoxib 60mg tablets		28		2296		C	Arcoxia
Etoricoxib 90mg tablets		28		2296		C	Arcoxia
Eucalyptus oil liquid		500	ml	970		C	Loveridge
Exemestane 25mg tablets		30		8880		C	Aromasin
Ezetimibe 10mg tablets		28		2631		C	Ezetrol

VIII

BASIC PRICES OF DRUGS

Drug		Quantity		Basic Price	Category	
Famciclovir 125mg tablets		10		3712	C	*Famvir*
Famciclovir 250mg tablets		15		11135	C	*Famvir*
		21		15587	C	*Famvir*
		56		41567	C	*Famvir*
Famciclovir 500mg tablets		14		20786	C	*Famvir*
		30		44528	C	*Famvir*
		56		83146	C	*Famvir*
Famciclovir 750mg tablets	♦	7		14879	C	*Famvir*
Famotidine 20mg tablets		28		642	M	
Famotidine 40mg tablets		28		843	M	
Felbinac 3% gel	■	30	g	226	C	*Traxam Pain Relief Gel*
	■	100	g	700	C	*Traxam*
Felbinac 3.17% foam	■	100	g	700	C	*Traxam*
Felodipine 10mg modified-release tablets	♦	28		601	C	*Plendil*
Felodipine 2.5mg modified-release tablets	♦	28		670	C	*Plendil*
Felodipine 5mg modified release / Ramipril 5mg tablets		28		3226	C	*Triapin*
Felodipine 5mg modified-release tablets	♦	28		447	C	*Plendil*
Fenbufen 300mg capsules	♦	84		2071	C	*Lederfen CP*
Fenbufen 300mg tablets	♦	84		764	M	
Fenbufen 450mg tablets	♦	56		1549	M	
Fenofibrate micronised 160mg tablets	♦	28		1475	C	*Supralip 160*
Fenofibrate micronised 200mg capsules	♦	28		1423	C	*Lipantil Micro 200*
Fenofibrate micronised 267mg capsules	♦	28		2175	C	*Lipantil Micro 267*
Fenofibrate micronised 67mg capsules		90		2330	C	*Lipantil Micro 67*
Fentanyl 100micrograms/hour patches		5		8646	C	
Fentanyl 12 micrograms/hour patches		5		1885	C	
Fentanyl 25micrograms/hour patches		5		2694	C	
Fentanyl 50micrograms/hour patches		5		5032	C	
Fentanyl 75micrograms/hour patches		5		7015	C	
Ferric chloride solution		500	ml	410	C	*Loveridge*
Ferrous fumarate 140mg/5ml oral solution		200	ml	300	C	*Fersamal Syrup*
Ferrous fumarate 140mg/5ml oral solution sugar free		300	ml	486	C	*Galfer Syrup*
Ferrous fumarate 210mg tablets		100		144	C	*Fersamal*
Ferrous fumarate 305mg / Folic acid 350microgram capsules		100		200	C	*Galfer F.A.*
Ferrous fumarate 305mg capsules		100		180	C	*Galfer*

BASIC PRICES OF DRUGS

Drug		Quantity		Basic Price		Category
Ferrous fumarate 322mg tablets	♦	28		66	C	Fersaday
Ferrous gluconate 300mg tablets		1000		3655	A	
Ferrous sulphate 200mg tablets	♦	28		181	M	
Ferrous sulphate 325mg / Folic acid 350microgram modified-release tablets		30		132	C	Ferrograd Folic
Ferrous sulphate 325mg modified-release tablets		30		118	C	Ferrograd
Fexofenadine 120mg tablets		30		623	C	Telfast 120
Fexofenadine 180mg tablets		30		789	C	Telfast 180
Fexofenadine 30mg tablets		60		568	C	Telfast 30
Finasteride 5mg tablets	♦	28		1394	C	Proscar
Flavoxate 200mg tablets		90		1187	C	Urispas 200
Flecainide 100mg tablets		60		2304	M	
Flecainide 50mg tablets		60		1772	M	
Flexible collodion methylated		500	ml	1100	▽ A	
Flucloxacillin 125mg/5ml oral solution	●	100	ml	564	M	
Flucloxacillin 125mg/5ml oral suspension	●	100	ml	325	C	Floxapen Syrup
Flucloxacillin 250mg capsules		28		320	M	
Flucloxacillin 250mg/5ml oral solution	●	100	ml	658	▽ A	
Flucloxacillin 250mg/5ml oral suspension	●	100	ml	648	C	Floxapen Syrup
Flucloxacillin 500mg capsules		28		553	M	
Fluconazole 150mg capsules	■	1		160	M	
Fluconazole 150mg capsules and Clotrimazole 2% cream	■	1		718	C	Canesten Oral & Cream Duo
Fluconazole 200mg capsules	♦	7		437	M	
Fluconazole 200mg/5ml oral suspension	●	35	ml	6642	C	Diflucan
Fluconazole 50mg capsules	♦	7		189	M	
Fluconazole 50mg/5ml oral suspension	●	35	ml	1661	C	Diflucan
Fludrocortisone 100microgram tablets		56		250	C	Florinef
Flunisolide 25micrograms/actuation nasal spray	■	24	ml	505	C	Syntaris
Fluocinolone 0.0025% cream	■	50	g	325	C	Synalar 1 in 10 Dilution
Fluocinolone 0.00625% cream	■	50	g	343	C	Synalar 1 in 4 Dilution
Fluocinolone 0.00625% ointment	■	50	g	343	C	Synalar 1 in 4 Dilution
Fluocinolone 0.025% cream	■	30	g	293	C	Synalar
	■	100	g	834	C	Synalar
Fluocinolone 0.025% gel	■	30	g	434	C	Synalar
Fluocinolone 0.025% ointment	■	30	g	293	C	Synalar
	■	100	g	834	C	Synalar
Fluocinonide 0.05% cream	■	25	g	257	C	Metosyn FAPG
	■	100	g	868	C	Metosyn FAPG

VIII

BASIC PRICES OF DRUGS

Drug		Quantity		Basic Price	Category	
Fluocinonide 0.05% ointment	■	25	g	228	C	*Metosyn*
	■	100	g	856	C	*Metosyn*
Fluorouracil 5% cream	■	20	g	1772	C	*Efudix*
Fluoxetine 20mg capsules		30		184	M	
Fluoxetine 20mg/5ml oral solution	■	70	ml	1453	M	
Fluoxetine 60mg capsules		30		4761	A	
Flupentixol 1mg tablets		60		486	C	*Fluanxol*
Flupentixol 3mg tablets		100		1392	C	*Depixol*
Flupentixol 500microgram tablets		60		288	C	*Fluanxol*
Fluphenazine 1mg tablets		100		530	C	*Moditen*
Fluphenazine decanoate 100mg/ 1ml solution for injection ampoules		5		4395	A	
Fluphenazine decanoate 25mg/1ml solution for injection ampoules		10		2346	C	*Modecate*
Flurbiprofen 100mg tablets		100		5139	M	
Flurbiprofen 200mg modified-release capsules		30		784	C	*Froben SR*
Flurbiprofen 50mg tablets		100		2684	M	
Flurbiprofen 8.75mg lozenges		16		208	C	*Strefen*
Flutamide 250mg tablets	♦	84		2781	M	
Fluticasone 0.005% ointment	■	15	g	241	C	*Cutivate*
	■	50	g	711	C	*Cutivate*
Fluticasone 0.05% cream	■	15	g	241	C	*Cutivate*
	■	50	g	711	C	*Cutivate*
Fluticasone 100micrograms/dose / Salmeterol 50micrograms/dose dry powder inhaler	■	60	dose	3119	C	*Seretide 100 Accuhaler*
Fluticasone 100micrograms/dose dry powder inhaler	■	60	dose	893	C	*Flixotide Accuhaler*
Fluticasone 125micrograms/dose / Salmeterol 25micrograms/dose inhaler CFC free	■	120	dose	3665	C	*Seretide 125 Evohaler*
Fluticasone 125micrograms/dose inhaler CFC free	■	120	dose	2126	C	*Flixotide Evohaler*
Fluticasone 250micrograms/dose / Salmeterol 25micrograms/dose inhaler CFC free	■	120	dose	6229	C	*Seretide 250 Evohaler*
Fluticasone 250micrograms/dose / Salmeterol 50micrograms/dose dry powder inhaler	■	60	dose	3665	C	*Seretide 250 Accuhaler*
Fluticasone 250micrograms/dose dry powder inhaler	■	60	dose	2126	C	*Flixotide Accuhaler*
Fluticasone 250micrograms/dose inhaler CFC free	■	120	dose	3614	C	*Flixotide Evohaler*
Fluticasone 500micrograms/dose / Salmeterol 50micrograms/dose dry powder inhaler	■	60	dose	4092	C	*Seretide 500 Accuhaler*
Fluticasone 500micrograms/dose dry powder inhaler	■	60	dose	3614	C	*Flixotide Accuhaler*
Fluticasone 50micrograms/dose / Salmeterol 25micrograms/dose inhaler CFC free	■	120	dose	1814	C	*Seretide 50 Evohaler*

BASIC PRICES OF DRUGS

Drug		Quantity		Basic Price	Category	
Fluticasone 50micrograms/dose dry powder inhaler	■	60	dose	638	C	*Flixotide Accuhaler*
Fluticasone 50micrograms/dose inhaler CFC free	■	120	dose	544	C	*Flixotide Evohaler*
Fluticasone 50micrograms/dose nasal spray	■	150	dose	1169	C	*Flixonase*
Fluvastatin 20mg capsules	♦	28		1526	C	*Lescol*
Fluvastatin 40mg capsules	♦	28		1526	C	*Lescol*
Fluvastatin 80mg modified-release tablets		28		1920	C	*Lescol XL*
Fluvoxamine 100mg tablets		30		1279	M	
Fluvoxamine 50mg tablets		60		1140	M	
Folic acid 2.5mg/5ml oral solution sugar free		150	ml	916	C	*Lexpec Syrup*
Folic acid 400microgram tablets		90		224	C	*Preconceive*
Folic acid 5mg tablets		28		147	M	
Formaldehyde solution		2	litre	526	A	
		500	ml	330	C	*Loveridge*
Formoterol 12microgram inhalation powder capsules with device	■	60		2923	C	*Foradil*
Formoterol 12micrograms/dose dry powder inhaler	■	60	dose	2480	C	*Oxis Turbohaler 12*
Formoterol 6micrograms/dose dry powder inhaler	■	60	dose	2480	C	*Oxis Turbohaler 6*
Fosinopril 10mg tablets	♦	28		379	M	
Fosinopril 20mg tablets	♦	28		489	M	
Frovatriptan 2.5mg tablets		6		1667	C	*Migard*
Furosemide 20mg tablets		28		128	M	
		250		276	M	
Furosemide 20mg/5ml oral solution sugar free		150	ml	1207	A	
Furosemide 40mg tablets	♦	28		134	M	
Furosemide 40mg/5ml oral solution sugar free		150	ml	1558	A	
Furosemide 500mg tablets		28		711	M	
Furosemide 50mg/5ml oral solution sugar free		150	ml	1684	A	
Fusidic acid 1% modified-release eye drops	■	5	g	209	C	*Fucithalmic Viscous Drops*
Fusidic acid 2% / Betamethasone valerate 0.1% cream	■	30	g	562	C	*Fucibet*
	■	60	g	1123	C	*Fucibet*
Fusidic acid 2% / Hydrocortisone acetate 1% cream	■	30	g	530	C	*Fucidin H*
	■	60	g	1060	C	*Fucidin H*
Fusidic acid 2% cream	■	15	g	200	C	*Fucidin*
	■	30	g	379	C	*Fucidin*
Gabapentin 100mg capsules		100		1526	M	
Gabapentin 300mg capsules		100		1892	M	

BASIC PRICES OF DRUGS

Drug		Quantity		Basic Price	Category	
Gabapentin 400mg capsules		100		2837	M	
Gabapentin 600mg tablets		100		10600	A	
Gabapentin 800mg tablets		100		23475	M	
Galantamine 12mg tablets	♦	56		8400	C	*Reminyl*
Galantamine 16mg modified-release capsules	♦	28		6832	C	*Reminyl XL*
Galantamine 24mg modified-release capsules	♦	28		8400	C	*Reminyl XL*
Galantamine 8mg modified-release capsules	♦	28		5460	C	*Reminyl XL*
Galantamine 8mg tablets	♦	56		6832	C	*Reminyl*
Gemfibrozil 300mg capsules		112		4431	M	
Gemfibrozil 600mg tablets		30		1341	M	
	♦	56		5098	M	
Gentamicin 0.3% ear/eye drops	■	10	ml	178	C	*Genticin*
Gentian compound infusion concentrated		500	ml	1395	C	*Loveridge*
Ginger syrup		500	ml	117	E	
Ginger tincture strong		500	ml	813	A	
Glibenclamide 2.5mg tablets	♦	28		143	M	
Glibenclamide 5mg tablets	♦	28		144	M	
Gliclazide 30mg modified-release tablets		28		308	C	*Diamicron*
		56		616	C	*Diamicron*
Gliclazide 80mg tablets		28		191	M	
		60		208	M	
Glimepiride 1mg tablets		30		418	△ A	
Glimepiride 2mg tablets		30		692	△ A	
Glimepiride 3mg tablets		30		1040	△ A	
Glimepiride 4mg tablets		30		1386	△ A	
Glipizide 2.5mg tablets		28		148	C	*Minodiab 2.5*
Glipizide 5mg tablets		28		126	C	*Minodiab 5*
		56		512	M	
Glucose 50% solution for injection 50ml vials	■	1		440	A	
Glucose liquid BPC1963		140	g	55	A	
Glutaraldehyde 10% solution	■	10	ml	217	C	*Glutarol*
Glycerol 1g suppositories		12		85	△ A	
Glycerol 2g suppositories		12		86	△ A	
Glycerol 4g suppositories		12		226	M	
Glycerol liquid		100	ml	69	A	
Glyceryl trinitrate 0.4% rectal ointment	■	30	g	3280	C	*Rectogesic*
Glyceryl trinitrate 2% ointment	■	60	g	955	C	*Percutol*
Glyceryl trinitrate 2mg modified-release buccal tablets sugar free		100		1270	C	*Suscard Buccal*
Glyceryl trinitrate 300microgram sublingual tablets	■	100		271	C	*GTN*

BASIC PRICES OF DRUGS

Drug		Quantity		Basic Price		Category	
Glyceryl trinitrate 3mg modified-release buccal tablets sugar free		100		1833		C	Suscard Buccal
Glyceryl trinitrate 400micrograms/dose sublingual spray	■	180	dose	263		C	Nitromin
	■	200	dose	313		C	Coro-Nitro
Glyceryl trinitrate 500microgram sublingual tablets	■	100		561		M	
Glyceryl trinitrate 5mg modified-release buccal tablets sugar free		100		2496		C	Suscard Buccal
Glyceryl trinitrate 600microgram sublingual tablets	■	100		976		M	
Goserelin 10.8mg implant pre-filled syringes	■	1		26748		C	Zoladex LA
Goserelin 3.6mg implant pre-filled syringes	■	1		8414		C	Zoladex
Griseofulvin 125mg tablets		100		3380		A	
Griseofulvin 500mg tablets		100		8760		A	
Halibut-liver oil 4000unit capsules		100		96		C	AAH
Haloperidol 1.5mg tablets		28		280		M	
Haloperidol 10mg tablets		28		744		M	
Haloperidol 20mg tablets		28		1415		M	
Haloperidol 500microgram capsules		30		98		C	Serenace
Haloperidol 5mg tablets		28		561		M	
		100		765		C	Haldol
Haloperidol 5mg/1ml solution for injection ampoules		5		152		C	Haldol
Hamamelis water		500	ml	194 ▽		C	Unichem
Heparinoid 0.3% cream	■	50	g	399		C	Hirudoid
Heparinoid 0.3% gel	■	50	g	399		C	Hirudoid
Hexetidine 0.1% mouthwash sugar free	■	100	ml	131		C	Oraldene
		200	ml	202		C	Oraldene
Homatropine 1% eye drops	■	10	ml	214		A	
Homatropine 2% eye drops	■	10	ml	226		A	
Hydralazine 25mg tablets		56		495		M	
Hydralazine 50mg tablets		56		920		M	
Hydrochloric acid dilute liquid		500	ml	295		C	Unichem
Hydrochlorothiazide 12.5mg / Quinapril 10mg tablets	♦	28		1175		C	Accuretic
Hydrocortisone 0.1% cream	■	15	g	165		C	Dermacort
	■	30	g	250		C	Dioderm
Hydrocortisone 0.5% cream	■	15	g	508		M	
	■	30	g	61		C	Efcortelan
Hydrocortisone 0.5% ointment	■	15	g	591		M	
	■	30	g	61		C	Efcortelan

BASIC PRICES OF DRUGS

Drug		Quantity		Basic Price		Category	
Hydrocortisone 1% cream	■	15	g	417		M	
	■	30	g	925		M	
	■	50	g	1750		M	
Hydrocortisone 1% ointment	■	15	g	514		M	
	■	30	g	797		M	
	■	50	g	2211		M	
Hydrocortisone 10mg tablets		30		70		C	Hydrocortone
Hydrocortisone 2.5% cream	■	15	g	2251		M	
Hydrocortisone 2.5% eye ointment	■	3	g	244		C	Martindale
Hydrocortisone 2.5% ointment	■	15	g	1993		M	
	■	30	g	170		C	Efcortelan
Hydrocortisone 2.5mg oromucosal tablets		20		254		C	Corlan Pellets
Hydrocortisone 20mg tablets		30		107		C	Hydrocortone
Hydrocortisone acetate 1% / Gentamicin 0.3% ear drops	■	10	ml	369		C	Gentisone HC
Hydrocortisone butyrate 0.1% cream	■	30	g	229		C	Locoid
	■	100	g	705		C	Locoid
Hydrocortisone butyrate 0.1% ointment	■	30	g	229		C	Locoid
	■	100	g	705		C	Locoid
Hydrocortisone butyrate 0.1% scalp lotion	■	100	ml	976		C	Locoid
Hydrocortisone powder		5	g	1455		A	
Hydrocortisone sodium succinate 100mg powder and solvent for solution for injection vials	■	1		116		C	Solu - Cortef
Hydrogen peroxide 1.5% ear drops		10	ml	2	△	E	
Hydrogen peroxide 6% solution		2	litre	385	△	A	
Hydrotalcite 500mg/5ml oral suspension		500	ml	196		C	Peckforton Pharmaceuticals Ltd
Hydrous ointment		500	g	199		A	
Hydrous wool fat		500	g	580		C	Loveridge
Hydroxocobalamin 1mg/1ml solution for injection ampoules		5		1231		A	
Hydroxycarbamide 500mg capsules		100		1111		C	Hydrea
Hydroxychloroquine 200mg tablets		60		546		C	Plaquenil
Hydroxyzine 10mg tablets		84		182		C	Atarax
Hydroxyzine 10mg/5ml oral solution		200	ml	178		C	Ucerax
Hydroxyzine 25mg tablets		28		122		C	Atarax
Hyoscine butylbromide 10mg tablets		56		259		C	Buscopan
Hyoscine hydrobromide 400micrograms/1ml solution for injection ampoules		10		2692	▽	A	
Hypromellose 0.3% eye drops	■	10	ml	203		M	
Hypromellose 0.5% eye drops	■	10	ml	85		C	Isopto Plain
Hypromellose 1% eye drops	■	10	ml	99		C	Isopto Alkaline

BASIC PRICES OF DRUGS

Drug		Quantity		Basic Price		Category	
Ibandronic acid 150mg tablets	■	1		2145		C	Bonviva
		3		6435		C	Bonviva
Ibuprofen 100mg/5ml oral suspension		500	ml	888		C	Brufen Syrup
Ibuprofen 100mg/5ml oral suspension sugar free		100	ml	296		M	
		150	ml	271		C	Nurofen
Ibuprofen 200mg tablets		84		288		M	
Ibuprofen 400mg tablets		84		345		M	
Ibuprofen 5% cream	■	30	g	268		C	Proflex Pain Relief Cream
	■	100	g	621		C	Proflex
Ibuprofen 5% gel	■	30	g	210		C	Fenbid
	■	50	g	246		A	
	■	100	g	531		A	
Ibuprofen 600mg effervescent granules sachets		20		680		C	Brufen
Ibuprofen 600mg tablets		84		437		M	
		100		567		M	
Ibuprofen 800mg modified-release tablets	♦	56		674		C	Brufen Retard
Ichthammol glycerin liquid		500	ml	692	△	A	
Ichthammol liquid		100	g	405		A	
Imidapril 10mg tablets		28		766		C	Tanatril
Imidapril 20mg tablets		28		920		C	Tanatril
Imidapril 5mg tablets		28		678		C	Tanatril
Imipramine 10mg tablets		28		216		M	
Imipramine 25mg tablets		28		203		M	
Imiquimod 5% cream 250mg sachet		12		5132		C	Aldara
Indapamide 1.5mg modified-release tablets		30		450		C	Natrilix SR
Indapamide 2.5mg tablets		28		280		M	
		56		534		M	
Indometacin 100mg suppositories		10		1091		A	
Indometacin 25mg capsules		28		230		M	
Indometacin 50mg capsules		28		270		M	
Indoramin 20mg tablets		60		1868		M	
Indoramin 25mg tablets		84		900		C	Baratol
Industrial methylated spirit 95%		500	ml	195		C	Loveridge
Inositol nicotinate 500mg tablets		100		3076		C	Hexopal
Inositol nicotinate 750mg tablets	♦	112		5103		C	Hexopal Forte
Iodine aqueous oral solution		100	ml	195		C	Thornton & Ross
		500	ml	595		A	
Iodine crystals		100	g	810		C	Loveridge
Ipecacuanha tincture		500	ml	878	△	A	
Ipratropium bromide 20micrograms/ dose inhaler CFC free	■	200	dose	421		C	Atrovent
Ipratropium bromide 21micrograms/ dose nasal spray	■	15	ml	455		C	Rinatec Aqueous

BASIC PRICES OF DRUGS

Drug		Quantity		Basic Price	Category	
Irbesartan 150mg / Hydrochlorothiazide 12.5mg tablets	♦	28		1257	C	CoAprovel
Irbesartan 150mg tablets	♦	28		1257	C	Aprovel
Irbesartan 300mg / Hydrochlorothiazide 12.5mg tablets	♦	28		1691	C	CoAprovel
Irbesartan 300mg tablets	♦	28		1691	C	Aprovel
Irbesartan 75mg tablets	♦	28		1029	C	Aprovel
Isoniazid 100mg tablets		28		577	A	
Isoniazid 50mg tablets		56		578	A	
Isopropyl myristate 15% / Liquid paraffin 15% gel	■	100	g	277	C	Doublebase
	■	500	g	609	C	Doublebase
Isosorbide dinitrate 10mg tablets		56		534	M	
Isosorbide dinitrate 20mg tablets		56		711	M	
Isosorbide mononitrate 10mg tablets		56		169	M	
Isosorbide mononitrate 20mg tablets		56		182	M	
Isosorbide mononitrate 25mg modified-release capsules	♦	28		659	C	Elantan LA 25
Isosorbide mononitrate 40mg tablets		56		253	M	
Isosorbide mononitrate 50mg modified-release capsules	♦	28		1054	C	Elantan LA 50
Isosorbide mononitrate 50mg modified-release tablets	♦	28		675	C	Isotard 50 XL
Isosorbide mononitrate 60mg modified-release capsules	♦	28		903	C	Monomax SR 60
Isosorbide mononitrate 60mg modified-release tablets	♦	28		1114	C	
Isotretinoin 0.05% gel	■	30	g	618	C	Isotrex
Ispaghula husk 3.4g oral powder sachets sugar free		30		254	C	Regulan
Ispaghula husk 3.5g / Mebeverine 135mg effervescent granules sachets sugar free		10		250	C	Fybogel Mebeverine
Ispaghula husk 3.5g effervescent granules sachets gluten free sugar free		30		212	C	Fybogel
Ispaghula husk 3.5g granules sachets gluten free		10		123	C	Fibrelief Orange
		30		207	C	Fibrelief Orange
Ispaghula husk 3.5g granules sachets gluten free sugar free		10		123	C	Fibrelief
		30		207	C	Fibrelief
Ispaghula husk 90% granules sugar free		200	g	267	C	Isogel
Isradipine 2.5mg tablets		56		1654	C	Prescal
Itraconazole 100mg capsules		4		390	C	Sporanox
		15		1992	M	
		60		5849	C	Sporanox

BASIC PRICES OF DRUGS

Drug		Quantity		Basic Price	Category	
Kaolin and Morphine mixture		200	ml	42	C	Unichem
Kaolin light powder		1	kg	440	C	Loveridge
Kaolin mixture		200	ml	52	A	
Kaolin mixture paediatric		100	ml	45	C	Thornton & Ross
Kaolin poultices	■	200	g	215 ▽	A	
	■	500	g	360	C	K/L
Ketoconazole 2% cream	■	30	g	354	C	Nizoral
Ketoconazole 2% shampoo	■	120	ml	628	M	
Ketoconazole 200mg tablets		30		1459	C	Nizoral
Ketoprofen 100mg capsules		56		944	M	
Ketoprofen 2.5% gel	■	30	g	249 ▽	A	
	■	50	g	306	C	Powergel
	■	100	g	333	M	
Ketoprofen 50mg capsules		28		645	M	
		112		1607	C	Orudis
Ketorolac 0.5% eye drops	■	5	ml	500	C	Acular
Ketotifen 1mg/5ml oral solution sugar free		300	ml	1273	C	Zaditen Elixir
Labetalol 100mg tablets		56		1172	M	
Labetalol 200mg tablets		56		1786	M	
Labetalol 400mg tablets		56		2414	M	
Labetalol 50mg tablets	♦	56		379	C	Trandate
Lacidipine 2mg tablets	♦	28		951	C	Motens
Lacidipine 4mg tablets	♦	28		1423	C	Motens
Lactic acid liquid		250	ml	415	C	Loveridge
Lactose powder		500	g	295	C	Loveridge
Lactulose 3.1-3.7g/5ml oral solution		300	ml	310	M	
		500	ml	384	M	
Lamotrigine 100mg dispersible tablets		56		2370	M	
Lamotrigine 100mg tablets		56		1300	M	
Lamotrigine 200mg tablets	♦	56		2744	M	
Lamotrigine 25mg dispersible tablets		56		811	M	
Lamotrigine 25mg tablets		21		765	C	Lamictal
		42		1530	C	Lamictal
		56		486	M	
Lamotrigine 2mg dispersible tablets		30		871	C	Lamictal Dispersible
Lamotrigine 50mg tablets		56		750	M	
Lamotrigine 5mg dispersible tablets		28		494	M	
Lansoprazole 15mg gastro-resistant capsules	♦	28		324	M	

VIII

BASIC PRICES OF DRUGS

Drug		Quantity		Basic Price	Category	
Lansoprazole 15mg orodispersible tablets	♦	28		597	C	Zoton FasTab
Lansoprazole 30mg gastro-resistant capsules	♦	28		555	M	
Lansoprazole 30mg gastro-resistant granules sachets		28		3397	C	Zoton
Lansoprazole 30mg orodispersible tablets	♦	14		547	C	Zoton FasTab
	♦	28		1100	C	Zoton FasTab
Latanoprost 50micrograms/ml eye drops	■	2.5	ml	1314	C	Xalatan
Leflunomide 10mg tablets	■	30		5113	C	Arava
Leflunomide 20mg tablets	■	30		5113	C	Arava
Lemon spirit		100	ml	584	△ A	
Lercanidipine 10mg tablets	♦	28		580	C	Zanidip
Lercanidipine 20mg tablets	♦	28		1100	C	Zanidip
Letrozole 2.5mg tablets	♦	14		4158	C	Femara
	♦	28		8316	C	Femara
Levetiracetam 100mg/ml oral solution sugar free	■	300	ml	7100	C	Keppra
Levetiracetam 1g tablets		60		10110	C	Keppra
Levetiracetam 250mg tablets		60		2970	C	Keppra
Levetiracetam 500mg tablets		60		5230	C	Keppra
Levetiracetam 750mg tablets		60		8910	C	Keppra
Levobunolol 0.5% eye drops	■	5	ml	380	M	
Levocetirizine 5mg tablets		30		745	C	Xyzal
Levofloxacin 250mg tablets		5		723	C	Tavanic
		10		1445	C	Tavanic
Levofloxacin 500mg tablets		5		1293	C	Tavanic
		10		2585	C	Tavanic
Levomepromazine 25mg tablets		84		2026	C	Nozinan
Levomepromazine 25mg/1ml solution for injection ampoules		10		2013	C	Nozinan
Levonorgestrel 1.5mg tablets	■	1		511	C	Levonelle 1500
Levothyroxine sodium 100microgram tablets		28		136	M	
		1000		481	M	
Levothyroxine sodium 100micrograms/5ml oral solution sugar free		100	ml	5275	C	Evotrox
Levothyroxine sodium 25microgram tablets		28		161	M	
		500		938	M	
Levothyroxine sodium 25micrograms/5ml oral solution sugar free		100	ml	4275	C	Evotrox
Levothyroxine sodium 50microgram tablets		28		136	M	
		1000		824	M	
Levothyroxine sodium 50micrograms/5ml oral solution sugar free		100	ml	4490	C	Evotrox

BASIC PRICES OF DRUGS

Drug	Quantity		Basic Price		Category
Lidocaine 100mg/10ml (1%) solution for injection ampoules	10		347		A
Lidocaine 100mg/5ml (2%) solution for injection ampoules	10		255	△	A
Lidocaine 2% / Chlorhexidine 0.25% gel 11ml pre-filled syringes	10		1576		C	Instillagel
Lidocaine 2% / Chlorhexidine 0.25% gel 6ml pre-filled syringes	10		1405		C	Instillagel
Lidocaine 200mg/20ml (1%) solution for injection ampoules	10		622		A
Lidocaine 20mg/2ml (1%) solution for injection ampoules	10		213		A
Lidocaine 400mg/20ml (2%) solution for injection ampoules	10		607		A
Lidocaine 40mg/2ml (2%) solution for injection ampoules	10		277		A
Lidocaine 5% ointment ■	15	g	88		A
Lidocaine 50mg/5ml (1%) solution for injection ampoules	10		226	▽	A
Linseed oil liquid	500	ml	215		C	Unichem
Liothyronine 20microgram tablets	100		1592		C	Tertroxin
Liquid paraffin / Magnesium hydroxide oral emulsion	2	litre	633		A
	150	ml	98	△	A
Liquid paraffin 50% / White soft paraffin 50% ointment	500	g	394		C	Unichem
Liquid paraffin light liquid	500	ml	275		C	Loveridge
Liquid paraffin liquid	2	litre	454	△	A
Liquid paraffin oral emulsion	500	ml	320		C	Loveridge
Liquorice liquid extract	500	ml	507	△	A
Lisinopril 10mg / Hydrochlorothiazide 12.5mg tablets ♦	28		1054	△	A
Lisinopril 10mg tablets ♦	28		167		M
Lisinopril 2.5mg tablets ♦	28		138		M
Lisinopril 20mg / Hydrochlorothiazide 12.5mg tablets ♦	28		531		M
Lisinopril 20mg tablets ♦	28		213		M
Lisinopril 5mg tablets ♦	28		143		M
Lithium carbonate 200mg modified-release tablets	100		239		C	Priadel 200
Lithium carbonate 250mg tablets	100		322		C	Camcolit 250
Lithium carbonate 450mg modified-release tablets	60		288		C	Liskonum
Lodoxamide 0.1% eye drops ■	10	ml	548		C	Alomide Ophthalmic Solution
Lofepramine 70mg tablets ♦	56		2892		M
Loperamide 1mg/5ml oral solution sugar free	100	ml	98		C	Imodium Syrup
Loperamide 2mg capsules	30		185		M

VIII

BASIC PRICES OF DRUGS

Drug		Quantity		Basic Price		Category	
Loperamide 2mg tablets		30		215		C	Norimode
Loprazolam 1mg tablets		28		558		C	Winthrop Pharm
Loratadine 10mg tablets		30		206		M	
Loratadine 5mg/5ml oral solution		100	ml	529	▽	A	
Lorazepam 1mg tablets		28		694		M	
Lorazepam 2.5mg tablets		28		1144		M	
Lormetazepam 1mg tablets		30		3782		M	
Lormetazepam 500microgram tablets		30		3178		M	
Losartan 100mg / Hydrochlorothiazide 25mg tablets	♦	28		2420		C	Cozaar-Comp
Losartan 100mg tablets	♦	28		2420		C	Cozaar
Losartan 25mg tablets	♦	28		1809		C	Cozaar
Losartan 50mg / Hydrochlorothiazide 12.5mg tablets	♦	28		1809		C	Cozaar-Comp
Losartan 50mg tablets	♦	28		1809		C	Cozaar
Lumiracoxib 100mg tablets		30		1724		C	Prexige
Lumiracoxib 400mg tablets		5		346		C	Prexige
Lymecycline 408mg capsules	♦	28		716		C	Tetralysal 300
	♦	56		1426		C	Tetralysal 300
Macrogol 4000 10g oral powder sachets sugar free		20		484		C	Idrolax
Macrogol compound 13.8g oral powder sachets NPF sugar free		20		463		C	Movicol
		30		695		C	Movicol
Magnesium carbonate light powder		500	g	470		C	Loveridge
Magnesium hydroxide oral suspension		500	ml	215	△	A	
Magnesium sulphate 50% solution for injection 2ml ampoules		10		2913	△	A	
Magnesium sulphate dried powder		1	kg	565		C	Loveridge
Magnesium sulphate paste		25	g	60		A	
		50	g	74		A	
Magnesium sulphate powder		500	g	90		C	Loveridge
Magnesium trisilicate oral suspension		200	ml	77		A	
Magnesium trisilicate powder		500	g	650		C	Loveridge
Malathion 0.5% alcoholic lotion	■	50	ml	222		C	Prioderm
	■	200	ml	570		C	Prioderm
Malathion 0.5% aqueous liquid	■	50	ml	227		C	Derbac-M
	■	200	ml	570		C	Derbac-M
Malathion 1% cream shampoo	■	40	g	277		C	Prioderm
Mebendazole 100mg chewable tablets		6		142		C	Vermox
Mebendazole 100mg/5ml oral suspension	■	30	ml	165		C	Vermox

BASIC PRICES OF DRUGS

Drug	Quantity		Basic Price		Category
Mebeverine 135mg tablets	100		982		M
Mecysteine 100mg gastro-resistant tablets	100		1765		C Visclair
Medroxyprogesterone 100mg tablets	100		4994		C Provera
Medroxyprogesterone 10mg tablets	10		247		C Provera
	90		2216		C Provera
Medroxyprogesterone 150mg/1ml ■ suspension for injection 1ml pre-filled syringes	1		501		C Depo-Provera
Medroxyprogesterone 2.5mg / ♦ Estradiol valerate 1mg tablets	84		2149		C Indivina
Medroxyprogesterone 2.5mg tablets	30		184		C Provera
Medroxyprogesterone 200mg tablets	30		2965		C Provera
Medroxyprogesterone 400mg tablets	30		5867		C Provera
Medroxyprogesterone 5mg / ♦ Estradiol valerate 1mg tablets	84		2149		C Indivina
Medroxyprogesterone 5mg / ♦ Estradiol valerate 2mg tablets	84		2149		C Indivina
Medroxyprogesterone 5mg tablets	10		123		C Provera
Mefenamic acid 250mg capsules	100		469		M
Mefenamic acid 500mg tablets	28		341		M
	100		892		M
Megestrol 160mg tablets	30		2725		C Megace
Megestrol 40mg tablets	120		2835		C Megace
Meloxicam 15mg suppositories	12		558		C Mobic
Meloxicam 15mg tablets	30		868	▽	A
Meloxicam 7.5mg suppositories	12		372		C Mobic
Meloxicam 7.5mg tablets	30		640	▽	A
Memantine 10mg tablets	28		3450		C Ebixa
	56		6901		C Ebixa
	112		13801		C Ebixa
Menthol 0.5% cream	500	g	1530		C Arjun
Menthol 1% cream	500	g	1530		C Arjun
Menthol 2% cream	500	g	1530		C Arjun
Menthol and Eucalyptus inhalation	100	ml	70		A
Menthol crystals	5	g	70		C AAH
Meptazinol 200mg tablets	112		2211		C Meptid
Mesalazine 1g suppositories	28		4155		C Pentasa
Mesalazine 400mg gastro-resistant tablets	90		3122		C Asacol
	120		4162		C Asacol
Metformin 1g / Rosiglitazone 2mg tablets	56		2771		C Avandamet
Metformin 1g / Rosiglitazone 4mg tablets	56		5245		C Avandamet
Metformin 500mg / Rosiglitazone 2mg tablets	112		5245		C Avandamet

VIII

BASIC PRICES OF DRUGS

Drug	Quantity		Basic Price		Category
Metformin 500mg tablets	28		160		M
	84		233		M
Metformin 500mg/5ml oral solution sugar free	100	ml	5990		C	Metsol
Metformin 850mg tablets	56		236		M
★	300		672		M
Methadone 10mg/1ml solution for injection ampoules	10		859		A
Methadone 1mg/ml oral solution	30	ml	44		C	Unichem
	50	ml	73		C	Unichem
	100	ml	135		C	Physeptone Mixture
	500	ml	745		A
Methadone 1mg/ml oral solution sugar free	30	ml	44		C	Rosemont Pharm
	50	ml	73		C	Rosemont Pharm
	100	ml	145		A
	500	ml	737		A
Methadone 20mg/2ml solution for injection ampoules	10		1450		A
Methadone 2mg/5ml linctus	500	ml	543		A
Methadone 35mg/3.5ml solution for injection ampoules	10		1783		A
Methadone 50mg/5ml solution for injection ampoules	10		1923		A
Methadone 5mg tablets	50		297		C	Physeptone
Methadone hydrochloride powder	2	g	959		A
Methenamine hippurate 1g tablets	60		658		C	Hiprex
Methocarbamol 750mg tablets	100		1265		C	Robaxin 750
Methotrexate 10mg tablets	100		5507		A
Methotrexate 2.5mg tablets	28		327		A
	100		1411 △		A
Methyl salicylate 25% liniment	500	ml	345		A
Methyl salicylate 50% ointment	500	g	510		A
Methyl salicylate liquid	500	ml	530		A
Methylcellulose 500mg tablets	112		269		C	Celevac
Methylcellulose powder	500	g	2300		C	Loveridge
Methyldopa 125mg tablets	56		482		M
Methyldopa 250mg tablets	56		369		M
Methyldopa 500mg tablets	56		608		M
Methylphenidate 10mg modified-release capsules	30		2500		C	Equasym XL
Methylphenidate 10mg tablets	30		482 ▽		A
Methylphenidate 18mg modified-release tablets	30		2970		C	Concerta XL
Methylphenidate 20mg modified-release capsules	30		3000		C	Equasym XL
Methylphenidate 20mg tablets	30		998		C	Equasym
Methylphenidate 30mg modified-release capsules	30		3500		C	Equasym XL
Methylphenidate 36mg modified-release tablets	30		4043		C	Concerta XL

BASIC PRICES OF DRUGS

Drug		Quantity		Basic Price	Category	
Methylphenidate 5mg tablets		30		278	C	Equasym
Metoclopramide 10mg tablets		28		152	M	
Metoclopramide 10mg/2ml solution for injection ampoules		10		259	A	
Metoclopramide 15mg modified-release capsules		56		701	C	Maxolon SR
Metolazone 5mg tablets		100		1894	C	Metenix 5
Metoprolol 100mg tablets		28		459	M	
	♦	56		403	M	
		100		937	M	
Metoprolol 50mg tablets		28		334	M	
	♦	56		285	M	
		100		553	M	
Metronidazole 0.75% cream	■	30	g	1000	C	Rozex
	■	40	g	1528	C	Rozex
Metronidazole 0.8% gel	■	15	g	459	C	Metrotop
	■	30	g	810	C	Metrotop
	■	60	g	1430	C	Metrotop
Metronidazole 200mg tablets		21		183	M	
Metronidazole 200mg/5ml oral suspension		100	ml	770	A	
Metronidazole 400mg tablets		21		205	M	
		100		389	M	
Metronidazole 500mg tablets		21		1364	M	
Mianserin 10mg tablets		28		552	M	
Mianserin 30mg tablets		28		995	M	
Miconazole 1.2g vaginal capsules	■	1		312	C	Gyno-Daktarin
Miconazole 100mg pessaries		14		312	C	Gyno-Daktarin
Miconazole 2% / Hydrocortisone 1% cream	■	15	g	273	C	Daktacort Hydrocortisone
	■	30	g	190	C	Daktacort
Miconazole 2% / Hydrocortisone 1% ointment	■	30	g	209	C	Daktacort
Miconazole 2% cream	■	30	g	193	C	Daktarin
Miconazole 20mg/g oromucosal gel sugar free	■	15	g	245	C	Daktarin
	■	80	g	465	C	Daktarin
Minocycline 100mg capsules	♦	28		1309	C	Aknemin
Minocycline 100mg modified-release capsules	♦	56		2114	C	
Minocycline 100mg tablets		28		1206	M	
Minocycline 50mg capsules	♦	56		1527	C	Aknemin 50
Minocycline 50mg tablets		28		755	M	
Minoxidil 10mg tablets		60		3068	C	Loniten
Minoxidil 2.5mg tablets		60		888	C	Loniten
Minoxidil 5mg tablets		60		1583	C	Loniten
Mirtazapine 15mg orodispersible tablets		30		1919	C	Zispin SolTab
Mirtazapine 15mg tablets		28		1947 △	A	
Mirtazapine 30mg orodispersible tablets		30		1919	C	Zispin SolTab

VIII

BASIC PRICES OF DRUGS

Drug		Quantity		Basic Price		Category	
Mirtazapine 30mg tablets	♦	28		1302		M	
Mirtazapine 45mg orodispersible tablets		30		1919		C	Zispin SolTab
Mirtazapine 45mg tablets		28		2034	△	A	
Misoprostol 200microgram tablets		60		1003		C	Cytotec
Mizolastine 10mg modified-release tablets		30		577		C	Mizollen
Moclobemide 150mg tablets		30		377		M	
Moclobemide 300mg tablets		30		561		M	
Modafinil 100mg tablets		30		5580		C	Provigil
Modafinil 200mg tablets		30		11160		C	Provigil
Mometasone 0.1% cream	■	30	g	454		C	Elocon
	■	100	g	1307		C	Elocon
Mometasone 0.1% ointment	■	30	g	454		C	Elocon
	■	100	g	1307		C	Elocon
Mometasone 0.1% scalp lotion	■	30	ml	454		C	Elocon
Mometasone 200micrograms/dose dry powder inhaler	■	30	dose	1600		C	Asmanex Twisthaler
	■	60	dose	2400		C	Asmanex Twisthaler
Mometasone 400micrograms/dose dry powder inhaler	■	30	dose	2220		C	Asmanex Twisthaler
	■	60	dose	3675		C	Asmanex Twisthaler
Mometasone 50micrograms/dose nasal spray	■	140	dose	783		C	Nasonex
Montelukast 10mg tablets	♦	28		2697		C	Singulair
Montelukast 4mg chewable tablets	♦	28		2569		C	Singulair
Montelukast 4mg granules sachets		28		2569		C	Singulair
Montelukast 5mg chewable tablets	♦	28		2569		C	Singulair
Morphine 100mg modified-release tablets		60		4066		C	MST Continus
Morphine 10mg modified-release capsules		60		408		C	Zomorph
Morphine 10mg modified-release tablets		60		548		C	MST Continus
Morphine 10mg tablets		56		561		C	Sevredol
Morphine 15mg modified-release tablets		60		961		C	MST Continus
Morphine 200mg modified-release capsules		60		6035		C	Zomorph
Morphine 200mg modified-release tablets		60		8134		C	MST Continus
Morphine 20mg tablets		56		1121		C	Sevredol
Morphine 30mg modified-release capsules		60		977		C	Zomorph
Morphine 30mg modified-release tablets		60		1317		C	MST Continus
Morphine 50mg tablets		56		2802		C	Sevredol
Morphine 5mg modified-release tablets		60		329		C	MST Continus
Morphine 60mg modified-release capsules		60		1906		C	Zomorph

BASIC PRICES OF DRUGS

Drug	Quantity		Basic Price		Category	
Morphine 60mg modified-release tablets	60		2569	C	MST Continus	
Morphine hydrochloride powder	2	g	1359	A		
Morphine sulphate 10mg/1ml solution for injection ampoules	5		362	A		
Morphine sulphate 15mg suppositories	12		714	A		
Morphine sulphate 15mg/1ml solution for injection ampoules	5		420	A		
Morphine sulphate 30mg suppositories	12		1038	A		
Morphine sulphate 30mg/1ml solution for injection ampoules	5		545	A		
Morphine sulphate powder	2	g	1120	C	Martindale	
	5	g	2800	A		
Mouthwash solution tablets ■	100		919	M		
Moxifloxacin 400mg tablets	5		1195	C	Avelox	
Moxisylyte 40mg tablets	112		7998	C	Opilon	
Moxonidine 200microgram tablets	28		490	M		
Moxonidine 300microgram tablets ♦	28		814	△ A		
Moxonidine 400microgram tablets ♦	28		569	M		
Mupirocin 2% cream ■	15	g	438	C	Bactroban	
Mupirocin 2% nasal ointment ■	3	g	580	C	Bactroban Nasal	
Mupirocin 2% ointment ■	15	g	438	C	Bactroban	
Nabumetone 500mg tablets	56		1033	M		
Nabumetone 500mg/5ml oral suspension sugar free	300	ml	2890	C	Relifex	
Naftidrofuryl 100mg capsules ♦	84		872	M		
	100		1023	C	Praxilene	
	500		4975	C	Praxilene	
Naltrexone 50mg tablets ♦	28		3953	C	Nalorex	
Naproxen 250mg gastro-resistant tablets	56		643	M		
Naproxen 250mg tablets	28		197	M		
	250		200	M		
Naproxen 500mg gastro-resistant tablets	56		1007	M		
Naproxen 500mg tablets	28		251	M		
	100		293	M		
Naproxen sodium 275mg tablets	60		754	C	Synflex	
Naratriptan 2.5mg tablets	6		2455	C	Naramig	
Nateglinide 120mg tablets	84		2250	C	Starlix	
Nateglinide 180mg tablets	84		2250	C	Starlix	
Nateglinide 60mg tablets	84		1975	C	Starlix	
Nebivolol 5mg tablets ♦	28		923	C	Nebilet	
Nedocromil 2% eye drops ■	5	ml	512	C	Rapitil	
Nefopam 30mg tablets	90		1118	C	Acupan	

BASIC PRICES OF DRUGS

Drug		Quantity		Basic Price	Category	
Neomycin 0.5% / Betamethasone valerate 0.1% cream	■	30	g	176	C	*Betnovate-N*
	■	100	g	488	C	*Betnovate-N*
Neomycin 0.5% / Betamethasone valerate 0.1% ointment	■	30	g	176	C	*Betnovate-N*
	■	100	g	488	C	*Betnovate-N*
Neomycin 0.5% / Chlorhexidine hydrochloride 0.1% cream	■	15	g	158	C	*Naseptin*
Nicardipine 20mg capsules		56		985	M	
Nicardipine 30mg capsules		56		1020	M	
Nicardipine 30mg modified-release capsules		56		1021	C	*Cardene SR*
Nicardipine 45mg modified-release capsules		56		1486	C	*Cardene SR*
Nicorandil 10mg tablets		60 (6x■10)		818	C	*Ikorel*
Nicorandil 20mg tablets		60 (6x■10)		1554	C	*Ikorel*
Nicotine 10mg inhalation cartridges with device	■	6		399	C	*Nicorette Inhalator*
	■	42		1281	C	*Nicorette Inhalator*
Nicotine 10mg/16hours patches		7		907	C	*Nicorette*
Nicotine 15mg/16hours patches		7		907	C	*Nicorette*
Nicotine 21mg/24hours patches		7		997	C	
Nicotine 2mg lozenges sugar free		36		512	C	*Niquitin CQ*
		72		997	C	*Niquitin CQ*
Nicotine 2mg medicated chewing gum sugar free		30		325	C	*Nicorette*
		96		826	C	*Nicotinell*
		105		889	C	*Nicorette*
		210		1482	C	*Nicorette*
Nicotine 2mg sublingual tablets		105		1112	C	*Nicorette Microtabs*
Nicotine 4mg lozenges sugar free		36		512	C	*Niquitin CQ*
		72		997	C	*Niquitin CQ*
Nicotine 4mg medicated chewing gum sugar free		30		399	C	*Nicorette*
		96		1026	C	*Nicotinell*
		105		1083	C	*Nicorette*
		210		1824	C	*Nicorette*
Nicotine 500micrograms/actuation nasal spray	■	10	ml	1226	C	*Nicorette*
Nicotine 5mg/16hours patches		7		907	C	*Nicorette*
Nicotine bitartrate 1mg lozenges sugar free		96		912	C	*Nicotinell*
Nicotine bitartrate 2mg lozenges sugar free		36		495	C	*Nicotinell*
		96		1060	C	*Nicotinell*
Nifedipine 10mg capsules		84		529	M	
Nifedipine 10mg modified-release capsules		60		427	C	*Coracten SR*
Nifedipine 20mg modified-release capsules		60		593	C	*Coracten SR*

BASIC PRICES OF DRUGS

Drug	Quantity		Basic Price	Category	
Nifedipine 5mg capsules	84		455	M	
Nifedipine 60mg modified-release tablets ♦	28		969	C	
Nitrazepam 2.5mg/5ml oral suspension	150	ml	530	C	*Somnite*
Nitrazepam 5mg tablets	28		147	M	
Nitrofurantoin 100mg capsules	30		576	C	*Macrodantin*
Nitrofurantoin 100mg modified-release capsules	14		489	C	*Macrobid*
Nitrofurantoin 100mg tablets	28		419	A	
	100		855	M	
Nitrofurantoin 50mg capsules	30		305	C	*Macrodantin*
Nitrofurantoin 50mg tablets	28		231	A	
	100		547	M	
Nizatidine 150mg capsules	30		517	M	
Nizatidine 300mg capsules	30		673	M	
Norethisterone 1mg tablets	36 (3x■12)		349	C	*Micronor HRT*
Norethisterone 5mg tablets	30		402	M	
Norfloxacin 400mg tablets	6		364	M	
	14		542	M	
Nortriptyline 10mg tablets	100		1206	C	*Allegron*
Nortriptyline 25mg tablets	100		2402	C	*Allegron*
Nystatin 100,000unit pastilles ■	28		301	C	*Nystan*
Nystatin 100,000units/4g application vaginal cream ■	60	g	258	C	*Nystan*
Nystatin 100,000units/g cream ■	30	g	203	C	*Nystan*
Nystatin 100,000units/g ointment ■	30	g	163	C	*Nystan*
Nystatin 100,000units/ml oral suspension ■	30	ml	191	C	*Nystan*
Nystatin 500,000unit tablets	56		437	C	*Nystan*
Ofloxacin 0.3% eye drops ■	5	ml	217	C	*Exocin*
Ofloxacin 200mg tablets	10		774	M	
	20		1566	C	*Tarivid*
Ofloxacin 400mg tablets	5		707	M	
	10		1106	M	
	50		7799	C	*Tarivid 400*
Olanzapine 10mg oral lyophilisates	28		9137	C	*Zyprexa Velotab*
Olanzapine 10mg tablets	28		7945	C	*Zyprexa*
Olanzapine 15mg oral lyophilisates	28		13706	C	*Zyprexa Velotab*
Olanzapine 15mg tablets	28		11918	C	*Zyprexa*
Olanzapine 2.5mg tablets	28		3329	C	*Zyprexa*
Olanzapine 20mg oral lyophilisates	28		18274	C	*Zyprexa Velotab*
Olanzapine 20mg tablets	28		15890	C	*Zyprexa*
Olanzapine 5mg oral lyophilisates	28		5610	C	*Zyprexa Velotab*
Olanzapine 5mg tablets	28		4878	C	*Zyprexa*
Olanzapine 7.5mg tablets	56		14634	C	*Zyprexa*

VIII

BASIC PRICES OF DRUGS

Drug	Quantity		Basic Price	Category	
Oleic acid liquid	500	ml	440	C	*Loveridge*
Olive oil liquid	2	litre	1450	C	*Thornton & Ross*
Olmesartan medoxomil 10mg tablets	28		1095	C	*Olmetec*
Olmesartan medoxomil 20mg tablets	28		1295	C	*Olmetec*
Olmesartan medoxomil 40mg tablets	28		1750	C	*Olmetec*
Olopatadine 0.1% eye drops ■	5	ml	411	C	*Opatanol*
Olsalazine 250mg capsules	112		2057	C	*Dipentum*
Olsalazine 500mg tablets	60		2204	C	*Dipentum*
Omeprazole 10mg dispersible ♦ gastro-resistant tablets	28		1934	C	*Losec MUPS*
Omeprazole 10mg gastro-resistant capsules	28		363	M	
Omeprazole 10mg gastro-resistant tablets	28		1023	M	
Omeprazole 20mg dispersible ♦ gastro-resistant tablets	28		2922	C	*Losec MUPS*
Omeprazole 20mg gastro-resistant capsules	28		445	M	
Omeprazole 20mg gastro-resistant tablets	28		1164	M	
Omeprazole 40mg dispersible ♦ gastro-resistant tablets	7		1461	C	*Losec MUPS*
Omeprazole 40mg gastro-resistant capsules	7		360	M	
Omeprazole 40mg gastro-resistant tablets	7		895	M	
Ondansetron 4mg tablets	30		10125	A	
Ondansetron 8mg tablets	10		6748	A	
Orange syrup	500	ml	595	C	*Loveridge*
Orange tincture BP 2001	100	ml	670	C	*Loveridge*
Orciprenaline 10mg/5ml oral solution sugar free	300	ml	226	C	*Alupent Syrup*
Orlistat 120mg capsules	84		3951	C	*Xenical*
Orphenadrine 50mg tablets	100		3540	M	
Oxazepam 10mg tablets	28		372	M	
Oxazepam 15mg tablets	28		393	M	
Oxcarbazepine 150mg tablets	50		1000	C	*Trileptal*
Oxcarbazepine 300mg tablets	50		2000	C	*Trileptal*
Oxcarbazepine 600mg tablets	50		4000	C	*Trileptal*
Oxerutins 250mg capsules	120		1305	C	*Paroven*
Oxprenolol 20mg tablets	56		186	C	*Trasicor*
Oxprenolol 40mg tablets	56		373	C	*Trasicor*
Oxprenolol 80mg tablets	56		620	C	*Trasicor*
Oxybutynin 2.5mg tablets	56		669	M	
Oxybutynin 2.5mg/5ml oral solution	150	ml	574	C	*Ditropan*
Oxybutynin 3.9mg/24hours patches	8		2720	C	*Kentera*
Oxybutynin 3mg tablets	56		915	C	*Cystrin*

BASIC PRICES OF DRUGS

Drug	Quantity		Basic Price	Category	
Oxybutynin 5mg tablets	56		413	M	
	84		361	M	
Oxycodone 10mg capsules	56		2218	C	OxyNorm
Oxycodone 10mg/ml oral solution sugar free	120	ml	4525	C	OxyNorm
Oxycodone 20mg capsules	56		4435	C	OxyNorm
Oxycodone 5mg capsules	56		1109	C	OxyNorm
Oxycodone 5mg/5ml oral solution sugar free	250	ml	943	C	OxyNorm
Oxytetracycline 250mg tablets	28		168	M	
Pantoprazole 20mg gastro-resistant tablets	28		1231	C	Protium
Pantoprazole 40mg gastro-resistant tablets	28		2140	C	Protium
Paracetamol 120mg suppositories	10		925	A	
Paracetamol 120mg/5ml oral solution paediatric	500	ml	194	A	
Paracetamol 120mg/5ml oral solution paediatric sugar free	2	litre	596	A	
	500	ml	160	C	AAH
Paracetamol 120mg/5ml oral suspension paediatric	500	ml	194	C	Paldesic
Paracetamol 120mg/5ml oral suspension paediatric sugar free	1	litre	340	C	AAH
	150	ml	65	C	Medinol
	200	ml	86	C	Medinol
Paracetamol 125mg suppositories	10		1150	C	Alvedon
Paracetamol 240mg suppositories	10		950	A	
Paracetamol 250mg suppositories	10		2300	C	Alvedon
Paracetamol 250mg/5ml oral suspension	500	ml	366	A	
Paracetamol 250mg/5ml oral suspension sugar free	200	ml	113	A	
Paracetamol 325mg / Tramadol 37.5mg tablets	60		1007	C	Tramacet
Paracetamol 500mg / Dihydrocodeine 20mg tablets	56		511	C	Remedeine
	112		1021	C	Remedeine
Paracetamol 500mg / Dihydrocodeine 30mg tablets	56		631	C	Remedeine Forte
Paracetamol 500mg / Metoclopramide 5mg tablets	42		803	C	Paramax
Paracetamol 500mg capsules	32		239	M	
Paracetamol 500mg soluble tablets	60		565	M	
Paracetamol 500mg suppositories	10		990	M	
Paracetamol 500mg tablets	16		17	A	
	32		172	M	
	100		212	M	

VIII

BASIC PRICES OF DRUGS

Drug	Quantity		Basic Price		Category	
Paracetamol 60mg suppositories	10		996		C	Alvedon
Paraffin hard MP 43-46°C solid	500	g	325		C	Loveridge
Paraffin hard solid	500	g	275		A	
Paroxetine 10mg/5ml oral suspension sugar free	150	ml	949		C	Seroxat Liquid
Paroxetine 20mg tablets	30		657		M	
Paroxetine 30mg tablets	30		895		M	
Penciclovir 1% cream ■	2	g	420		C	Vectavir Cold Sore Cream
Penicillamine 125mg tablets	56		1210		M	
Penicillamine 250mg tablets	56		2101		M	
Pentazocine 25mg tablets	28		340	△	A	
Pentazocine 30mg/1ml solution for injection ampoules	10		1671		C	Winthrop Pharm
Pentazocine 50mg capsules	28		640	△	A	
Pentazocine 60mg/2ml solution for injection ampoules	10		3214		C	Winthrop Pharm
Pentoxifylline 400mg modified-release tablets	90		2048		C	
Peppermint emulsion concentrated	250	ml	380		C	Loveridge
Peppermint oil 0.2ml gastro-resistant capsules	84		704		C	Mintec
Peppermint oil 0.2ml gastro-resistant modified-release capsules	20		275		C	Colpermin
	100		1205		C	Colpermin
Peppermint oil liquid	100	ml	677	△	A	
Peppermint water concentrated	100	ml	473	△	A	
Pergolide 1mg tablets	100		2970		M	
Pergolide 250microgram tablets	100		1102		M	
Pergolide 50microgram tablets	100		1526		M	
Pericyazine 10mg tablets	84		2495		C	Neulactil
Pericyazine 2.5mg tablets	84		923		C	Neulactil
Perindopril 2mg tablets	30		1136		C	Coversyl
Perindopril 4mg / Indapamide 1.25mg tablets	30		1449		C	Coversyl Plus
Perindopril 4mg tablets	30		1136		C	Coversyl
Perindopril 8mg tablets	30		1136		C	Coversyl
Permethrin 1% scalp application ■	59	ml	238		C	Lyclear Creme Rinse
■	118	ml	432		C	Lyclear Creme Rinse
Permethrin 5% cream ■	30	g	552		A	
Perphenazine 2mg tablets	100		1865		C	Fentazin
Perphenazine 4mg tablets	100		2195		C	Fentazin
Pethidine 100mg/2ml solution for injection ampoules	10		556		A	
Pethidine 50mg tablets	50		492		A	
Pethidine 50mg/1ml solution for injection ampoules	10		526		A	
Phenelzine 15mg tablets	100		1995		C	Nardil
Phenindione 10mg tablets	100		1450		A	
Phenindione 25mg tablets	100		1657		A	

BASIC PRICES OF DRUGS

Drug		Quantity		Basic Price		Category	
Phenindione 50mg tablets		100		2114		A	
Phenobarbital 15mg tablets		28		76	△	A	
Phenobarbital 15mg/5ml elixir		500	ml	386		A	
Phenobarbital 30mg tablets		28		60		A	
Phenobarbital 60mg tablets		28		71		A	
Phenol crystals		25	g	400		C	Loveridge
Phenol liquefied		200	ml	2573	△	E	
Phenothrin 0.2% lotion	■	50	ml	222		C	Full Marks
	■	200	ml	570		C	Full Marks
Phenothrin 0.5% liquid	■	50	ml	222		C	Full Marks
	■	200	ml	570		C	Full Marks
Phenoxymethylpenicillin 125mg/5ml oral solution	●	100	ml	130	△	A	
Phenoxymethylpenicillin 125mg/5ml oral solution sugar free	●	100	ml	190	△	A	
Phenoxymethylpenicillin 250mg tablets		28		316		M	
Phenoxymethylpenicillin 250mg/5ml oral solution	●	100	ml	156	△	A	
Phenoxymethylpenicillin 250mg/5ml oral solution sugar free	●	100	ml	253	△	A	
Phenylephrine 10% eye drops	■	10	ml	338		A	
Phenytoin 30mg/5ml oral suspension		500	ml	427		C	Epanutin
Phenytoin sodium 100mg capsules		84		283		C	Epanutin
Phenytoin sodium 100mg tablets		28		4858		M	
Phenytoin sodium 25mg capsules		28		66		C	Epanutin
Phenytoin sodium 300mg capsules		28		283		C	Epanutin
Phenytoin sodium 50mg capsules		28		67		C	Epanutin
Pholcodine 10mg/5ml linctus strong sugar free		2	litre	656		A	
Pholcodine 2mg/5ml oral solution sugar free		2	litre	352		C	Galenphol Paediatric
	■	90	ml	111		C	Galenphol Paediatric
Pholcodine 5mg/5ml linctus		200	ml	59		C	Unichem
Pholcodine 5mg/5ml linctus sugar free		2	litre	485		A	
Phosphates enema (Formula B) 128ml long tube	■	128	ml	57		C	Fletchers
Phosphates enema (Formula B) 128ml standard tube	■	128	ml	41		C	Fletchers
Phytomenadione 10mg tablets		10		165		C	Konakion
Phytomenadione 10mg/1ml solution for injection ampoules		10		401		C	Konakion MM
Pilocarpine 5mg tablets		84		5143		C	Salagen
Pilocarpine hydrochloride 0.5% eye drops	■	10	ml	139		A	
Pilocarpine hydrochloride 1% eye drops	■	10	ml	303		M	
Pilocarpine hydrochloride 2% eye drops	■	10	ml	289		M	

VIII

BASIC PRICES OF DRUGS

Drug		Quantity		Basic Price	Category	
Pilocarpine hydrochloride 3% eye drops	■	10	ml	144	A	
Pilocarpine hydrochloride 4% eye drops	■	10	ml	387	M	
Pimecrolimus 1% cream	■	30	g	1969	C	Elidel
	■	60	g	3741	C	Elidel
	■	100	g	5907	C	Elidel
Pimozide 4mg tablets		100		2852	C	Orap
Pindolol 10mg / Clopamide 5mg tablets	♦	28		670	C	Viskaldix
Pioglitazone 15mg tablets	♦	28		2414	C	Actos
Pioglitazone 30mg tablets	♦	28		3354	C	Actos
Pioglitazone 45mg tablets	♦	28		3696	C	Actos
Piperazine 4g / Senna 15.3mg oral powder sachets	■	2		147	C	Pripsen
Piroxicam 0.5% gel	■	60	g	272	M	
	■	112	g	472	M	
Piroxicam 10mg capsules		56		416	M	
Piroxicam 10mg dispersible tablets		56		998 △	A	
Piroxicam 20mg capsules		28		427	M	
Piroxicam 20mg dispersible tablets		28		2533	M	
Pizotifen 1.5mg tablets	♦	28		556	M	
Pizotifen 250micrograms/5ml oral solution sugar free		300	ml	451	C	Sanomigran
Pizotifen 500microgram tablets		28		282	M	
		60		257	C	Sanomigran
Podophyllin paint		10	ml	79	E	
Podophyllotoxin 0.15% cream	■	5	g	1546	C	Warticon
Podophyllum resin powder		25	g	770	C	Loveridge
Potassium (potassium 6.5mmol) effervescent tablets BPC 1968	■	56		1893	M	
Potassium bromide powder		500	g	650	C	Loveridge
Potassium chlorate powder		500	g	950	C	Loveridge
Potassium chloride (potassium 6.7mmol) effervescent tablets sugar free	■	50		271	C	Kloref
Potassium chloride 600mg (potassium 8mmol) modified-release tablets		100		268	C	Slow K
Potassium chloride 600mg / Potassium bicarbonate 400mg effervescent tablets		100 (5x■20)		765	C	Sando-K
Potassium chloride powder		500	g	335	C	Loveridge
Potassium citrate mixture		200	ml	85	A	
Potassium citrate powder		500	g	395	C	Loveridge
Potassium iodide powder		250	g	1350	C	Loveridge
Potassium nitrate powder		500	g	775	C	Loveridge
Potassium permanganate 0.1% solution		100	ml	1	E	
Potassium permanganate 400mg solution tablets		30		848	C	Permitabs

BASIC PRICES OF DRUGS

Drug		Quantity		Basic Price	Category	
Potassium permanganate powder		500	g	385	A	
Povidone K25 eye drops 0.4ml unit dose preservative free		20		340	C	*Oculotect*
Povidone-Iodine 1% mouthwash		250	ml	107	C	*Betadine Gargle & Mouthwash*
Povidone-Iodine 1.14% dry powder spray	■	50	ml	239	C	*Savlon Dry*
Povidone-Iodine 10% paint	■	8	ml	93	C	*Betadine*
Povidone-Iodine 4% shampoo	■	250	ml	209	C	*Betadine*
Pramipexole 180microgram tablets		30		1850	C	*Mirapexin*
		100		6167	C	*Mirapexin*
Pramipexole 700microgram tablets		30		5889	C	*Mirapexin*
		100		19632	C	*Mirapexin*
Pramipexole 88microgram tablets		30		925	C	*Mirapexin*
Pravastatin 10mg tablets		28		268	M	
Pravastatin 20mg tablets		28		368	M	
Pravastatin 40mg tablets		28		611	M	
Prazosin 1mg tablets		56		323	C	*Hypovase*
Prazosin 500microgram tablets		56		251	C	*Hypovase*
Prednisolone 1mg tablets		28		148	M	
Prednisolone 2.5mg gastro-resistant tablets	★	30		160	M	
		100		68	C	*Deltacortril*
Prednisolone 20mg/100ml enema standard tube		7		750	C	*Predsol*
Prednisolone 25mg tablets		56		1451	A	
Prednisolone 5mg gastro-resistant tablets	★	30		188	M	
		100		122	C	*Deltacortril*
Prednisolone 5mg soluble tablets		30		220	A	
Prednisolone 5mg tablets		28		172	M	
Prednisolone acetate 1% eye drops	■	5	ml	152	C	*Pred Forte*
	■	10	ml	305	C	*Pred Forte*
Prednisolone sodium phosphate 0.5% ear/eye drops	■	10	ml	200	C	*Predsol Ear / Eye Drops*
Pregabalin 100mg capsules		84		9660	C	*Lyrica*
Pregabalin 150mg capsules		56		6440	C	*Lyrica*
Pregabalin 200mg capsules		84		9660	C	*Lyrica*
Pregabalin 25mg capsules		56		6440	C	*Lyrica*
Pregabalin 300mg capsules		56		6440	C	*Lyrica*
Pregabalin 50mg capsules		84		9660	C	*Lyrica*
Pregabalin 75mg capsules		56		6440	C	*Lyrica*
Primidone 250mg tablets		100		1260	C	*Mysoline*
Prochlorperazine 12.5mg/1ml solution for injection ampoules		10		544	C	*Stemetil*
Prochlorperazine 3mg buccal tablets		50		575	C	*Buccastem*
Prochlorperazine 5mg suppositories		10		874	C	*Stemetil*
Prochlorperazine 5mg tablets		28		205	M	
		84		307	M	

VIII

BASIC PRICES OF DRUGS

Drug		Quantity		Basic Price		Category	
Prochlorperazine 5mg/5ml oral solution		100	ml	348		C	Stemetil Syrup
Procyclidine 2.5mg/5ml oral solution sugar free		150	ml	422		C	Arpicolin Syrup
Procyclidine 5mg tablets		28		276		M	
Procyclidine 5mg/5ml oral solution sugar free		150	ml	754		C	Arpicolin Syrup
Proflavine 0.1% cream		100	ml	90		C	Loveridge
	★	500	ml	305	△	A	
Proflavine 0.1% solution		100	ml	14	△	E	
Proflavine hemisulphate powder		25	g	1790		C	Loveridge
Progesterone 200mg pessaries		15		746		C	Cyclogest
Progesterone 400mg pessaries		15		1080		C	Cyclogest
Proguanil 100mg tablets	♦	98		743		C	Paludrine
Promazine 25mg tablets		100		570		A	
Promazine 25mg/5ml oral solution		150	ml	367	▽	A	
Promazine 50mg tablets		250		4346		M	
Promazine 50mg/5ml oral solution		150	ml	377	△	A	
Promethazine 5mg/5ml oral solution		100	ml	193		C	Phenergan Elixir
Promethazine hydrochloride 10mg tablets		56		205		C	Phenergan
Promethazine hydrochloride 25mg tablets		56		306		C	Phenergan
Promethazine teoclate 25mg tablets		28		313		C	Avomine
Propafenone 150mg tablets		90		737		C	Arythmol
Propafenone 300mg tablets		60		934		C	Arythmol
Propiverine 15mg tablets		56		2445		C	Detrunorm
Propranolol 10mg tablets		28		147		M	
Propranolol 160mg tablets		56		395		M	
Propranolol 40mg tablets		28		153		M	
Propranolol 80mg tablets		56		230		M	
Propylene glycol liquid		500	ml	330		C	Loveridge
Propylthiouracil 50mg tablets		56		3024		A	
		100		4896		A	
Pseudoephedrine 30mg/5ml oral solution sugar free		2	litre	1375		C	Galpseud
Pseudoephedrine 60mg tablets		100		528		C	Sudafed
Purified talc powder		500	g	360		C	Loveridge
Purified water		5	litre	318	△	A	
Pyridostigmine bromide 60mg tablets	■	200		4812		C	Mestinon
Pyridoxine 50mg tablets		28		54	△	A	
Quetiapine 100mg tablets		60		11310		C	Seroquel
Quetiapine 150mg tablets		60		11310		C	Seroquel
Quetiapine 200mg tablets		60		11310		C	Seroquel
Quetiapine 25mg tablets		60		2980		C	Seroquel
Quetiapine 300mg tablets		60		17000		C	Seroquel
Quinapril 10mg tablets	♦	28		303		M	

BASIC PRICES OF DRUGS

Drug		Quantity		Basic Price	Category	
Quinapril 20mg tablets	♦	28		372	M	
Quinapril 40mg tablets	♦	28		446	M	
Quinapril 5mg tablets	♦	28		250	M	
Quinine bisulphate 300mg tablets		28		272	M	
		500		3479	M	
Quinine sulphate 200mg tablets		28		261	M	
Quinine sulphate 300mg tablets	♦	28		297	M	
		500		1832	A	
Rabeprazole 10mg gastro-resistant tablets	♦	28		1156	C	Pariet
Rabeprazole 20mg gastro-resistant tablets	♦	28		2116	C	Pariet
Raloxifene 60mg tablets	♦	28		1706	C	Evista
	♦	84		5959	C	Evista
Ramipril 1.25mg capsules		28		184	M	
Ramipril 1.25mg tablets	♦	28		366	M	
Ramipril 10mg capsules		28		282	M	
Ramipril 10mg tablets	♦	28		712	M	
Ramipril 2.5mg capsules		28		213	M	
Ramipril 2.5mg tablets	♦	28		441	M	
Ramipril 5mg capsules		28		238	M	
Ramipril 5mg tablets	♦	28		572	M	
Ranitidine 150mg effervescent tablets		60 (4x■15)		2080	M	
Ranitidine 150mg tablets	♦	60		216	M	
Ranitidine 300mg effervescent tablets		30 (2x■15)		1133	M	
Ranitidine 300mg tablets	♦	30		241	M	
Ranitidine 75mg/5ml oral solution sugar free		300	ml	2153 ▽	A	
Rasagiline 1mg tablets		28		7072	C	Azilect
Raspberry syrup		500	ml	505	C	Loveridge
Reboxetine 4mg tablets		60		1891	C	Edronax
Repaglinide 1mg tablets		30		392	C	
		90		1176	C	
Repaglinide 2mg tablets		90		1176	C	
Repaglinide 500microgram tablets		30		392	C	
		90		1176	C	
Rifampicin 150mg capsules		100		4361	M	
Rifampicin 300mg capsules		100		8553	M	
Riluzole 50mg tablets		56		24239	C	Rilutek
Rimexolone 1% eye drops	■	5	ml	595	C	Vexol
Rimonabant 20mg tablets		28		5520	C	Acomplia
Risedronate sodium 30mg tablets	♦	28		15281	C	Actonel
Risedronate sodium 35mg tablets	■	4		2030	C	Actonel Once Weekly
Risedronate sodium 5mg tablets	♦	28		1910	C	Actonel

VIII

BASIC PRICES OF DRUGS

Drug		Quantity		Basic Price	Category	
Risperidone 1mg orodispersible tablets sugar free		28		1839	C	*Risperdal Quicklet*
Risperidone 1mg tablets		20		1161	C	*Risperdal*
Risperidone 1mg/ml oral liquid	■	100	ml	5612	C	*Risperdal*
Risperidone 2mg orodispersible tablets sugar free		28		3466	C	*Risperdal Quicklet*
Risperidone 2mg tablets		60		6869	C	*Risperdal*
Risperidone 3mg tablets		60		10101	C	*Risperdal*
Risperidone 4mg tablets		60		13334	C	*Risperdal*
Risperidone 500microgram orodispersible tablets sugar free		28		1143	C	*Risperdal Quicklet*
Risperidone 500microgram tablets		20		706	C	*Risperdal*
Risperidone 6mg tablets		28		9428	C	*Risperdal*
Rivastigmine 1.5mg capsules	♦	28		3912	C	*Exelon*
Rivastigmine 3mg capsules	♦	28		3912	C	*Exelon*
Rivastigmine 4.5mg capsules	♦	28		3912	C	*Exelon*
Rivastigmine 6mg capsules	♦	28		3912	C	*Exelon*
Rizatriptan 10mg oral lyophilisates sugar free	■	3		1337	C	*Maxalt Melt*
	■	6		2674	C	*Maxalt Melt*
Ropinirole 1mg tablets		84		4726	C	*Requip*
Ropinirole 2mg tablets		84		9453	C	*Requip*
Ropinirole 5mg tablets		84		16327	C	*Requip*
Rosiglitazone 4mg tablets		28		2474	C	*Avandia*
		56		4948	C	*Avandia*
Rosiglitazone 8mg tablets		28		5078	C	*Avandia*
Rosuvastatin 10mg tablets	♦	28		1803	C	*Crestor*
Rosuvastatin 20mg tablets	♦	28		2969	C	*Crestor*
Rosuvastatin 40mg tablets	♦	28		2969	C	*Crestor*
Rosuvastatin 5mg tablets	♦	28		1803	C	*Crestor*
Saccharin sodium powder		25	g	395	C	*Loveridge*
Salbutamol 100micrograms/dose / Ipratropium 20micrograms/ dose inhaler	■	200	dose	645	C	*Combivent*
Salbutamol 100micrograms/dose inhaler CFC free	■	200	dose	288	A	
Salbutamol 1mg/ml nebuliser liquid 2.5ml unit dose vials		20		199	C	*Salamol*
Salbutamol 200microgram inhalation powder capsules		120		899	C	*Salbutamol 200 Cyclocaps*
Salbutamol 200micrograms/dose dry powder inhaler	■	60	dose	512	C	*Ventolin Accuhaler*
	■	100	dose	505	C	*Pulvinal Salbutamol*
Salbutamol 2mg tablets		28		513	M	
Salbutamol 2mg/5ml oral solution sugar free		150	ml	201	M	
Salbutamol 2mg/ml nebuliser liquid 2.5ml unit dose vials		20		398	C	*Salamol*

BASIC PRICES OF DRUGS

Drug		Quantity		Basic Price		Category	
Salbutamol 400microgram inhalation powder capsules		120		1299		C	Salbutamol 400 Cyclocaps
Salbutamol 4mg modified-release tablets	♦	56		981		C	Volmax
Salbutamol 4mg tablets		28		627		M	
Salbutamol 8mg modified-release tablets	♦	56		1177		C	Volmax
Salbutamol 95micrograms/dose dry powder inhaler	■	200	dose	588		C	Asmasal Clickhaler
Salicylic acid 12% / Lactic acid 4% gel	■	8	g	312		C	Salatac
Salicylic acid 2% / Betamethasone dipropionate 0.05% scalp application	■	100	ml	1050		C	Diprosalic
Salicylic acid 2% lotion		500	ml	211	△	E	
Salicylic acid 2% ointment		450	g	345		A	
Salicylic acid 26% solution	■	10	ml	339		C	Occlusal
Salicylic acid 3% / Betamethasone dipropionate 0.05% ointment	■	30	g	330		C	Diprosalic
	■	100	g	950		C	Diprosalic
Salicylic acid 3% / Sulphur 3% ointment		500	g	217	△	E	
Salicylic acid powder		500	g	660	△	A	
Salmeterol 25micrograms/dose inhaler CFC free	■	120	dose	2926		C	Serevent Evohaler
Salmeterol 50micrograms/dose dry powder inhaler	■	60	dose	2926		C	Serevent Accuhaler
Selegiline 10mg tablets	♦	28		585		M	
		30		965		M	
Selegiline 5mg tablets	♦	56		642		M	
		60		655		M	
Senna 15mg/5ml granules		100	g	310		C	Senokot
Senna 7.5mg tablets		60		250		M	
		500		738		C	Senokot
Senna 7.5mg/5ml oral solution sugar free		500	ml	269		C	Senokot Pharmacy
Senna fruit 12.4% / Ispaghula 54.2% granules	■	400	g	745		C	Manevac
Sertraline 100mg tablets	♦	28		216		M	
Sertraline 50mg tablets	♦	28		324		M	
Sevelamer 800mg tablets		180		12276		C	Renagel
Sibutramine 10mg capsules	♦	28		3690	▽	C	Reductil
Sibutramine 15mg capsules	♦	28		4365	▽	C	Reductil
§ Sildenafil 100mg tablets		4		2350		C	Viagra
§		8		4699		C	Viagra
§ Sildenafil 25mg tablets		4		1659		C	Viagra
§		8		3319		C	Viagra
§ Sildenafil 50mg tablets		4		2127		C	Viagra
§		8		4254		C	Viagra
Silver nitrate 95% caustic pencils	■	1		194		C	Avoca Wart Treatment Set
Simple eye ointment	■	4	g	268		A	

BASIC PRICES OF DRUGS

Drug		Quantity		Basic Price		Category	
Simple linctus		2	litre	361		A	
Simple linctus paediatric		200	ml	67		C	Thornton & Ross
Simple linctus sugar free		2	litre	330		C	Unichem
		200	ml	64		A	
Simvastatin 10mg tablets	♦	28		166		M	
Simvastatin 20mg / Ezetimibe 10mg tablets		28		3342		C	Inegy
Simvastatin 20mg tablets	♦	28		202		M	
Simvastatin 40mg / Ezetimibe 10mg tablets		28		3898		C	Inegy
Simvastatin 40mg tablets	♦	28		354		M	
Simvastatin 80mg / Ezetimibe 10mg tablets		28		4121		C	Inegy
Simvastatin 80mg tablets	♦	28		1210		M	
Soap liniment methylated		500	ml	241		A	
Soap spirit methylated		500	ml	205		A	
Sodium bicarbonate 500mg capsules		56		1641		M	
Sodium bicarbonate powder		2	kg	260		C	Unichem
Sodium chloride 0.9% eye drops	■	10	ml	237		A	
Sodium chloride 0.9% solution		100	ml	7	△	E	
Sodium chloride 0.9% solution for injection 10ml ampoules		10		466	▽	A	
Sodium chloride 0.9% solution for injection 20ml ampoules		10		1036		A	
Sodium chloride 0.9% solution for injection 2ml ampoules		10		244		A	
Sodium chloride 0.9% solution for injection 50ml ampoules		10		2009		C	Martindale
Sodium chloride 0.9% solution for injection 50ml vials	■	1		208		A	
Sodium chloride 0.9% solution for injection 5ml ampoules		10		326		A	
Sodium chloride powder		500	g	235		C	Loveridge
Sodium citrate powder		500	g	410		C	Loveridge
Sodium clodronate 400mg capsules		120		16197		C	Bonefos
Sodium clodronate 520mg tablets		60		16199		C	Loron 520
Sodium clodronate 800mg tablets		60		16962		C	Bonefos
Sodium cromoglicate 100mg capsules		100		6217		C	Nalcrom
Sodium cromoglicate 2% eye drops	■	13.5	ml	288		M	
Sodium cromoglicate 2% nasal spray	■	15	ml	856		C	Vividrin
Sodium cromoglicate 4% nasal spray	■	22	ml	1776		C	Rynacrom
Sodium cromoglicate 5mg/dose inhaler	■	112	dose	1530		C	Cromogen
Sodium dihydrogen phosphate dihydrate powder		500	g	595		C	Loveridge
Sodium feredetate 190mg/5ml oral solution sugar free		500	ml	446		C	Sytron Elixir

BASIC PRICES OF DRUGS

Drug		Quantity		Basic Price		Category
Sodium fluoride 0.37% oral drops sugar free	■	60	ml	182	C	En-De-Kay Fluodrops
Sodium fluoride 1.1mg chewable tablets		200		191	C	Fluor-A-Day
Sodium fluoride 1.1mg tablets		200		180	C	En-De-Kay Fluotabs 3-6 years
Sodium fluoride 2.2mg chewable tablets		200		191	C	Fluor-A-Day
Sodium fluoride 2.2mg tablets		200		180	C	En-De-Kay Fluotabs 6+ years
Sodium fusidate 2% / Hydrocortisone acetate 1% ointment	■	30	g	326	C	Fucidin-H
	■	60	g	653	C	Fucidin-H
Sodium fusidate 2% ointment	■	15	g	223	C	Fucidin
	■	30	g	379	C	Fucidin
Sodium fusidate 250mg tablets		10		602	C	Fucidin
		100		5722	C	Fucidin
Sodium metabisulphite powder		500	g	400	C	Loveridge
Sodium picosulfate 5mg/5ml oral solution sugar free		100	ml	185	C	Laxoberal Liquid
		300	ml	440	C	Laxoberal Liquid
Sodium salicylate powder		250	g	415	C	Loveridge
Sodium valproate 100mg tablets		100		467	C	Epilim
Sodium valproate 200mg gastro-resistant tablets		100		908	M	
Sodium valproate 200mg/5ml oral solution		300	ml	778	C	Epilim Syrup
Sodium valproate 200mg/5ml oral solution sugar free		300	ml	920	M	
Sodium valproate 500mg gastro-resistant tablets		100		2049	M	
Solifenacin 10mg tablets		30		3591	C	Vesicare
Solifenacin 5mg tablets		30		2762	C	Vesicare
Sotalol 160mg tablets	♦	28		395	M	
Sotalol 200mg tablets		28		250	C	Beta-Cardone
Sotalol 40mg tablets		56		134	C	Beta-Cardone
		100		239	C	Beta-Cardone
Sotalol 80mg tablets		56		199	C	Beta-Cardone
		100		354	C	Beta-Cardone
Spironolactone 100mg tablets		28		605	M	
Spironolactone 25mg tablets		28		365	M	
Spironolactone 50mg tablets		28		519	M	
		30		429	A	
Squill oxymel		2	litre	1823 △	A	
Stearic acid crystals		500	g	660	C	Loveridge
Sterculia 62% / Frangula 8% granules 7g sachets gluten free		60		556	C	Normacol Plus
Sterculia 62% / Frangula 8% granules gluten free		500	g	660	C	Normacol Plus
Sterculia 62% granules 7g sachets gluten free		60		519	C	Normacol

VIII

BASIC PRICES OF DRUGS

Drug	Quantity		Basic Price		Category	
Sterculia 62% granules gluten free	500	g	618		C	Normacol
Strontium ranelate 2g granules sachets sugar free	28		2560		C	Protelos
Sucralfate 1g tablets	50		437		C	Antepsin
Sucralfate 1g/5ml oral suspension sugar free	250	ml	437		C	Antepsin
Sucrose	1	kg	72		C	
Sulfadiazine silver 1% cream ■	50	g	385		C	Flamazine
Sulfasalazine 500mg gastro-resistant tablets	100		5007		M	
	112		1870		M	
Sulfasalazine 500mg tablets	112		1873		M	
Sulfinpyrazone 100mg tablets	84		566		C	Anturan
Sulfinpyrazone 200mg tablets	84		1125		C	Anturan
Sulindac 100mg tablets	56		1593		M	
Sulindac 200mg tablets	56		3076		M	
Sulphur precipitated powder	500	g	325		C	Loveridge
Sulphur sublimed powder	500	g	230		A	
Sulphuric acid dilute liquid	500	ml	580		C	Loveridge
Sulpiride 200mg tablets	30		468		M	
	56		708		M	
Sulpiride 400mg tablets	30		1081		A	
	100		3629		C	Dolmatil
Sumatriptan 100mg tablets	6		3004	▽	A	
Sumatriptan 10mg unit dose nasal spray	2 (2x■1)		1228		C	Imigran
Sumatriptan 20mg unit dose nasal spray	2 (2x■1)		1228		C	Imigran
	6 (6x■1)		3683		C	Imigran
Sumatriptan 50mg tablets	6		1879	▽	A	
	12		5248		C	Imigran 50
Sumatriptan 6mg/0.5ml solution for injection pre-filled syringes ■	2		4419		C	Imigran Subject
Sumatriptan 6mg/0.5ml solution for injection syringe refill ■	2		4205		C	Imigran Subject
	6 (3x■2)		12613		C	Imigran Subject
Surgical spirit	2	litre	396		A	
Syrup	2	litre	322		A	
Tacalcitol 4micrograms/g ointment ■	30	g	1340		C	Curatoderm
■	60	g	2314		C	Curatoderm
■	100	g	3086		C	Curatoderm
Tacrolimus 0.03% ointment ■	30	g	1944		C	Protopic
■	60	g	3694		C	Protopic
Tacrolimus 0.1% ointment ■	30	g	2160		C	Protopic
■	60	g	4104		C	Protopic

BASIC PRICES OF DRUGS

Drug		Quantity		Basic Price		Category	
Tacrolimus 1mg capsules		50 (5x■10)		8522		C	Prograf
Tacrolimus 500microgram capsules		50 (5x■10)		6569		C	Prograf
Tacrolimus 5mg capsules		50 (5x■10)		31484		C	Prograf
§ Tadalafil 10mg tablets		4		2499		C	Cialis
§ Tadalafil 20mg tablets		4		2499		C	Cialis
§		8		4997		C	Cialis
Tamoxifen 10mg tablets		30		243		M	
Tamoxifen 20mg tablets		30		282		M	
Tamoxifen 40mg tablets		30		660		M	
Tamsulosin 400microgram modified-release capsules		30		824	▽	A	
Tamsulosin 400microgram modified-release tablets		30		1755		C	Flomaxtra XL
Tartaric acid powder		500	g	810		C	Loveridge
Telmisartan 20mg tablets	♦	28		1134		C	Micardis
Telmisartan 40mg / Hydrochlorothiazide 12.5mg tablets	♦	28		1134		C	MicardisPlus
Telmisartan 40mg tablets	♦	28		1134		C	Micardis
Telmisartan 80mg / Hydrochlorothiazide 12.5mg tablets	♦	28		1418		C	MicardisPlus
Telmisartan 80mg tablets	♦	28		1418		C	Micardis
Temazepam 10mg tablets		28		208		M	
		500		1124		A	
Temazepam 10mg/5ml oral solution sugar free		300	ml	995		A	
Temazepam 20mg tablets		28		146	▽	A	
		250		992		A	
Tenoxicam 20mg tablets		28		1286	△	A	
Terazosin 10mg tablets		28		1734		M	
Terazosin 2mg tablets		28		505		M	
Terazosin 5mg tablets		28		686		M	
Terbinafine 1% cream	■	15	g	486		C	Lamisil
	■	30	g	876		C	Lamisil
Terbinafine 1% spray	■	15	ml	313		C	Lamisil AT
Terbinafine 250mg tablets		14		226		M	
	♦	28		283		M	
Terbutaline 1.5mg/5ml oral solution sugar free		300	ml	260		C	Bricanyl
Terbutaline 500micrograms/dose dry powder inhaler	■	100	dose	692		C	Bricanyl Turbohaler
Terbutaline 5mg tablets		100		409		C	Bricanyl
Testosterone 2.5mg/24hours patches		60		4910		C	Andropatch
Testosterone 40mg capsules		28		830		C	Restandol
		56		1660		C	Restandol
Testosterone 50mg gel sachets		30		3300		C	Testogel

VIII

BASIC PRICES OF DRUGS

Drug	Quantity		Basic Price	Category	
Testosterone 5mg/24hours patches	30		4910	C	Andropatch
Tetrabenazine 25mg tablets	112		10000	C	Xenazine
Tetracycline 250mg tablets	28		489	M	
Theophylline 125mg modified-release capsules	56		348	C	Slo-Phyllin
Theophylline 175mg modified-release tablets	60		319	C	Nuelin SA
Theophylline 250mg modified-release capsules	56		434	C	Slo-Phyllin
Theophylline 250mg modified-release tablets	60		446	C	Nuelin SA-250
Theophylline 400mg modified-release tablets	56		565	C	Uniphyllin Continus
Theophylline 60mg modified-release capsules	56		276	C	Slo-Phyllin
Thiamine 100mg tablets	100		616	C	Benerva
Thiamine 50mg tablets	100		398	C	Benerva
Thymol glycerin compound mouthwash	200	ml	57	C	Thornton & Ross
Tiaprofenic acid 300mg modified-release capsules	♦ 56		1556	C	Surgam SA
Tibolone 2.5mg tablets	♦ 28		1077	C	Livial
Timolol 0.1% gel eye drops	■ 5	ml	285	C	Nyogel
Timolol 0.25% eye drops	■ 5	ml	387	M	
Timolol 0.25% eye gel	■ 2.5	ml	312	C	Timoptol-LA
Timolol 0.5% eye drops	■ 5	ml	338	M	
Timolol 0.5% eye gel	■ 2.5	ml	312	C	Timoptol-LA
Timolol 10mg tablets	30		208	C	Betim
Timolol 5mg/ml / Brimonidine 2mg/ml eye drops	■ 5	ml	1000	C	Combigan
Timolol 5mg/ml / Latanoprost 50micrograms/ml eye drops	■ 2.5	ml	1507	C	Xalacom
Tinidazole 500mg tablets	20		1380	C	Fasigyn
Tioconazole 28.3% nail solution	■ 12	ml	2738	C	Trosyl
Tiotropium bromide 18microgram inhalation powder capsules	30 (6x■5)		3440	C	Spiriva
Tiotropium bromide 18microgram inhalation powder capsules with device	■ 30		3762	C	Spiriva
Tizanidine 2mg tablets	120		4030	M	
Tizanidine 4mg tablets	120		4977	M	
Tolbutamide 500mg tablets	28		254	M	
Tolfenamic acid 200mg tablets	10		1500	C	Clotam Rapid
Tolterodine 1mg tablets	56		2903	C	Detrusitol
Tolterodine 2mg tablets	56		3056	C	Detrusitol
Tolterodine 4mg modified-release capsules	28		2903	C	Detrusitol XL
Topiramate 100mg tablets	60		5531	C	Topamax
Topiramate 15mg capsules	60		1570	C	Topamax Sprinkle
Topiramate 200mg tablets	60		10280	C	Topamax
Topiramate 25mg capsules	60		2355	C	Topamax Sprinkle

BASIC PRICES OF DRUGS

Drug	Quantity		Basic Price	Category	
Topiramate 25mg tablets	60		1908	C	Topamax
Topiramate 50mg capsules	60		3557	C	Topamax Sprinkle
Topiramate 50mg tablets	60		3212	C	Topamax
Torasemide 10mg tablets	28		808	A	
Torasemide 2.5mg tablets ♦	28		378	C	Torem 2.5
Torasemide 5mg tablets	28		551	A	
Tragacanth powder	500	g	4995	C	Loveridge
Tramadol 100mg modified-release tablets	60		1826	C	Zydol SR 100
Tramadol 150mg modified-release tablets	60		2739	C	Zydol SR 150
Tramadol 200mg modified-release tablets	60		3652	C	Zydol SR 200
Tramadol 50mg capsules	30		267	M	
	100		442	M	
Tramazoline 120micrograms/dose / ■ Dexamethasone 20micrograms/dose nasal spray	110	dose	215	C	Dexa-Rhinaspray Duo
Trandolapril 2mg capsules ♦	28		686	C	Gopten
Trandolapril 4mg capsules ♦	28		1164	C	Gopten
Trandolapril 500microgram capsules ♦	14		140	C	Gopten
Tranexamic acid 500mg tablets	60		1111	M	
Tranylcypromine 10mg tablets	28		1650 △	A	
Travoprost 40micrograms/ml eye ■ drops	2.5	ml	1106	C	Travatan
Trazodone 100mg capsules	56		2948	M	
Trazodone 150mg tablets ♦	28		2028	M	
Trazodone 50mg capsules	84		2566	M	
Trazodone 50mg/5ml oral solution sugar free	120	ml	1114	C	Molipaxin
Tretinoin 0.01% gel ■	60	g	561	C	Retin-A
Tretinoin 0.025% cream ■	60	g	561	C	Retin-A
Tretinoin 0.025% gel ■	60	g	561	C	Retin-A
Triamcinolone 0.1% oromucosal ■ paste	10	g	118	C	Adcortyl in Orabase
Triamcinolone 55micrograms/dose ■ nasal spray	120	dose	739	C	Nasacort
Triamcinolone acetonide 40mg/1ml ■ suspension for injection pre-filled syringes	1		196	C	Kenalog
Triamcinolone acetonide 40mg/1ml suspension for injection vials	5		791	C	Kenalog
Triamcinolone acetonide 80mg/2ml ■ suspension for injection pre-filled syringes	1		340	C	Kenalog
Triamterene 50mg / Furosemide ♦ 40mg tablets	56		454	C	Frusene
	100		810	C	Frusene
Triamterene 50mg capsules	30		1735	C	Dytac
Triclofos 500mg/5ml oral solution	300	ml	2823	A	

VIII

BASIC PRICES OF DRUGS

Drug	Quantity		Basic Price		Category
Trifluoperazine 10mg modified-release capsules	30		283	C	Stelazine
Trifluoperazine 15mg modified-release capsules	30		427	C	Stelazine
Trifluoperazine 1mg tablets	100		430	M	
Trifluoperazine 1mg/5ml oral solution sugar free	200	ml	295	C	Stelazine
Trifluoperazine 5mg tablets	100		464	M	
	112		489	C	Stelazine
Trifluoperazine 5mg/5ml oral solution sugar free	150	ml	877 △	A	
Trihexyphenidyl 2mg tablets	84		450	M	
	100		810	M	
Trihexyphenidyl 5mg tablets	100		507	M	
Trimethoprim 100mg tablets	28		158	M	
Trimethoprim 200mg tablets	14		150	M	
Trimethoprim 50mg/5ml oral suspension sugar free	100	ml	168	A	
Trimipramine 10mg tablets	84		1069	C	Surmontil
Trimipramine 25mg tablets	84		1410	A	
Trimipramine 50mg capsules	28		791	A	
Trospium chloride 20mg tablets	60		2600	C	Regurin
Turpentine oil liquid	500	ml	440	C	Loveridge
Urea 10% / Hydrocortisone 1% cream ■	30	g	198	C	Alphaderm
■	100	g	586	C	Alphaderm
Urea 10% / Lactic acid 5% cream ■	100	g	684	C	Calmurid
■	500	g	2578	C	Calmurid
Ursodeoxycholic acid 150mg tablets	60		1851	A	
Ursodeoxycholic acid 250mg capsules	60		3511	A	
Ursodeoxycholic acid 300mg tablets	60		2650	C	Urdox
Valaciclovir 250mg tablets	60		13087	C	Valtrex
Valaciclovir 500mg tablets	10		2186	C	Valtrex
	42		9161	C	Valtrex
Valproic acid 250mg gastro-resistant tablets	90		1217	C	Depakote
Valproic acid 500mg gastro-resistant tablets	90		2429	C	Depakote
Valsartan 160mg / Hydrochlorothiazide 12.5mg tablets	28		2166	C	Co-Diovan
Valsartan 160mg / Hydrochlorothiazide 25mg tablets	28		2166	C	Co-Diovan
Valsartan 160mg capsules ♦	28		2166	C	Diovan

BASIC PRICES OF DRUGS

Drug	Quantity	Basic Price	Category	
Valsartan 40mg capsules ♦	7	411	C	Diovan
Valsartan 80mg / Hydrochlorothiazide 12.5mg tablets	28	1644	C	Co-Diovan
Valsartan 80mg capsules ♦	28	1644	C	Diovan
§ Vardenafil 10mg tablets	4	2224	C	Levitra
§	8	4447	C	Levitra
§ Vardenafil 20mg tablets	4	2350	C	Levitra
§	8	4699	C	Levitra
§ Vardenafil 5mg tablets	4	1659	C	Levitra
§	8	3319	C	Levitra
Varenicline 1mg tablets	28	2730	C	Champix
Varenicline 500microgram tablets	56	5460	C	Champix
Venlafaxine 150mg modified-release capsules ♦	28	3903	C	Efexor XL
Venlafaxine 37.5mg tablets ♦	56	2341	C	Efexor
Venlafaxine 75mg modified-release capsules ♦	28	2341	C	Efexor XL
Venlafaxine 75mg tablets ♦	56	3903	C	Efexor
Verapamil 120mg modified-release capsules ♦	28	751	C	Univer
Verapamil 120mg modified-release tablets ♦	28	818	C	Half - Securon SR
Verapamil 120mg tablets	28	245	M	
Verapamil 160mg tablets	56	677	M	
Verapamil 180mg modified-release capsules ♦	56	1815	C	Univer
Verapamil 240mg modified-release capsules ♦	28	1224	C	Univer
Verapamil 240mg modified-release tablets ♦	28	589	C	Securon SR
Verapamil 40mg tablets	84	266	M	
Verapamil 80mg tablets	84	290	M	
Vigabatrin 500mg oral powder sachets sugar free	50	1708	C	Sabril
Vigabatrin 500mg tablets	100	3084	C	Sabril
Vitamin B compound strong tablets	28	241	M	
Vitamins A and D capsules	84	267	A	
Vitamins B and C high potency intramuscular solution for injection 5ml and 2ml ampoules	10	1959	C	Pabrinex
Vitamins B and C high potency intravenous solution for injection 5ml and 5ml ampoules	10	1959	C	Pabrinex
Vitamins capsules	1000	1131	A	
Warfarin 1mg tablets	28	146	M	
Warfarin 3mg tablets	28	150	M	

VIII

BASIC PRICES OF DRUGS

Drug		Quantity		Basic Price		Category	
Warfarin 500microgram tablets		28		81	▽	A	
Warfarin 5mg tablets		28		162		M	
Water for injection 100ml vials	■	1		226		A	
Water for injection 10ml ampoules		10		311		A	
Water for injection 1ml ampoules		10		177		A	
Water for injection 20ml ampoules		10		545		C	Martindale
Water for injection 2ml ampoules		10		173		A	
Water for injection 5ml ampoules		10		282		A	
White liniment		2	litre	556		A	
		500	ml	280		C	Loveridge
White soft paraffin solid		500	g	396		M	
Wild cherry syrup		2	litre	1856	△	C	AAH
Wool alcohols ointment		450	g	395		C	Thornton & Ross
Wool fat solid		500	g	830		C	Loveridge
Xipamide 20mg tablets	♦	140		1946		C	Diurexan
Xylometazoline 0.05% nasal drops	■	10	ml	159		C	Otrivine
Xylometazoline 0.1% nasal drops	■	10	ml	191		C	Otrivine
Xylometazoline 0.1% nasal spray	■	10	ml	191		C	Otrivine
Yellow soft paraffin solid		500	g	165		A	
Zafirlukast 20mg tablets	♦	56		2826		C	Accolate
Zaleplon 10mg capsules		14		376		C	Sonata
Zaleplon 5mg capsules		14		312		C	Sonata
Zinc and Castor oil ointment		500	g	286		A	
Zinc and Salicylic acid paste		500	g	340		A	
Zinc compound paste		500	g	306		A	
Zinc ointment		500	g	380		C	Loveridge
Zinc oxide 12.5% / Dimeticone 1.04% spray	■	115	g	354		C	Sprilon
Zinc oxide powder		500	g	300		C	Loveridge
Zinc sulphate 0.25% eye drops	■	10	ml	315		A	
Zolmitriptan 2.5mg orodispersible tablets sugar free		6		2400		C	Zomig Rapimelt
Zolmitriptan 2.5mg tablets		6		2400		C	Zomig
		12		4800		C	Zomig
Zolmitriptan 50mg/ml nasal spray 0.1ml unit dose		6 (6x■1)		4050		C	Zomig
Zolmitriptan 5mg orodispersible tablets sugar free		6		2616		C	Zomig Rapimelt
Zolpidem 10mg tablets		28		323		M	
Zolpidem 5mg tablets		28		321		M	

BASIC PRICES OF DRUGS

Drug	Quantity	Basic Price	Category	
Zopiclone 3.75mg tablets	28	299	M	
Zopiclone 7.5mg tablets	28	305	M	
Zuclopenthixol 10mg tablets	100	806	C	*Clopixol*
Zuclopenthixol 25mg tablets	100	1612	C	*Clopixol*
Zuclopenthixol 2mg tablets ■	100	299	C	*Clopixol*
Zuclopenthixol acetate 100mg/2ml solution for injection ampoules	5	4663	C	*Clopixol Acuphase*
Zuclopenthixol acetate 50mg/1ml solution for injection ampoules	5	2420	C	*Clopixol Acuphase*
Zuclopenthixol decanoate 200mg/ 1ml solution for injection ampoules	10	3151	C	*Clopixol*
Zuclopenthixol decanoate 500mg/ 1ml solution for injection ampoules	5	3718	C	*Clopixol-Conc*

VIII

BASIC PRICES OF DRUGS

Drug	Quantity	Basic Price	Category

This Page is Intentionally Blank

APPROVED LIST OF APPLIANCES
See Part II, Clause 8A (page 6)

The price listed in respect of an appliance specified in the following list is the basic price (see Part II, Clause 8) on which payment will be calculated pursuant to Part II, Clause 6 in respect of the dispensing of appliances.

NOTES

1. **Definition** - The appliances that may be supplied against orders on Forms FP10 are listed below and must conform with the specifications shown. See Part 1, Clause 2 (page 3). These specifications include published official standards ie BP, BPC or relevant British, European or International Standards or the Drug Tariff Technical Specification. It should be emphasized that any appliance must conform with the entry in this part of the Tariff as well as the official standard or technical specification quoted therein. Other dressings and appliances which may be necessary will normally be provided through the Hospital Services.

2. **Sealed Packets** - These are those which are "tamper-evident" - sealed with an easily detachable device that prevents removal of the contents without the seal being broken. Additionally in the case of sterile products: once a sealed package has been opened it should not be possible to re-seal it easily. Where an appliance, other than a bandage, required by the Tariff to be supplied in a sealed packet is ordered of a quantity or weight not listed in the Tariff, the quantity ordered should be made up as nearly as possible with the smallest numbers of sealed packets available for the purpose. Where the quantity ordered is less than the smallest quantity/weight, supply the smallest pack. The quantity of material in each packet supplied should be recorded on the prescription form.

3. **Quality Systems** - Non CE marked sterile products shall be manufactured in accordance with the requirements and guidance given in the Department of Health "Quality Systems for Sterile Medical Devices and Surgical Products - Good Manufacturing Practice" (HMSO, ISBN0-11-321341-7), which is the basis of the DH Manufacturer Registration Scheme (MRS) for such products.

   Details of this scheme may be obtained from the MRS Registration Officer, Medicines and Health products Regulatory Agency, Hannibal House, Elephant & Castle, London SE1 6TQ.

   Manufacturers who have received approval to CE mark their sterile products have demonstrated that these meet the essential requirements of the Medical Devices Regulations 2002, which incorporate quality system requirements.

4. **Weights** - All weights specified in the Tariff in respect of appliances are exclusive of wrappings and packing material.

5. **Invoice price** - This is the price chargeable for the appliance to the contractor by the manufacturer, wholesaler or supplier.

6. **Technical Specifications** - Numbered Technical Specifications for the items in Part IXA/B/C were published separately in 1981 in loose leaf volume and a revised list was published in 1983. The Specifications will not be reprinted annually but individual specifications will be introduced, amended and reprinted, or withdrawn, as necessary. A list of Technical Specifications is given on page 136. CE marked Devices have shown that they meet the essential requirements of the Medical Devices Regulations 2002 and there is no further need for them to demonstrate compliance with other specifications, such as those referred to above.

7. **Nurse Prescribing** - See Part XVIIB for details of Nurse Prescribing.

IX

APPLIANCES (LIST OF TECHNICAL SPECIFICATIONS)

LIST OF TECHNICAL SPECIFICATIONS

These specifications are available from:
NHS Business Services Authority,
Prescription Pricing Division
Bridge House
152 Pilgrim Street
Newcastle upon Tyne
NE1 6SN

	Spec No.	Date of last revision
Absorbent Cotton, Hospital Quality	1	1981
Bandages		
High Compression (Extensible)	52	5/1992
Contraceptive Devices		
Vaginal Contraceptive Caps (Pessaries)	8	1981
Dressings		
Povidone Iodine Fabric	43	1988
Sterile Dressing Pack	10	1981
Sterile Dressing Pack with NW Pads	35	1/1991
Elastic Hosiery		
Graduated Compression	40	1988
Suspender Belt	13	1981
Gauze Tissues		
Gauze and Cotton Tissue	14	1983
Hypodermic Equipment		
Non-Sterile		
Hypodermic Needles (Luer Fitting)	15	1981
Hypodermic Syringes (Luer Fitting)	16	12/1990
Latex Foam Adhesive	19	1981
Pessaries	20	1981
Protectives		
EMA Film Gloves, Disposable	21	1981
Stockinette		
Elasticated Surgical Tubular, Foam Padded	25	1983
Swabs		
Non-Woven Fabric	28	3/1993
Non-Woven Fabric, Filmated	29	1981
Trusses		
Spring	31a	1981
Elastic Band	31b	1981

APPLIANCES

Appliance	Size or Weight	Basic Price p
ABSORBENT COTTONS		**each**
Absorbent Cotton BP 1988	25g	66
Where no quantity is stated on the prescription the 25g pack is	100g	151
to be supplied.	500g	510
Absorbent Cotton, Hospital Quality	100g	105
Specification 1	500g	332
To be supplied only where specifically ordered.		

APPLICATORS - VAGINAL
Type 1. *(Ortho)*		75
Type 2. *(Durex)*		75

N.B.

1. *Where an Ortho pack ordered by the prescriber does not include an applicator, and the contractor considers that one is required, an Ortho Vaginal Applicator should be supplied and the prescription form endorsed accordingly.*
2. *Where Duragel Spermicide Jelly is ordered by the prescriber without an applicator and the contractor considers that one is required, a Durex Vaginal Applicator should be supplied and the prescription form endorsed accordingly.*
3. *For details of prescription charges payable, See Part XVI, Sub paragraph 12.13.8.*

ARM SLINGS
Web, Adjustable	178

ATOMIZERS, HAND OPERATED
Nebulizers
(a) Inhalers.
    (i) Type specified by the prescriber:

Brovon Midget Inhaler	596
Rybar Standard Inhaler No. 1 (without mask)	929
Rybar Standard Inhaler No. 2 (without mask)	929
Other inhalers conforming to this specification may be supplied if specifically ordered and endorsed providing the *invoice price does not exceed	929
(ii) Type not specified by the prescriber	
The invoice price must not exceed	596
Spare Parts for above	*Invoice Price

*   For invoice price see Note 5 (page 135)

(b) Devices for use with Pressurised Aerosols.
Spacer/Holding Chamber Devices

Able Spacer	420
Able Spacer with either small (infant), medium (child) or large (adult) mask	686
Aerochamber Plus	443
Aerochamber Plus with adult, child or infant face mask	740
NebuChamber with child mask	856
Nebuhaler	428
Nebuhaler with paediatric mask	428
Optichamber	428
Pocket Chamber	418
Pocket Chamber with neonatal, child, teenager or adult mask	975
Volumatic	275
Volumatic paediatric with mask	275

AUTO INFLATION DEVICE (for the treatment of Glue Ear)
Otovent	424

APPLIANCES

Appliance	Size or Weight	Basic Price p
BANDAGES		**each**

1. The term "bandage" used in a prescription form without qualification is to be interpreted to mean an Open-Wove Bandage, Type 1 BP 5cm x 5m. All bandages supplied are to be of the lengths and widths specified in the Tariff. Where a bandage longer than those specified in the Tariff is ordered, the number of bandages which will, in total, provide the length nearest to that ordered should be supplied. Where a bandage in a width other than those specified is ordered, the next wider specified width should be supplied.

2. All bandages to be supplied completely wrapped as received from the manufacturer or wholesaler. Elastic Adhesive Bandages and Plaster of Paris Bandages to be supplied sealed in containers as received from the manufacturer or wholesaler. Except where otherwise stated all bandages possessing elasticity to be not less than 4.5m in length when fully stretched.

Conforming Bandage (Synthetic)

Hospiform	6cm x 4m (stretched)	12
	8cm x 4m	15
	10cm x 4m	17
	12cm x 4m	21

Cotton Conforming Bandage BP 1988

Type A

Crinx	5cm x 3.5m	62
	7.5cm x 3.5m	76
	10cm x 3.5m	94
	15cm x 3.5m	128

Cotton Crêpe Bandage

Hospicrepe 229	5cm	41
	7.5cm	57
	10cm	74
	15cm	108
Hospicrepe 239	5cm	44
	7.5cm	62
	10cm	80
	15cm	117

Cotton Crêpe Bandage BP 1988

	7.5cm	270
	10cm	347

Cotton, Polyamide and Elastane Bandage

Neosport	5cm	54
	7.5cm	73
	10cm	91
	15cm	112
Setocrepe	*10cm	110
Soffcrepe	5cm	63
	7.5cm	89
	10cm	114
	15cm	164

Cotton Stretch Bandage BP 1988

Hospicrepe 233	5cm	52
	7.5cm	72
	10cm	96
	15cm	136

Crêpe Bandage BP 1988

	5cm	86
	7.5cm	121
	10cm	158
	15cm	229

APPLIANCES

Appliance	Size or Weight	Basic Price p
BANDAGES		**each**
Elastic Adhesive Bandage BP 1993	5cm	318
(Syn: Zinc Oxide Elastic Adhesive Bandage)	7.5cm	460
Where no size is stated by the prescribed 7.5cm size should be supplied.	10cm	612
Elastomer and Viscose Bandage, Knitted		
BS compression type 2, for light support		
K-Lite	5cm x 4.5m	49
4.5m stretched	7cm x 4.5m	68
	*10cm x 4.5m	89
	15cm x 4.5m	129
K-Lite Long		
5.25m stretched	*10cm x 5.25m	104
Knit-Firm	5cm	36
	7cm	51
	10cm	66
	15 cm	96
BS compression type 3a, for light compression		
Elset		
6m stretched	*10cm x 6m	239
	15cm x 6m	259
8m stretched	*10cm x 8m	306
Elset S		
12m stretched	15cm x 12m	513
K-Plus		
8.7m stretched	*10cm x 8.7m	200
K-Plus Long		
10.25m stretched	*10cm x 10.25m	236
HIGH COMPRESSION BANDAGES (Extensible)		
Specification No. 52		
P.E.C. High Compression Bandage		
Syns: Polyamide, Elastane, and Cotton Compression (High) Extensible Bandage; "PECCHE" Bandage		
Setopress	7.5cm x 3.5m unstretched	251
	10cm x 3.5m unstretched	325
V.E.C. High Compression Bandage		
Syns: Polyamide, Elastane, and Cotton Compression (High) Extensible Bandage; "VECCHE" Bandage		
Tensopress	7.5cm x 3m unstretched	248
	10cm x 3m unstretched	319
HIGH COMPRESSION BANDAGE (Extensible)		
Adva-Co	10cm x 3.5m unstretched	179
SurePress	10cm x 3m unstretched	320

* see also Multi Layer Compression Bandaging

IXA

APPLIANCES

Appliance	Size or Weight	Basic Price p
BANDAGES		**each**
Multi-layer Compression Bandaging		
3M Health Care Ltd		
Coban - multi-layer compression bandage kit	one size	808
Coban Self-Adherent Bandage	10cm x 6m (stretched)	276
BSN medical Ltd		
Velband Absorbent Padding Bandage - listed on page 143	10cm x 4.5m	66
ConvaTec Limited		
SurePress Absorbent Padding - listed on page 143	10cm x 3m	53
Molnlycke (formerly SSL International Plc)		
System 4 - multi-layer compression bandage kit	18-25cm	777
System 4 kits contain a combination of the following components:		
Setoprime (wound contact layer - listed on page 164)	9.5cm x 9.5cm	26
Softexe (layer #1 - listed on page 143)	10cm x 3.5m (unstretched)	58
Setocrepe (layer #2 - listed on page 138)	10cm x 4.5m (stretched)	110
Elset (layer #3 - listed on page 139)	10cm x 6m (stretched)	239
	10cm x 8m (stretched)	306
Coban Self-Adherent Bandage (layer #4 - 3M Health Care Ltd)	10cm x 6m (stretched)	276
Robinson Healthcare		
(Ultra Four Non-latex Bandages)		
Ultra Four - multi-layer compression bandage kit	up to 18cm	641
	18-25cm	567
Ultra Four RC - multi-layer compression bandage kit	18-25cm	414
Ultra Four kits contain a combination of the following components:		
Ultra Soft Wadding Bandage (layer #1 - listed on page 143)	10cm x 3.5m (unstretched)	39
Ultra Lite (layer #2)	10cm x 4.5m (stretched)	85
Ultra Plus (layer #3)	10cm x 8.7m (stretched)	189
Ultra Fast Cohesive Bandage (layer #4)	10cm x 6.3m (stretched)	259
Smith & Nephew Healthcare Ltd		
Profore - multi-layer compression bandage kit	up to 18cm	896
	18-25cm	835
	25-30cm	693
	above 30cm	1038
Profore Lite - multi-layer compression bandage kit	above 18cm	482
Profore kits contain a combination of the following components:		
Profore Wound Contact Layer	14cm x 20cm	28
Profore #1 - listed on page 143	10cm x 3.5m (unstretched)	62
Profore #2	10cm x 4.5m (stretched)	119
Profore #3	10cm x 8.7m (stretched)	346
Profore #4	10cm x 2.5m (unstretched)	286
Profore +	10cm x 3m (unstretched)	324

APPLIANCES

Appliance	Size or Weight	Basic Price p
BANDAGES		**each**
Smith & Nephew Healthcare Ltd		
Profore Latex Free - multi-layer compression bandage kit	18-25cm	892
Profore Lite Latex Free - multi-layer compression bandage kit	above 18cm	524
Profore Latex Free kits contain a combination of the following components:		
Profore #1 Latex-free	10cm x 3.5m (unstretched)	67
Profore #2 Latex-free	10cm x 4.5m (stretched)	126
Profore #3 Latex-free	10cm x 8.7m (stretched)	376
Profore #4 Latex-free	10cm x 2.5m (unstretched)	311
Profore + Latex-free	10cm x 3m (unstretched)	346
ProGuide - multi-layer compression bandage kit	18-22cm (Red)	864
	22-28cm (Yellow)	912
	28-32cm (Green)	958
ProGuide kits contain a combination of the following components:		
ProGuide Wound Contact Layer	10cm x 10cm	192
ProGuide #1	10cm x 4m	143
ProGuide #2		
(Red)	10cm x 3m (unstretched)	516
(Yellow)	10cm x 3m (unstretched)	563
(Green)	10cm x 3m (unstretched)	610
Urgo Ltd		
K-Four - multi-layer compression bandage kit	18-25cm	626
K-Four kits contain a combination of the following components:		
Paratex (wound contact layer - listed on page 164)	9.5cm x 9.5cm	24
K-Soft (layer #1 - listed on page 143)	10cm x 3.5m (unstretched)	40
K-Lite (layer #2 - listed on page 139)	10cm x 4.5m (stretched)	89
K-Plus (layer #3 - listed on page 139)	10cm x 8.7m (stretched)	200
Ko-Flex (layer #4)	10cm x 6m (stretched)	271
Please note the following components are only available individually and not as part of a kit:		
K-Soft Long (layer #1 - listed on page 143)	10cm x 4.5m (unstretched)	51
K-Lite Long (layer #2 - listed on page 139)	10cm x 5.25m (stretched)	104
K-Plus Long (layer #3 - listed on page 139)	10cm x 10.25m (stretched)	236
Ko-Flex Long (layer #4)	10cm x 7m (stretched)	316
Vernon-Carus Ltd		
Cellona Undercast Padding - listed on page 143	5cm x 2.75m	28
	7.5cm x 2.75m	34
	10cm x 2.75m	42
	15cm x 2.75m	54
Open-Wove Bandage, Type 1 BP 1988	2.5cm x 5m	29
(Syn: White open-wove bandage)	5cm x 5m	49
	7.5cm x 5m	69
	10cm x 5m	90
Plaster of Paris Bandage BP 1988		
Gypsona	7.5cm x 2.7m	156
	10cm x 2.7m	206

IXA

APPLIANCES

BANDAGES
Polyamide and Cellulose Contour Bandage, BP 1988
(Nylon & Viscose Stretch Bandage)
Length 4m stretched

Size	Basic Price (p) each				
	Acti-Wrap (Cohesive/ Latex Free)	Easifix	Kontour	Slinky	Stayform
5cm	-	33	28	39	29
6cm	41	-	-	-	-
7.5cm	-	40	35	55	36
8cm	60	-	-	-	-
10cm	71	47	40	66	40
15cm	-	80	66	95	68

Appliance	Size or Weight	Basic Price p each
Polyamide and Cellulose Contour Bandage, Knitted BP 1988		
K-Band		
For dressing retention - Length 4m stretched	5cm	18
	7cm	23
	10cm	25
	15cm	44
Knit-Band		
For dressing retention - Length 4m stretched	5cm	10
	7cm	15
	10cm	17
	15cm	30
Knit Fix		
For dressing retention - Length 4m stretched	5cm	12
	7cm	17
	10cm	17
	15cm	33
Short Stretch Compression Bandage		
Indications: Venous leg ulcers and lymphoedema		
Actiban	8cm x 5m	296
	10cm x 5m	318
	12cm x 5m	387
Actico (Cohesive)	4cm x 6m	211
	6cm x 6m	247
	8cm x 6m	284
	10cm x 6m	295
	12cm x 6m	376
Comprilan	6cm x 5m	247
	8cm x 5m	290
	10cm x 5m	312
	12cm x 5m	380
Rosidal K	4cm x 5m	170
	6cm x 5m	237
	8cm x 5m	283
	10cm x 5m	309
	10cm x 10m	538
	12cm x 5m	375
Silkolan	8cm x 5m	300
	10cm x 5m	339

APPLIANCES

Appliance	Size or Weight	Basic Price p each
BANDAGES		
Sub-compression Wadding Bandage		
Advasoft		
3.5m unstretched	10cm x 3.5m	36
Cellona Undercast Padding	*5cm x 2.75m	28
2.75m unstretched	*7.5cm x 2.75m	34
	*10cm x 2.75m	42
	*15cm x 2.75m	54
Flexi-Ban		
3.5m unstretched	10cm x 3.5m	44
K-Soft		
3.5m unstretched	*10cm x 3.5m	40
K-Soft Long		
4.5m unstretched	*10cm x 4.5m	51
Ortho-Band Plus		
3.5m unstretched	10cm x 3.5m	37
Profore #1 (100% Natural Fleece)		
3.5m unstretched	*10cm x 3.5m	62
Softexe		
3.5m unstretched	*10cm x 3.5m	58
SurePress Absorbent Padding	*10cm x 3m	53
Ultra Soft Wadding Bandage		
3.5m unstretched	*10cm x 3.5m	39
Velband Absorbent Padding Bandage		
4.5m unstretched	*10cm x 4.5m	66
Suspensory Bandage, Cotton		
Note: type supplied to be endorsed.		
Type 1	Small	149
Cotton net bag with draw tapes and webbing waistband	Medium	149
	Large	149
	Ex-large	158
Type 2	Small	165
Cotton net bag with elastic edge and webbing waistband	Medium	170
	Large	176
	Ex-large	183
Type 3	Small	178
Cotton net bag with elastic edge and webbing waistband with	Medium	178
insertion of elastic centre-front	Large	178
	Ex-large	184
Triangular Calico Bandage BP 1980	Sides - 90cm	108
	Base - 127cm	
Zinc Paste Bandages		
Zinc Paste Bandage BP 1993		
Benefoot Zinc Paste (10%)	7.5cm x 6m	285
Viscopaste PB7 (10%)	7.5cm x 6m	322
Zinc Paste and Ichthammol Bandage BP 1993		
Ichthopaste (6/2%)	7.5cm x 6m	325

* see also Multi-layer Compression Bandaging

APPLIANCES

Appliance	Size or Weight	Basic Price p
BREAST RELIEVER		**each**
Plasticised PVC polymer bulb with glass or polycarbonate receiver	60ml approx.	428
BREAST SHIELDS		**per pair**
Plastic circular - (Not to be confused with Nipple Shields)		402
CATHETERS, ACCESSORIES		**pack of 5**
Bard Comfasure Catheter Retainer Strap	Small	1386
	Adult	1386
	Abdominal	1442
P. Grip Catheter Retaining Strap		**each**
CS.01 1 x leg strap (38mm x 600mm)		245
1 x green velcro tab (20mm x 130mm)		
2 x self adhesive micro hooktabs (43mm x 25mm)		
CS.02 1 x abdominal strap (38mm x 900mm)		260
1 x green velcro tab (20mm x 130mm)		
2 x self adhesive micro hooktabs (43mm x 25mm)		
CS.TABS		219
1 x green velcro tab (20mm x 130mm)		
10 x self adhesive micro hooktabs (43mm x 25mm)		
CATHETER MAINTENANCE SOLUTIONS		
OptiFlo G	(CSG50)	50ml	340
3.23% Citric Acid (Suby G)	(CSG100)	100ml	340
OptiFlo R	(CSR50)	50ml	340
6.0% Citric Acid (Solution R)	(CSR100)	100ml	340
OptiFlo S	(CSS50)	50ml	320
0.9% Saline	(CSS100)	100ml	320
Uriflex G	(GR076)	100ml	329
3.23% Citric Acid		
Uriflex R	(GR086)	100ml	329
6% Citric Acid		
Uriflex S	(GR066)	100ml	329
NaCl 0.9%		
Uriflex SP	(GR027)	50ml	329
NaCl 0.9%	(GR026)	100ml	329
Uriflex W	(GR056)	100ml	329
Sterile Water		
Uro-Tainer NaCl 0.9%	(FB99849)	50ml	311
	(FB99833)	100ml	311
Uro-Tainer Twin Solutio R	(9746625)	2 x 30ml	425
6.0% Citric Acid		
Uro-Tainer Twin Suby G	(9746609)	2 x 30ml	425
3.23% Citric Acid		

APPLIANCES

CATHETERS, URINARY, URETHRAL

1. Catheter sizes are designated by the Charrière (Ch) gauge system - even numbers only. (The equivalent metric sizes for Charrière gauges 6-30 are 2.0mm-10.0mm, rising in 0.66mm). Where size is not stated by the prescriber, size 14 or 16 should be supplied.

2. If a balloon size is not stated by the prescriber when ordering a Foley catheter, a 10ml balloon catheter should be supplied - a 5ml balloon in the case of a paediatric catheter.

3. Where the brand is not stated by the prescriber, the basic price of each listed catheter supplied must not exceed:

	Basic Price p
Nélaton (Male)	41
Nélaton (Female)	38
Nélaton (Paediatric)	38
Foley (Male)	210
Foley (Female)	210
Foley (Paediatric)	418

4. 5-units of plastic catheters, for example, represents on average one month's supply for patients practising intermittent catheterisation.

5. *For names and addresses of suppliers see pages 255-256*

6. *The rate of use of single use Nélaton catheters is approximately between 6 and 45 times greater than reusable Nélaton catheters for patients practising intermittant catheterisation.*

Appliance		Gauge (Ch) (See Note 1 - page 145)	Basic Price p
(A)(i) Nélaton Catheter ('ordinary' cylindrical Catheter)			**pack of 5**
Bard Reliacath PTFE Coated Latex			
	(DO159C)	14	779
			($\equiv$156 each)
Bard Reliacath Plastic (Male)	(D5030)	12-18	718
			($\equiv$144 each)
(Female)	(D5031)	12-18	718
			($\equiv$144 each)
(Paediatric)	(D5032)	8-10	718
			($\equiv$144 each)
Coloplast Ltd PVC			
(Male)	(T1010-T1018)	10-18	567
			($\equiv$113 each)
(Female)	(T2012-T2018)	12-18	603
			($\equiv$121 each
(Paediatric)	(T3006-T3010)	6-10	603
			($\equiv$121 each)
Hunter Urology Ltd SafetyCat non-coated ISC			**pack of 30**
(Male)	(SCM08-SCM18)	8-18	4542
			($\equiv$151 each)
(Female)	(SCF08-SCF18)	8-18	4542
			($\equiv$151 each)
(Paediatric)	(SCP06-SCP10)	6-10	4542
			($\equiv$151 each)

APPLIANCES

Appliance		Gauge (Ch) (See Note 1 - page 145)	Basic Price p
(A)(i) Nelaton Catheter ('ordinary' cylindrical Catheter)			**pack of 30**
Mentor Medical Ltd			
Mentor Self-Cath			
(Male)	(408-418)	8-18	3233 ($\equiv$108 each)
(Female)	(208-214)	8-14	3233 ($\equiv$108 each)
(Paediatric)	(305-310)	5-10	3233 ($\equiv$108 each)
(Male Coude Taper Tip)	(608-614)	8-14	4500 ($\equiv$150 each)
(Male Coude Olive Tip)	(806-816)	6-16	4500 ($\equiv$150 each)
PVC			**pack of 5**
(Male)	(WS 850/8-14)	8-14	843 ($\equiv$169 each)
(Female)	(WS 854/8-14)	8-14	813 ($\equiv$163 each)
Pennine			**pack of 10**
(Male)	(NC-1212/FP-1216/FP)	12-16	412 ($\equiv$ 41 each)
(Female)	(FC-1410/FP-1414/FP)	10-14	376 ($\equiv$ 38 each)
(Paediatric)	(NC-1206/FP/25-1210/ FP/25)	6-10	376 ($\equiv$ 38 each)
Pennine Pre-Lube catheter with integral PVC capsule containing lubragel			
(Male)	(NC1608/FP-NC1616/ FP)	8-16	985 ($\equiv$ 99 each)
(Male)	(NC1608/BG/FP- NC1616/BG/FP) (including 1 litre integral bag)	8-16	1140 ($\equiv$ 114 each)
(Female)	(FC1608/FP-FC1616/ FP)	8-16	984 ($\equiv$98 each)
Teleflex Medical			**pack of 5**
Rusch PVC Riplex Jaques			
(Male)	(DT6115-5)	8-18	727 ($\equiv$145 each)
(Female)	(DT6114-5)	8-18	663 ($\equiv$133 each)
Rusch PVC Riplex Extra Long (76cm)			
(Male/Female)	(DT6116)	8-18	737 ($\equiv$147 each)
Rusch Soft Rubber Jaques			**pack of 1**
	(DT5143-1/5)	8-18	150
			pack of 5
			632 ($\equiv$126 each)

APPLIANCES

Appliance		Gauge (Ch) (See Note 1 - page 145)	Basic Price p
(A)(i) Nélaton Catheter ('ordinary' cylindrical Catheter)			**pack of 5**
Unomedical Ltd			
(Male)	(ZT01007182- ZT01013182)	10-16	547 (≡109 each)
(Male Paediatric)	(ZT01004182)	8	547 (≡109 each)
(Female)	ZT02015182- ZT02017182)	10-14	547 (≡109 each)
(A)(ii) Nélaton Catheter ('ordinary' cylindrical Catheter) Single use			**pack of 25**
Astra Tech LoFric Plus (non PVC)			
(Male)	(903800-905400)	8-24	3274 (≡131 each)
(Female)	(943800-944800)	8-18	3274 (≡131 each)
(Female 15cm)	(983800-984800)	8-18	3274 (≡131 each)
(Paediatric)	(923600-924000)	6-10	3274 (≡131 each)
(Paediatric 30cm)	(993600-994000)	6-10	3274 (≡131 each)
Astra Tech LoFric			
(Male)	(900800-902400)	8-24	3274 (≡131 each)
(Female)	(940800-941800)	8-18	3274 (≡131 each)
(Female 15cm)	(980800-981400)	8-14	3274 (≡131 each)
(Paediatric)	(920600)	6	3274 (≡131 each)
	(990600-991000)	6-10	3274 (≡131 each)
(Tiemann Tip)	(961000-962000)	10-20	3274 (≡131 each)
Astra Tech LoFric H$_2$0 with integral water sachet			
(Male)	(9900800-9901600)	8-16	3649 (≡146 each)
(Female)	(9940800-9941600)	8-16	3649 (≡146 each)
(Paediatric)	(9920600-9921000)	6-10	3649 (≡146 each)
Astra Tech LoFric Insti-Cath			
(Male)	(800800-801400)	8-14	3441 (≡138 each)
(Female)	(810800-811400)	8-14	3441 (≡138 each)
(Paediatric)	(812800-813000)	8-10	3441 (≡138 each)
(Tiemann)	(821000-821400)	10-14	3441 (≡138 each)

IXA

APPLIANCES

Appliance	Gauge (Ch) (See Note 1 - page 145)		Basic Price p
(A)(ii) Nelaton Catheter ('ordinary' cylindrical Catheter) Single use			**pack of 30**
Astra Tech LoFric Primo with integrated water pocket			
(Male)	(9600800)	8	4374
			(≡146 each)
	(9601000-9601800)	10-18	4374
			(≡146 each)
(Female 15cm)	(9680800-9681400)	8-14	4374
			(≡146 each)
(Female 20cm)	(9640800-9641800)	8-18	4374
			(≡146 each)
(Paediatric)	(9620600)	6	4374
			(≡146 each)
	(9620800-9621000)	8-10	4374
			(≡146 each)
Bard Interglide Coated Intermittent Catheter			**pack of 25**
(Male)	(D6030)	8-18	3390
			(≡136 each)
(Female)	(D6031)	8-18	3390
			(≡136 each)
(Paediatric)	(D6032)	8-10	3390
			(≡136 each)
B.Braun Medical Actreen Glys Cath			**pack of 30**
(Male)	(225208E-225218E)	8-18	4230
			(≡141 each)
(Female)	(225306E-225316E)	6-16	4230
			(≡141 each)
(Male Tiemann)	(225108E-225118E)	8-18	4230
			(≡141 each)
B.Braun Medical Actreen Glys Luer Lock			**pack of 10**
(Male)	(227208E-227216E)	8-16	1380
			(≡138 each)
(Female)	(227308E-227316E)	8-16	1380
			(≡138 each)
(Male Olive Tip Tiemann)	(227408E-227416E)	8-16	1380
			(≡138 each)
Coloplast Ltd			
Speedicath (Pre-Hydrated Polyurethane)			**pack of 30**
(Male)	(28408)	8	4230
			(≡141 each)
	(28410-28414)	10-14	4230
			(≡141 each)
	(28416-28418)	16-18	4230
			(≡141 each)
(Female)	(28506)	6	4230
			(≡141 each)
	(28508)	8	4230
			(≡141 each)
	(28510-28514)	10-14	4230
			(≡141 each)
	(28516)	16	4230
			(≡141 each)

APPLIANCES

Appliance		Gauge (Ch) (See Note 1 - page 145)	Basic Price p
(A)(ii) Nélaton Catheter ('ordinary' cylindrical Catheter) Single use			**pack of 30**
(Paediatric)	(28706)	6	4230 (≡141 each)
	(28708-28710)	8-10	4230 (≡141 each)
(Speedicath 30cm)	(28606)	6	4230 (≡141 each)
	(28608-28612)	8-12	4230 (≡141 each)
(Tiemann)	(28490-28494)	10-14	4230 (≡141 each)
Speedicath Compact			
(Female)	(28578-28584)	8-14	4374 (≡146 each)
Conveen EasiCath			**pack of 25**
(Male Nélaton)	(5348-5362)	8-22	2940 (≡118 each)
(Female)	(5368-5376)	8-16	2940 (≡118 each)
(Paediatric)	(5006-5010)	6-10	2940 (≡118 each)
(Easicath 30cm)	(5086-5092)	6-12	2888 (≡116 each)
(Tiemann Tip)	(5380-5388)	10-18	2940 (≡118 each)
EMS Medical Ltd			**pack of 100**
Intex Drainage Catheter			
(Female)	(13002-13004)	10-14	11000 (≡110 each)
GTA (UK) Ltd Idrocath			**pack of 20**
(Male)	(50010)	8-24	1980 (≡ 99 each)
(Female)	(50011)	8-18	1980 (≡ 99 each)
(Paediatric)	(50012)	6-10	1980 (≡ 99 each)
(Child)	(50013)	8-10	1980 (≡ 99 each)
(Tiemann)	(50014)	10-20	1980 (≡ 99 each)
			pack of 25
Hollister Advance Hydro Soft Hydrophilic Intermittent Catheter with integral sterile water			
(Male 40cm)	(82108-82188)	10-18	3398 (≡136 each)
(Female 15cm)	(82103-82143)	10-14	3398 (≡136 each)
(Paediatric 25cm)	(82085-82105)	8-10	3398 (≡136 each)

IXA

APPLIANCES

Appliance		Gauge (Ch) (See Note 1 - page 145)	Basic Price p
(A)(ii) Nélaton Catheter ('ordinary' cylindrical Catheter) Single use			**pack of 25**
Hollister Advance Intermittent catheters with protective tip			
(Male)	(92084-92184)	8-18	3408
			(≡136 each)
(Female)	(92062-92142)	6-14	3408
			(≡136 each)
Hollister InstantCath			
(Male)	(9670-9673)	10-16	3166
			(≡127 each)
(Female)	(9674-9676)	10-14	3166
			(≡127 each)
(Paediatric)	(9677-9678)	6-8	3166
			(≡127 each)
Hunter Urology Ltd AntiBac			**pack of 30**
(Male)	(ABM08-ABM18)	8-18	4132
			(≡138 each)
(Female)	(ABF08-ABF18)	8-18	4132
			(≡138 each)
(Paediatric)	(ABP06-ABP10)	6-10	4132
			(≡138 each)
Hunter Urology Ltd AntiBac AV			
(Male)	(AVM08-AVM18)	8-18	4132
			(≡138 each)
(Female)	(AVF08-AVF18)	8-18	4132
			(≡138 each)
(Paediatric)	(AVP06-AVP10)	6-10	4132
			(≡138 each)
Manfred Sauer iQ Cath			
(Male)	(IQ2014.12-IQ2014.16)	12-16	4350
			(≡145 each)
Mentor Medical Ltd			**pack of 25**
Self-Cath HydroGel	(9410-9416)	10-16	3450
			(≡138 each)
Self-Cath plus			
(Male)	(USCC8M-USCC16M)	8-16	3461
			(≡138 each)
(Female)	(USCC8F-USCC16F)	8-16	3461
			(≡138 each)
(Paediatric)	(USCCO6P)	6	3461
			(≡138 each)
Rochester Medical Silicone Personal Catheter			**pack of 30**
(Male)	(63310-63318)	10-18	3388
			(≡113 each)
(Female)	(61310-61318)	10-18	3388
			(≡113 each)
(Paediatric)	(62308-62310)	8-10	3388
			(≡113 each)

APPLIANCES

Appliance		Gauge (Ch) (See Note 1 - page 145)	Basic Price p
(A)(ii) Nélaton Catheter ('ordinary' cylindrical Catheter) Single use			**pack of 30**
Rochester Medical Silicone Hydrophilic Personal			
Catheter with integral water pack			
(Male)	(63610-63618)	10-18	4029
			(≡134 each)
(Female)	(61610-61618)	10-18	4029
			(≡134 each)
(Paediatric)	(62608-62610)	8-10	4029
			(≡134 each)
Shiloh Healthcare Conticath Bluelite Coated			
(Male)	CCNM8-CCNM18	8-18	3206
			(≡107 each)
(Female)	CCNF8-CCNF16	8-16	3206
			(≡107 each)
(Paediatric)	CCNP6-CCNP10	6-10	3206
			(≡107 each)
Teleflex Medical			
Rusch Flocath Hydro Gel			
(Female)	(851121)	8-16	3480
			(≡116 each)
(Female Olive Tip)	(851122)	8-16	3900
			(≡130 each)
(Paediatric)	(851131)	6-10	3480
			(≡116 each)
(Paediatric Olive Tip)	(851132)	8-10	3900
			(≡130 each)
(Male)	(851141)	8-20	3480
			(≡116 each)
(Male Olive Tip)	(851142)	8-18	3900
			(≡130 each)
(Male Tiemann Tip)	(851143)	10-18	3480
			(≡116 each)
Rusch Flocath quick, with integral 0.9% sterile saline solution			
(Female)	(851221)	8-14	3600
			(≡120 each)
(Male)	(851241)	8-18	3600
			(≡120 each)
(A)(iii) Dilatation Catheter without drainage eyes			**pack of 25**
Not indicated for bladder emptying			
Astra Tech LoFric Dila-Cath	(891600/800)	16-18	3274
			(≡131 each)
GTA(UK) Ltd			
Idrocath Dilatation	(50316-18)	16-18	3000
			(≡120 each)
Hunter Urology Ltd			**pack of 30**
AntiBac D	(ABD16-ABD18)	16-18	3791
			(≡126 each)
(A)(iv) Nélaton Catheter with Urine Drainage Bag			**pack of 20**
Astra Tech			
LoFric Cath-Kit			
(Male)	(910800-911800)	8-18	3222
			(≡161 each)
(Female)	(950800-951800)	8-18	3222
			(≡161 each)
(Paediatric)	(930600-931000)	6-10	3222
			(≡161 each)
(Tiemann)	(971000-971800)	10-18	3222
			(≡161 each)

APPLIANCES

Appliance		Gauge (Ch) (See Note 1 - page 145)	Basic Price p
(A)(iv) Nelaton Catheter with Urine Drainage Bag			
B.Braun Medical Actreen Glys Set			**pack of 30**
(Male)	(226208E-226218E)	8-18	5707 (≡190 each)
(Female)	(226306E-226316E)	6-16	5707 (≡190 each)
(Male Tiemann)	(226108E-226116E)	8-16	5707 (≡190 each)
(A)(v) Nélaton Catheter with Water Container and Urine Drainage Bag			**pack of 20**
Astra Tech			
LoFric Hydro-Kit II			
(Male)	(9830800-9831800)	8-18	3613 (≡181 each)
(Female)	(9850800-9851800)	8-18	3613 (≡181 each)
(Paediatric)	(9840600-9841000)	6-10	3613 (≡181 each)
(Tiemann)	(9871000-9871800)	10-18	3613 (≡181 each)
GTA(UK) Ltd			
Idrocath Kit			
(Male)	(50110)	8-24	3300 (≡165 each)
(Female)	(50111)	8-18	3300 (≡165 each)
(Paediatric)	(50112)	6-10	3300 (≡165 each)
(Child)	(50113)	8-10	3300 (≡165 each)
(Tiemann)	(50114)	10-18	3300 (≡165 each)
(B) Scott Catheter (short curved tubular catheter for women and girls)			**pack of 5**
Mentor Medical Ltd			
Polythene	(WS852/8-14)	8-14	1321 (≡264 each)

APPLIANCES

Appliance		Balloon Size (ml)	Gauge (Ch)	Basic Price p
		(See Note 2 - page 145)	(See Note 1 - page 145)	

(C)(i)(a) Foley Catheter - 2 Way (indwelling Nélaton catheter with balloon)   pack of 1
For Short/Medium Term Use - Adult

Note: Average period of use is 1 to 3 weeks

Appliance		Balloon Size (ml)	Gauge (Ch)	Basic Price p
Bard PTFE Coated Latex				
(Male)	(D1265LV)	10	12-26	261
	(D1266LV)	30	16-26	261
(Female)	(D0169LV)	10	12-22	390
# Bard PTFE Aquamatic Coated Latex				
	(D1265AL)	10	12-22	298

\# Pre-filled with sterile water

Appliance		Balloon Size (ml)	Gauge (Ch)	Basic Price p
Mentor Medical Ltd				
Freedom Folatex Silicone Coated Latex				
(Male)	(HA1412-HA1418)	10	12-18	236
	(HA1424)	10	24	236
(Female)	(HA3112-HA3118)	10	12-18	236

Appliance		Balloon Size (ml)	Gauge (Ch)	Basic Price p
Teleflex Medical				
Rüsch PTFE AquaFlate. PTFE Coated Latex with sterile water filled syringe for balloon inflation and empty syringe for balloon deflation				
(Male)	(DP310112 - DP310124)	10	12-24	210
(Female)	(DP210112 - DP210124)	10	12-24	210
Universal Hospital Supplies Ltd				
Silicone Elastomer				
(Male)	(UN51161210-UN51162610)	10	12-26	280

(C)(i)(b) Foley Catheter - 2 Way (indwelling Nélaton catheter with balloon)
For Short/Medium Term Use - Paediatric

Note: Average period of use is 1 to 3 weeks

Appliance		Balloon Size (ml)	Gauge (Ch)	Basic Price p
Bard				
PTFE Coated Latex				
	(D0165PV)	5	8-10	721
Mentor Medical Ltd				
Freedom Folatex Silicone Coated Latex				
	(AP1408-AP1410)	5	8-10	418

APPLIANCES

Appliance		Balloon Size (ml) (See Note 2 - page 145)	Gauge (Ch) (See Note 1 - page 145)	Basic Price p
(C)(ii)(a)Foley Catheter - 2 Way For Long Term Use - Adult				**pack of 1**
Note: Average period of use is 3 to 12 weeks				
Bard Bardex I.C. with silver alloy coating and a pre-filled syringe of sterile water				
(Standard)	(D236512S-D236522S)	10	12-22	941
(Female)	(D236912S-D236916S)	10	12-16	941
Bard Biocath Hydrogel Coated				
(Male)	(D2265)	10	12-26	806
	(D2266)	30	12-26	816
(Female)	(D2269)	10	12-22	816
# Bard Biocath Aquamatic Hydrogel Coated				
(Male)	(D2264)	10	12-22	829
(Female)	(D2268)	10	12-22	833
Bard Lubri-Sil Aquafil Hydrogel Coated Silicone with pre-filled syringe of sterile water				
(Male)	(D1758)	10	12-22	926
(Female)	(D1761)	10	12-16	926
Bard Lubri-Sil Hydrogel Coated Silicone				
(Male)	(D1768)	30	16-22	911
Bard Silicone Elastomer Coated Latex				
(Male)	(D1657)	10	12-22	886
	(D1667)	30	16-22	886
(Female)	(D1647)	30	16-22	886
# Bard Silicone Elastomer Coated Latex				
(Male)	(D1657AL)	10	12-22	957
(Female)	(D1637AL)	10	12-22	957
Bard All Silicone				
(Male/Standard)	(D1658)	10	12-22	914
(Male/Standard)	(D1668)	30	16-22	914
(Female)	(D1661)	10	12-16	877
Bard Silastic Silicone Coated	(336)	10	12-24	836
	(334)	30	16-28	889
# Pre-filled with sterile water				
Coloplast Ltd				
All Silicone				
(Male)	(367312-367314)	10	12-14	898
	(367516-367520)	10	16-20	898
	(367216-367218)	20	16-18	898
	(367220)	30	20	898
(Female)	(366312-366314)	10	12-14	889
	(366516-366518)	10	16-18	889
	(366220)	30	20	889
Folysil X-tra silicone	100% silicone with pre-filled syringe			
(Male)	(AA8112-AA8120)	10	12-20	597
(Female)	(AA8512-AA8518)	10	12-18	597

APPLIANCES

Appliance	Balloon Size (ml) (See Note 2 - page 145)	Gauge (Ch) (See Note 1 - page 145)	Basic Price p
(C)(ii)(a)Foley Catheter - 2 Way For Long Term Use - Adult			**pack of 1**
Note: Average period of use is 3 to 12 weeks			
L.IN.C Medical			
All Silicone Catheter with integral balloon			
(Male) (08501205)	5	12	550
(08501405)	5	14	550
(08501610)	10	16	550
(08501810)	10	18	550
(Female) (085012051)	5	12	550
(085014051)	5	14	550
(085016101)	10	16	550
2 Way Foley All Silicone			
(Male) (08501430)	30	14	550
(08501630)	30	16	550
(08501830)	30	18	550
(08502030)	30	20	550
(08502230)	30	22	550
(08502430)	30	24	550
(08502630)	30	26	550
Medasil (Surgical) Ltd All Silicone			
(Male) (84M)	10	12-26	462
(85M)	30	16-26	462
(Female) (86F)	10	12-26	462
(87F)	30	16-26	462
Mentor Medical Ltd			
Freedom Folysil All Silicone Catheter			
(Male) (open ended) (AA74)	10	12-18	597
(Male) (AA71)	10	12-24	597
(Female) (AA75)	10	12-16	597
Rochester Medical All Silicone 2-way			
(Male) (14212-14224)	10	12-24	865
(24216-24226)	30	16-26	865
Teleflex Medical			
Rüsch Brilliant AquaFlate All-Silicone with sterile water filled syringe for balloon inflation and empty syringe for balloon deflation			
(Male) (DA310112 - DA310124)	10	12-24	595
(Female) (DA210112 - DA210124)	10	12-24	595
Rüsch Brilliant SilFlate All-Silicone with glycerine filled syringe for balloon inflation and empty syringe for balloon deflation			
(Male) (DG310112 - DG310124)	10	12-24	699
(Female) (DG210112 - DG210124)	10	12-24	699
Rüsch Sympacath AquaFlate Hydrogel Coated Latex with sterile water filled syringe for balloon inflation and empty syringe for balloon deflation.			
(Male) (DH310112 - DH310124)	10	12-24	595
(Female) (DH210112 - DH310124)	10	12-24	595

IXA

APPLIANCES

Appliance	Balloon Size (ml) (See Note 2 - page 145)	Gauge (Ch) (See Note 1 - page 145)	Basic Price p
(C)(ii)(a)Foley Catheter - 2 Way For Long Term Use - Adult			**pack of 1**
Note: Average period of use is 3 to 12 weeks			
The Kendall Company (UK) Ltd see Tyco Healthcare			
Tyco Healthcare (formerly The Kendall Company (UK) Ltd)			
Argyle All Silicone			
(Male) (8887-805128-805227)	10	12-22	583
(8887-830167)	20	16	583
(8887-830183-830266)	30	18-26	583
(Female) (8887-815127-815184)	10	12-18	583
Dover Silver			
(Male) (605122IC-605247IC)	10	12-24	898
Ultramer			
(Male) (1612-1M/1620-1M)	5	12-20	625
(1624-1M/1626-1M)	5	24-26	625
(Female) (1712-1F/1722-1F)	5	12-22	625
(Male) (1416-1M/1418-1M)	30	16-18	625
(1422-1M/1426-1M)	30	22-26	625
(Female) (1216-1F/1220-1F)	30	16-20	625
Universal Hospital Supplies Ltd			
All Silicone			
(Male) (UN41151205-UN41152005)	10	12-20	420
Lubricious			
(Male) (UN51181210-UN51182610)	10	12-26	515
Unomedical Ltd			
2 Way Foley All Silicone			
(Male) (MMS41151205-MMS41152605)	10	12-26	510
(Male) (MMS41151630-MMS41152630)	30	16-26	510
2 Way Silicone Elastomer Coated Latex			
(Male) (MMS51161210-MMS51162610)	10	12-26	490
(Male) (MMS51161230-MMS51162630)	30	12-26	490
(Female) (MMS54161210-MMS54162410)	10	12-24	490

APPLIANCES

Appliance		Balloon Size (ml)	Gauge (Ch)	Basic Price p
		(See Note 2 - page 145)	(See Note 1 - page 145)	
(C)(ii)(b) Foley Catheter - 2 Way For Long Term Use - Paediatric				**pack of 1**
Note: Average period of use is 3 to 12 weeks				
Bard Biocath Hydrogel Coated				
	(D2263)	5	8-10	816
Bard Lubri-Sil Hydrogel Coated Silicone				
	(D1758)	5	8-10	911
Coloplast Ltd				
All Silicone	(367308-367310)	5	8-10	897
Folysil X-tra silicone	100% silicone with pre-filled syringe			
(Paediatric)	(AP8106-AP8110)	1.5	6-10	597
L.IN.C Medical				
2 Way Foley All Silicone				
	(08580803)	3	8	795
	(08581003)	3	10	795
	(08500601)	5	6	795
	(08500803)	5	8	795
	(08501003)	5	10	795
Medasil (Surgical) Ltd				
All Silicone	(83P)	5	8-10	462
Mentor Medical Ltd				
Freedom Folysil All Silicone Catheter				
	(AA7106, AA7108, AA7110)	1.5-3	6-10	650
The Kendall Company (UK) Ltd see Tyco Healthcare				
Tyco Healthcare (formerly The Kendall Company (UK) Ltd)				
Argyle All Silicone	(8887-803081-803107)	5	8-10	629
+ Unomedical Ltd				
2 Way Silicone Elastomer Coated Latex				
(Paediatric)	(MMS53160605-MMS53161005)	5	6-10	540

(D) Intermittent Catheter with finger grip and lid				**pack of 30**
Engineers & Doctors Ltd				
Emteva	46F12-30-UK		12	3900
				(≡130 each)

(E) Intermittent Catheter with introducer tip and urine bag				**pack of 25**
Hollister Advance Plus				
(Nélaton)	(94064-94184)		6-18	6593
				(≡264 each)
(Tiemann Tip)	(95124-95164)		12-16	6593
				(≡264 each)
Hollister InstantCath Protect				
(Nélaton)	(9690-9696)		6-18	6720
				(≡269 each)
(Tiemann Tip)	(9697-9699)		12-16	6720
				(≡269 each)

(F) Intermittent Catheter with lubricant, insertion aid and urine bag				
Coloplast Ltd				**pack of 20**
Speedicath Complete				
(Female)	(28430-28434)		10-14	4400
				(≡220 each)
(Male)	(28460-28464)		10-14	4400
				(≡220 each)

+to be deleted 1 June 2007

IXA

APPLIANCES

Appliance		Balloon Size (mL)	Gauge (Ch)	Basic Price p
		(See Note 2 - page 145)	(See Note 1 - page 145)	
(F) Intermittent Catheter with lubricant, insertion aid and urine bag				
Teleflex Medical				**pack of 30**
Rusch Flocath Intro Gel				
(Female)	(851621)		8-16	6600
				(≡220 each)
(Female Olive Tip)	(851622)		8-16	7320
				(≡244 each)
(Paediatric)	(851631)		8-10	6600
				(≡220 each)
(Paediatric Olive Tip)	(851632)		8-10	7320
				(≡244 each)
(Male)	(851641)		8-18	6600
				(≡220 each)
(Male Olive Tip)	(851642)		8-18	7320
				(≡244 each)
(Male Tiemann Tip)	(851643)		10-18	6600
				(≡220 each)
(G) Silver Female Reusable Catheter				**pack of 1**
For Long Term Use, Reusable For Intermittent Self Catheterisation				
S G & P Payne				
Incontiaid Silver Female Catheter				
	(1315-1318)		8-14	3978
(H) Stainless Steel Catheter				**pack of 6**
For Long Term Use, Reusable For Intermittent Self Catheterisation				
Malvern Medical Developments Ltd				
Biscath System	Comprises of 6 stainless steel catheters with case, brushes, scraper and hard and soft carrying case.			
(Female)	(BISC001)		8	24875
	(BISC002)		10	24875
	(BISC003)		12	24875
	(BISC004)		14	24875
(I) Urinary Suprapubic Catheters				**pack of 1**
L.IN.C Medical				
2 Way All Silicone Suprapubic Catheter with integral balloon & central opening				
(Paediatric)	(08471003)	3	10	1095
(Short)	(08471205)	5	12	1095
	(08471405)	5	14	1095
	(08471610)	10	16	1095
	(08471810)	10	18	1095
	(08472010)	10	20	1095
	(08472210)	10	22	1095
	(08472410)	10	24	1095
(Long)	(08451205)	5	12	1095
	(08451405)	5	14	1095
	(08451610)	10	16	1095
	(08451810)	10	18	1095
	(08452010)	10	20	1095
	(08452210)	10	22	1095
	(08452410)	10	24	1095
2 Way All Silicone Suprapubic Catheter with integral balloon, central opening and shaped tip				
	(084612051)	5	12	1095
	(084614051)	5	14	1095
	(084616101)	10	16	1095
	(084618101)	10	18	1095
	(084620101)	10	20	1095

APPLIANCES

Appliance		Size or Weight	Basic Price p
CELLULOSE WADDING BP 1988			**each**
Cellosene		500g	220
CERVICAL COLLAR, SOFT FOAM			
Clini Cervical Collar			
Small (44cm)	OA8009		240
Medium (48cm)	OA8016		240
Large (53cm)	OA8023		240
Eesiness Soft Cervical Foam Collar			
Small	23562000		250
Medium	23562100		250
Large	23562200		250
CHIROPODY APPLIANCES			
Adhesive Felt		10.5cm x 8.3cm x 5mm thick	90
Zinc oxide or acrylic adhesive, spread		10cm x 22.5cm x 5mm thick	183
on semi-compressed surgical			
Animal Wool BP 1988		25g	86
(Syn: Animal Wool for Chiropody)			
(Long Strand Lamb's Wool for Chiropody)			
			box
Bunion Rings			88
Self-adhesive, semi-compressed felt			
(in box of 4 pieces)			
Corn Rings		5 mm thick	88
Self-adhesive, semi-compressed felt in			
a box of 9 pieces			
			pair
Metatarsal Arch Supports			685
(Price of a single article is half that of a pair)			
CONTRACEPTIVE DEVICES			**each**
Fertility (Ovulation) Thermometer			186

A mercury-in-glass thermometer, conforming to BS691-1987 and BS 6834 - 1991.
To be supplied in a re-usable screw capped plastics protective case.
NB: *TEMPERATURE CHARTS (Form FP 1004) and advice on their use are given by the prescribing doctor;
they are also available from pharmacists.*

Intrauterine Contraceptive Device	
Flexi-T 300	911
Flexi-T+380	1006
GyneFix intrauterine contraceptive implant (formerly GyneFixIN implant and insertion system)	2562
GyneFixIN implant and insertion system see GyneFix intrauterine contraceptive implant	
✖ Gyne-T380S	993
Load 375	800
● Multiload CU 250	713
Multiload CU 375	924
Multi-Safe 375	847

✖**to be deleted 1 May 2007**

●**These products are no longer available from the manufacturer but will remain reimbursable until such time that stocks run out or the product expiry dates are passed.**

IXA

APPLIANCES

Appliance	Size or Weight	Basic Price p
CONTRACEPTIVE DEVICES		**each**
Neo-Safe T380		1258
† Nova - T		1045
Nova-T 380		1350
T-Safe 380A see T-Safe 380A QL		
T-Safe 380A QL (formerly T-Safe 380A)		990
TT380 Slimline		1170
UT380 Short		1053
UT380 Standard		1053

The type of device and the size (where more than one is listed above) must be specified by the prescriber.

Vaginal Contraceptive Caps (Pessaries)
1. Rubber
Specification 8

Type A (*Dumas* Vault Cap)	Numbers 1 - 5	672
Translucent rubber pessary		
(plus postage 65p)		
Type B (*Prentif* Cavity Rim Cervical Cap)	22, 25, 28, 31mm	795
Opaque rubber pessary		
(plus postage 65p)		
Type C *(Vimule Cap)*	Numbers 1 - 3	672
Translucent rubber pessary		
(plus postage 65p)		

The size of the pessary and the type must be specified by the prescriber.
2. Silicone
CE Marked

FemCap	22, 26, 30mm	1500
Soft Silicone Cap		

Vaginal Contraceptive Diaphragm
1. Complies with British Standard 4028:1989

Reflexions Flat Spring Diaphragm	55-95mm (rising in 5 mm)	588
Type B (BS 4028, Type 1) Diaphragm with a coil spring.	60-100 mm (rising in 5 mm)	646
Type C (BS 4028, Type 3) Diaphragm with an arcing spring (flat and coiled steel combination spring).	60-95 mm (rising in 5 mm)	735

The size of the diaphragm, and the type must be specified by the prescriber.
2. CE Marked
Milex Silicone Diaphragm

Omniflex - Coil Spring (Type B)	60-90mm (rising in 5mm)	835
Arcing - Arcing Spring (Type C)	60-90mm (rising in 5mm)	835

DOUCHES
With Rectal and Vaginal fittings

Plastic Douche - Rigid plastics container, with 2m approx. flexible plastics tubing, a tap and vulcanite or rigid platics rectal pipe and plastics vaginal pipe.	1 litre approx	613
Spare Plastics Tubing	2m approx.	99

Where type not specified by the prescriber, plastics tubing to be supplied

†to be deleted 1 April 2007

APPLIANCES

Appliance	Size or Weight	Basic Price p
DRESSINGS		**each**

Note for all dressings: The exact number of pieces, ordered by the prescriber is to be dispensed.

Absorbent Cellulose Dressing with Fluid Repellent Backing
CE
Indications: Primary or secondary dressing for medium to heavily exuding wounds.

Appliance	Size or Weight	Basic Price p
Eclypse	15cm x 15cm	95
	20cm x 30cm	210
	60cm x 40cm	799
Eclypse Adherent	10cm x 10cm	299
	10cm x 20cm	375
	15cm x 15cm	499
	20cm x 30cm	999
Exu-Dry	10cm x 15cm	99
	15cm x 23cm	203
	23cm x 38cm	471
Mesorb	10cm x 10cm	56
	10cm x 15cm	72
	10cm x 20cm	89
	15cm x 20cm	127
	20cm x 25cm	200
	20cm x 30cm	227
Telfa Max	15cm x 22.8cm	196
	22.8cm x 38cm	453
	38cm x 45.7cm	550
	38cm x 60.9cm	800
Zetuvit E (Sterile)	10cm x 10cm	19
	10cm x 20cm	22
	20cm x 20cm	35
	20cm x 40cm	98

Packed in outer container not exceeding 10 units.

Absorbent Dressing Pads, Sterile

Appliance	Size or Weight	Basic Price p
Drisorb Dressing Pad	10cm x 20cm	17
Xupad Dressing Pad	10cm x 20cm	17
	20cm x 20cm	28
	20cm x 40cm	40

Absorbent, Perforated Dressing with Adhesive Border
Cosmopor E

Size	Description	Price
5 x 7.2cm	(wound contact pad 2.7cm x 4cm + border 1.15 - 1.6cm)	7
6 x 10cm	(wound contact pad 2.7cm x 6.5cm + border 1.65 - 1.75cm)	13
8 x 10cm	(wound contact pad 4cm x 6.5cm + border 1.75 - 2.0cm)	16
6 x 15cm	(wound contact pad 2.7cm x 11cm + border 1.65cm - 2.0cm)	18
8 x 15cm	(wound contact pad 4cm x 11cm + border 2.0cm)	25
8 x 20cm	(wound contact pad 4cm x 16cm + border 2.0cm)	33
10 x 20cm	(wound contact pad 5.5cm x 16cm + border 2.0cm - 2.25cm)	40
10 x 25cm	(wound contact pad 5.5cm x 20cm + border 2.25cm - 2.5cm)	50
10 x 35cm	(wound contact pad 5.5cm x 30cm + border 2.25cm - 2.5cm)	69

APPLIANCES

Appliance	Size or Weight	Basic Price p
DRESSINGS		**each**
Medipore + Pads		
5 x 7.2cm	(wound contact pad 2.8cm x 3.8cm + border 1 - 2 cm)	7
10 x 10cm	(wound contact pad 5cm x 5.5cm + border 2 - 2.5cm)	15
10 x 15cm	(wound contact pad 5cm x 10.5cm + border 2 - 2.5cm)	23
10 x 20cm	(wound contact pad 5cm x 15.5cm + border 2 - 2.5cm)	36
10 x 25cm	(wound contact pad 5cm x 20.5cm + border 2 - 2.5cm)	44
10 x 35cm	(wound contact pad 5cm x 30.4cm + border 2 - 2.5cm)	61
Medisafe		
6 x 8cm	(wound contact pad 3cm x 5cm + border 1.5cm)	8
8 x 10cm	(wound contact pad 4cm x 6cm + border 2cm)	13
8 x 12cm	(wound contact pad 4cm x 8cm + border 2cm)	23
9 x 15cm	(wound contact pad 4cm x 10cm + border 2.5cm)	29
9 x 20cm	(wound contact pad 4cm x 14cm + border 2.5 - 3cm)	34
9 x 25cm	(wound contact pad 4cm x 19cm + border 2.5 - 3cm)	36
Mepore		
7 x 8cm	(wound contact pad 4cm x 5cm + border 1.5cm)	10
10 x 11cm	(wound contact pad 6cm x 6cm + border 2cm - 2.5cm)	19
11 x 15cm	(wound contact pad 6cm x 10cm + border 2.5cm)	32
9 x 20cm	(wound contact pad 5cm x 15cm + border 2.0 - 2.5cm)	40
9 x 25cm	(wound contact pad 5cm x 20cm + border 2.0 - 2.5cm)	54
9 x 30cm	(wound contact pad 5cm x 25cm + border 2.0 - 2.5cm)	62
9 x 35cm	(wound contact pad 5cm x 30cm + border 2.0 - 2.5cm)	68
Primapore		
6 x 8.3cm	(wound contact pad 3.4cm x 5.7cm + border 1.3cm)	16
8 x 10cm	(wound contact pad 4.5cm x 5cm + border 1.75 - 2.5cm)	17
8 x 15cm	(wound contact pad 4.5cm x 10cm + border 1.75 - 2.5cm)	29
10 x 20cm	(wound contact pad 5cm x 14cm + border 2.5 - 3cm)	38
10 x 25cm	(wound contact pad 5cm x 18cm + border 2.5 - 3.5cm)	44
10 x 30cm	(wound contact pad 5cm x 23cm + border 2.5 - 3.5cm)	55
10 x 35cm	(wound contact pad 5.1cm x 28cm + border 2.45-3.5cm)	85
Softpore		
6 x 7cm	(wound contact pad 3cm x 4cm + border 1.5cm)	6
10 x 10cm	(wound contact pad 5cm x 6cm + border 2-2.5cm)	13
10 x 15cm	(wound contact pad 5cm x 10cm + border 2.5cm)	20
10 x 20cm	(wound contact pad 5cm x 15cm + border 2.5cm)	35
10 x 25cm	(wound contact pad 5cm x 20cm + border 2.5cm)	40
10 x 30cm	(wound contact pad 5cm x 25cm + border 2.5cm)	49
10 x 35cm	(wound contact pad 5cm x 30cm + border 2.5cm)	58
Sterifix (with two adhesive strips)		
5 x 7cm	(wound contact pad 5cm x 5cm + border 1.0cm)	18
7 x 10cm	(wound contact pad 5cm x 10cm + border 1.0cm)	29
10 x 14cm	(wound contact pad 8cm x 14cm + border 1.0cm)	52
Telfa AMD Island		
10 x 12.5cm	(wound contact pad 5cm x 8cm + border 2.5-2.25cm)	57
10 x 20cm	(wound contact pad 5cm x 15.5cm + border 2.5-2.25cm)	83
10 x 25.5cm	(wound contact pad 5cm x 20.5cm + border 2.5cm)	94
10 x 35cm	(wound contact pad 5cm x 30.5cm + border 2.25-2.5 cm)	117
Telfa Island (Non adherent dressing pad)		
5 x 10cm	(wound contact pad 3.3cm x 4.8cm + border 0.85-2.6cm)	8
10 x 12.5cm	(wound contact pad 5cm x 8.5cm + border 2.0-2.5cm)	26
10 x 20cm	(wound contact pad 5cm x 15cm + border 2.5cm)	34
10 x 25.5cm	(wound contact pad 5cm x 20cm + border 2.5-2.75cm)	43
10 x 35cm	(wound contact pad 5cm x 30cm + border 2.5cm)	60

APPLIANCES

Appliance	Size or Weight	Basic Price p
DRESSINGS		**each**
Absorbent, Perforated Plastic Film Faced, Dressing		
Interpose	5cm x 5cm	9
	10cm x 10cm	15
	10cm x 20cm	32
Melolin	5cm x 5cm	15
	10cm x 10cm	24
	20cm x 10cm	47
Release	5cm x 5cm	14
	10cm x 10cm	22
	20cm x 10cm	42
Skintact	5cm x 5cm	10
	10cm x 10cm	17
	20cm x 10cm	34
Solvaline N	5cm x 5cm	9
	10cm x 10cm	16
	10cm x 20cm	32
Telfa (Non adherent dressing pad)	7.5cm x 5cm	12
	10cm x 7.5cm	15
	15cm x 7.5cm	17
	20cm x 7.5cm	28
Telfa AMD	7.5cm x 10cm	17
	7.5cm x 20cm	27

Where not specified by the prescriber, the 5cm size to be supplied.
Where the brand is not specified by the prescriber, for the sizes listed below, the Basic Price must not exceed:

	5cm x 5cm	9
	10cm x 10cm	15
	20cm x 10cm	32

	Size or Weight	per pack
Gauze Dressings (Impregnated)		
Activon Tulle		
(Impregnated with manuka honey)		
Sterile one-piece pack containing a single piece of impregnated	5cm x 5cm	175
gauze	10cm x 10cm	295

Note: The exact number of pieces (ie packs) ordered by the prescriber are to be dispensed.
Where not specified by the prescriber, the 5cm size to be supplied.

	Size or Weight	
Chlorhexidine Gauze Dressing BP	5cm x 5cm	26
(Syn: Chlorhexidine Tulle Gras)	10cm x 10cm	54

Where not specified by the prescriber, the 5cm size to be supplied.

	Size or Weight	
Cutisorb Sorbact Dressing Pad	7cm x 9cm	320
(Impregnated with dialkylcarbamoyl chloride)	10cm x 10cm	500
	10cm x 20cm	780

IXA

APPLIANCES

Appliance	Size or Weight	Basic Price p
DRESSINGS		**each**
Cutisorb Sorbact Swab	4cm x 6cm	150
(Impregnated with dialkylcarbamoyl chloride)	7cm x 9cm	250
Paraffin Gauze Dressing BP Sterile (Syn: Tulle Gras)		
Light Loading - 90-130g/m^2		
Paranet	10cm x 10cm	25
Normal Loading - 175-220g/m^2		
Jelonet	10cm x 10cm	36
Neotulle	10cm x 10cm	29
Knitted Polyester Primary Dressing Impregnated with Neutral Triglycerides		
Atrauman	5cm x 5cm	24
	7.5cm x 10cm	25
	10cm x 20cm	56
	20 x 30cm	154
Knitted Viscose Primary Dressing BP Type 1		
(Sterile Knitted Viscose Dressing)		
N-A Dressing	9.5cm x 9.5cm	33
	19cm x 9.5cm	63
N-A Ultra	9.5cm x 9.5cm	32
	19cm x 9.5cm	60
Paratex	* 9.5cm x 9.5cm	24
Setoprime	* 9.5cm x 9.5cm	26
Tricotex	9.5cm x 9.5cm	30

* **See also Multi-layer Compression Bandaging**

Multiple Pack Dressing No. 1		377
Carton containing:		
Absorbent Cotton BP 1988 (interleaved)	25g	
Absorbent Cotton Gauze. Type 13 Light BP, sterile	90 cm x 1 m	
Open-Wove Bandages BP 1988 (banded)	3 x 5 cm x 5 m	

Perforated Film Absorbent Dressing BP - See Absorbent, Perforated Plastic Film Faced, Dressing (P.F.A. Dressing).

Povidone–Iodine Fabric Dressing, Sterile
Specification 43

Inadine	5cm x 5cm	30
	9.5cm x 9.5cm	45

Where not specified by the prescriber, the 5cm size is to be supplied.

Standard Dressings
No. 16 Eye Pad with Bandage BPC, sterile   60

APPLIANCES

Appliance	Size or Weight	Basic Price p
DRESSINGS		**each**

STERILE DRESSING PACKS *The exact number of pieces, ordered by the prescriber is to be dispensed.*
Drug Tariff Specification Sterile Dressing Packs

Sterile Dressing Pack Specification 10		47
Sterile Pack containing:		
Gauze and Cotton Tissue Pad	8.5cm x 20cm	
Gauze Swabs 12 ply	4 x 10 x 10cm	
Absorbent Cotton Balls, large	4 x 0.9g approx	
Absorbent Paper Towel	45cm x 50cm	
Water Repellent Inner Wrapper opens out as a sterile working field	50cm x 50cm	
Sterile Dressing Pack with Non-Woven Pads Specification 35		46
Sterile Pack containing:		
Non-woven Fabric Covered Dressing Pad	10cm x 20cm	
Non-woven Fabric Swabs	4 x 10cm x 10cm	
4 Absorbent Cotton Wool Balls		
Absorbent Paper Towel	50cm x 45cm	
Water Repellent Inner Wrapper opens out as a sterile working field	50cm x 50cm	

Non Drug Tariff Specification CE marked Sterile Dressing Packs

Dress-it		60
Sterile Pack containing:		
1 Pair Vitrex Gloves	small/medium, medium/large	
1 Large Apron		
1 Disposable Bag	26cm x 46cm	
1 Paper Towel	45cm x 50cm	
4 Softswabs 4 ply	10cm x 10cm	
1 Absorbent Pad	10cm x 20cm	
1 Sterile field	50cm x 50cm	
Polyfield Soft Vinyl Patient Pack (formerly Premier Polyfield Patient Pack)		52
Sterile Pack containing:		
1 Pair Powder Free sterile soft vinyl gloves	small, medium or large	
1 Polythene Sheet	50cm x 45cm	
7 Non Woven Swabs	10cm x 10cm	
1 Towel	43cm x 38cm	
1 White Polythene Disposable Bag		
1 Apron		
Propax SDP		45
Sterile Pack Containing:		
1 Paper Towel	45cm x 50cm	
1 Disposable bag	35cm x 47cm	
4 Gauze Swabs 12 ply	10cm x 10cm	
1 Dressing Pad	10cm x 20cm	
1 Sterile Field	50cm x 50cm	

Vapour-permeable Adhesive Film Dressing
(Syn: Semipermeable Adhesive Dressing)

ActivHeal	6cm x 7cm	31
	10cm x 12.7cm	73
	15cm x 17.8cm	178
Bioclusive	10.2cm x 12.7cm	145
Blisterfilm	5cm x 8cm	40
	9cm x 10cm	70
	10cm x 13cm	90
	14cm x 15cm	123

IXA

APPLIANCES

Appliance	Size or Weight	Basic Price p
DRESSINGS		**each**
Central Gard (Intravenous/Sub-Cutaneous Therapy)		
	16cm x 7cm central line	90
	16cm x 8.8cm central line	99
C-View	6cm x 7cm	37
	10cm x 12cm	104
	12cm x 12cm	120
	15cm x 20cm	238
Hydrofilm	6cm x 9cm	50
	10cm x 15cm	132
	12cm x 25cm	237
IV3000 (Intravenous/Sub-Cutaneous Therapy)		
	6cm x 7cm Non-winged peripheral	49
	7cm x 9cm Ported peripheral	64
	9cm x 12cm PICC line	129
	10cm x 12cm Central line	123
Mefilm see Mepore Film		
Mepore Film (formerly Mefilm)	6cm x 7cm	41
	10cm x 12cm	110
	10cm x 25cm	215
	15cm x 20cm	272
Niko Fix IV (Ported and non ported peripheral)	7cm x 8.5cm	37
OpSite Flexifix (non sterile)	5cm x 1m	345
	10cm x 1m	582
OpSite Flexigrid	6cm x 7cm	35
	12cm x 12cm	100
	15cm x 20cm	252
Pharmapore-PU.-I.V		
	6cm x 7cm ported cannula	8
	7cm x 9cm one hand application	17
	8.5cm x 7cm for cannula	7
Polyskin II	4cm x 4cm	35
	5cm x 7cm	38
	10cm x 12cm	99
	10cm x 20cm	196
	15cm x 20cm	226
	20cm x 25cm	395
ProtectFilm	6cm x 7cm	11
	10cm x 12cm	20
	15cm x 20cm	40

APPLIANCES

Appliance	Size or Weight	Basic Price p
DRESSINGS		**each**
Suprasorb F	5cm x 7cm	30
	10cm x 12cm	72
	15cm x 20cm	225
Tegaderm	6cm x 7cm	38
	12cm x 12cm	123
	15cm x 20cm	234
Tegaderm IV with securing tapes (Intravenous/Sub-cutaneous Therapy)		
	7cm x 8.5cm peripheral line	57
	8.5cm x 10.5cm central line	111
	10cm x 15.5cm PICC line	160
Vacuskin	6cm x 7cm	40
	10cm x 12cm	106
	10cm x 25cm	206
	15cm x 20cm	219

Vapour-permeable Adhesive Film Dressing - with absorbent pad
(Syn: Semipermeable Adhesive Dressing)

Appliance	Size or Weight	Basic Price p
Alldress	10cm x 10cm	85
	15cm x 15cm	185
	15cm x 20cm	228
Mepore Ultra	6cm x 7cm	27
	9cm x 10cm	59
	9cm x 15cm	89
	9cm x 20cm	134
	9cm x 25cm	148
	9cm x 30cm	244
OpSite Plus	5cm x 5cm (wound contact pad 2.5cm x 2.5cm + border 1.25cm)	28
	8.5cm x 9.5cm (wound contact pad 3.7cm x 7.3cm + border 2.4cm - 1.1cm)	78
	10cm x 12cm (wound contact pad 5cm x 7.5cm + border 2.5cm - 2.25cm)	106
	10cm x 20cm (wound contact pad 5.5cm x 15cm + border 2.25cm - 2.5cm)	178
	10 cm x 35cm (wound contact pad 5.7cm x 30cm + border 2.15cm - 2.5cm)	295
Pharmapore-PU	8.5cm x 15.5cm	20
	10cm x 25cm	38
	10cm x 30cm	58
PremierPore VP	6cm x 7cm	21
	10cm x 10cm	45
	10cm x 15cm	68
	10cm x 25cm	115
Tegaderm +Pad	5 cm x 7cm (wound contact pad 2.5cm x 4cm + border 1.25cm - 1.5cm)	24
	9cm x 10cm (wound contact pad 4.5cm x 6cm + border 2.25cm - 2cm)	61
	9cm x 15cm (wound contact pad 4.5cm x 10cm + border 2.25cm - 2.5cm)	90
	9cm x 20cm (wound contact pad 4.5cm x 15cm + border 2.25cm - 2.5cm)	132
	9cm x 25cm (wound contact pad 4.5cm x 20cm + border 2.25cm - 2.5cm)	148
	9cm x 35cm (wound contact pad 4.5cm x 30cm + border 2.25cm - 2.5cm)	250

IXA

APPLIANCES

Appliance	Size or Weight	Basic Price
DRESSINGS		**each**

WOUND MANAGEMENT DRESSINGS

Note for all wound management dressings: The exact number of pieces, ordered by the prescriber is to be dispensed.

Activated Charcoal Absorbent Dressing

Carboflex	10cm x 10cm	284
	8cm x 15cm (Oval)	341
	15cm x 20cm	646
Lyofoam C	10cm x 10cm	274
	15cm x 20cm	623
Sorbsan Plus Carbon	7.5cm x 10cm	232
	10cm x 15cm	452
	10cm x 20cm	540
	15cm x 20cm	622

Activated Charcoal Non-Absorbent Dressing

Carbopad VC	10cm x 10cm	159
	10cm x 20cm	215
CliniSorb	10cm x 10cm	168
	10cm x 20cm	224
	15cm x 25cm	361
Legius	10cm x 10cm	160
	10cm x 20cm	218
	15cm x 25cm	350

Activated Charcoal Cloth with Silver

Actisorb Silver 220	6.5cm x 9.5cm	155
	10.5cm x 10.5cm	244
	10.5cm x 19cm	443

Alginate Dressing - Sterile

Indications: Medium to heavily exuding wounds.
Precautions: Not the dressing of choice for infected wounds; not suitable for those which are very dry or covered with hard necrotic tissue.

ActivHeal	5cm x 5cm	57
	10cm x 10cm	111
	10cm x 20cm	273
Algisite M	5cm x 5cm	82
	10cm x 10cm	169
	15cm x 20cm	453
Algivon	5cm x 5cm	205
	10cm x 10cm	346
Algosteril	5cm x 5cm	81
	10cm x 10cm	185
	10cm x 20cm	313

APPLIANCES

Appliance	Size or Weight	Basic Price
DRESSINGS		**each**
WOUND MANAGEMENT DRESSINGS		
Curasorb	5cm x 5cm	69
	10cm x 10cm	146
	10cm x 14cm	236
	10cm x 20cm	287
	15cm x 25cm	505
	30cm x 61cm	2650
Curasorb Plus	10cm x 10cm	200
Curasorb Zn	5cm x 5cm	78
	10cm x 10cm	165
	10cm x 20cm	324
Kaltostat	5cm x 5cm	84
	7.5cm x 12cm	183
	10cm x 20cm	363
	15cm x 25cm	623
Melgisorb	5cm x 5cm	80
	10cm x 10cm	168
	10cm x 20cm	315
Sorbalgon	5cm x 5cm	73
	10cm x 10cm	152
Sorbsan see Sorbsan Flat		
Sorbsan Flat (formerly Sorbsan)	5cm x 5cm	75
	10cm x 10cm	158
	10cm x 20cm	296
Suprasorb A	5cm x 5cm	56
	10cm x 10cm	110
Tegaderm Alginate (formerly Tegagen)	5cm x 5cm	76
	10cm x 10cm	161
Tegagen see Tegaderm Alginate		
Trionic	5cm x 10cm	119
	10cm x 15cm	268
	10cm x 20cm	332
Alginate Dressing with Absorbent Backing - Sterile		
Sorbsan Plus	7.5cm x 10cm	160
	10cm x 15cm	282
	10cm x 20cm	360
	15cm x 20cm	500

Sorbsan Plus SA (with adhesive border)

11.5cm x 14cm	(wound contact pad 10cm x 7.5cm + border 2cm)	278
14cm x 19cm	(wound contact pad 10cm x 15cm + border 2cm)	406
14cm x 24cm	(wound contact pad 10cm x 20cm + border 2cm)	490
19cm x 24cm	(wound contact pad 15cm x 20cm + border 2cm)	616

IXA

APPLIANCES

Appliance		Size or Weight	Basic Price p
DRESSINGS			**each**
WOUND MANAGEMENT DRESSINGS			
Alginate containing Hydrocolloid Dressing - Sterile			
Indications: Medium to heavily exuding wounds.			
SeaSorb Soft		5cm x 5cm	86
		10cm x 10cm	205
		15cm x 15cm	390
Urgosorb Pad		5cm x 5cm	78
		10cm x 10cm	186
		10cm x 20cm	341
Capillary Action Absorbent Wound Dressing			
Indications: Low to heavily exuding wounds.			
Precautions: Avoid any arterial bleeds or very vascular wounds eg fungating wounds			
Advadraw		5cm x 7.5cm	55
		10cm x 10cm	85
		10cm x 15cm	115
Advadraw Spiral		0.5cm x 40cm	79
Sumar Lite		10cm x 10cm	159
		10cm x 15cm	212
Sumar Max		10cm x 10cm	161
		10cm x 15cm	215
Vacutex		5cm x 5cm	94
		10cm x 10cm	166
		10cm x 15cm	223
		10cm x 20cm	268
		15cm x 20cm	314
		20cm x 20cm	428
Cavity Dressing			
Indications: Medium/heavily exuding cavity wounds			
Acticoat Absorbent		2cm x 30cm	1140
ActivHeal		2cm x 30cm	205
Algisite M-Rope		2cm x 30cm	306
Algosteril Rope		30cm/2g	334
Allevyn Cavity	circular	5cm diameter	371
		10cm diameter	886
	tubular	9cm x 2.5cm	360
		12cm x 4cm	634
Allevyn Plus Cavity		5cm x 6cm	167
		10cm x 10cm	278
		15cm x 20cm	557

APPLIANCES

Appliance	Size or Weight	Basic Price p
DRESSINGS		**each**
WOUND MANAGEMENT DRESSINGS		
Aquacel Ribbon	2cm x 45cm	249
Aquacel Ag Ribbon	2cm x 45cm	417
Contreet Foam Filler	5cm x 8cm	358
Curasorb Rope	30cm	278
	61cm	488
	91cm	525
Cutisorb Sorbact Tupfer	3cm/5 pieces	300
Kaltostat	2g	340
Melgisorb Cavity	2.2cm x 32cm	317
PermaFoam Cavity	10cm x 10cm	180
SeaSorb Soft Filler	44cm	242
Sorbalgon T	30cm/2g	311
Sorbsan Packing	2g	328
Sorbsan Ribbon (with probe)	40cm	191
Suprasorb A	30cm/2g	204
Tegaderm Alginate (formerly Tegagen)	2cm x 30cm	268
Tegagen see Tegaderm Alginate		
Tielle Packing	9.5cm x 9.5cm	200
Trionic Rope	2cm x 30cm	360
Urgosorb Rope	30cm	248
Collagen Dressing		
Catrix	1g sachet	380
Conforming Foam Cavity Wound Dressing		
Cavi-Care	20g	1743
Honey Based Topical Application		
Activon Medical Grade Manuka Honey	25g	195
Medihoney Antibacterial Medical Honey	20g	396
Medihoney Antibacterial Wound Gel	10g	269
	20g	402
Mesitran Ointment	15g	334
	50g	918
Mesitran Ointment S	15g	333

IXA

APPLIANCES

Appliance	Size or Weight	Basic Price p
		each

DRESSINGS
WOUND MANAGEMENT DRESSINGS
Hydrocolloid Dressing - Semi-permeable - Sterile - With Adhesive Border
Indications: Light to medium exudating wounds.
Precautions: Not suitable for infected wounds. Heavy exudate leads to too frequent changes of dressing.
Dressing should seal round the borders of a wound.
Sterile one-piece pack:
Comfeel Plus Contour Dressing

These dressings are contoured to facilitate application to difficult areas, such as elbows and heels.

6cm x 8cm	(wound contact pad 6cm x 8cm + irregular border)	196
9cm x 11cm	(wound contact pad 9cm x 11cm + irregular border)	340

Comfeel Plus Pressure Relieving Dressing
Circular

7cm diameter	(wound contact pad 7cm diameter + irregular border)	306
10cm diameter	(wound contact pad 10cm diameter + irregular border)	410
15cm diameter	(wound contact pad 15cm diameter + irregular border)	617

Granuflex Bordered
Square

6cm x 6cm	(wound contact pad 6cm x 6cm + border 2cm)	156
10cm x 10cm	(wound contact pad 10cm x 10cm + border 2.0 - 2.5cm)	294
15cm x 15cm	(wound contact pad 15cm x 15cm + border 2.5cm)	566

Triangular

10cm x 13cm	(wound contact pad 10cm x 13cm + border 2.0 - 2.5cm)	347
15cm x 18cm	(wound contact pad 15cm x 18cm + border 2.0 - 2.5cm)	540

Hydrocoll Border (Bevelled Edge)
Square

5cm x 5cm	(wound contact pad 3.5cm x 3.5cm + border 0.75cm)	90
7.5cm x 7.5cm	(wound contact pad 4.5cm x 4.5cm + border 1.5cm)	148
10cm x 10cm	(wound contact pad 7.75cm x 7.75cm + border 1.25cm)	215
15cm x 15cm	(wound contact pad 12.5cm x 12.5cm + border 1.5cm)	405

Concave

These dressings are contoured to facilitate application to difficult areas such as elbows and heels.

8cm x 12cm	(wound contact pad 9.3cm x 4.7cm + irregular border)	190

Sacral (previously measured as 15cm x 18cm)

12cm x 18cm	(wound contact pad 14cm x 11cm + irregular border)	322

Suprasorb H
Square

14cm x 14cm	(wound contact pad 10cm x 10cm + border 2cm)	223

Tegaderm Hydrocolloid (formerly Tegasorb)
Oval

10cm x 12cm	(wound contact pad 7cm x 9cm + border 1.5cm)	224
13cm x 15cm	(wound contact pad 10cm x 12cm + border 1.5cm)	419

Sacral

17.1cm x 16.1cm	(wound contact pad 13.9cm x 12.3cm + irregular border)	468

Tegasorb see Tegaderm Hydrocolloid

Ultec Pro
Square

10.5cm x 10.5cm	(wound contact pad 6.4cm x 6.4cm + 2.05cm border)	139
14cm x 14cm	(wound contact pad 10.5cm x 10.5cm + 1.75cm border)	224
21cm x 21cm	(wound contact pad 15.2cm x 15.2cm + 2.9cm border)	449

Sacral

15cm x 18cm	(wound contact pad 10cm x 12.5cm + irregular border)	317
19.5cm x 23cm	(wound contact pad 15cm x 17.5cm + irregular border)	488

APPLIANCES

Appliance	Size or Weight	Basic Price p each
DRESSINGS		
WOUND MANAGEMENT DRESSINGS		
Hydrocolloid Dressing - Semi-permeable - Sterile - Without Adhesive Border		
ActivHeal		
Square	10cm x 10cm	152
	15cm x 15cm	331
Sacral	15cm x 18cm	384
Rectangular	5cm x 7.5cm	75
Comfeel Plus Ulcer Dressing (Bevelled Edge)		
Square	10cm x 10cm	216
	15cm x 15cm	464
	20cm x 20cm	668
Rectangular	4cm x 6cm	85
Triangular	18cm x 20cm	505
DuoDERM Signal		
Square	10cm x 10cm	189
	14cm x 14cm	332
	20cm x 20cm	659
Heel	18.5cm x 19.5cm	464
Sacral	22.5cm x 20cm	542
Oval	11cm x 19cm	287
Flexigran		
Square	10cm x 10cm	219
Granuflex (modified)		
Square	10cm x 10cm	247
	15cm x 15cm	468
	20cm x 20cm	704
Rectangular	15cm x 20cm	507
Hydrocoll Basic		
Square	10cm x 10cm	219
NU-DERM		
Square	5cm x 5cm	80
	10cm x 10cm	150
	15cm x 15cm	300
	20cm x 20cm	600
Heel/Elbow	8cm x 12cm	300
Sacral	15cm x 18cm	420
Suprasorb H		
Square	10cm x 10cm	151
	15cm x 15cm	330
Tegaderm Hydrocolloid (formerly Tegasorb)		
Square	10cm x 10cm	229
	15cm x 15cm	442
Tegasorb see Tegaderm Hydrocolloid		
Ultec Pro		
Square	10cm x 10cm	219
	15cm x 15cm	427
	20cm x 20cm	643

IXA

APPLIANCES

Appliance	Size or Weight	Basic Price p
DRESSINGS		**each**
WOUND MANAGEMENT DRESSINGS		
Hydrocolloid Dressing, Thin - Semi-permeable - Sterile		
With Adhesive Border		
Tegaderm Hydrocolloid Thin (formerly Tegasorb Thin)		
Oval		
10cm x 12cm (wound contact pad 7cm x 9cm + border 1.5cm)		149
13cm x 15cm (wound contact pad 10cm x 12cm + border 1.5cm)		279
Tegasorb Thin see Tegaderm Hydrocolloid Thin		
Without Adhesive Border		
Askina Biofilm Transparent		
Square	10cm x 10cm	102
	15cm x 15cm	231
	20cm x 20cm	302
Comfeel Plus Transparent Dressing		
Square	10cm x 10cm	113
	15cm x 15cm	295
	20cm x 20cm	301
Rectangular	5cm x 7 cm	59
	5cm x 15cm	140
	5cm x 25cm	228
	9cm x 14cm	215
	9cm x 25cm	305
	15cm x 20cm	299
Sacral	17cm x 17cm	331
DuoDERM Extra Thin		
Rectangular	5cm x 10cm	68
	9cm x 15cm	157
	9cm x 25cm	251
	9cm x 35cm	351
Square	7.5cm x 7.5cm	70
	10cm x 10cm	116
	15cm x 15cm	251
Flexigran Thin		
Square	10cm x 10cm	108
Hydrocoll Thin Film		
Square	7.5cm x 7.5cm	62
	10cm x 10cm	103
	15cm x 15cm	232
NU-DERM	10cm x 10cm	100
Suprasorb H		
Rectangular	5cm x 10cm	65
Square	10cm x 10cm	99
	15cm x 15cm	226
Tegaderm Hydrocolloid Thin (formerly Tegasorb Thin)		
Square	10cm x 10cm	150
Tegasorb Thin see Tegaderm Hydrocolloid Thin		

APPLIANCES

Appliance	Size or Weight	Basic Price p
DRESSINGS		**each**

WOUND MANAGEMENT DRESSINGS

Hydrocolloid Dressing - Semi-permeable - Sterile - Chronic and acute exudating wounds

With Adhesive Border

Alione

Square			
10cm x 10cm	(wound contact pad 6cm x 6cm + border 2cm)		284
12.5cm x 12.5cm	(wound contact pad 8.5cm x 8.5cm + border 2cm)		391
15cm x 15cm	(wound contact pad 10cm x 10cm + border 2.5cm)		495
20cm x 20cm	(wound contact pad 14cm x 14cm + border 3cm)		738
Rectangular			
12cm x 20cm	(wound contact pad 8cm x 16cm + border 2cm)		514

CombiDERM

Square			
10cm x 10cm	(wound contact pad 5cm x 5cm + border 2.5cm)		147
14cm x 14cm	(wound contact pad 7.5cm x 7.5cm + border 3.5cm)		204
20cm x 20cm	(wound contact pad 13cm x 13cm + border 3.5cm)		392
Triangular			
15cm x 18cm	(wound contact pad 8cm x 11cm + border 3cm)		352
20cm x 23cm	(wound contact pad 12cm x 15cm + border 4cm)		473

Versiva

Square			
9cm x 9 cm	(wound contact pad 5cm x 5cm + border 2cm)		235
14cm x 14cm	(wound contact pad 10cm x 10cm + border 2cm)		438
19cm x 19cm	(wound contact pad 15cm x 15cm + border 2cm)		681
Rectangular			
19cm x 24cm	(wound contact pad 15cm x 20cm + border 2cm)		823
Sacral			
19cm x 17.7cm	(wound contact pad 12cm x 13cm + irregular border)		580
21cm x 22.5cm	(wound contact pad 14cm x 15cm + irregular border)		823
Heel			
19.5cm x 18.5cm	(wound contact pad 11.5cm x 15.5cm + irregular border)		699
Oval			
11cm x 19cm	(wound contact pad 7cm x 15cm + border 2cm)		408

With Non-Adhesive Border

Alione

Square			
10cm x 10cm	(wound contact pad 6cm x 6cm + border 2cm)		284
12.5cm x 12.5cm	(wound contact pad 8.5cm x 8.5cm + border 2cm)		391
15cm x 15cm	(wound contact pad 10cm x 10cm + border 2.5cm)		495
20cm x 20cm	(wound contact pad 14cm x 14cm + border 3cm)		738
Rectangular			
12cm x 20cm	(wound contact pad 8cm x 16cm + border 2cm)		514

CombiDERM-N

Square			
7.5cm x 7.5cm	(wound contact pad 5.5cm x 5.5cm + border 1cm)		115
14cm x 14cm	(wound contact pad 11cm x 11cm + border 1.5cm)		205
Rectangular			
15cm x 25cm	(wound contact pad 13cm x 23cm + border 1cm)		418

IXA

APPLIANCES

Appliance			Size or Weight	Basic Price p
DRESSINGS				**each**
WOUND MANAGEMENT DRESSINGS				
Hydrocolloid Dressing - Fibrous - Silver Impregnated - Sterile				
Silvercel	Square		5cm x 5cm	158
			11cm x 11cm	390
	Rectangular		2.5cm x 30.5cm	420
			10cm x 20cm	724
Hydrocolloid Dressing - Silver Impregnated - Sterile				
Without Adhesive Border				
Contreet Hydrocolloid	Square		10cm x 10cm	646
			15cm x 15cm	1292
Hydrocolloid Paste				
Comfeel Paste			50g	608

Hydrogel Dressing - Sterile

Indications:Dry "sloughy" or necrotic wounds; lightly exudating wounds; granulating wounds.
Precautions: Not suitable for infected or heavily-exudating wounds. Care should be taken to choose the appropriate secondary dressing.

ActivHeal	15g	136
AquaForm Hydrogel	8g	151
	15g	184
Citrugel	15g	135
Flexigran Gel	15g	190
Granugel Hydrocolloid Gel	15g	205
IntraSite Conformable - See Hydrogel Sheet Without Adhesive Border page 177		
IntraSite Gel	8g	159
	15g	213
	25g	316
Nu-Gel	15g	197
Prontosan Wound Gel	30ml	585
Purilon Gel	8g	155
	15g	202
Suprasorb G	6g	110
	20g	180

APPLIANCES

Appliance		Size or Weight	Basic Price p
DRESSINGS			**each**
WOUND MANAGEMENT DRESSINGS			
Hydrogel Sheet			
With Adhesive Border			
Curagel Island	Rectangular	7.5cm x 10cm	247
	Square	12.5cm x 12.5cm	358
Hydrosorb Comfort	Square	12.5cm x 12.5cm	373
	Rectangular	4.5cm x 6.5cm	166
		7.5cm x 10cm	259
Mesitran Border			
Square			
10cm x 10cm	(wound contact pad 5.8cm x 5.8cm + border 2.1cm)		251
15cm x 15cm	(wound contact pad 10cm x 10cm + border 2.5cm)		444
Sacral			
15cm x 13cm	(wound contact pad 10cm x 8cm + border 2.5cm)		425
Without Adhesive Border			
ActiFormCool	Square	10cm x 10cm	233
	Rectangular	5cm x 6.5cm	159
		10cm x 15cm	335
Aquaflo	Discs	7.5cm	250
		12cm	516
Coolie	Disc	7cm Diameter	196 ▽
Curagel	Rectangular	5cm x 7.5cm	174
	Square	10cm x 10cm	271
Gel FX	Square	10cm x 10cm	160
		15cm x 15cm	320
	Rectangular	10cm x 15cm	220
Geliperm	Square	10cm x 10cm	227
Hydrosorb	Square	10cm x 10cm	284
		20cm x 20cm	684
	Rectangular	5cm x 7.5cm	180
IntraSite Conformable	Square	10cm x 10cm (7.5g)	159
	Rectangular	10cm x 20cm (15g)	215
		10cm x 40cm (30g)	384
Mesitran	Square	10cm x 10cm	241
	Rectangular	10cm x 17.5cm	435
		15cm x 20cm	502
Mesitran Mesh	Square	10cm x 10cm	232
Novogel	Square	10cm x 10cm	301
		30cm x 30cm (0.15cm thickness)	1203
		30cm x 30cm (0.30cm thickness)	1274
	Rectangular	5cm x 7.5cm	191
		15cm x 20cm	574
		20cm x 40cm	1094
	Circular	7.5cm Diameter	273
Suprasorb G	Rectangular	5cm x 7.5cm	173
	Square	10cm x 10cm	222
		20cm x 20cm	671
Vacunet	Square	10cm x 10cm	193
	Rectangular	10cm x 15cm	286

IXA

APPLIANCES

Appliance	Size or Weight	Basic Price p
DRESSINGS		**each**

WOUND MANAGEMENT DRESSINGS

Polyurethane Foam Dressing BP - Sterile

Indications: Light to medium exudating wounds.

Precautions: Not recommended for dry superficial wounds. Dressings should be secured at the edge by adhesive tape. Dressing should not be covered by occlusive tape or film. Secondary absorbent dressing is not required.

	Size or Weight	Basic Price p
Lyofoam	7.5cm x 7.5cm	98
	10cm x 10cm	114
	17.5cm x 10cm	181
	20cm x 15cm	245

Polyurethane Foam Film Dressing - Sterile - With Adhesive Border
Light to medium exudating wounds

Lyofoam Extra Adhesive

Square

	9cm x 9cm	(wound contact pad 5cm x 5cm + border 2cm)	122
	15cm x 15cm	(wound contact pad 10cm x 10cm + border 2.5cm)	229
	22cm x 22cm	(wound contact pad 15cm x 15cm + border 3.5cm)	452

Sacral

	15cm x 13cm	(wound contact pad 10cm x 8cm + border 2.5cm)	188
	22cm x 26cm	(wound contact pad 15cm x 19cm + border 3.5cm)	356

Suprasorb P

Square

	7.5cm x 7.5cm	(wound contact pad 4cm x 4cm + border 1.75cm)	116
	10cm x 10cm	(wound contact pad 6.3cm x 6.3cm + border 1.85cm)	125
	15cm x 15cm	(wound contact pad 10.3cm x 10.3cm + border 2.35cm)	224

Tielle

Square

	11cm x 11cm	(wound contact pad 7cm x 7cm + border 2cm)	224
	15cm x 15cm	(wound contact pad 11cm x 11cm + border 2cm)	366
	18cm x 18cm	(wound contact pad 14cm x 14cm + border 2cm)	467

Rectangular

	7cm x 9cm	(wound contact pad 3cm x 5cm + border 2cm)	121
	15cm x 20cm	wound contact pad 11cm x 16cm + border 2cm)	459

Tielle Sacrum

Square

	18cm x 18cm	(wound contact pad 12cm x 10cm + border 3 - 5cm)	339

APPLIANCES

Appliance		Size or Weight	Basic Price p
DRESSINGS			**each**

WOUND MANAGEMENT DRESSINGS

Polyurethane Foam Film Dressing - Sterile - Without Adhesive Border
Light to medium exudating wounds

Appliance	Shape	Size or Weight	Basic Price p each
Allevyn Lite	Square	5cm x 5 cm	100
		10cm x 10cm	181
	Rectangular	10cm x 20cm	310
		15cm x 20cm	386
Allevyn Thin (adhesive)	Square	10cm x 10cm	190
		15cm x 15cm	314
	Rectangular	5cm x 6cm	94
		15cm x 20cm	380
Flexipore (adhesive)	Square	10cm x 10cm	173
		20cm x 20cm	506
	Rectangular	6cm x 7cm	93
		10cm x 30cm	360
		15cm x 20cm	370
Lyofoam Extra (non adhesive)	Square	10cm x 10cm	195
	Rectangular	10cm x 17.5cm	329
		15cm x 20cm	427
Suprasorb M	Square	10cm x 10cm	172
		20cm x 20cm	505
	Rectangular	10cm x 20cm	303
Suprasorb P	Square	5cm x 5cm	90
		7.5cm x 7.5cm	96
		10cm x 10cm	113
		15cm x 15cm	301
Tielle Borderless	Square	11cm x 11cm	260
		15cm x 15cm	420
Transorbent (adhesive)	Square	10cm x 10cm	182
		15cm x 15cm	334
		20cm x 20cm	533
	Rectangular	5cm x 7cm	96

Polyurethane Foam Film Dressing - Sterile - With Adhesive Border
Lightly to non-exuding wounds
Tielle Lite

Shape	Size	Description	Basic Price p each
Square	11cm x 11cm	(wound contact pad 7cm x 7cm + border 2cm)	215
Rectangular	7cm x 9cm	(wound contact pad 3cm x 5cm + border 2cm)	114
	8cm x 15cm	(wound contact pad 4cm x 11cm + border 2cm)	265
	8cm x 20cm	(wound contact pad 4cm x 16cm + border 2cm)	280

APPLIANCES

Appliance	Size or Weight	Basic Price p
DRESSINGS		**each**

WOUND MANAGEMENT DRESSINGS
Polyurethane Foam Film Dressing - Sterile - With Adhesive Border
Moderate to heavily exuding wounds
3M Foam Adhesive Dressing see Tegaderm Foam Adhesive

ActivHeal
  Square

10cm x 10cm	(wound contact pad 5cm x 5cm + border 2.5cm)	157
12.5cm x 12.5cm	(wound contact pad 7.5cm x 7.5cm + border 2.5cm)	150
15cm x 15cm	(wound contact pad 11cm x 11cm + border 2cm)	192
20cm x 20cm	(wound contact pad 13.5cm x 13.5cm + border 3cm)	434

Allevyn Adhesive (Adhesive faced pad)
  Square

7.5cm x 7.5cm	(wound contact pad 5cm x 5cm + border 1.25cm)	134
10cm x 10cm	(wound contact pad 7.5cm x 7.5cm + border 1.25cm)	197
12.5cm x 12.5cm	(wound contact pad 10cm x 10cm + border 1.25cm)	241
17.5cm x 17.5cm	(wound contact pad 15cm x 15cm + border 1.25cm)	474
22.5cm x 22.5cm	(wound contact pad 20cm x 20cm + border 1.25cm)	691

  Rectangular

12.5cm x 22.5cm	(wound contact pad 10cm x 20cm + border 2cm)	374

  Anatomically Shaped Sacral Dressing

17cm x 17cm	(wound contact pad 13cm x 13cm + border 2cm)	356
22cm x 22cm	(wound contact pad 18cm x 18cm + border 2cm)	512

Allevyn Plus Adhesive
  Square

12.5cm x 12.5cm	(wound contact pad 10cm x 10cm + border 1.25cm)	296
17.5cm x 17.5cm	(wound contact pad 15cm x 15cm + border 1.25cm)	571

  Rectangular

12.5cm x 22.5cm	(wound contact pad 10cm x 20cm + border 2cm)	524

  Anatomically Shaped Sacral Dressing

17cm x 17cm	(wound contact pad 13cm x 13cm + border 2cm)	431
22cm x 22cm	(wound contact pad 18cm x 18cm + border 2cm)	624

Biatain Adhesive
  Square

10cm x 10cm	(circular wound contact pad 6cm diameter + irregular border)	156
12cm x 12cm	(wound contact pad 8cm x 8cm + border 2cm)	229
18cm x 18cm	(wound contact pad 13cm x 13cm + border 2.5cm)	459

  Sacral

23cm x 23cm	(wound contact pad 13cm x 13cm + border 5cm)	392

  Heel Dressing

19cm x 20cm	(wound contact pad 12cm x 13cm + border 3.5cm)	458

  Contour

17cm diameter	(wound contact pad 8cm diameter + irregular border)	441

  Rectangular

18cm x 28cm	(wound contact pad 10cm x 20cm + border 4cm)	679

  Circular   see under 'Square' with circular pad

Comfifoam
  Square

7.5cm x 7.5cm	(wound contact pad 4cm x 4cm + border 1.75cm)	113
10cm x 10cm	(wound contact pad 5cm x 5cm + border 2.5cm)	165
12.5cm x 12.5cm	(wound contact pad 7.5cm x 7.5cm + border 2.5cm)	203
17.5cm x 17.5cm	(wound contact pad 12.5cm x 12.5cm + border 2.5cm)	401

PermaFoam
  Concave

16.5cm x 18cm	(wound contact pad 10.5cm x 12cm + border 3cm)	360

  Sacral

18cm x 18cm	(wound contact pad 11cm x 9.5cm + border 3-4.25cm)	296
22cm x 22cm	(wound contact pad 14.5cm x 12.5cm + border 3.75-4.75cm)	340

APPLIANCES

Appliance	Size or Weight	Basic Price p
DRESSINGS		**each**
WOUND MANAGEMENT DRESSINGS		
PermaFoam Comfort		
Square		
8cm x 8cm	(wound contact pad 3.5cm x 3.5cm + border 2.25cm)	100
11cm x 11cm	(wound contact pad 6cm x 6cm + border 2.5cm)	190
15cm x 15cm	(wound contact pad10cm x 10cm + border 2.5cm)	310
20cm x 20cm	(wound contact pad 14cm x 14cm + border 3cm)	450
Rectangular		
10cm x 20cm	(wound contact pad 5cm x 14cm + border 2.5-3cm)	300
PolyMem		
Square		
15cm x 15cm	(wound contact pad 9cm x 9cm + border 3cm)	272
Rectangular		
10cm x 13cm	(wound contact pad 5cm x 8cm + border 2.5cm)	202
Oval		
5cm x 7.6cm	(wound contact pad 2.5cm x 5cm + irregular border)	107
8.8cm x 12.7cm	(wound contact pad 5cm x 7.6cm + irregular border)	190
16.5cm x 20.9cm	(wound contact pad 10.1cm x 14.6cm + irregular border)	625
Sacral		
18.4cm x 20cm	(wound contact pad 11.4cm x 12cm + border 3.5-4cm)	420
Tegaderm Foam Adhesive (formerly 3M Foam Adhesive Dressing)		
Square		
14cm x 14cm	(wound contact pad 10cm x 10cm + border 2cm)	337
Oval		
10cm x 11cm	(wound contact pad 6cm x 7.6cm + border 1.7-2cm)	228
14cm x 15cm	(wound contact pad 10cm x 11cm + border 2cm)	405
19cm x 22.2cm	(wound contact pad 14cm x 17.1cm + border 2.5cm)	664
Circular (Heel)		
14cm x 14cm	(wound contact pad 7.6cm x 7.6cm + border 3.2cm)	406
Tielle Plus		
Square		
11cm x 11cm	(wound contact pad 7cm x 7cm + border 2cm)	248
15cm x 15cm	(wound contact pad 11cm x 11cm + border 2cm)	405
Rectangular		
15cm x 20cm	(wound contact pad 11cm x 16cm + border 2cm)	508
Sacrum		
15cm x 15cm	(wound contact pad 7.2cm x 10cm + border 2.5-5.3cm)	295
Tielle Plus Heel Hydropolymer Adhesive Dressing		
Heel Dressing		
20cm x 26.5cm	(wound contact pad 14.5cm x 14.5cm + irregular border)	420
Trufoam		
Square		
11cm x 11cm	(wound contact pad 7cm x 7cm + border 2cm)	208
15cm x 15cm	(wound contact pad 11cm x 11cm + border 2cm)	348
Rectangular		
7cm x 9cm	(wound contact pad 3cm x 5cm + border 2cm)	109
15cm x 20cm	(wound contact pad 11cm x 15cm + border 2.5cm)	436
V.A.C. (Vacuum Assisted Closure) Therapy		
(The following items are to be used as part of the V.A.C. Therapy system)		
V.A.C. GranuFoam dressing kit		
Small		2100
Medium		2500
Large		2900
V.A.C. Freedom Canister with Gel		2600
For use with the V.A.C. Freedom		

APPLIANCES

Appliance	Size or Weight		Basic Price p
DRESSINGS			**each**

WOUND MANAGEMENT DRESSINGS
   Polyurethane Foam Film Dressing - Sterile - Without Adhesive Border
   Moderate to heavily exuding wounds
     3M Foam Dressing see Tegaderm Foam

ActivHeal	Square	5cm x 5cm	72
		10cm x 10cm	109
		20cm x 20cm	378
	Rectangular	10cm x 17.8cm	226
† *Advazorb*	Square	10cm x 10cm	80
	Rectangular	5cm x 7.5cm	45
		10cm x 20cm	120
		15cm x 20cm	160
Allevyn Compression	Square	10cm x 10cm	227
		15cm x 15cm	386
	Rectangular	5cm x 6cm	110
		15cm x 20cm	432
Allevyn Non-Adhesive	Square	5cm x 5cm	113
		10cm x 10cm	225
		20cm x 20cm	603
	Rectangular	10cm x 20cm	361
	Heel (Cup Shaped)	10.5cm x 13.5cm	450
Biatain Non-Adhesive	Circular	5cm diameter	109
		8cm diameter	153
	Square	10cm x 10cm	211
		15cm x 15cm	390
		20cm x 20cm	578
	Rectangular	10cm x 20cm	349
Biatain Soft Hold Dressing	Square	10cm x 10cm	230
		15cm x 15cm	382
	Rectangular	10cm x 20cm	349
Comfifoam	Square	5cm x 5cm	96
		10cm x 10cm	190
		20cm x 20cm	509
	Rectangular	10cm x 20cm	305
Kerraboot	Boot Shaped	Extra Small (Clear)	1427
		Extra Small (White)	1427
		Small (Clear)	1427
		Small (White)	1427
		Large (Clear)	1427
		Large (White)	1427
		Extra Large (Clear)	1427
		Extra Large (White)	1427
PermaFoam	Circular	6cm diameter	98
	Square	8cm x 8cm (fenestrated)	112
		10cm x 10cm	190
		15cm x 15cm	360
		20cm x 20cm	550
	Rectangular	10cm x 20cm	325
PolyMem	Square	8cm x 8cm	147
		10cm x 10cm	229
		13cm x 13cm	382
	Rectangular	17cm x 19cm	564
	Roll	10cm x 61cm	1215

†to be deleted 1 April 2007

APPLIANCES

Appliance	Size or Weight		Basic Price p each
DRESSINGS			
WOUND MANAGEMENT DRESSINGS			
PolyMem Max	Square	11cm x 11cm	275
Tegaderm Foam	Square	8.8cm x 8.8cm (Fenestrated)	213
(formerly 3M Foam Dressing)		10cm x 10cm	209
		20cm x 20cm	565
	Rectangular	10cm x 20cm	354
		10cm x 60cm	1196
Tielle Plus Borderless	Square	11cm x 11cm	298
	Rectangular	15cm x 20cm	540
Trufoam NA	Square	5cm x 5cm	104
		10cm x 10cm	197
		15cm x 15cm	363

Packed in outer container not exceeding 10 units.

Polyurethane Matrix Dressing
Indications: Light to medium exudating wounds

† **With Adhesive Border**

Cutinova Hydro Border

Square	15cm x 15cm	(wound contact pad 10cm x 10cm + border 2.5cm)	275
Rectangular	10cm x 11cm	(wound contact pad 5cm x 6cm + border 2.5cm)	121
	17cm x 20cm	(wound contact pad 12cm x 15cm + border 2.5cm)	422

Without Adhesive Border

Cutinova Hydro	Square	10cm x 10cm	224
	Rectangular	5cm x 6cm	112
		15cm x 20cm	475

Protease Modulating Matrix - Sterile

Aquacel	Square	5cm x 5cm	103
		10cm x 10cm	244
		15cm x 15cm	460
	Rectangular	4cm x 10cm	133
		4cm x 20cm	196
		4cm x 30cm	294
Aquacel Ag	Square	5cm x 5cm	174
		10cm x 10cm	415
		15cm x 15cm	782
	Rectangular	4cm x 10cm	255
		4cm x 20cm	332
		4cm x 30cm	498
		20cm x 30cm	1940
Cadesorb		10g tube (approximate coverage 60cm^2)	477
		20g tube (approximate coverage 120cm^2)	814
Epi-Max		5cm x 6cm	475
		8cm x 10cm	975
Flaminal		15g tube (approximate coverage 40cm^2)	699
Flaminal Hydro		15g tube (approximate coverage 40cm^2)	699
Promogran		28cm^2 (matrix is hexagonal in shape)	489
		123cm^2 (matrix is hexagonal in shape)	1473
Promogran Prisma		28cm^2 (matrix is hexagonal in shape)	595
		123cm^2 (matrix is hexagonal in shape)	1695

†to be deleted 1 April 2007

IXA

APPLIANCES

Appliance	Size or Weight		Basic Price p
DRESSINGS			**each**
WOUND MANAGEMENT DRESSINGS			
Suprasorb C		4cm x 6cm	255
		6cm x 8cm	390
		8cm x 12cm	765
Silicone Gel Sheet			
Indications: For prevention treatment - Keloid and Hypertrophic scars.			
Advasil	Square	10cm x 10cm	510
Cica-Care	Rectangular	6cm x 12cm	1291
		15cm x 12cm	2516
Mepiform	Rectangular	5cm x 7.5cm	329
		10cm x 18cm	1338
		4cm x 30cm	942
Oleeva Clear	Square	13cm x 13cm	1517
	Rectangular	4cm x 13cm	661
		13cm x 25cm	2741
		20cm x 30cm	4992
Oleeva Fabric	Square	13cm x 13cm	1517
	Rectangular	4cm x 13cm	661
		13cm x 25cm	2741
		20cm x 30cm	4992
Silgel	Square	10cm x 10cm	1350
		20cm x 20cm	4000
		40cm x 40cm	14400
	Rectangular	10cm x 5cm	750
		15cm x 10cm	1950
		30cm x 5cm	1950
		10cm x 30cm	3150
	Shaped	5cm Diameter	400
		5.5cm Diameter	400
		25cm x 15cm	2112
		46cm x 8.5cm	3946
Silicone Topical Cream & Gel			
Indications: For prevention treatment - Keloid and Hypertrophic scars.			
Dermatix		15g tube	1900
		60g tube	5700
Silgel STC-SE (gel)		20ml tube	1900
Silver Coated Barrier Dressings - Sterile			
Acticoat	Square	5cm x 5cm	309
		10cm x 10cm	755
	Rectangular	10cm x 20cm	1181
		20cm x 40cm	4040
Acticoat Absorbent	Square	5cm x 5cm	472
	Rectangular	10cm x 12.5cm	1133
Acticoat 7	Square	5cm x 5cm	537
		15cm x 15cm	2878
	Rectangular	10cm x 12.5cm	1601
Acticoat Moisture Control	Square	5cm x 5cm	633
		10cm x 10cm	1480
	Rectangular	10cm x 20cm	2884

APPLIANCES

Appliance	Size or Weight		Basic Price p each

DRESSINGS
WOUND MANAGEMENT DRESSINGS
  Silver Impregnated Polyurethane Foam Film Dressings
  With Adhesive Border
  Avance A

<u>Square</u>	9cm x 9cm	(wound contact pad 5cm x 5cm + border 2cm)	222
	12cm x 12cm	(wound contact pad 8cm x 8cm + border 2cm)	368
	15cm x 15cm	(wound contact pad 10cm x 10cm + border 2.5cm)	451
<u>Sacral</u>	15cm x 13cm	(wound contact pad 10cm x 8cm + border 2.5cm)	332

  Contreet Foam

<u>Square</u>	12.5cm x 12.5cm	(wound contact pad 8cm x 8cm + border 2.25cm)	822
	18cm x 18cm	(wound contact pad 13cm x 13cm + border 2.5cm)	1649
<u>Heel</u>	19cm x 20cm	(wound contact pad 12cm x 13cm + border 3.5cm)	1626
<u>Sacral</u>	23cm x 23cm	(wound contact pad 13cm x 13cm + border 5cm)	1728

  Without Adhesive Border
  Avance

	<u>Square</u>	10cm x 10cm	264
	<u>Rectangular</u>	10cm x 17.5cm	421
		15cm x 20cm	582

  Contreet Foam

	<u>Square</u>	10cm x 10cm	718
		15cm x 15cm	1442
		20cm x 20cm	2034
	<u>Rectangular</u>	10cm x 20cm	1320
	<u>Circular</u>	5cm diameter	301

  Soft Polymer Wound Contact Dressing
  CE
  Physiotulle

	10cm x 10cm	202
	15cm x 20cm	613

  Tegaderm Contact (formerly Tegapore)

	7.5cm x 10cm	213
	7.5cm x 20cm	417
	20cm x 25cm	1016

  Tegapore see Tegaderm Contact

  Urgotul

†	10cm x 12cm	292
	10cm x 40cm	951
	11cm x 11cm	292
†	15cm x 20cm	738
	16cm x 21cm	826

  UrgotulDuo

	5cm x 10cm	220
	10cm x 12cm	340
	15cm x 20cm	790

  Soft Polymer Wound Contact Dressing Impregnated with Silver
  Atrauman Ag

	5cm x 5cm	46
	10cm x 10cm	112
	10cm x 20cm	219

  Physiotulle Ag

	10cm x 10cm	202

  Urgotul SSD

†	10cm x 12cm	289
	11cm x 11cm	289
†	15cm x 20cm	731
	16cm x 21cm	819

  Soft Polymer Wound Contact Dressing with Polyurethane Foam Film Backing - Sterile
  CE
  UrgoCell

	(adhesive)	13cm x 13cm	427
		15cm x 20cm	865
	(non-adhesive)	10cm x 12cm	427
		15cm x 20cm	865

†to be deleted 1 April 2007

IXA

APPLIANCES

Appliance	Size or Weight	Basic Price p
		each

DRESSINGS
WOUND MANAGEMENT DRESSINGS
Soft Polymer Wound Contact Dressing with Polyurethane Foam Film Backing Impregnated with Silver

UrgoCell Silver	6cm x 6cm	400
	10cm x 10cm	550
	15cm x 20cm	990

Soft Silicone Wound Contact Dressing - Sterile
CE
Indications: Non-exuding to heavily exuding wounds.Should be covered with a simple absorbent secondary dressing.
Precautions: Dressing should be used with care in heavily bleeding wounds.

Mepilex Transfer	15cm x 20cm	951
	20cm x 50cm	2430
Mepitel	5cm x 7cm	147
	8cm x 10cm	293
	12cm x 15cm	593
	20cm x 30cm	1528
Silon-TSR	13cm x 13cm	352
	13cm x 25cm	547
	28cm x 30cm	737

Soft Silicone Wound Contact Dressing with Polyurethane Foam Film Backing - Sterile
CE
Precautions: Dressing should be used with care in heavily bleeding wounds.

Mepilex	10cm x 10cm	237
	10cm x 20cm	391
	15cm x 15cm	440
	20cm x 20cm	652
Mepilex Heel	13cm x 20cm	495
Mepilex Lite	6cm x 8.5cm	163
	10cm x 10cm	194
	15cm x 15cm	377
	20cm x 50cm	2382
Mepilex Border	7.5cm x 7.5cm	138
	10cm x 10cm	249
	15cm x 15cm	407
	15cm x 20cm	511
Mepilex Border Lite	4cm x 5cm	85
	7.5cm x 7.5cm	128
	5cm x 12.5cm	185
	10cm x 10cm	233
	15cm x 15cm	380

Wound Drainage Pouch
CE
Indications: Suitable for wounds with a low volume of exudate

Biotrol Draina S Fistula for wound drainage and fistula management		**pack of 30**
Mini (Cut to 20mm) 150ml Capacity	(H0856OE)	7035

Oakmed Option Wound Manager		
cut-to-fit:		
10mm - 30mm Small	(OM-S)	6444
10mm - 50mm Medium	(OM-M)	7139
10mm - 50mm Large	(OM-L)	7477

APPLIANCES

Appliance	Size or Weight		Basic Price p

DRESSINGS
WOUND MANAGEMENT DRESSINGS

Indications: Suitable for wounds with a high volume of exudate

ADI Medical Dermasure   **each**

For wounds up to:			
Small (9cm x 16cm)	7OS3010		1529
Medium (15cm x 27cm)	7OS3020		2039

Biotrol Draina S Fistula for wound drainage and fistula management   **pack of 20**

Medium (Cut to 50mm) 350ml Capacity	(H28555E)		7014
Large (Cut to 88mm) 500ml Capacity	(H28556E)		8626

ConvaTec Wound Manager   **each**

For wounds up to:			
Small (7.6cm x 7.6cm)			946
Medium (7.6cm x 18cm)			1577
Large (10cm x 23cm)			2081

Eakin Wound Pouches

Fold and Tuck closure for wounds up to:			**pack of 10**
Small (45 x 30mm)	839250		4500
Medium (110 x 75mm)	839251		6500
Large (175 x 110mm)	839252		8500
Extra Large (horizontal wounds upto 245 x 160mm)			**pack of 5**
	839253		7500
Bung Closure for wounds up to:			**pack of 10**
Small (45 x 30mm)	839260		5000
Medium (110 x 75mm)	839261		7000
Large (175 x 110mm)	839262		9500
Extra Large (horizontal wounds upto 245 x 160mm)			**pack of 5**
	839263		8500
Extra Large (vertical wounds upto 245 x 160mm)			
	839265		8500
Extra Large (vertical incision wounds upto 290 x 130mm)			
	839266		8500
Bung Closure and access window for wounds up to:			
Extra Large (horizontal wounds upto 245 x 160mm)			
	839264		9500
Eakin access windows for use with Eakin pouches			
	839280		3500

Oakmed Option Wound Manager   **pack of 10**

Extra Small (wounds upto 90mm x 180mm)		10700
(WWM-XS)		
Small (horizontal wounds upto 245mm wide x 160mm high)		11674
(WWM-S)		
Medium (vertical wounds upto 90mm wide x 260mm high)		11933
(WWM-M)		
Large (wounds upto 160mm x 260mm)		14500
(WWM-L)		
Square (vertical wounds upto 160mm wide x 200mm high)		12452
(WWM-SQ)		
Extra Small with Access Port (wounds upto 90mm x 180mm)		11700
(WWM-XSA)		
Small with Access Port (horizontal wounds upto 245mm wide x 160mm high)		12192
(WWM-SA)		
Medium with Access Port (vertical wounds upto 90mm wide x 260mm high)		12452
(WWM-MA)		
Large with Access Port (wounds upto 160mm x 260mm)		15500
(WWM-LA)		
Square with Access Port (vertical wounds upto 160mm wide x 200mm high)		12971
(WWM-SQA)		

IXA

APPLIANCES

Appliance	Size or Weight	Basic Price p
		each
DROPPERS		30

Glass, with bull-nose or curved flat end fitted (each in box) with good quality rubber teat. Where appropriate, a dropper should be supplied with eye, ear and nasal drops (See Part IV, containers and Part XVI (11.1.6) for details of prescription charges payable).

DRY MOUTH PRODUCTS
Saliva Replacement

Salinum	300ml	1350

Saliva Stimulating

SST Saliva Stimulating Tablets	container of 100	486

EAR WAX SOFTENING MEDICAL DEVICES

Sodium Bicarbonate Ear Drops (Thornton & Ross)	10ml	125

ELASTIC HOSIERY
Graduated Compression Hosiery
Specification 40
Explanation of Garments
N.B. The "Class" can be expressed either with roman or arabic numerals.

Class I   Light (Mild) Support
                 Compression at ankle 14mm Hg - 17mm Hg
     Indications - Superficial or early Varices. Varicosis during pregnancy.
     Styles   - Thigh length or below knee with knitted in heel (reciprocated).

Class II   Medium (Moderate) Support
                 Compression at ankle 18mm Hg - 24mm Hg
     Indications - Varices of medium severity
                 - Ulcer Treatment and prevention of recurrence. Mild oedema
                 - Varicosis during pregnancy
                 - Anklets and kneecaps: for soft tissue support
     Styles   - Thigh length or below knee with knitted in heel (reciprocated)

Class III
         Strong support
         Compression at ankle 25mm Hg - 35mm Hg
     Indications - Gross varices
                 - Post Thrombotic Venous Insufficiency
                 - Gross Oedema
                 - Ulcer Treatment and prevention of recurrence
                 - Anklets and kneecaps: for soft tissue support
     Styles   - Thigh length or below knee open or knitted in heel (reciprocated)

General Notes
Prescribing
Before the prescription can be dispensed the following details must be given by the prescriber.
1.   Quantity - single or pair
2.   Article including any accessories (see pages 188-189 for knit, style and price)
3.   Compression Class I, II or III
Constructional Specification
The complete structural specification, as well as performance requirements are contained in Drug Tariff Specification No. 40.
Specially Made Garments
1.   In cases where stock sizes are not suitable for patients owing to irregular limb dimensions, surgical stockings in the prescribed compression class, to be made to the patient's individual measurements, should be specified.
2.   All such garments are specially shaped during manufacture and may have a knitted in or open heel and open or knitted in toe.
Sizing
All articles must conform to BS 6612:1985 with regard to size designation.

APPLIANCES

ELASTIC HOSIERY

Labelling

All articles must state clearly on the packaging that they conform with Drug Tariff Technical Specification No 40. The packaging should also provide clear washing instructions in conformity with handwashing at 40°C as defined in BS 2747 and washing instructions should be durably and clearly marked on each garment. The packaging should clearly define the garments percentage and fibre content.

DESCRIPTION OF ARTICLES AVAILABLE

Compression Class (See page 188)	Type of Garment		Standard Stock Sized Garments	* Made-to-Measure Garments
	Knit	Style	Price per pair in pence	Price per pair in pence
CLASS I	Circular	Thigh	714	3545
		B. Knee	652	2218
	Lt. Wt Elas. Net	Thigh		1912
		B. Knee		1492
CLASS II	Circular	Thigh	1061	3545
		B. Knee	953	2218
	Net	Thigh		1912
		B. Knee		1492
	Flat Bed	Thigh		3545
		B. Knee		2218
CLASS III	Circular	Thigh	1257	3545
		B. Knee	1081	2218
	Flat Bed	Thigh		3545
		B. Knee		2218

* All such garments are specially shaped during manufacture and many have a knitted in or open heel and open or knitted in toe with the following exceptions:
Class II/III - Flat Bed Knit can only be supplied with closed heel and open toe.
For Above Knee Stockings - see Thigh Length.

Accessories		Price per item in pence
Acti-Glide		1276
Additional Price for Fitted Suspender		62
Easy-Slide (application aid for open toe stockings)	(S,M,L,XL)	1099
Sockaid		1273
Spare Suspender for thigh stockings		62
Suspender Belt Drug Tariff Specification No. 13		476

DESCRIPTION OF ARTICLES AVAILABLE

Compression Class	Knit	Type of Garment	Standard Stock Sized Garments	Made-to-Measure Garments
			Price per pair in pence	Price per pair in pence
CLASS II	Circular	Anklet	625	625
		Kneecap	625	625
	Flat Bed	Anklet	1298	1298
		Kneecap	1298	1298
	Net	Anklet		1228
		Kneecap		1020
CLASS III	Circular	Anklet	872	872
		Kneecap	833	833
	Flat Bed	Anklet	872	1298
		Kneecap	833	1298

NB: The reimbursable price for one item is half the price of a pair.
.More than one prescription charge is payable when more than one piece of elastic hosiery is supplied. (see Part XVI sub paragraph 12.12)
Note: Prescriptions should be endorsed with the style, ie, fabric or knit supplied.

IXA

APPLIANCES

Appliance	Size or Weight	Basic Price p
EMOLLIENTS		**per tub**
Epaderm	125g	348
	500g	590
EYE BATHS		**each**
Squat shape, with finger grips, rigid plastics smooth inner surface and base, rounded rim		22
EYE DROPS DISPENSERS		
Opticare	(for 2.5, 5, 10, 15 & 20ml bottles)	492
Opticare Arthro 5	(for 2.5 & 5ml bottles)	492
Opticare Arthro 10	(for 10, 15, 20ml bottles)	492
EYE SHADES		28
Plastics, semi-rigid, non flam., perforation along top for ventilation, to fit either eye		
		per box
FINGER COTS Seamless latex	box of 10	30
FINGER STALLS		**each**
Simulated Leather	Small, Medium,	40
On a knitted fabric base, with adjustable elastic wrist band	Large & Extra Large	
GAUZES		
Absorbent Cotton Gauze, Type 13 Light BP 1988, sterile		
(Syn: Absorbent Gauze)	90cm x 1m	100
	90cm x 3m	208
Where no quantity is stated by the prescriber the 1m packet	90cm x 5m	324
should be supplied.	90cm x 10m	621
Absorbent Cotton Gauze, Type 13 Light BP 1988	25m roll	1422
not sterilised		
(Syn. Absorbent Gauze)		
Absorbent Cotton and Viscose Ribbon Gauze BP 1988 Sterile		
	1.25cm x 5m	75
	2.5cm x 5m	83
GAUZE PADS/SWABS - See SWABS		
GAUZE TISSUES		
Gauze and Cotton Tissue BP 1988	500g	646
(Absorbent Gauze Tissue; Gauze Tissue)		
Gauze and Cotton Tissue (Drug Tariff)	500g	472
Specification 14		
To be supplied only where specifically ordered.		
HEAD LICE DEVICE		
Bug Buster Kit		446
(Kit containing 3 Bug Buster combs,		
1 Nit Buster comb, 1 wide tooth comb plus a protective cape).		
The Bug Buster Kit works in combination with ordinary shampoo and hair conditioner - no additional medicated products are required.		
Nitty Gritty NitFree		567
Steel Nit comb with Microgrooved Teeth		

APPLIANCES

Appliance	Size or Weight	Basic Price p
HYPODERMIC EQUIPMENT		**each**
A. **Hypodermic Needles**		33

Specification 15

British Standard 3522 Luer Mount Needles

NB: The appropriate British Standard Needles must be supplied if the old "Hypo" sizes are ordered

B.   **Hypodermic Syringes**

Glass barrels with Luer taper conical fittings.

(i)   Syringes for use with drugs other than insulin

Ordinary Purpose Syringe	1ml	865
Specification 16	2ml	865

British Standard 1263 Luer mount syringe.

C.   **Single Patient-Use Products**

(i)   **U100 Insulin Syringes with Needle - Sterile, Single-use or Single Patient-use** for the injection of U100 Insulin by diabetics in the community.

Shall comply with the requirements of BS 7548:1992

COLOUR CODING: The colour orange is used to distinguish U100 insulin syringes.

Note: When the size is not specified by the prescriber the 0.5ml syringe with needle should be supplied. If the patient is known to inject more than 50 units of insulin per injection the 1.0ml syringe shall be supplied.

Needles 8mm long shall have a range of needle diameters as follows:
0.33mm (29G) and 0.3mm (30G)

Size	per 10
0.3ml syringe and needle	129
0.5ml syringe and needle	125
1.0ml syringe and needle	124

Needles not less than 12mm long shall have a range of needle diameters as follows:
0.45mm (26G), 0.4mm (27G), 0.36mm (28G) and 0.33mm (29G)

Size	
0.3ml syringe and needle	139
0.5ml syringe and needle	134
1.0ml syringe and needle	136

(ii)   **Hypodermic Needles-Sterile, Single-use**

Shall comply with the requirements of BS 5081: Part 2: 1987:

0.4mm size needles shall comply with the requirements of the above BS and the needle tube shall have the properties given in Annex D of BS 7548: 1992.

For use with the re-usable glass syringes listed in this Tariff on page 191.

The needles shall be of a length not less than 12mm and the following diameters may be supplied:

Size		each
0.5 mm (25G)	100	257
0.45 mm (26G)	100	257
0.4 mm (27G)	100	257

APPLIANCES

Appliance			Size or Weight	Basic Price p
HYPODERMIC EQUIPMENT				**each**
D. **Reusable Pens**	Cartridge Size		Dial up unit dose	
Autopen Classic	3.0ml		1 unit (1-21 units)	1518
(Owen Mumford)	3.0ml		2 unit (2-42 units)	1518
Autopen 24	3.0ml		1 unit (1-21 units)	1495
(Owen Mumford)	3.0ml		2 unit (2-42 units)	1495
HumaPen Ergo				
(Burgundy)	3.0ml		1 unit (1-60 units)	2239
(Teal)	3.0ml		1 unit (1-60 units)	2239
(Lilly)				
HumaPen Luxura	3.0ml		1 unit (1-60 units)	2636
(Lilly)				
NovoPen 3				
Classic	3.0ml		1 unit (2-70 units)	2407
Demi	3.0ml		0.5 unit (1-35 units)	2407
Fun	3.0ml		1 unit (2-70 units)	2407
(Novo Nordisk)				
NovoPen Junior				
(Green)	3.0ml		0.5 unit (1-35 units)	2366
(Yellow)	3.0ml		0.5 unit (1-35 units)	2366
(Novo Nordisk)				
Optipen Pro 1	3.0ml		1 unit (1-60 units)	2200
(Aventis)				

E. **Needles for Pre-filled and Reusable Pen Injectors**

<u>Screw On</u>		**100 pack**
BD Micro-Fine+	5mm/31 gauge	1208
	8mm/31 gauge	857
	12.7mm/29 gauge	857
Comfort Point (formerly Exel Comfort Point)	6mm/31 gauge	995
	8mm/31 gauge	695
	12mm/29 gauge	695
NovoFine	6mm/31 gauge	1229
	8mm/30 gauge	872
	12mm/28 gauge	872
Unifine Pentips	6mm/31 gauge	1229
	8mm/31 gauge	872
	12mm/29 gauge	872

<u>**Snap On**</u>		
Penfine	6mm/31 gauge	1202
	8mm/31 gauge	852
	10mm/29 gauge	852
	12mm/29 gauge	852

APPLIANCES

Appliance		Size or Weight	Basic Price p
HYPODERMIC EQUIPMENT			
F. **Lancets - Sterile, Single-Use**			**each**
Ascensia Microlet Lancets	0.5mm/28 gauge	100	355
(Bayer Diagnostics)		200	676
BD Micro-Fine +	0.20mm/33 gauge	100	316
(formerly Micro-Fine +)	0.30mm/30 gauge	200	613
(Becton Dickinson)			
Cleanlet Fine	0.36mm/28gauge	100	319
(Gainor Medical)		200	613
FinePoint	0.5mm/25 gauge	100	348
(LifeScan UK)			
Freestyle	0.5mm/25 gauge	200	663
(Abbott Labs Ltd)			
GlucoMen (Fine)	0.45mm/26 gauge	100	342
(A. Menarini Diagnostics)		200	661
MediSense Thin Lancets see Thin Lancets			
Micro-Fine + see BD Micro-Fine +			
Milward Steri-Let	0.66mm/23 gauge	100	300
(Entaco)		200	570
	0.36mm/28 gauge	100	300
		200	570
Monolet	0.8 mm/21gauge	100	328
(Tyco Healthcare formerly Sherwood		200	624
Medical)			
Monolet Extra	0.8 mm/21gauge	100	328
(Tyco Healthcare formerly Sherwood			
Medical)			
MPD Ultra Thin Lancets	0.46mm/26 gauge	100	330
(Medical Plastics Devices Inc)		200	650
Multiclix	0.3mm/30 gauge	204	867
(Roche Diagnostics)			
One Touch UltraSoft	0.4mm/28 gauge	100	349
(LifeScan UK)			
Softclix	0.4mm/28 gauge	200	693
(Roche Diagnostics Ltd)			
Softclix XL	0.8mm/21 gauge	50	173
(Roche Diagnostics Ltd)			
Thin Lancets	0.36mm/28 gauge	200	675
(formerly MediSense Thin Lancets)			
(Abbott Labs Ltd)			
Unilet ComforTouch	0.375mm/28gauge	100	346
(Owen Mumford Ltd)		200	657
Unilet General Purpose	0.81mm/21gauge	100	352
(Owen Mumford Ltd)		200	670

IXA

APPLIANCES

Appliance	Size or Weight	Basic Price p each
HYPODERMIC EQUIPMENT		
Unilet General Purpose Superlite	0.66mm/23 gauge	100 353
(Owen Mumford Ltd)		200 669
Unilet Superlite	0.66mm/23 gauge	100 353
(Owen Mumford Ltd)		200 669
Unistik 3 Comfort	1.8mm/28 gauge	100 624
(Owen Mumford Ltd)		200 1220
Unistik 3 Normal	1.8mm/23 gauge	100 624
(Owen Mumford Ltd)		200 1220
Unistik 3 Extra	2.0mm/21 gauge	100 624
(Owen Mumford Ltd)		200 1220
VitalCare	0.36mm/28 gauge	200 620
(VitalCare UK)		
† VitalCare Auto Safety Lancets	1.8mm/26 gauge	100 390
(VitalCare UK)	1.8mm/21 gauge	100 390
	2.4mm/21 gauge	100 390
	3.0mm/21 gauge	100 390
Vitrex Gentle	0.36mm/28gauge	100 319
(Vitrex Medical Ltd)		200 613
Vitrex Soft	0.65mm/23 gauge	100 300
(Vitrex Medical Ltd)		200 570

G. Accessories

Needle Clipping (Chopping) Device		126
Sharpsafe	1 litre	85
Sharpsbin	1 litre	85

H. Needle-Free Insulin Delivery Systems

Injex Starter Set	60500	14936
(Set includes 1 needle-free delivery system, reset box, transporter, 9 disposable 10ml vial adaptors, 165 ampoules)		
Injex 4 monthly Refill Pack	60504	2447
(Pack contains 6 disposable 10ml vial adaptors, 100 ampoules)		
Injex Ampoule Pack	60501	1228
(Contains 50 ampoules)		
Injex 10ml Vial Adaptor Pack	60502	1223
(Contains 20 10ml vial adaptors)		
mhi-500 Vial Adaptor Pack		
(Contains 6 sterile vial adaptors)		
3ml vial adaptor	MH79002-14	752
10ml vial adaptor	MH79002-09	766
mhi-500 3-month Consumable Kit (10ml vial adaptor)		
(Kit contains 13 nozzle assemblies, 5 disposable 10ml vial adaptors)		
Size 6 nozzle	MH79002-07	2298
Size 7 nozzle	MH79002-08	2298
mhi-500 3-month Consumable Kit (3ml vial adaptor)		
(Kit contains 13 nozzle assemblies, 15 disposable 3ml vial adaptors)		
Size 6 nozzle	MH79002-12	3512
Size 7 nozzle	MH79002-13	3512
mhi-500 nozzle pack (Contains 6 sterile nozzle assemblies)		
Size 6 nozzle	MH79002-10	766
Size 7 nozzle	MH79002-11	766

†to be deleted 1 April 2007

APPLIANCES

Appliance		Size or Weight	Basic Price p
HYPODERMIC EQUIPMENT			**each**
SQ-Pen Starter Pack			
(System includes 1 needle-free insulin injector, 1 practice nozzle,			
1 sterile nozzle, 1 sterile 3ml vial adaptor, 1 sterile 10ml vial adaptor)			
	SQ 001		14500
SQ-Pen Vial Adaptor Pack			
(Contains 6 sterile vial adaptors)			
3ml vial adaptor	SQ 003		751
10ml vial adaptor	SQ 005		751
SQ-Pen 3-month 3ml Consumable Pack			
(Pack contains 15 x 3ml vial adaptors and 7 nozzles)			
	SQ 004		3023
SQ-Pen 3-month 10ml Consumable Pack			
(Pack contains 5 x 10ml vial adaptors and 7 nozzles)			
	SQ 006		1773
SQ-Pen Nozzle Pack (Contains 6 sterile nozzle assemblies)			
	SQ 002		984
INHALERS			
Spare Tops - mouthpiece and cork			206
See also Atomizers, Hand Operated, Nebulizers			
INSPIRATORY PRESSURE THRESHOLD LOADING DEVICE			
POWERbreathe Medic			1790
INSUFFLATORS			
Cyclohaler (for use with Cyclocaps)			140
Exubera			
Kit (Consists of 1 inhaler, 1 spare chamber, 6 insulin release units)			5268
Insulin Release Units (Box of 6)			910
Chamber			1011
Intal Spinhaler (for use with Intal Spincaps)			192
IRRIGATION SOLUTIONS			
Prontosan	Pod	6 x 40ml	334
(B Braun Medical Ltd)	Bottle	350ml	438
Sodium Chloride 0.9% Irrigation Solution - Sterile			
Flowfusor	Bellows Pack	1 x 120ml	150
(Fresenius Kabi)			
Fresenius Kabi	Pour Bottle	1 x 1000ml	95
Irriclens	Aerosol	1 x 240ml	312
(ConvaTec)			
Irripod	Pod	25 x 20ml	550
(C D Medical Ltd)			
MiniVersol	Bottle	30 x 45ml	1500
(Aguettant Ltd)	Bottle	30 x 100ml	2130
Nine Lives	Can	1 x 200ml	265
(Nine Lives)			
Normasol	Sachet	25 x 25ml	575
(Seton)		10 x 100ml	699
Stericlens	Aerosol	100ml	194
(C D Medical Ltd)		240ml	295
Steripod	Pod	25 x 20ml	708
(Seton)			

APPLIANCES

Appliance		Size or Weight	Basic Price p
IRRIGATION SOLUTIONS			**each**
Water for Irrigation - Sterile			
Baxter Healthcare	Pour Bottle	1 x 500ml	70
	Pour Bottle	1 x 1000ml	80
Fresenius Kabi	Pour Bottle	1 x 1000ml	95
MiniVersol	Bottle	30 x 45ml	1500
(Aguettant Ltd)			
Sterets Aquasol	Sachets	10 x 100ml	825
(Molnlycke Health Care)			
Versol	Bottle	1 x 500ml	90
(Aguettant Ltd)	Bottle	1 x 1000ml	95

Note: *The exact number of containers (ie aerosols, bellows packs, bottles, cans, pods, pour bottles or sachets) ordered by the prescriber is to be dispensed.*

LARYNGECTOMY PROTECTORS - See "Tracheostomy and Laryngectomy Protectors" on page 211.

			per piece
LATEX FOAM, ADHESIVE, raised cotton backed		22.5cm x 45cm	442
Specification 19		7mm thick	
		Box of 4	

Cervical Collar - now listed in Part IXA

LEG ULCER WRAP		**each**
4UlcerCare	28-35cm	1380
	35-43cm	1380
	43-51cm	1380
	51-61cm	1380
	61cm+	1380

LINT

Absorbent Lint BPC		
	25g	82
(Syn: Absorbent Cotton Lint; Cotton Lint; Plain Lint; White Lint)	100g	252
Where no quantity is stated on the prescription form the 25g	500g	1062
pack is to be supplied.		

LUBRICANT GELS

Aquagel Lubricating Jelly (sterile until opened)	5g sachet	18
	42g tube	108
	82g tube	179
Cathejell with Lidocaine	8.5g	120
	12.5g	125
Elite Lubricating Jelly	50ml pump	225
K-Y Jelly (sterile until opened)	42g tube	142
	82g tube	224
Sutherland Lubricating Jelly (sterile until opened)	5g sachet	18
	42g tube	124
	82g tube	194

APPLIANCES

LYMPHOEDEMA GARMENTS

ActiLymph

Style	Lengths	Sizes	
Class 1(18-21mmHg)			**Price per pair**
Below Knee Closed Toe No Top Band	Standard,Petite	S,M,L,XL	2550
Thigh Closed Toe With Top Band	Standard	S,M,L,XL	4900
			Price per piece
Armsleeve No Top Band	Standard	S,M,L	1350
Armsleeve With Top Band	Standard	S,M,L	1800
Combined Armsleeve No Top Band	Standard	S,M,L	2450
Combined Armsleeve With Top band	Standard	S,M,L	2900
Class 2 (23-32mmHg)			**Price per pair**
Below Knee Closed Toe No Top Band	Standard, Petite	S, M, L, XL	2550
Thigh Closed Toe with Top Band	Standard	S, M, L, XL	4900
Below Knee Open Toe No Top Band	Standard, Petite	S, M, L, XL	2550
Thigh Open Toe with Top Band	Standard	S, M, L, XL	4900
			Price per piece
Armsleeve No Top Band	Standard	S, M, L	1450
Armsleeve With Top Band	Standard	S, M, L	1900
Combined Armsleeve No Top Band	Standard	S, M, L	2550
Combined Armsleeve With Top Band	Standard	S, M, L	3000
Class 3 (34-46mmHg)			**Price per pair**
Below Knee Open Toe No Top Band	Standard, Petite	S, M, L, XL	2800
Thigh Open Toe with Top Band	Standard	S, M, L, XL	5100

Jobst Bellavar - Sahara

Style	Lengths	Sizes	
Class 2 (23-32mmHg)			**Price per pair**
Knee High, Open Toe	Short, Long	I, II, III, IV, V, VI	2550
Thigh High, Open Toe, With Knitted Band	Standard	I, II, III, IV, V, VI	4900
Thigh High, Open Toe, With Silicone Band	Standard	I, II, III, IV, V, VI	4900
Class 3 (34-46mmHg)			**Price per pair**
Knee High, Open Toe	Short, Long	I, II, III, IV, V, VI	2800

APPLIANCES

LYMPHOEDEMA GARMENTS
Jobst Elvarex Custom Fit - For lower extremities

Garment Type	Class 1 (18-21mmHg)	Class 2 (23-32mmHg)	Class 3 (34-46mmHg)	Class 3 forte (34-46mmHg)	Class 4 (49-70mmHg)	Class 4 Super (60-90mmHg)
(a) Foot Cap with toes						
Code	L1-01-02	L2-02-02	L3-03-02			
Price per piece	4057	4224	4402			
(b) Knee High						
Code	L1-01-04	L2-02-04	L3-03-04	L3-04-04	L4-05-04	L5-06-04
Price per piece	3165	3314	3610	3714	3866	4046
(c) Thigh High						
Code	L1-01-06	L2-02-06	L3-03-06	L3-04-06	L4-05-06	L5-06-06
Price per piece	3684	4069	4384	4577	4945	5102
(d) Body Bandage						
Code	L1-01-08	L2-02-08	L3-03-08	L3-04-08	L4-05-08	L5-06-08
Price per piece	6507	7198	7487	7534	7836	8089

NB: The above garments are available with additional options. These are priced separately. See below

	Code	Price
Closed Toe	L-A001	10
2 Ankle pads	L-A002	1988
Zipper	L-A003	2043
Silicone band	L-A004	737
Waist attachment with garter belt	L-A005	1577
Leg extension	L-A007	565
Non-standard colour	L-A008	295

NB: *Where Jobst Elvarex garments are prescribed including specifically prescribed additional options, the dispenser must ensure that full details including order codes are clearly endorsed on the FP10. The additional options for the base garments do not attract any additional prescription charges.*

One prescription charge is payable where one or more of the same base garment is supplied. More than one prescription charge is payable if different base garments (including different compression of the same garment type) are ordered
(See Part XVI sub-paragraph 12.13)

Jobst Elvarex Custom Fit - For upper extremities

Garment Type	Class 1 (14-18mmHg)	Class 2 (20-25mmHg)	Class 3 (25-30mmHg)
(a) Gauntlet to Wrist			
Code	U1-01-01	U2-02-01	U3-03-01
Price per piece	3330	3487	3558
(b) Gauntlet to Elbow			
Code	U1-01-03	U2-02-03	U3-03-03
Price per piece	3776	3804	3897
(c) Armsleeve to Axilla with Gauntlet			
Code	U1-01-05	U2-02-05	U3-03-05
Price per piece	6470	6584	6631
(d) Armsleeve from Wrist to Axilla			
Code	U1-01-07	U2-02-07	U3-03-07
Price per piece	2994	3570	3606

NB: The above garments are available with additional options. These are priced separately. See below

	Code	Price
Zipper	U-A001	2043
Silicone band	U-A002	437
Shoulder cap	U-A003	1258
Non-Standard colour	U-A007	295
1finger 14-18mmHg	U1-A009	372
1finger 20-25mmHg	U2-A011	480
1finger 25-30mmHg	U3-A013	495

NB: *Where Jobst Elvarex garments are prescribed including specifically prescribed additional options, the dispenser must ensure that full details including order codes are clearly endorsed on the FP10. The additional options for the base garments do not attract any additional prescription charges.*

One prescription charge is payable where one or more of the same base garment is supplied. More than one prescription charge is payable if different base garments (Including different compression of the same garment type) are ordered.
(See Part XVI sub-paragraph 12.13)

APPLIANCES

LYMPHOEDEMA GARMENTS
Jobst MedicalWear

Garment Type	Class 1 (15-20mmHg)	Class 2 (20-30mmHg)
(a) Armsleeve with Knitted Band		
Small	77149-00003	78608-00001
Medium	77159-00003	78613-00001
Large	77191-00003	78614-00001
Price per piece	1350	1450
(b) Armsleeve with Silicone Band		
Small	77149-00006	78608-00006
Medium	77159-00006	78613-00006
Large	77191-00006	78614-00006
Price per piece	1800	1900
(c) Gauntlet with Thumb		
Small	77192-00003	78609-00001
Medium	77199-00003	78636-00001
Large	77272-00003	78637-00001
Price per piece	1250	1300

Jobst Opaque

Style	Colour	Lengths	Sizes	
Class 1 (18-21mmHg)				**Price per pair**
Knee High Closed Toe	Black, Sand	Short, Long	I, II, III, IV, V, VI	2550
Knee High Open Toe	Black, Sand	Short, Long	I, II, III, IV, V, VI	2550
Thigh High Open Toe with Silicone Band Standard Width	Black, Sand	Short, Long	I, II, III, IV, V, VI	4900
Thigh High Open Toe with Silicone Band Wide Width	Black, Sand	Short, Long	I, II, III, IV, V, VI	4900
Class 2 (23-32mmHg)				**Price per pair**
Knee High Closed Toe	Black, Sand	Short, Long	I, II, III, IV, V, VI	2550
Knee High Open Toe	Black, Sand	Short, Long	I, II, III, IV, V, VI	2550
Thigh High Open Toe with Silicone Band Standard Width	Black, Sand	Short, Long	I, II, III, IV, V, VI	4900
Thigh High Open Toe with Silicone Band Wide Width	Black, Sand	Short, Long	I, II, III, IV, V, VI	4900

Sigvaris
Arm Sleeves

	Lengths	Sizes	Codes	**Price per piece**
Low Compression (12-16mmHg)				
with Grip Top/no Hand Piece	Short, Long	S,M,L	25206-25212	1670
no Grip Top/no Hand Piece	Short, Long	S,M,L	16096-16101	1510
no Grip Top with Hand Piece	Short, Long	S,M,L	16102-16107	2450
with Grip Top/with Hand Piece	Short, Long	S,M,L	25213-25218	2600
Medium Compression (18-22mmHg)				
with Grip Top/no Hand Piece	Short, Long	S,M,L	18718-18723	1670
no Grip Top/no Hand Piece	Short, Long	S,M,L	11040-11045	1510
no Grip Top with Hand Piece	Short, Long	S,M,L	11046-11051	2450
with Grip Top/with Hand Piece	Short, Long	S,M,L	18724-18729	2600
with Shoulder Cap/no Hand Piece	Short, Long	S,M,L	10218-10223	1795
with Shoulder Cap/with Hand Piece	Short, Long	S,M,L	23840-23845	2835

Appliance		Size or Weight	Basic Price p
NASAL DEVICE			**pack of 2**
Nozovent (Anglian Pharma)		Small	500
Nasal dilator to reduce snoring		Medium	500
		Large	500
NASAL DROPS - SODIUM CHLORIDE 0.9%			**each**
Almus Pharmaceuticals	Dropper Bottle	10ml	99
Orbis Consumer Products Ltd	Dropper Bottle	10ml	95
RX Farma	Dropper Bottle	10ml	99
Sandoz	Dropper Bottle	10ml	99
Tubilux Pharma (Tubilux Brand)	Dropper Bottle	10ml	99

IXA

APPLIANCES

Appliance		Size or Weight	Basic Price p
			each
NIPPLE SHIELDS, PLASTICS			58
(Not to be confused with Breast Shields)			
ORAL FILM FORMING AGENTS			
Gelclair		21 x 15ml Sachets	2984
Gengigel	Gel	20ml tube	370
	Mouthrinse	150ml bottle	455
Orabase Paste		30g	198
(Carmellose Gelatin Paste DPF)		100g	440
(This product is also used as a stoma protective)			

PEAK FLOW METERS
syn: P.F.M.
(Non-powered; hand-held)
Portable meters intended for single-patient use.
The standard range is suitable for use by both adults and children.
The low range model is for adults or children with severely restricted airflow.

The Medicines and Healthcare products Regulatory Agency (MHRA) has announced the introduction of a new standard for Peak Flow Meters and published a Medical Device Alert providing further information in June 2004. The Peak Flow Meters standard range will conform to the EU standard EN 13826.
The Peak Flow Meters low range will be CE marked and comply with EN 13826 in all aspects except for a reduced measurement range.
The new products will be available on 1 September 2004.
Contractors should note that the Drug Tariff Specification 51 standard and low range Peak Flow Meters were deleted on 1 September 2004 and are replaced with devices conforming to the new standard.
From 1 September 2004 only those Peak Flow Meters meeting the new standard can be prescribed, dispensed and reimbursed.
The Department of Health has been closely monitoring the continuity of supply of Drug Tariff Specification 51 Peak Flow Meters. This monitoring has indicated that there is no need for additional guidance on the reimbursement of these meters.

Manufacturer	Order No.	Basic Price p
		each
Standard Range EN 13826		
Clement Clarke	3103388	686
Ferraris PiKo-1	346005-EU	950
Ferraris Pocket Peak	208(EU)/F	653
Micro Medical	MPE8200EU	650
Respironics	755EU	686
Vitalograph	43602	475
Vitalograph Child	43703	475
Low Range CE marked (must comply with the EN 13826 except for scale range)		
Clement Clarke	3104708	690
Ferraris Pocket Peak	209(EU)/F	653
Respironics	756EU	690

N.B:
1. *"Low range" to be supplied only where specifically ordered.*
2. *Where the brand or manufacturer is not stated by the prescriber and has not been endorsed, the basic price must not exceed 475p (Standard range) and 653p (Low Range).*
3. *Replacement recording charts (FP1010) are given by the prescribing doctor; they are also available from pharmacists.*

Replacement Mouthpiece (Plastics)
(Not interchangeable between brands or manufacturers)

Replacement mouthpiece - suitable for both standard and low range models for use by adults or children	
Clement Clarke	38
Ferraris	38
Micro Medical	38
Vitalograph	40

APPLIANCES

Appliance	Size or Weight	Basic Price p
PESSARIES		**each**
Ring		
Polythene	7.5mm thick, 50-80mm	
Specification 20(ii)	(rising in 3mm)	
	7.5mm thick, 80-100mm	181
	(rising in 5mm)	
	7.5mm thick, 110mm	
PVC	1.25cm thick, 50-80mm	
Specification 20(iii)	(rising in 3mm)	
	1.25cm thick, 85-100mm	196
	(rising in 5mm)	
	1.25cm thick, 110mm	
PLASTERS		
Belladonna Adhesive Plaster BP 1980	Medium	
(Syn: Belladonna Self-Adhesive Plaster;	19cm x 12.5cm	81
Belladonna Plaster)	Large	
	28cm x 17.5cm	140
PROTECTIVES		
Hand		
EMA Film Gloves-Disposable Specification 21		
Dispos-A-Gloves (non-sterile)	Small, Medium, Large	**pack of 30**
		230
		pack of 100
		314
		pack of 25
Gloves - Polythene, 100 gauge		53
(Polythene Occlusives, Disposable For use as occlusives with medicated creams.)		
Limb		**each**
LIMBO Waterproof Protector - Adult 1/2 leg		
MP80	Normal build	1020
MP80S	Normal build, short leg	1020
MP180	Large build	1020
MP180S	Large build, short leg	1020
Seal-Tight wound care protector		
CV27105	Adult foot/ankle	1050
CV27103	Adult short leg	1050
CV27106	Adult wide short leg	1050
SODIUM HYALURONATE CREAM		
Xclair	50g	1700

IXA

APPLIANCES

Appliance	Size or Weight	Basic Price p

STOCKINETTE

When Elasticated Stockinette is ordered or prescribed without qualification, the term is to be interpreted as Elasticated Tubular Bandage.

		each
Cotton Stockinette, Bleached BP 1988 Heavyweight	2.5cm x 1m	32
(Syn: Cotton Stockinette)	5cm x 1m	49
	7.5cm x 1m	60
	10cm x 6m	406

Elasticated Tubular Bandage BP
(Elasticated Surgical Tubular Stockinette; ESTS; Elasticated Stockinette)

Size	6.25 cm		6.75 cm		7.5 cm		8.75 cm		10.0 cm		12.0 cm	
Ref	B	B	C	C	D	D	E	E	F	F	G	G
Quantity	0.5m (p)	1m (p)	0.5m (p)	1m (p)	0.5m (p)	1m (p)	0.5m (p)	1m (p)	0.5m (p)	1m (p)	0.5m (p)	1m (p)
Comfigrip	63	114	67	121	67	121	76	130	76	130	79	153
easiGRIP	61	110	65	117	65	117	74	126	74	126	77	147
Eesiban ESTS	79	143	86	151	86	151	95	164	95	164	99	190
Sigma ETB	61	110	65	117	66	119	74	126	74	126	77	147
Tubigrip	88	159	96	168	96	168	106	182	106	182	110	211

1. Where the quantity is not stated by the prescriber the 0.5 metre length should be supplied.
2. Where the size is not stated by the prescriber, the size supplied should be endorsed.
3. Where the brand is not stated by the prescriber the basic price of this stockinette must not exceed:

Size and Quantity	each (p)		each (p)		each (p)
6.25cm x 0.5m	61	7.5cm x 0.5m	65	10.00cm x 0.5m	74
6.25cm x 1.0m	110	7.5cm x 1.0m	117	10.00cm x 1.0m	126
6.75cm x 0.5m	65	8.75cm x 0.5m	74	12.00cm x 0.5m	77
6.75cm x 1.0m	117	8.75cm x 1.0m	126	12.00cm x 1.0m	147

Appliance		Size or Weight	Basic Price p
Elasticated Surgical Tubular Stockinette Foam Padded			each
(Tubipad)			
Specification 25			
Heel, Elbow,Knee			
	small 'P4'	6.5cm x 60cm	268
	medium 'P4X'	7.5cm x 60cm	289
	large 'P5'	10cm x 60cm	309
Sacral			
	medium 'P9'	28cm x 27cm	1382
	large 'P9'	35cm x 27cm	1382

APPLIANCES

STOCKINETTE

Elasticated Viscose Stockinette - Bandage
(Lightweight Elasticated Viscose Tubular Bandage)

Size		Basic Price (p) Each				
		Acti-Fast	Comfifast	Coverflex	Easifast	Tubifast
Small Limb 3.5cm (Red Line)	1m	62	64	73	65	82
Medium Limb 5.0cm (Green Line)	1m	65	68	76	69	88
	3m	190	194	224	195	252
	5m	330	333	387	340	431
Large Limb 7.5cm (Blue Line)	1m	90	92	107	94	118
	3m	250	256	254	260	332
	5m	440	447	504	450	579
Trunk (Child) 10.75cm (Yellow Line)	1m	145	146	168	150	189
	3m	410	417	483	425	541
	5m	710	716	850	720	928
Trunk (Adult) 17.5cm (Beige Line)	1m	215	184	224	190	238
Trunk (Large Adult) 25cm (Purple Line)	1m	-	-	-	-	390
	5m	-	-	-	-	1911

Elasticated Viscose Stockinette - Garments

Appliance	Size	Basic Price p	
		Comfifast Easywrap	Tubifast
		each	
Clava	6 months-5 years	650	-
	5-14 years	750	-
Vest	6-24 months	792	1027
	2-5 years	1056	1369
	5-8 years	1188	1540
	8-11 years	1320	1711
	11-14 years	1320	1711
		per pair	
Tights	6-24 months	792	1027
Leggings	2-5 years	1056	1369
	5-8 years	1188	1540
	8-11 years	1320	1711
	11-14 years	1320	1711
Socks	One Size	-	428
	Up to 8 years	330	-
	8-14 years	330	-
Mittens	Up to 24 months	330	-
	2-8 years	330	-
	8-14 years	330	-
Gloves	Medium Child	-	525
	Large Child, Small Adult	-	525
	Medium Adult	-	525
	Large Adult	-	525

APPLIANCES

Appliance	Size or Weight	Basic Price p
STOCKINETTE		**each**
Ribbed Cotton and Viscose Surgical Tubular Stockinette BP 1988		
(Syn: Ribbed Cotton and Viscose Stockinette)		
Type A Lightweight (Molnlycke) (formerly Seton)		
Arm/leg (child); arm (adult)	5cm x 5m	230
Arm (OS adult); leg (adult)	7.5cm x 5m	302
Leg (OS adult)	10cm x 5m	401
Trunk (child)	15cm x 5m	577
Trunk (adult)	20cm x 5m	667
Trunk (OS adult)	25cm x 5m	797

Type B Heavyweight (Eesiban) (see Ribbed Cotton Surgical Tubular Stockinette - Eesiban)

Ribbed Cotton Surgical Tubular Stockinette
Eesiban

Arm/leg (child); arm (adult)	5cm x 5m	230
Arm (OS adult); leg (adult)	7.5cm x 5m	302
Leg (OS adult)	10cm x 5m	401
Trunk (child)	15cm x 5m	577
Trunk (adult)	20cm x 5m	667
Trunk (OS adult)	25cm x 5m	797

NB:
One 5m length of the relevant width is sufficient to provide two sets of dressing for a pair of limbs or a trunk.
Two full suits for an OS adult are provided from one pack each of the 7.5cm, 10cm and 25cm widths.
Two full suits for a standard sized adult are provided from one pack each of the 5cm, 7.5cm and 20cm widths.
Two full suits for a young child are provided from one pack each of the 5cm and 15cm widths.

SUPRAPUBIC BELTS: Replacements Only   Invoice Price
                                                        (see note 5) (page 135)

    N.B Original Belts are supplied by the Hospital Service.

       Prescription ordering replacement of a complete Belt or Outfit may only be accepted by a pharmacy or appliance contractor who will carry out the actual measurement, fitting and supply of the belt.

       Orders for replacement of "a belt" are to be taken as being for the belt alone and the prescription referred back to the prescriber to specify orders for a Complete Belt or Outfit where such appears to be required.

       Parts may include the following:

       Rubber Flaps

       Rubber Shields

       Rubber Understraps

       Rubber Urinal, single or double-chambered (See Incontinence Appliances)

       Belt Webbing

       Night Drainage Bag, Plastics (See Incontinence Appliances)

       Night Tube and Glass or Plastics Connector

APPLIANCES

Appliance	Size or Weight	Basic Price p
SURGICAL ADHESIVE TAPES		**each**
Elastic Adhesive Tape BP 1988	2.5cm x 4.5m	158
(Syn: Elastic Surgical Adhesive Tape)	stretched	
	5cm x 4.5m	
	(See Elastic Adhesive Bandage)	
Impermeable Plastic Adhesive Tape BP 1988	2.5cm x 3m	125
(Syn: Impermeable Plastic Surgical Adhesive Tape)	2.5cm x 5m	187
	5cm x 5m	237
	7.5cm x 5m	345
Impermeable Plastic Synthetic Adhesive Tape BP 1988	2.5cm x 5m	172
(Syn: Impermeable Plastic Surgical Synthetic Adhesive Tape)	5cm x 5m	327
(Blenderm)		
Permeable Woven Synthetic Adhesive Tape BP 1988	1.25cm x 5m	74
(Syn: Permeable Woven Surgical Synthetic Adhesive Tape)	2.5cm x 5m	107
(Leukosilk)	5cm x 5m	187

Permeable Non-Woven Synthetic Adhesive Tape BP 1988
(Syn: Permeable Non-Woven Surgical Synthetic adhesive Tape)l

Size	1.25 cm		2.5 cm		5 cm		7.5 cm	
Quantity	5m	10m	5m	10m	5m	10m	5m	10m
	(p)	(p)	(p)	(p)	(p)	(p)	(p)	(p)
Clinipore	35	-	59	-	99	-	-	-
Leukofix	51	-	81	-	142	-	-	-
Leukopore	45	-	70	-	123	-	-	-
Mediplast	30	-	50	-	-	-	-	-
Micropore	60	-	89	-	157	-	-	-
Scanpor	40	52	64	86	111	164	-	240

Where no brand is stated by the prescriber, the basic price of the tape supplied must not exceed

	1.25cm x 5m	30
	2.5cm x 5m	50
	5cm x 5m	99

Permeable, Apertured Non-Woven Synthetic Adhesive Tape BP 1988
(Syn:Permeable Non-Woven Surgical Synthetic Adhesive Tape)

Hypafix	2.5cm x 10m	153
	5cm x 10m	244
	10cm x 10m	425
	15cm x 10m	630
	20cm x 10m	835
	30cm x 10m	1207
Mefix	2.5cm x 5m	91
	5cm x 5m	161
	10cm x 5m	258
	15cm x 5m	352
	20cm x 5m	451
	30cm x 5m	647
Omnifix	5cm x 10m	215
	10cm x 10m	362
	15cm x 10m	534

IXA

APPLIANCES

Appliance	Size or Weight	Basic Price p
SURGICAL ADHESIVE TAPES		**each**
Soft Silicone Fixation Tape		
Mepitac	2cm x 3m	614
	4cm x 1.5m	614
Zinc Oxide Adhesive Tape		
(Zinc Oxide Surgical Adhesive Tape)		
Mediplast - Zinc Oxide Plaster	1.25cm x 5m	82
	2.5cm x 5m	119
	5cm x 5m	199
	7.5cm x 5m	299
Strappal	1.25cm x 5m	87
	2.5cm x 5m	126
	5cm x 5m	213
	7.5cm x 5m	321
Zinc Oxide Adhesive Tape BP 1988	1.25cm x 5m	89
(Syn: Zinc Oxide Surgical Adhesive Tape)	2.5cm x 5m	129
	5cm x 5m	219
	7.5cm x 5m	329

SURGICAL SUTURES

Ethicon Code No.	Metric Gauge	Length	Needle	Basic Price p

Absorbable Sutures
Sterile Synthetic

Ethicon Monocryl Poliglecaprone absorbable sutures composed of a copolymer of glycolide ε-caprolactone:

Ethicon Code No.	Metric Gauge	Length	Needle	pack of 12
W3650	2.0	70cm	60mm straight cutting	2752

Ethicon Vicryl-polyglactin 910 absorbable sutures composed of copolymer of glycolide and lactide

				pack of 36
W9505H	1.0	45cm	16mm P needle curved cutting	10191
				pack of 12
W9074	1.5	45cm	16mm curved round bodied	2364
				pack of 36
W9570H	1.5	75cm	19mm P needle curved cutting	10124
W9525H	2.0	45cm	26mm P needle curved reverse cutting	9707

Ethicon Vicryl Rapide-polyglactin 910 absorbable sutures composed of copolymer of glycolide and lactide which have been specially treated to give rapid strength loss and absorption profiles:

				pack of 12
W9915	1.0	45cm	12mm P needle curved reverse cutting	4344
W9922	1.5	75cm	19mm P needle curved reverse cutting	3941
W9918	1.5	75cm	16mm P needle curved cutting	3487
W9932	2.0	75cm	26mm P needle curved reverse cutting	3665
W9923	2.0	75cm	19mm P needle curved reverse cutting	3641
W9962	3.0	90cm	35mm tapercut half circle	3694

APPLIANCES

Ethicon Code No.	Metric Gauge	Length		Needle	Basic Price p
Non Absorbable Sutures					
Sterile Braided Silk Suture					
W501H	1.5	75cm	(black) 16mm curved cutting		**pack of 36** 3906
W321H	3.0	45cm	(black) 26mm curved reverse cutting		3793
W2511T	2.0	45cm	(black) 26mm P needle curved reverse cutting		**pack of 24** 3290
Sterile Polyamide Synthetic Suture					
W1618T	1.0	45cm	19mm P needle curved reverse cutting		3866
Sterile Polyamide 6 Suture, Monofilament					
W319	1.5	45cm	(blue) 19mm curved reverse cutting		**pack of 12** 1302
W320	2.0	45cm	(blue) 26mm curved reverse		1346
W1615T	0.7	45cm	(black) 16mm P needle curved cutting		**pack of 24** 3780
Sterile Polyamide 66 Suture, Braided					
W5414	3.5	1m	(black) 50mm tapercut half circle heavy		**pack of 12** 1863
Sterile Polypropylene Suture, Monofilament					
W8020T	1.5	45cm	(blue) 26mm P needle curved cutting		**pack of 24** 4461

Appliance	Size or Weight	Basic Price p
Skin Adhesives, Sterile		**each**
● Dermabond	0.5ml	1036
Dermabond ProPen	0.5ml pen	1838
● Epiglu	Four vials (containing approx 80 applications)	9500
Histoacryl	0.2g	641
	0.5g	650
Histoacryl L	0.2g	620
	0.5g	672
Indermil	0.5g	650
LiquiBand - Adhesive	0.5g	550
- Flow Control Tissue Adhesive	0.5g	550

Note:These items are specifically for personal administration by the prescriber.

● This product is no longer available from the manufacturer but will remain reimbursable until such time that stocks run out or the product expiry dates are passed.

Skin Closure Strips, Sterile

Leukostrip	Code No. 2952	6.4mm x 76mm 3 strips per env.	**10 envelopes** 557
Steri-strip	Code No.GP 41	6mm x 75mm 3 strips per env.	**12 envelopes** 852

Note:These items are specifically for personal administration by the prescriber.

APPLIANCES

Appliance	Size or Weight	Basic Price p
SWABS (see note * below on sterile swabs)		

N.B. *The exact number of single swabs ordered by the prescriber is to be dispensed.(see also Note (ii) below)*

Gauze Swabs   **pkt**

Gauze Swab Type 13 Light BP 1988, Sterile*   7.5cm sq   36
Sterile swabs of folded 8-ply undyed gauze   5 pads per pkt

Gauze Swab Type 13 Light BP 1988, Non Sterile   10cm sq   126
Swabs of folded 8-ply undyed gauze   100 pads per pkt

Filmated Gauze Swab BP 1988 Non Sterile   10cm sq   338
A thin layer of absorbent cotton enclosed within Absorbent   100 pads per pkt
Cotton Gauze Type 13 Light BP 1988 8-ply

Non-Woven Fabric Swabs
The labelling of each pack shall include:
> The Title
> "Drug Tariff Specification" and number

Non-Woven Fabric Swab, Sterile*   7.5cm sq   23
Specification 28   5 pads per pkt
Sterile swabs of folded 4-ply non-woven fabric. These swabs are an alternative to gauze swabs, Type 13
Light BP 1988 sterile.

Non-Woven Fabric Swab, Non Sterile   10cm sq   73
Specification 28   100 pads per pkt
Swabs of folded 4-ply non woven fabric. These swabs are an alternative to gauze swabs, Type 13 Light
BP 1988, for general and cleansing purposes.

Filmated Non-Woven Fabric Swab Non-Sterile   10cm sq   338
(Regal)   100 pads per pkt
Specification 29
Swabs of folded 8-ply non-woven viscose fabric containing a film of viscose fibres to increase absorbency.
These swabs are an alternative to Filmated Gauze Swabs BP 1988 for general swabbing and cleansing
purposes.

*Notes: Sterile Swabs
*(i) These sterile dressings are to be supplied in packs of 5 swabs 7.5cm square in a sealed packs as
received from the manufacturer, supplier or wholesaler. They should not be confused with the non-sterile
10cm size in packets of 100 swabs used for general swabbing purposes.*
*(ii) The exact number of sterile swabs ordered are to be supplied except for orders not in multiples of 5
(See Note 2 page 135). A packet to be used for each sterile dressing operation; unused swabs to be
discarded as unsterile.*

SYNOVIAL FLUID   **each**

Durolane	Box containing 1 pre-filled 3ml syringe	19200
Fermathron	Box containing 1 pre-filled 20mg/2ml syringe	3900
Orthovisc	Box containing 1 pre-filled 2ml syringe	6500
Ostenil	Box containing 1 pre-filled 20mg/2ml syringe	3000
Suplasyn	Box containing 1 pre-filled 20mg/2ml syringe	3550
	Box containing 1 vial 20mg/2ml	3550
Synocrom	Box containing 1 pre-filled 20mg/2ml syringe	3000
Synvisc (Hylan G-F20)	Box containing 3 pre-filled 2ml syringes (1 treatment)	20500

SYRINGES

Bladder/Irrigating	100ml	400
Ear Syringe	60ml approx	181
Enema Higginson's:		584
Spare Vaginal Pipes Plastics	15cm	47
or rubber, straight		

APPLIANCES

Appliance		Order No.	Basic Price p
TRACHEOSTOMY AND LARYNGECTOMY APPLIANCES			**each**
Tracheostomy Breathing Aids			
Blom-Singer Hands-Free ATSV II System (formerly Blom-Singer Truseal HumidiFilter system)			
Blom-Singer ATSV II Cap & 7 Foam Filters		BE1010	1731
Replacement Foam Filters for ATSV II		BE1020/1030	97
Silicone Adhesive (for use with baseplates)		BE6067	2400
Blom-Singer HumidiFilter HME System (formerly Blom-Singer Truseal HumidiFilter System)			
Adhesive Housing (Baseplates) see TruSeal Adhesive Housing			
Blom-Singer HumidiFilter Starter Kit		BE1050	3450
Blom-Singer HumidiFilter Holder		BE1060	1324
Replacement Foam Filters (normal resistance)		BE1070/1080	97
TruSeal Adhesive Housing (formerly Adhesive Housing (Baseplates))		BE6053/6054	207
Tracheostoma Valve Housing	Standard	BE6038	600
	Large	BE6039	600
Adhesive Tape Discs	Standard Regular	BE6041	40
	Large Regular	BE6042	43
	Standard Thin	BE6043	53
	Large Thin	BE6044	57
	Standard Heavy Duty	BE6034	53
	Large Heavy Duty	BE6035	57
Adhesive Foam Discs	Standard Regular	BE6045	80
	Large Regular	BE6046	100
	Standard Thin	BE6047	100
	Large Thin	BE6049	110

Blom-Singer Truseal HumidiFilter System
  see Blom-Singer HumidiFilter HME System and Blom-Singer Hands-Free ATSV II System

Humistom Stoma Button/Stud and HPC Filter (Nasal Restoration System)			
HPC Filter Normal to low resistance		HSF1	290
Humistom Stoma Button/Stud	size 10	HS1-L10	1000
Standard Length 20mm	size 12	HS1-L12	1000
	size 14	HS1-L14	1000
Short Length 14mm	size 10	HS1-S10	1000
	size 12	HS1-S12	1000
	size 14	HS1-S14	1000

Provox FreeHands HME System			
Filter Cassette		7712	211
Replacement Kit	Light	7716	20150
(Device & Fitted Membrane)	Medium	7717	20150
	Strong	7721	20150
Replacement Membrane	Light	7713	4615
	Medium	7714	4615
	Strong	7715	4615
Silicone Glue (for use with Flexiderm adhesive)		7720	2340

Provox HME System ("Stomafilter")			
Flexiderm adhesive round	(Transparent with strong	7253	271
Flexiderm adhesive oval	adhesive)	7254	271
Optiderm adhesive round	(Skin coloured,	7255	446
Optiderm adhesive oval	hydrocolloid for sensitive	7256	446
	skin)		
Regular adhesive round	(Transparent, normal	7251	175
Regular adhesive oval	adhesive)	7252	175

IXA

APPLIANCES

Appliance		Order No.	Basic Price p
TRACHEOSTOMY AND LARYNGECTOMY APPLIANCES			**each**
Normal filter cassette	(Normal resistance)	7240	164
Hiflow filter cassette	(Low resistance for sport and first time users)	7241	175
Purifoam Laryngectomy Filters		CR3853	36
Saint Marina Safety Net Air filter and humidifier		SMSN	160
Trachi-Naze Nasal Restoration System			
Blue Filter (Night filter)	resistance level -2 to -3kPas 1^{-1}	LANNZ 0001A	158
Green Filter (Day filter)	resistance level -1 to 2kPas 1^{-2}	LANNZ 0002A	158
Orange Filter (Active filter)	resistance level less than -1kPas 1^{-1}	LANNZ 0003A	158
Baseplate			
Hydrocolloid	(small)	LANNZ 0004A	249
Hydrocolloid	(large)	LANNZ 0005	266
Non-Woven Adhesive	(large)	LANNZ 0006	266
Clear Adhesive Waterproof Film	(round)	LANNZ 0007	260
Hands Free Valve 'Type A' (for replacement only)		LATNV 1001	8000
Hands Free Valve 'Type B' (for replacement only)		LATNV 2001	8000
			pack of 3
Occlusion Cap		LATNV 3001	1000
Trachi-Naze Plus Nasal Restoration System			**each**
Trachi-Naze Plus Filters			
Blue (Night Filter)	resistance level -2 to 3kPas 1^{-1}	LATNP 1001	158
Green (Day Filter)	resistance level -1 to 2kPas 1^{-2}	LATNP 1002	158
Orange (Active Filter)	resistance level -1kPas 1^{-1}	LATNP 1003	158
Trachi-Naze Plus Stoma Stud			
Short Length 14.5mm	size 8	LATNP 2001	1053
	size 10	LATNP 2002	1053
	size 12	LATNP 2003	1053
	size 14	LATNP 2004	1053
	size 16	LATNP 2005	1053
Long Length 22.5mm	size 8	LATNP 3001	1053
	size 10	LATNP 3002	1053
	size 12	LATNP 3003	1053
	size 14	LATNP 3004	1053
	size 16	LATNP 3005	1053
Tracheostomy Cleaning Devices			
Tracheostomy Cannula Cleaning Swabs			**pack of 10**
(Insight Medical Products Ltd)			
	Small	TCS/950	170
	Large	TCS/900	170
Tracheo Cleaning Brush			**pack of 2**
(Kapitex)	8mm	TR ACC 0001	345
	10mm	TR ACC 0002	345
	12mm	TR ACC 0003	345
	14mm	TR ACC 0004	345

APPLIANCES

Appliance			Order No.	Basic Price p
TRACHEOSTOMY AND LARYNGECTOMY APPLIANCES				**each**
Tracheostomy Dressings - Sterile				
Advadress 'T'		80mm x 80mm	CR3854	64
Excilon AMD IV Sponges		5cm x 5cm	7089	9
		10cm x 10cm	7088	23
Note: This dressing is in 2 pieces but is a single dressing				
Metalline		8cm x 9cm		49
Trachi-Dress	Small	60mm x 82mm	TR DRE 0001	67
	Large	80mm x100mm	TR DRE 0002	67
Tracheostomy Tube Holders				
EMS Adjustable Tracheostomy Tube Holder with Elasticated Cough Strip			T550	265
Insight 2 Piece Adjustable Latex Free Tracheostomy Tube Holder				
	Adult		TH100	240
	Child		TH150	240
Trachi-Hold	Adult		TR ACC 0012	295
	Child		TR ACC 0014	295
Tracheostomy and Laryngectomy Protectors				
Buchanan Protector				
(Laryngectomy - Permanent tracheostomy)				**pack of 10**
	Small			3257
	Large			3533
Buchanan DeltaNex Protector				
(Laryngectomy - Permanent tracheostomy)				
	Small			3291
Cascade Shower Protector				**pack of 2**
			AS/3835	740
Hirst Protector				**pack of 10**
				2885
Laryngofoam				**pack of 30**
flesh or white	5.1cm x 6.2cm 4mm thick			1166
flesh	6.3cm x 6.5cm			1166
				each
				39
Sofnex Laryngectomy Shield				**pack of 10**
(contains 2 neckbands)				
	Beige		CR3860	3020
	Blue		CR3859	3020
	White		CR3856	2900
Sofshield Laryngectomy Protectors				
(Laryngectomy - Permanent tracheostomy)				
White	Small		AS3698	2890
	Large		AS3669	3200
Beige	Small		AS3778	3016
	Large		AS3765	3400
Blue	Small		AS3777	3016
	Large		AS3764	3400
Wet Protect				**pack of 2**
			TWP2	852
Voice Prosthesis Cleaning Brush				**pack of 10**
Insight			PB/50	720
Voiceline			LA PCB 0003	800

IXA

APPLIANCES

Appliance	Size or Weight	Basic Price p
TRUSSES		**each**

(See Part 1, Clause 2 page 3)
Before the prescription can be dispensed three details must be given by the prescriber:
(i) Single, or double, and the side, if single
(ii) Position, eg. Inguinal; Scrotal
(iii) Type, eg. truss; Elastic band truss

In the event of a dispute between the patient and the pharmacy or the appliance contractor about whether the truss supplied is satisfactory, the doctor's decision shall be binding.

Spring Truss

		each
Specification 31(a)		
Spring Trusses shall conform to the British Standard 2930: 1970 for Surgical Spring Trusses		
Inguinal	Single	2967
	Double	4140
Inguinal Rat-tail	Single	3653
	Double	5459
Femoral	Single	3277
	Double	5070
Scrotal	Single	3653
	Double	5459
Double Inguinal/Scrotal		5250
Back Pad, fixed or sliding (if ordered)	extra	842
Slotted, polished Spring Ends (if ordered)	Single Extra	428
	Double Extra	862
"Special" Trusses	Single Extra	945
- conforming to the requirements in Specification 31b	Double Extra	1866

NB:Requirement for a "Special" Truss should normally be confirmed by the prescriber.

Replacements and repairs:-

Understrap for Inguinal or Femoral Trusses		260

Elastic Band Truss

Specification 31b		
Elastic Band Trusses shall conform to the British Standard 3271: 1970 for Surgical Elastic Band Trusses		
Inguinal	Single	2015
	Double	3356
Scrotal	Single	2097
	Double	3416
Umbilical, Single Belt	Single	2288
Double Belt where specified by prescriber	Double	3115
"Special" Trusses	Single Extra	592
- conforming to the requirements in Specification 31b	Double Extra	858

NB:Requirement for a "Special" Truss should normally be confirmed by the prescriber

APPLIANCES

Appliance	Order No.	Basic Price p

VACUUM PUMPS AND CONSTRICTOR RINGS FOR ERECTILE DYSFUNCTION

The following products may be ordered on a prescription form (ie prescribed "on the NHS") only if the patient is a person of a description mentioned in column 1 of the prescribing restrictions note below, and for the purpose specified in column 2 of that note, and if the prescriber endorses the face of the prescription form with the reference "SLS".

Vacuum Pumps

Euro Surgical Ltd

Pos-T-Vac	AVP1000 Battery Operated	12700
	MVP 700 Manual	9800

Farnhurst Medical Ltd

Elite	ES101	13500
Elite Plus with gauge	EG105	16000
Elite Plus 2 with limiter	EL108	16000

Genesis Medical Ltd

Active II with limiter	0100 Battery Operated	14900
Impulse with limiter	0102 Manual	11900

Healthcare 2000 Ltd

E.I.D. Erection Inducer Device		14900

iMedicare Ltd

SomaCorrect	15080	15900
SomaCorrect Xtra	15111	17900
SomaErect Response II	15019	16081
SomaErect Response II - XL	15888	16081
SomaErect Touch II	15013	16900

Mediplus Ltd (formerly Osbon Medical UK)

Osbon ErecAid Classic	XX-02	9900
Osbon ErecAid Esteem	XX-50	17900

Mediwatch UK Ltd

ErectEase	S0001	9400

Osbon Medical UK see Mediplus Ltd

Owen Mumford Ltd

Rapport Classic	SM2000	10511
Rapport Premier	SM2200	16030

Vetco UK

Vetex Pump System	001 Manual	9500

Constrictor Rings - to maintain an erection

Euro Surgical Ltd

Constrictor Ring		968

Farnhurst Medical Ltd

Constriction Rings (pack of 5 rings)	Sizes 1-5	ECR01	2000
	Size 1	ECR01/1	2000
	Size 2	ECR01/2	2000
	Size 3	ECR01/3	2000
	Size 4	ECR01/4	2000
	Size 5	ECR01/5	2000
Applicator and cone set with 5 different sized rings		ECA02	2400

Genesis Medical Ltd

Asset

Set of 5 different rings, loading cone, and holding cylinder for maintaining an erection	0105	2400

Genesis constriction ring

Single ring for use with erection assistance devices 0110B, 0110C, 0110D, 0110E, 0110F,	Sizes B,C,D,E,F	700

IXA

APPLIANCES

Appliance		Order No.	Basic Price p
VACUUM PUMPS AND CONSTRICTOR RINGS FOR ERECTILE DYSFUNCTION			
Healthcare 2000 Ltd			
Confidence Rings			
Starter pack of 2 Rings (1x Regular, 1x Firm)			2400
Firm x 2 Rings (Pink)			2900
Regular x 2 Rings (Natural)			2900
iMedicare Ltd			
Assist Erection Maintenance System		15109	2700
Select Erection Maintenance Ring Set (Set of 3 rings)		15230	2900
SureEase Erection Maintenance Ring Set		15085	3200
Ultimate Erection Maintenance Ring Set		15222	3400
Ultra Erection Maintenance Ring Set		15444	3400
Mediwatch UK Ltd			
ErectAssist			
Set of 3 retention rings, loading cone, transfer collar and lubricating gel		S0007	2300
Retention Rings			
Set of 3 retention rings			
25mm		S0101A	2100
32mm		S0101B	2100
40mm		S0101C	2100
1 of each of the above sizes		S0101	2100
Owen Mumford Ltd			
Rapport Ring Loading System			
Set of 5 different sized rings, loading cone and transfer sleeves for maintaining an erection		SM2220	2101
Vetco UK Constriction Rings			
White C-Flex	(small, medium, large)	VA005	650
Mentor	(medium, large)	VA006	1000
Comfort	(one size fits all)	VA007	1000

PRESCRIBING RESTRICTIONS APPLYING TO VACUUM PUMPS AND CONSTRICTOR RINGS FOR ERECTILE DYSFUNCTION

The products listed may be ordered on a prescription form (ie prescribed "on the NHS") only if the patient is a person of a description mentioned in column 1 below, and for the purpose specified in column 2, and if the prescriber endorses the face of the prescription form with the reference "SLS".

Patient	Purpose
(a) a man who is suffering from any of the following -	Treatment of erectile dysfunction.

    diabetes
    multiple sclerosis
    Parkinson's disease
    poliomyelitis
    prostate cancer
    severe pelvic injury
    single gene neurological disease
    spina bifida
    spinal cord injury; or

(b) a man who is receiving treatment for renal failure by dialysis; or

(c) a man who has had the following surgery -
    prostatectomy
    radical pelvic surgery
    renal failure treated by transplant.

Appliance		Size or Weight	Basic Price p
VAGINAL DILATORS			**per kit**
Amielle Comfort		SM2100	3400
(Owen Mumford Ltd)			
Femmax		MDTi4006	1500
(Medical Devices Technology International Ltd)			

VAGINAL MOISTURISERS

			per pack
● *Replens MD*		3 dose pack	282
		6 dose pack	452
		35g tube	452

● Please note: For reimbursement purposes Replens MD should not be confused with the product Replens listed in Drug Tariff Part XVIIIA - Drugs and other substances not to be prescribed under the NHS Pharmaceutical Services

VENOUS ULCER COMPRESSION SYSTEM

Activa Leg Ulcer	Medical Stocking & Compression Liner		
Hosiery Kit	(pack contains 1 stocking and 2 liners)		
(Activa Healthcare)	Small, Medium, Large, Extra Large, Extra Extra Large		1999
	Compression Liner pack (formerly Liner pack)		
	(pack contains 3 liners)		
	Small, Medium, Large, Extra Large, Extra Extra Large		1499
Jobst UlcerCARE	Medical Stocking & Compression Liner	Small	2961
(BSN medical Ltd)	(pack contains 1 stocking and 1 liner)	Medium	2961
		Large	2961
		Extra Large	2961
	Compression Liner pack	Small	1788
	(pack contains 3 liners)	Medium	1788
		Large	1788
		Extra Large	1788
Jobst UlcerCARE Custom	Medical Stocking		6000
(BSN medical Ltd)	Compression Liner pack (pack contains 2 liners)		3000

SurePress Comfort Pro Graduated Compression System
(ConvaTec Ltd) (pack contains 1 stocking and 1 liner)

Size	Ankle Circ	Calf Circ	
A	18-20cm	25.5-33cm	2801
B	20-22.5cm	30.5-38cm	2801
C	22.5-25.5cm	35.5-43cm	2801
D	25.5-28cm	40.5-48.5cm	2801
E	28-30.5cm	45.5-53cm	2801

Ulcertec	Medical Stocking & Compression Liner		
(Bauerfeind UK)	(pack contains 1 stocking & 2 liners)		
	Short (Small, Medium or Large)		2710
	Long (Small, Medium or Large)		2710

IXA

APPLIANCES

This Page is Intentionally Blank

INCONTINENCE APPLIANCES

1. Prescribers and suppliers should note that products not included in the list are not prescribable (See Part 1 Clause 2). Attention is drawn particularly to the information on the average life-in-use of each type of product which, together with the pack size, should enable prescribers to calculate their patients' requirements with reasonable accuracy.

2. Only basic information on each product has been provided and prescribers may on occasions wish to seek further information about certain products eg when assessing a patient for the first time. If so, this is always available from the manufacturers (addresses and telephone numbers are given at the end of the entry). Information may also be sought from community nurses and community pharmacists. Where possible manufacturers'/suppliers' order code numbers have been shown but prescribers should note that the order numbers shown are not necessarily the full codes for the appliances they wish to order. This is particularly true of urinal systems where additional code numbers are usually necessary to denote variations from the basic design and individual sizes.

3. Prescribers are reminded that incontinence pads (including products not necessarily described as such but using the absorption principle), incontinence garments, skin wipes and occlusive devices such as female vaginal devices and male penile clamps are not prescribable under the Drug Tariff provisions.

IXB

INCONTINENCE APPLIANCES

ANAL PLUGS

Warning: This product should not be used without assessment by an appropriate medical professional.

Manufacturer	Appliance	Order No.	Quantity	List Price p
Coloplast Ltd	Peristeen Anal Plug			
	Small	1450	20	4378
	Large	1451	20	4288

CATHETER VALVES

Warning: This product should not be used without assessment of bladder function by an appropriate medical professional.

Indications: For use with an indwelling urethral catheter.

Contraindications:
Reduced bladder capacity
No bladder sensation
Cognitive impairment
Insufficient manual dexterity to operate the Catheter Valve

Note: *It is recommended that the Catheter Valve is changed every 5 - 7 days.*

The following symbols are used in this section

     S   Sterile

Manufacturer		Appliance	Order No.	Quantity	List Price p
Bard Ltd		Flip-Flo catheter valve	BFF5	5	1293
Coloplast Ltd		Simpla Catheter Valve	T180	5	1269
Flexicare Medical Ltd	S	E-Z Flow Catheter Valve	00-0060	5	1101
Jade- Euro-Med Ltd	S	Euro Catheter Valve	JECV	5	1197
+L.IN.C. Medical Systems Ltd	S	CareVent Duo Catheter Valve	08.9801	5	1186
Manfred Sauer UK Ltd	S	Smartflow Catheter Valve	CVS	5	1095
Mentor Medical Ltd		Uro-Flo Catheter Valve	WS856-01-A	5	1246

Catheter Valve with Integral Bag

Jade-Euro-Med Ltd	S	Euro Bag with duel tap	JEDT	10	2884

+to be deleted 1 June 2007

INCONTINENCE APPLIANCES

DRAINABLE DRIBBLING APPLIANCES

Bags or pouches which use absorptive material to soak up urine are not prescribable.

Note: The appliances listed below may be re-used, on average, for at least a month.

Manufacturer	Appliance	Order no	Quantity	List Price p
Jade-Euro-Med	Dribbling bag with loops and tapes	Fig 18	1	1853
Ltd	Drip Male Urinal with tap	M 100	1	4979
	Replacement belt for M100	JB 100	1	1228
Ward Surgical	Male Dribbling bag with diaphragm and belt	WM60	1	2792
Appliance Co				

FAECAL COLLECTORS

Manufacturer	Appliance	Order No.	Quantity	List Price p
Hollister Ltd	Hollister Faecal Collector			
	500ml	9822	10	4310
	1000ml	9821	10	4310

INCONTINENCE BELTS

Note: Average Life-in-Use - 6 Months

Manufacturer	Appliance		Order No.	Quantity	List Price p
DBT Medical Ltd	Waist and support for Kipper bag		LM 886103	1	697
Jade-Euro-Med Ltd	Waist belt for Kipper bags		KBWB	1	592
(including products	37mm webbing/elastic waistbelt for		WB	1	613
formerly listed under	use with Jade-Euro-Med appliances				
Mentor Medical Ltd)	Web belt				
		86cm	WS105-91-34	1	1225
		91cm	WS105-91-36	1	1225
		97cm	WS105-91-38	1	1225
		107cm	WS105-91-42	1	1225
		112cm	WS105-91-44	1	1225
		86cm	WS106-01-34	1	1225
		91cm	WS106-01-36	1	1225
		97cm	WS106-01-38	1	1225
		107cm	WS106-01-42	1	1225
		91cm	WS107-01-G	1	1225
Mentor Medical Ltd see Jade-Euro-Med Ltd					
Ward Surgical	Waist belt for black Kipper bag		WM62	1	513
Appliance Co	Rubber belt for PP Urinal		WM63	1	444

INCONTINENCE APPLIANCES

INCONTINENCE SHEATHS

The incontinence sheaths (also known as penile sheaths and external catheters) listed below, are, except where indicated, of the soft, flexible, latex type. Sheaths are available with and without fixing devices which may be applied externally (around the outside of the sheath) or internally (around the penis between the skin and the sheath). A list of fixing devices and other adhesion products is included in 'Incontinence Sheath Fixing Strips & Adhesives'.

Note: Each Sheath may be left in place for 1 to 3 days between changes.

The following symbols are used in this section

⊗	Non-adhesive sheath without liner
⊙	Sheath with self-adhesive liner
↕	Sheath with separate double-sided adhesive strip
≐	Sheath with separate single-sided adhesive strip

Manufacturer	Appliance		Order No.	Quantity	List Price p
Bard Ltd	Encompass				
	Latex free self-adhesive penile sheath				
		24mm	BLFS24	30	4560
		28mm	BLFS28	30	4560
		30mm	BLFS30	30	4560
		32mm	BLFS32	30	4560
		35mm	BLFS35	30	4560
	Reliasheath latex free penile sheath (including adhesive strip)				
		24mm	D523LF	30	4465
		28mm	D524LF	30	4465
		30mm	D525LF	30	4465
		32mm	D526LF	30	4465
		35mm	D527LF	30	4465
	Latex free penile sheath				
		24mm	U523LF	30	2747
		28mm	U524LF	30	2747
		30mm	U525LF	30	2747
		32mm	U526LF	30	2747
		35mm	U527LF	30	2747
	⊗ Uro sheath (washable - may be re-used many times) small (32mm), medium (38mm) large (41mm)		1502	1	593
Beambridge Medical ↕	Beambridge Urinary Sheath				
	Small		6-65(20mm)	30	4537
	Medium		6-65(25mm)	30	4537
	Large		6-65(30mm)	30	4537
	Extra Large		6-65(35mm)	30	4537
CliniMed Ltd	BioDerm ECD (Circular)				
	†		20006	1	790
			20006/starter	5	3950
			20006/10	10	7900
	BioDerm XLS (Oval)				
	†		20026	1	790
			20026/starter	5	3950
			20026/10	10	7900

†to be deleted 1 April 2007

INCONTINENCE APPLIANCES

INCONTINENCE SHEATHS

Manufacturer	Appliance	Order No.	Quantity	List Price p
Coloplast Ltd	Conveen Optima (non-latex) self-sealing Urisheath			
	(Shorter Length)			
	21mm	22121	30	4890
	25mm	22125	30	4890
	30mm	22130	30	4890
	35mm	22135	30	4890
	(Standard Length)			
	25mm	22025	30	4890
	30mm	22030	30	4890
	35mm	22035	30	4890
	40mm	22040	30	4890
⊙	Conveen Security + self-sealing Urisheath (non-latex) with Anti-kink Design			
	extra small	5221	30	4922
	small	5225	30	4922
	medium	5230	30	4922
	large	5235	30	4922
	extra large	5240	30	4922
⊙	Conveen Security + Easifit Shorter length self sealing			
	Urisheath (non-latex) with Anti-kink Design			
	extra small (dia 21mm)	22011	30	4866
	small (dia 25mm)	22012	30	4866
	medium (dia 30mm)	22013	30	4866
	large (dia 35mm)	22014	30	4866
↕	Conveen Security + Sheath (non-latex) with Anti-kink Design			
	(including Uriliner adhesive strip)			
	extra small	5021	30	4974
	small	5025	30	4974
	medium	5030	30	4974
	large	5035	30	4974
	extra large	5040	30	4974
⊙	Conveen self-sealing Urisheath			
	extra small	5212	30	4926
	small	5200	30	4926
	medium	5205	30	4926
	large	5210	30	4926
	extra large	5215	30	4926
↕	Conveen Urisheath/Uriliner			
	very small	5120	30	4980
	small	5125	30	4980
	medium	5130	30	4980
	large	5135	30	4980
	ex- large	5140	30	4980
Coloplast Ltd also see Rochester Medical Ltd				
DBT Medical Ltd ↕	Dryaid Penile Sheath (including adhesive strip)			
	small	AL834021	20	2901
	medium	AL834022	20	2901
	large	AL834023	20	2901
	ex-large	AL834024	20	2901
⊗	Dryaid Penile Sheath (without adhesive strip)			
	small	AL861021	20	1681
	medium	AL861022	20	1681
	large	AL861023	20	1681
	ex-large	AL861024	20	1681

IXB

INCONTINENCE APPLIANCES

INCONTINENCE SHEATHS

Manufacturer		Appliance	Order No.	Quantity	List Price p
Hollister Ltd	☉	CV (non-latex, self-adhesive sheath)			
		(Standard Length)			
		25mm	9306	30	4747
		29mm	9307	30	4747
		32mm	9309	30	4747
		36mm	9308	30	4747
		41mm	9305	30	4747
		(Brief Length)			
		25mm	9316	30	4747
		29mm	9317	30	4747
		32mm	9319	30	4747
		36mm	9318	30	4747
		41mm	9315	30	4747
	☉	Self Adhesive Sheath			
		22-25mm	9636	30	4774
		26-30mm	9637	30	4774
		31-35mm	9639	30	4774
		36-39mm	9638	30	4774
Hospital Management	≐	Macrodom (including adhesive strip)			
and Supplies Ltd		with O 51mm tube	GS7654	30	2230
		with O 127mm tube	GS7655	25	2333
Jade-Euro-Med Ltd	⊗	Incontinence Sheath			
(including products		Small	WS165-01-F	1	164
formerly listed under		Medium	WS165-03-K	1	164
Mentor Medical Ltd)		Large	WS165-05-P	1	164
		Ex-large	WS165-07-T	1	164
	⊗	Jade Naturaflex Clear Non-Adhesive sheath			
		25mm (small)	M410	30	4471
		29mm (medium)	M420	30	4471
		32mm (intermediate)	M430	30	4471
		36mm (large)	M440	30	4471
	☉	Jade Ultra Flex Clear Sheath (Self-adhesive))			
		small	M510	30	4471
		medium	M520	30	4471
		intermediate	M530	30	4471
		large	M540	30	4471
		ex-large	M550	30	4471
Manfred Sauer UK Ltd	☉	Comfort Plus Latex Free Urinary Sheath with hydrocolloid double sided			
(formerly Manfred		adhesive liner			
Sauer GmbH)		Dia 18	56.18	30	4617
		Dia 20	56.20	30	4617
		Dia 22	56.22	30	4617
		Dia 24	56.24	30	4617
		Dia 26	56.26	30	4617
		Dia 28	56.28	30	4617
		Dia 30	56.30	30	4617
		Dia 32	56.32	30	4617
		Dia 35	56.35	30	4617
		Dia 37	56.37	30	4617
		Dia 40	56.40	30	4617

INCONTINENCE APPLIANCES

INCONTINENCE SHEATHS

Manufacturer	Appliance	Order No.	Quantity	List Price p
Manfred Sauer UK Ltd ⊗ (formerly Manfred Sauer GmbH)	Comfort Sheath (in 11 sizes) + Residual Free removal and Anti-Blow-Back system			
	Paediatric (dia 18mm)	53.18	30	2335
	Small - (dia 20mm)	53.20	30	2335
	Small (dia 22mm)	53.22	30	2335
	Small + (dia 24mm)	53.24	30	2335
	Medium - (dia 26mm)	53.26	30	2335
	Medium (dia 28mm)	53.28	30	2335
	Medium + (dia 30mm)	53.30	30	2335
	Large - (dia 32mm)	53.32	30	2335
	Large (dia 35mm)	53.35	30	2335
	Large + (dia 37mm)	53.37	30	2335
	Extra Large (dia 40mm)	53.40	30	2335
⊗	Comfort Sheath Extra Thin for male retraction + Residual Free removal and Anti-Blow-Back system.			
	Medium - (dia 26mm)	53.26D	30	2335
	Medium + (dia 30mm)	53.30D	30	2335
	Large (dia 35mm)	53.35D	30	2335
	Extra Large (dia 40mm)	53.40D	30	2335
⊗	K+ICS Sheath (plus 5 Sheath tip connectors) have special removable tips which enable the sheath to be expanded over the penis with a special sheath expander tool, to allow for clean intermittent self catheterisation (see Tubing and Accessories section of this publication for Manfred Sauer Sheath Expander order no. 100.01).			
	18mm	103.18	30	4698
	20mm	103.20	30	4698
	22mm	103.22	30	4698
	24mm	103.24	30	4698
	26mm	103.26	30	4698
	28mm	103.28	30	4698
	30mm	103.30	30	4698
	32mm	103.32	30	4698
	35mm	103.35	30	4698
	37mm	103.37	30	4698
	40mm	103.40	30	4698
	P-SURE Latex Free self-adhesive with Residual Free removal and Anti-Blow-Back system. Includes 1 free pubic hair protective cloth.			
	Paediatric (dia 18mm)	97.18	30	4389
	Small - (dia 20mm)	97.20	30	4389
	Small (dia 22mm)	97.22	30	4389
	Small + (dia 24mm)	97.24	30	4389
	Medium - (dia 26mm)	97.26	30	4389
	Medium (dia 28mm)	97.28	30	4389
	Medium + (dia 30mm)	97.30	30	4389
	Large - (dia 32mm)	97.32	30	4389
	Large (dia 35mm)	97.35	30	4389
	Large + (dia 37mm)	97.37	30	4389
	Extra Large (dia 40mm)	97.40	30	4389

IXB

Manfred Sauer GmbH see Manfred Sauer UK Ltd

Mentor Medical Ltd see Jade-Euro-Med Ltd & Rochester Medical Ltd

INCONTINENCE APPLIANCES

INCONTINENCE SHEATHS

Manufacturer		Appliance	Order No.	Quantity	List Price p
North West Medical	⊗	Uridrop Incontinence Sheath			
Supplies Ltd		Size 1 (70mm)	30/80	30	1270
		Size 2 (80mm)	30/81	30	1270
		Size 3 (100mm)	30/82	30	1270
		Size 4 (107mm)	30/83	30	1270
		Size Paed 42mm	30/60	30	1270
		Size Paed 55mm	30/61	30	1270
	↕	Uridrop Incontinence Sheath and Uristrip Adhesive Strip			
		Size 1 (70mm)	8480	30	2540
		Size 2 (80mm)	8481	30	2540
		Size 3 (100mm)	8482	30	2540
		Size 4 (107mm)	8483	30	2540
		Size Paed 42mm	8460	30	2540
		Size Paed 55mm	8461	30	2540
S G & P Payne	⊗	Incontiaid Penile Sheath			
		20mm	1111	1	97
		25mm	1112	1	97
		30mm	1113	1	97
		35mm	1114	1	97
		40mm	1115	1	97
	↕	with adhesive strip			
		20mm	1116	10	1542
		25mm	1117	10	1542
		30mm	1118	10	1542
		35mm	1119	10	1542
		40mm	1120	10	1542
Rochester Medical Ltd	☉	Clear Advantage with Aloe silicone sheath, style 1			
(formerly Coloplast Ltd,		Standard			
Mentor Medical Ltd &		24mm	1243	30	4722
Rochester Medical		28mm	1283	30	4722
Corporation)		32mm	1323	30	4722
		36mm	1363	30	4722
		40mm	1403	30	4722
	☉	Clear Advantage with Aloe silicone sheath, style 2			
		Pop-On			
		24mm	2243	30	4722
		28mm	2283	30	4722
		32mm	2323	30	4722
		36mm	2363	30	4722
		40mm	2403	30	4722
	☉	Clear Advantage with Aloe silicone sheath, style 3			
		Wideband			
		24mm	3243	30	4722
		28mm	3283	30	4722
		32mm	3323	30	4722
		36mm	3363	30	4722
		40mm	3403	30	4722
	☉	Freedom Transfix Silicone Sheath, Style 1 self adhering, standard sheath			
		25mm	TF12530	30	4562
		29mm	TF12930	30	4562
		32mm	TF13230	30	4562
		36mm	TF13630	30	4562
		41mm	TF14130	30	4562
	☉	Freedom Transfix Silicone Sheath, Style 2 self adhering, short sheath			
		25mm	TF22530	30	4562
		29mm	TF22930	30	4562
		32mm	TF23230	30	4562
		36mm	TF23630	30	4562
		41mm	TF24130	30	4562

INCONTINENCE APPLIANCES

INCONTINENCE SHEATHS

Manufacturer		Appliance	Order No.	Quantity	List Price p
Rochester Medical Ltd	☉	Freedom Transfix Silicone Sheath, Style 3 self adhering - extra wide adhesive			
(formerly Coloplast Ltd,		band			
Mentor Medical Ltd &		25mm	TF32530	30	4562
Rochester Medical		29mm	TF32930	30	4562
Corporation)		32mm	TF33230	30	4562
		36mm	TF33630	30	4562
		41mm	TF34130	30	4562
	☉	Freedom Sheath (Self-adhesive) (formerly Aquadry Freedom Sheath (Self Adhesive))			
		small (dia 23mm)	786268	30	4746
		medium (dia 28mm)	786276	30	4746
		standard (dia 31mm)	786280	30	4746
		large (dia 35mm)	786284	30	4746
		extra large (dia 40mm)	786288	30	4746
	☉	Freedom Plus Sheath (Self-adhesive) (Shorter length) (formerly Aquadry Freedom Plus Sheath (Self Adhesive) (Shorter Length))			
		small (dia 23mm)	786292	30	4746
		medium (dia 28mm)	786306	30	4746
		standard (dia 31mm)	786310	30	4746
		large (dia 35mm)	786314	30	4746
		extra large (dia 40mm)	786318	30	4746
	☉	Clear Advantage Silicone Sheath (Self-adhesive)			
		small (dia 23mm)	786187	30	4722
		medium (dia 28mm)	786195	30	4722
		standard (dia 31mm)	786225	30	4722
		large (dia 35mm)	786233	30	4722
		extra large (dia 40mm)	786241	30	4722
	⊗	Natural Clear Non-Adhesive Sheath			
		25mm (small)	38301	30	4471
		29mm (medium)	38302	30	4471
		32mm (intermediate)	38303	30	4471
		36mm (large)	38304	30	4471
		Natural Silicone Sheath (self-adhesive) see UltraFlex Silicone Sheath (self-adhesive)			
	☉	Pop-On Silicone Sheath (self-adhesive)			
		25mm	32301	30	4471
		29mm	32302	30	4471
		32mm	32303	30	4471
		36mm	32304	30	4471
		41mm	32305	30	4471
	☉	UltraFlex Clear Sheath (Self-adhesive)			
		small	33101	30	4471
		medium	33102	30	4471
		intermediate	33103	30	4471
		large	33104	30	4471
		ex-large	33105	30	4471
	☉	UltraFlex Silicone Sheath (self-adhesive) (formerly Natural Silicone Sheath (self-adhesive)			
		25mm	31301	30	4471
		29mm	31302	30	4471
		32mm	31303	30	4471
		36mm	31304	30	4471
		41mm	31305	30	4471
	☉	Wide Band Silicone Sheath (self-adhesive)			
		25mm	36301	30	4471
		29mm	36302	30	4471
		32mm	36303	30	4471
		36mm	36304	30	4471
		41mm	36305	30	4471

IXB

INCONTINENCE APPLIANCES

INCONTINENCE SHEATHS

Manufacturer	Appliance	Order No.	Quantity	List Price p
Salts Healthcare	⊗ Male Continence Sheath			
	17mm	ZL0028	10	891
	22mm	ZL0029	10	891
	25mm	ZL0030	10	891
	32mm	ZL0031	10	891
	34mm	ZL0032	10	891
Teleflex Medical	≐ Rusch Secure external catheter kit (including adhesive strip)			
	25mm diameter	4000025	10	950
	30mm diameter	4000030	10	950
	35mm diameter	4000035	10	950
The Kendall Company see Tyco Healthcare				
Tyco Healthcare (formerly The Kendall Company (UK) Ltd)	↕ Texas Catheter (including adhesive strip)	8884-731300	12	864

INCONTINENCE APPLIANCES

INCONTINENCE SHEATH FIXING STRIPS & ADHESIVES
(Available separately from sheaths)

The following symbols are used in this section

↕	Double-sided adhesive strip
≠	Foam and Velcro
⏀	For use with urinal systems
*	Safe for direct application on the skin

Manufacturer		Appliance	Order No.	Quantity	List Price p
Bio Diagnostics	↕	Urifix Tape 5m	SU1	1	490
Camp Ltd	≠	Posey Sheath Holder			
		Adult	90500	12	1325
		Paediatric	6555	12	1020
Coloplast Ltd	↕	Conveen Sheath Liners	5100	20	930
ConvaTec Ltd	↕	Urihesive Strips	S120	15	729
DBT Medical Ltd	↕	Dryaid Strip	AL832025	20	1220
Jade-Euro-Med Ltd	⏀	Jade Velcro Foam Strap	M450	10	1176
JLJ Healthcare Ltd	↕	Urifix Tape 5m	T115	1	634
Manfred Sauer UK Ltd (formerly Manfred Sauer GmbH)	*	Original Latex Skin Adhesive in a 28g tube with a long pipette/nozzle applicator	50.01	2	869
	*	Pure Latex Skin Adhesive without any skin care components giving a stronger bond, in a 28g tube with a long pipette/nozzle applicator.	50.00	2	854
	*	Lanolin Free Latex Skin Adhesive for people allergic to lanolin, in a 28g tube with a long pipette/nozzle applicator.	50.03	2	854
	*	50% reduction in skin care components, in a 28g tube with a long pipette/nozzle applicator.	50.05	2	854
	↕	Comfort Plus hydrocolloid adhesive tape	50.14	30	1402
	*	2% Resin giving a stronger bond than the original adhesive 50.01, in a 28g tube with a long pipette/nozzle applicator. Should only be tried after 50.01 is found to be too weak.	50.20	2	854

IXB

INCONTINENCE APPLIANCES

INCONTINENCE SHEATH FIXING STRIPS & ADHESIVES (Available separately from sheaths)

Manufacturer		Appliance	Order No.	Quantity	List Price p
Manfred Sauer UK Ltd (formerly Manfred Sauer GmbH)	*	12% Resin giving a stronger bond than the 2% resin adhesive 50.20, in a 28g tube with a long pipette/nozzle applicator. Should only be tried after 50.20 is found to be too weak.	50.22	2	854
	*	Synthetic Skin Adhesive in a 28g tube with a long pipette/nozzle applicator	50.36-2	2	1525
	*	Synthetic Skin Adhesive in a 45ml bottle with brush in the lid	50.36	1	1525
Manfred Sauer GmbH see Manfred Sauer UK Ltd					
North West Medical Supplies Ltd	↕	Uristrip Adhesive Strip	30/84	30	1270
S G & P Payne	≠	Incontiaid Sheath Holder	1123	1	113
		Incontiaid Single Sided Adhesive Strips	1004	10	453
	↕	Adhesive Strips	1002	10	501
Salts Healthcare	≠	Heritage Sheath Collar Pack	ZL0022	30	447

INCONTINENCE APPLIANCES

LEG BAGS

The leg bags listed are suitable for collection of urine from indwelling catheters or incontinence sheaths. They are intended for daytime use although the larger bags may have adequate capacity for overnight use by some patients. The bags may be worn in different positions on the leg and the intended position (eg thigh, knee or calf) will determine the length of the inlet tube. The bags are attached to the leg by means of straps (included with each pack) which are generally either latex or foam with velcro fasteners.

Note: *Plastic leg bags identified in the list with an asterisk* may on average be used for 5-7 days. With proper care and cleansing rubber leg bags are re-usable for 4-6 months.*

Symbols used in this section
S These leg bags are supplied sterile. This does not affect the guidance given in the note at the beginning.
* Plastics
W Due to the size and weight of these bags when full, this capacity of bag should be prescribed only for
    wheelchair-bound patients.

Manufacturer		Appliance	Order No.	Quantity	List Price p
Bard Ltd	S *	Uriplan Range: Shaped Leg Bags with tap outlet, overnight connector and elastic velcro straps			
	*	350ml, direct inlet	D3S	10	2841
	*	350ml, 30cm inlet tube	D3L	10	2816
	*	500ml, direct inlet	D5S	10	2863
	*	500ml, 10cm inlet tube	D5M	10	2874
	*	500ml, 30cm inlet tube	D5L	10	2874
	*	750ml, direct inlet	D7S	10	2884
	*	750ml, 10cm inlet tube	D7M	10	2884
	*	750ml, 30cm inlet tube	D7L	10	2884
	*	750ml, 38cm adjustable inlet tube	D7LX	10	2884
	S *	Urisac Range: Leg Bags with push/pull outlet and foam velcro straps			
	*	350ml, long tube	7660	10	1507
	*	350ml, short tube	7661	10	1463
	*	500ml, long tube	7662	10	1638
	*	500ml, short tube	7663	10	1593
	*	750ml, long tube	7664	10	1752
	*	750ml, short tube	7665	10	1680
Beambridge Medical		Beambridge Leg Bags with 1 pair of Flexible leg bag straps			
		500ml short tube (10cm)	6-70	10	2702
		500ml long tube (30cm)	6-75	10	2702
CliniSupplies Ltd	S	ProSys Sterile Leg Bags. Containing 1 pair of soft elasticated cotton velcro straps per box of 10			
		350ml short tube	P350S	10	2600
		350ml long tube	P350L	10	2600
		500ml short tube	P500S	10	2600
		500ml long tube	P500L	10	2600
		750ml short tube	P750S	10	2600
		750ml long tube	P750L	10	2600

IXB

INCONTINENCE APPLIANCES

LEG BAGS

Manufacturer		Appliance	Order No.	Quantity	List Price p
Coloplast Ltd	*	Conveen Security+ leg bag 350ml			
		25cm tube	5164	10	2375
		50cm tube	5165	10	2375
	*	Conveen Security+ leg bag 500ml			
		25cm tube	5160	10	2375
		50cm tube	5161	10	2375
	S	25cm tube	5162	10	2525
	S	50cm tube	5163	10	2525
	*	Conveen Security+ leg bag 750ml			
		25cm tube	5166	10	2375
		50cm tube	5167	10	2375
	*	Conveen Contour 600ml leg bag			
		(adjustable tube)	5170	10	2884
	S	5cm inlet tube	5172	10	2884
	S	30cm inlet tube	5173	10	2884
	*	Conveen Contour 800ml leg bag			
	S	45cm tube	5175	10	2884
S	*	Aquadry leg bag			
	*	350ml short tube	783463	10	2543
	*	350ml long tube Adjustable	783501	10	2543
	*	500ml short tube	783471	10	2543
	*	500ml long tube Adjustable	783528	10	2543
	*	750ml short tube	783498	10	2543
	*	750ml long tube Adjustable	783536	10	2543
		Simpla Plus leg bags with two-step safety lock tap and anti-kink tubing			
	S	350ml 6cm tube	21561	10	2836
	S	350ml 25cm tube	21562	10	2836
	S	500ml 6cm tube	21571	10	2836
	S	500ml 25cm tube	21572	10	2836
		500ml 50cm tube	21583	10	2774
	S	750ml 6cm tube	21591	10	2836
	S	750ml 25cm tube	21592	10	2836
		Simpla Plus knee bag with additional strap			
		(3 straps per box of 10)			
S W		1500ml	21577	10	2885
S		Simpla Plus Syphon Bags			
		750ml, 6cm tube	21566	10	2885
		750ml, 25cm tube	21567	10	2885
S		Simpla Trident T1 with slide action tap			
	*	350ml short tube	370802	10	2816
	*	500ml long tube	370817	10	2838
	*	500ml short tube	370807	10	2838
	*	750ml long tube	370819	10	2851
	*	750ml short tube	370809	10	2851
	*	750ml adjustable long tube	370904	10	2851
S		Simpla Trident T2 with lever action tap			
	*	350ml bag short tube	376137	10	2850
	*	500ml bag short tube	376138	10	2881
	*	500ml bag long tube	376139	10	2881
	*	750ml bag short tube	376140	10	2895
	*	750ml bag long tube	376142	10	2895
	*	750ml bag adjustable long tube	376141	10	2895

INCONTINENCE APPLIANCES

LEG BAGS

Manufacturer		Appliance	Order No.	Quantity	List Price p
ConvaTec Ltd	*	500ml Accuseal leg bag	S450	10	2137
DBT Medical Ltd		Kipper bag			
		Trans/white without strap and buckle	LM886000	1	2388
		Trans/white	LM886001	1	2914
		All black rubber	LM886002	1	2914
		All black plastic	LM886003	1	2914
Flexicare Medical Ltd		Flexicare leg bag with lever tap outlet, night drainage connector and velcro anti slip straps			
	S *	350ml short tube	00-1352	10	2260
	S *	500ml short tube	00-1502	10	2260
	S *	750ml short tube	00-1752	10	2260
	S *	350ml long tube	00-2352	10	2260
	S *	500ml long tube	00-2502	10	2260
	S *	750ml, long tube	00-2752	10	2260
	S *	500ml (60cm adjustable tube)	00-3502	10	2300
	*	500ml (60cm adjustable tube)	00-3501	10	2188
Hollister Ltd	S	Leg Bag 500ml/10cm inlet (Regular)	9621	10	2778
	S	Leg Bag 500ml/50cm inlet (Regular)	9624	10	2778
	S	Leg Bag 800ml/10cm inlet (Regular)	9631	10	2788
	S	Leg Bag 800ml/50cm variable inlet (Regular)	9632	10	2788
	*	Urinary Leg Bag 540ml with 37cm extension tube	9820	10	2824
	S *	Urinary Leg Bag 540ml with direct inlet connector	9814	10	2756
Jade-Euro-Med Ltd (including products formerly listed under Mentor Medical Ltd)	*	Catheter drainage bag -			
		Large	WP205-01-S	1	431
		Small	WP205-05-B	1	431
		Kipper bag, black	KB	1	2820
	+	Kipper bag, trans	KBT	1	2771
	S *	Leg Drainage bag/Direct Inlet 350ml S	LBWT/350	10	2419
	S *	Leg Drainage bag/30cm Inlet tube 350ml L	LBWT/350	10	2419
	S *	Leg Drainage bag/Direct Inlet 500ml S	LBWT/500	10	2419
	S *	Leg Drainage bag/10cm Inlet tube 500ml M	LBWT/500	10	2419
	S *	Leg Drainage bag/30cm Inlet tube 500ml L	LBWT/500	10	2419
	S *	Leg Drainage bag/Direct Inlet 750ml S	LBWT/750	10	2524
	S *	Leg Drainage bag/10cm Inlet tube 750ml M	LBWT/750	10	2524
	S *	Leg Drainage bag/30cm Inlet tube 750ml L	LBWT/750	10	2524
	S *	Leg Drainage bag/38cm Inlet tube 750ml XL	LBWT/750	10	2524
		Rubber bag with leg strap	WS111-05-U	1	4153

+to be deleted 1 June 2007

IXB

INCONTINENCE APPLIANCES

LEG BAGS

Manufacturer	Appliance	Order No.	Quantity	List Price p
Manfred Sauer UK Ltd (formerly Manfred Sauer GmbH)	Discreet Thigh Bag, overnight connector tube and fabric/velcro leg straps (1 pair per box of 10)			
S *	450ml diagonal direct inlet tube suitable for suprapubic catheter connection	70.04S	10	2323
S *	400ml straight direct inlet tube	70.06S	10	2323
	Bendi Bag leg bag with tap outlet, overnight connector tube and fabric/velcro leg straps (1 pair per box of 10)			
*	700ml Direct inlet tube, swing tap	70.33-04	10	2163
*	700ml 12cm inlet tube, swing tap	70.33-12	10	2163
*	700ml 20cm inlet tube, swing tap	70.33-20	10	2163
*	700ml 35cm adjustable inlet tube, swing tap	70.33-35adj	10	2163
*	700ml 35cm adjustable inlet tube, slide tap	70.33-35Padj	10	2163
S *	700ml Direct inlet tube, swing tap	70.33-04S	10	2498
S *	700ml 12cm inlet tube, swing tap	70.33-12S	10	2499
S *	700ml 20cm inlet tube, swing tap	70.33-20S	10	2499
S *	700ml 35cm adjustable inlet tube, swing tap	70.33-35Sadj	10	2498
* W	1300ml Direct inlet tube, swing tap	70.47-04	10	2163
* W	1300ml 12cm inlet tube, swing tap	70.47-12	10	2163
* W	1300ml 20cm inlet tube, swing tap	70.47-20	10	2163
* W	1300ml 35cm adjustable inlet tube, swing tap	70.47-35adj	10	2163
* W	1300ml 35cm adjustable inlet tube, slide tap	70.47-35Padj	10	2163
*S W	1300ml Direct inlet tube, swing tap	70.47-04S	10	2498
*S W	1300ml 12cm inlet tube, swing tap	70.47-12S	10	2499
*S W	1300ml 20cm inlet tube, swing tap	70.47-20S	10	2499
*S W	1300ml 35cm adjustable inlet tube, swing tap	70.47-35Sadj	10	2498
	Comfort Leg Bag 600ml with universal adapter, 2 straps and 1 latex connector			
	Direct inlet glued adapter, swing tap	710.1104	10	2331
	15cm inlet adjustable, swing tap	710.1315adj	10	2331
	45cm inlet adjustable, swing tap	710.1345adj	10	2331
	Direct inlet glued adapter, push valve/sliding tap	710.2104	10	2331
	15cm inlet adjustable, push valve/sliding tap	710.2315adj	10	2331
	45cm inlet adjustable, push valve/sliding tap	710.2345adj	10	2331
	Comfort Leg Bag 600ml with universal adapter, 1x 4cm wide top strap & 1 x 2cm wide bottom strap and 3 latex connectors.			
S *	Direct inlet glued adapter, swing tap	710.1204S	10	2515
S *	15cm inlet adjustable, swing tap	710.1415Sadj	10	2515
S *	45cm inlet adjustable, swing tap	710.1445Sadj	10	2515
S *	Direct inlet glued adapter, push valve/sliding tap	710.2204S	10	2515
S *	15cm inlet adjustable, push valve/sliding tap	710.2415Sadj	10	2515
S *	45cm inlet adjustable, push valve/sliding tap	710.2445Sadj	10	2515
	Comfort Leg Bag "R" 600ml with universal adapter, 2 straps and 10 latex adapters			
S *	45cm inlet adjustable, reverse swing tap, attached night bag adapter	R710.1445SOadj	10	2711
	Comfort Leg Bag "XR" 1000ml with universal adapter, 2 straps and 10 latex adapters			
S *	45cm inlet adjustable, reverse swing tap, attached night bag adapter.	R711.1445SOadj	10	2763
S	Smartflow Children's leg bag			
	210ml, direct inlet	CBDirectS	10	2748
	210ml, 30cm adjustable inlet	CB30S	10	2748

Manfred Sauer GmbH see Manfred Sauer UK Ltd

INCONTINENCE APPLIANCES

LEG BAGS

Manufacturer		Appliance	Order No.	Quantity	List Price p
Mentor	S	Freedom Triform Leg Bags			
Medical Ltd	*	350ml short tube	5350	10	2751
	*	350ml short tube with soft backing	5351	10	2751
	*	500ml short tube	5500	10	2755
	*	500ml short tube with soft backing	5501	10	2751
	*	500ml medium tube	5502	10	2787
	*	500ml medium tube with soft backing	5503	10	2783
	*	500ml long tube	5504	10	2811
	*	500ml long tube with soft backing	5505	10	2806
	*	500ml extra long adjustable tube with soft backing	5507	10	2898
	*	750ml short tube	5750	10	2941
	*	750ml short tube with softbacking	5751	10	2941
	*	750ml long tube	5754	10	2941
	*	750ml long tube with soft backing	5755	10	2941
	*	750ml extra long adjustable tube with soft backing	5757	10	2941
		Paediatric/Child 120ml leg bag with 1 pair of leg straps per pack	E120V	10	2355

Mentor Medical Ltd also see Jade-Euro-Med Ltd

S G & P Payne	*	Incontiaid leg bag			
		500ml	0830	1	288
		750ml	0831	1	288
		GU Black Butyl (or Latex) Rubber Kipper (SP, St. Peter's) Bags			
		Standard single chambered bag 568ml	0922/GU532	1	4561
		Ross type. As above, but with reinforced patches	0926/GU532/R	1	5206
		Standard 568ml bag with box outlet tap	0924/GU532/LT	1	5622
		Standard 568ml bag with short neck for females	0925/GU532/F	1	4561
		Standard 1136ml bag for night use	0923/GU532/40	1	6141
		Rubber bag for catheter drainage, short neck leg strap	SP/1	1	3126
		Female rubber drainage bag with conical mount	SP/5	1	2967
		As above with web belt and looped support strap	SP/5a	1	3499

Salts Healthcare	*	Heritage leg bag pack	ZL0020	5	1175

Shiloh		Contibag leg bag			
Healthcare	S	350ml short tube	CBS350	10	2544
Ltd	S	500ml short tube	CBS500	10	2595
	S	750ml short tube	CBS750	10	2646
	S	350ml long tube	CBL350	10	2544
	S	500ml long tube	CBL500	10	2595
	S	750ml long tube	CBL750	10	2646

IXB

INCONTINENCE APPLIANCES

LEG BAGS

Manufacturer		Appliance	Order No.	Quantity	List Price p
Universal	S	Unicorn leg bag			
Hospital	*	350ml short tube	UN222V	10	1760
Supplies	*	500ml short tube	UN333V	10	1780
	*	500ml long tube	UN333VL	10	1780
	*	750ml short tube	UN444V	10	1800
	*	750ml long tube	UN444VL	10	1800
Unomedical	S	Careline Leg Bag with tap outlet, overnight connection tube and elasticated			
Ltd		velcro straps (1 pair per box of 10)			
	*	350ml short tube	45-01 SVC	10	2478
	*	350ml long tube	45-02 LVC	10	2478
	*	500ml short tube	45-05 SVC	10	2543
	*	500ml long tube	45-06 LVC	10	2543
	*	750ml short tube	45-09 SVC	10	2597
	*	750ml long tube	45-10 LVC	10	2597
		Careline Leg Bag with lever tap			
	S *	500ml short tube	46-05-SVC	10	2543
	S *	500ml long tube	46-06-LVC	10	2543
	S *	750ml short tube	46-09-SVC	10	2597
	S *	750ml long tube	46-10-LVC	10	2597
Ward Surgical		Kipper bag, black trans or white rubber	WM64	10	2332
Appliance Co	*	Leg drainage bag			
		350ml	WM65	10	1126
		500ml	WM66	10	1161
		750ml	WM67	10	1230
		Ward's Comfort Range			
	*	Leg drainage bag			
		350ml	WM68	10	1131
		500ml	WM69	10	1163
		750ml	WM70	10	1223

NIGHT DRAINAGE BAGS

These bags are suitable for night-time use for the collection of urine from indwelling catheters or incontinence sheaths. They are generally used in conjunction with a bag hanger which, being a nursing aid, is not prescribable. Supply arrangements for bag hangers tend to vary throughout the country but they are normally supplied through the community nursing service.

Note: The drainage bags listed below except non-drainable bags, have a life-in-use of, on average 5-7 days.

Symbols used in this section
- # Non-drainable bags
- S These Night Drainage Bags are supplied sterile
- ❑ Single Use Only
- * Plastics

Manufacturer		Appliance	Order No.	Quantity	List Price p
A1 Pharmaceuticals	#	Uriline Non sterile 2 litre bag	A1	10	205
	#	Uriline Non sterile 2 litre bag with non-return valve	A2	10	220
	S	Uriline 2 litre bag with non-return valve and tap	A4	10	1100
Bard Ltd	#	Uriplan collection bag, 2 litre with 90cm inlet tube and non-return valve	D8420	10	256
		Uriplan drainage bag, 2 litre with 98cm inlet tube, non-return valve and tap outlet	D81-3131	10	1289
	❑	Uriplan One MT 2 litre bag with drainage tap	D1MT	10	326
CliniSupplies Ltd		ProSys Sterile 2 litre night bag with 90cm inlet tube, non-return valve, sample port connector and outlet tap	P2000	10	1220
		ProSys Non Sterile 2 litre night bag with 90cm inlet tube and non-return valve	P2	10	209
Coloplast Ltd	S	Conveen drainage bag 1.5 litre	5062	10	1457
		Assura 2 litre night bag with 120cm anti-kink tubing	21365	10	1646
	S	Simpla 2 litre S5 Urine drainage bag	346145	10	1220
		Simpla 2 litre S4 Urine drainage bag -			
	S	long tube	340805	10	1351
	S	short tube	340801	10	1307
	#	Simpla 2 litre S1 Urine drainage bag with standard size connector	311102	10	258
	#	Simpla 2 litre S2 Urine drainage bag with non-return valve with standard size connector	320902	10	272
	S	Simpla Plus 2 litre night bag with 120cm anti-kink tubing	21576	10	1681
ConvaTec Ltd		Accuseal drainage bag	S500	5	860
		Night drainage bag	S320	5	860
Dansac Ltd		Dansac night drainage bag 2 litre	420-00	10	1214
Flexicare Medical Ltd		Flexicare F4, sterile 2 litre drainage bag with 100cm inlet tube, non-return valve and tap outlet	00-1200	10	967
		Flexicare F4L, sterile 2 litre drainage bag with 100cm inlet tube, non-return valve and lever tap outlet	00-1201	10	987
	#	Flexicare F2, sterile 2 litre drainage bag with 100cm inlet tube and non-return valve	00-2202C	10	214

IXB

INCONTINENCE APPLIANCES

NIGHT DRAINAGE BAGS

Manufacturer		Appliance	Order No.	Quantity	List Price p
Flexicare Medical Ltd	❑	Flexicare F2 EZ 2 litre drainage bag with single use snap twist-off tap	00-2203C	10	327
Hollister Ltd	#	Night drainage bag 2000ml (Non-Drainable)	9651	10	246
	S	Night drainage bag 2000ml (Drainable)	9650	10	1245
		Hollister urostomy night drainage bag	5550	10	1154
Jade-Euro-Med Ltd	S	2 litre drainage bag with tap outlet	2LNB	1	158
	#	Jade J2 2 litre bag with 90cm inlet tube and non-return valve	J2	10	239
L.IN.C Medical Ltd	❑	2 litre overnight drainage bag with non-return valve	LM2LNS	10	210
	S ❑	2 litre overnight drainage bag with non-return valve	LM2LS	10	262
	S	2 litre drainage bag with tap, 120cm tube, non-return valve, antibacterial filter, Pasteur drip chamber and integral handle	TZ01	10	1600
	S	2 litre drainage bag with tap, 120cm tube, non-return valve, antibacterial filter and integral handle	TZ02	10	1200
Manfred Sauer UK Ltd (formerly Manfred Sauer GmbH)		Smartflow 2 litre drainable night bag, swing tap, 120cm inlet tube and non return valve	NB2	10	1559
	#	Smartflow 2.6L drainage bag non sterile with 90cm kink resistant inlet tube	NB26	10	490

Manfred Sauer GmbH see Manfred Sauer UK Ltd

Manufacturer		Appliance	Order No.	Quantity	List Price p
Mentor Medical Ltd	S	FreedomCysto-Care, 2 litre silver	2011	10	1336
		Inbeds 2 litre drainage bag with twist tap	IB2000C	10	1515
	*	Tri-Form 2 litre night drainage bag with 90cm inlet tube and non-return valve with universal connector	TFN2000	10	237
Neomedic Ltd	S	Neovac 2000ml urine drainage bag with 90cm inlet tube and non-return valve	NVB2	10	224
Salts Healthcare		2 litre urine drainage bags	ZL0400	10	1366
Shiloh Healthcare Ltd		Contibag sterile 2 litre storage bag (drainable)	CBN2L	10	1119
Unomedical Ltd	#	Careline E1, 2 litre urine drainage bag with 90cm inlet tube	45-30-LBC	10	218
	#	Careline E2, 2 litre urine drainage bag with 90cm inlet tube and non-return valve	45-40-LBC	10	233
		Careline E4, 2 litre urine drainage bag with 90cm inlet tube and non-return valve and tap outlet	45-20-IDC	10	1142
	S	Careline E4 Night Bag, 2 litre with lever tap	46-20-IDC	10	1123
	❑	Easi MT 2 litre drainage bag with 90cm inlet tube, non-return valve and single use twist off drainage outlet	47-60-LBH	10	318
Ward Surgical Appliance Co		2 litre drainage bag with outlet and non-outlet	WM71	10	1224

INCONTINENCE APPLIANCES

SUSPENSORY SYSTEMS

These appliances should not be confused with leg bag garments which are not prescribable. Each system comprises a drainage bag with its means of support.

Note: The bags may be used for 5-7 days, sometimes longer, but the support systems will have a much longer life.

Symbols used in this section
   * Plastics

Manufacturer	Appliance	Order No.	Quantity	List Price p
Bard Ltd	Urisac Portabag belt	7681	1	801
*	Urisac Portabag	7680	10	1368
Jade-Euro-Med Ltd	Portabag Left Hand Inlet	JEPB/L	10	1760
	Portabag Right Hand Inlet	JEPB/R	10	1760
	Portabelt	JEPB/B	1	895
Manfred Sauer UK Ltd (formerly Manfred Sauer GmbH)	NephSys: Nephrostomy drainage system			
	Contains 4x 500ml sterile drainage bags, 2x bag suspenders, 1x waist belt			
	Small belt (20cm inlet)	NephSys.01S	1	3401
	Small belt (30cm inlet)	NephSys.01L	1	3401
	Adult Belt (20cm inlet)	NephSys.02S	1	3401
	Adult Belt (30cm inlet)	NephSys.02L	1	3401
	NephSys: Replacement belts			
	Small	NSBelt.01	1	1835
	Adult	NSBelt.02	1	1835
	NephSys: 500ml sterile drainage bag			
	20cm inlet	NS721.1720S	10	3915
	30cm inlet	NS721.1730S	10	3915
Manfred Sauer GmbH see Manfred Sauer UK Ltd				
Mentor Medical Ltd	Leg bag holster			
	Small 61cm-76cm	WH6176	1	997
	Medium 76cm-91.5cm	WH7691	1	997
	Large 91.5cm - 112cm	WH91112	1	997
*	400ml Holster bag	400 H	10	2133
Teleflex Medical	Rusch Belly Bag (includes belt) (Each bag may be used for up to 28 days)	B1000	2	2100
	Rusch Belly Bag with extended drainage tubing	B1000CT	2	2100
	Rusch Belly Bag replacement belt	P0337	2	470
	Rusch Belly Bag with sample port	B1000P	2	2100

IXB

INCONTINENCE APPLIANCES

TUBING AND ACCESSORIES

Manufacturer	Appliance	Order No.	Quantity	List Price p
Bard Ltd	Leg bag straps (washable)	15LS	10	1421
	Leg bag straps, Latex	8440	20	291
	Leg bag straps, foam/velcro	8441	20	553
	Urisleeve leg bag holder			
	Small (24-39cm)	150111	4	793
	Medium (36-55cm)	150121	4	793
	Large (40-70cm)	150131	4	793
Beambridge Medical	Beambridge Funnel Male Urinal Director/Positioner	6-35	1	1223
	Beambridge Lady Funnel Female Urinal Director/Positioner	6-40	1	1273
	Beambridge Mini Funnel Male Urinal Director/Positioner	6-35M	1	1223
CliniSupplies Ltd	Soft elasticated cotton leg bag support straps with silicone leg grip	P10LS	10	1295
Coloplast Ltd	Velcrobands (washable)	5050	20	4065
	Aquasleeve			
	Small (leg circum. 24-33cm)	783678	4	796
	Standard (leg circum. 34-39cm)	783680	4	796
	Medium (leg circum. 40-46cm)	783686	4	796
	Large (leg circum. 47-64cm)	783694	4	796
	Extra Large (leg circum. 65cm+)	783708	4	780
	Leg bag extension tube	380303	10	528
	Elasticated leg bag straps (washable)	380812	10	1477
	Simpla G-Strap			
	short	383002	5	1352
	adult	383001	5	1352
	abdominal	383003	5	1492
	Simpla Plus Knee Bag Straps	21560	15	2172
ConvaTec Ltd	Accuseal leg bag extension tube	S455	10	788
DBT Medical Ltd	35.5cm connecting tube for drip urinal	LM754136	1	289
Flexicare Medical Ltd	Leg bag straps (pairs); washable, anti slip with velcro fastening	00-0032	10	1170
G F Products	Safehold Straps			
	+ Pack of 2 G Straps	G2	1	100
	Pack of 2 Body straps with tube holders	B	1	130

+to be deleted 1 June 2007

INCONTINENCE APPLIANCES

TUBING AND ACCESSORIES

Manufacturer	Appliance	Order No.	Quantity	List Price p
Hollister Ltd	Deluxe Leg bag straps			
	35cm (extra small)	9663	2	310
	38cm (small)	9660	2	310
	49cm (medium)	9661	2	310
	56cm (large)	9662	2	310
	Leg bag holsters			
	Small	9612	4	782
	Medium	9613	4	782
	Large	9614	4	782
	Leg bag straps,	9625	10	1326
	Elasticated and washable			
	Leg bag straps			
	35.5cm (calf)	9342	2	315
	58.5cm (thigh)	9343	2	315
Jade-Euro-Med	Euro J-strap	JEJS	5	1279
Ltd (including	Eurosleeve			
products formerly	Small (24-33cm)	JES1	4	762
listed under	Standard (34-39cm)	JES2	4	762
Mentor Medical	Medium (40-46cm)	JES3	4	762
Ltd)	Large (47-64cm)	JES4	4	762
	Eurosleeve All in One			
	Small (24-39cm Yellow)	JES6	4	763
	Medium (36-55cm Blue)	JES7	4	763
	Large (40-70cm Brown)	JES8	4	763
	Leg bag connecting tube with mount	LBCTM	1	265
	Leg bag connecting tube	LBCT	1	154
	Velcro leg straps	VLS	2	198
	Female connector for Mitcham bag	WH566-01-G	1	236
	Rubber extension tube (with mounts)	WS152-01-M	1	529
	Night bag connector	WH533-01-C	1	143
	Spare "O" rings for pp urinal	WR045-01-R	5	135
	Uro-Flo Elastic Velcro Leg Straps	WS167-35-H	10	486
JBOL Ltd	Whiz Urine Director	ATD2002.1	1	890
	Whiz Urine Director (with 10cm connecting tube)	ATD2004.10	1	1075
Manfred Sauer UK	K+ICS Sheath Expander	100.01	1	6669
Ltd (formerly	(can only be used to expand Manfred Sauer K+ICS Sheaths over the penis to allow			
Manfred Sauer	for clean intermittant self catheterisation - see Incontinence Sheaths section this			
GmbH)	publication for Manfred Sauer K+ICS Sheaths, order no. 103.nn).			
	K+ICS Sheath Tips	100.05	10	1665
	(can only be used with Manfred Sauer K+ICS Sheaths - see Incontinence Sheaths			
	section of this publication for Manfred Sauer K+ICS Sheaths, order no. 103.nn.)			
	Leg Bag Narrow Strap	LB.N	1	117
	20mm wide			
	Leg Bag Wide Strap	LB.W	1	196
	38mm wide			
	Leg Bag to Night Bag	55.38-10	10	275
	Latex Connectors			
	p.hold Penis Director/Positioner & Holder/Stretcher			
	Normal 2cm thick (blue)	PHN	1	345
	Wide 4cm thick (green)	PHW	1	345

Manfred Sauer GmbH see Manfred Sauer UK Ltd

IXB

INCONTINENCE APPLIANCES

TUBING AND ACCESSORIES

Manufacturer	Appliance	Order No.	Quantity	List Price p
Mentor Medical Ltd	Leg bag extension tube			
	30cm	ET30	10	2760
	60cm	ET60	10	3036
	Silgrip Elasticated leg strap	EC1	10	1405
	Silgrip side-fix leg strap (thigh fitting)	SF1	10	1405
	Silgrip side-fix leg strap (calf fitting)	SF2	10	1336
	Easisleeve			
	Small	5900	4	765
	Standard	5901	4	765
	Medium	5902	4	765
	Large	5903	4	765
	Extra Large	5904	4	765
Mentor Medical Ltd also see Jade-Euro-Med Ltd				
S G & P Payne	152mm Rubber extension tube	1201	1	386
	Non-Spill Adaptor	1351	1	673
	Velcro leg strap	1001	1	106
	Rubber leg strap	1003	1	135
Salts Healthcare	Heritage leg bag extension tube	ZL0021	2	235
The Kendall Company (UK) Ltd see Tyco Healthcare				
Tyco Healthcare (formerly The Kendall Company (UK) Ltd)				
	Argyle Foam and Velcro Abdomen strap 150cm (washable)	8887-600156	1	317
	Argyle Penrose Tubing			
	6mm ID, length 44cm	8888-514604	50	3075
	8mm ID, length 44cm	8888-514802	50	3075
	10mm ID, length 44cm	8888-515007	50	3075
	13mm ID, length 44cm	8888-515205	50	3075
	16mm ID, length 44cm	8888-515403	50	3075
	19mm ID, length 44cm	8888-515601	50	3075
	25mm ID, length 44cm	8888-515809	50	3075
Unomedical Ltd	Careline leg bag straps	45-85-EX	10	1362

INCONTINENCE APPLIANCES

URINAL SYSTEMS

The devices listed below are specialist appliances which comprise several components and need to be correctly fitted by someone competent to do so. Generally patients should have 2 appliances, one to wear and one to wash.

Note: *In general the individual components can be prescribed separately for replacement purposes. With proper care and cleansing, each appliance should last for 6 months.*

Manufacturer	Appliance	Order No.	Quantity	List Price p
Bard Ltd	Maguire urinal and adaptor			
	waist sizes			
	66-81 cm	050802	1	6942
	81-96 cm	050803	1	6942
	96-112 cm	050804	1	6942
	Maguire adaptor & tubing	600532		937
Beambridge	Bridge Saddle urinal	6-26	1	1324
Medical	Bridge urinal	6-18	1	1324
	Bridge urinal with tap	6-18T	1	1324
	Beambridge Drainage Bags for use with	6-55	10	1427
	Beambridge Urinals			
	Beambridge Lady Jug	6-45	1	1425
	Male Draining Jug	6-50	1	1324
	Male Draining Jug with tap	6-50T	1	1324
C S Bullen Ltd	Acti-Brief Uri-Drain System with 10 pouches			
	Sizes S, M, L, XL			
	Flange size 20mm	AB/18/20	1	2375
	25mm	AB/18/25	1	2375
	27.5mm	AB/18/27.5	1	2375
	30mm	AB/18/30	1	2375
	32.5mm	AB/18/32.5	1	2375
	35mm	AB/18/35	1	2375
	40mm	AB/18/40	1	2375
	Uri-Drain System with 10 pouches			
	Flange Size 20mm	LU18/20	1	2375
	25mm	LU18/25	1	2375
	27.5mm	LU/18/27.5	1	2375
	30mm	LU18/30	1	2375
	32.5mm	LU/18/32.5	1	2375
	35mm	LU18/35	1	2375
	40mm	LU18/40	1	2375
	Replacement pouches for LU18	SP18	15	2475

Coloplast Ltd see Jade-Euro-Med Ltd

IXB

INCONTINENCE APPLIANCES

URINAL SYSTEMS

Manufacturer	Appliance	Order No.	Quantity	List Price p
DBT Medical Ltd	Thames urinal with standard bag and connecting tube	LM751100	1	8465
	Thames urinal with long bag and connecting tube	LM751102	1	8465
	Severn urinal with standard bag and connecting tube	LM752120	1	8465
	Severn urinal with 5 plastic bags and connecting tube	LM752124	1	8465
	Mersey urinal with 5 plastic bags and connecting tube	LM753224	1	8465
	'55' male urinal	LM756200	1	8338
	Spare sheaths for' 55' urinal	LM756212	6	3781
	Stoke Mandeville Pattern			
	Male urinal			
	20mm sheath	LM754001	1	8465
	24mm sheath	LM754002	1	8465
	25mm sheath	LM754003	1	8465
	28mm sheath	LM754004	1	8465
	32mm sheath	LM754005	1	8465
	35mm sheath	LM754006	1	8465
	38mm sheath	LM754007	1	8465
	42mm sheath	LM754008	1	8465
	45mm sheath	LM754009	1	8465
	48mm sheath	LM754010	1	8465
	51mm sheath	LM754011	1	8465
	54mm sheath	LM754012	1	8465
	57mm sheath	LM754013	1	8465
	60mm sheath	LM754014	1	8465
	63mm sheath	LM754015	1	8465
	Spare sheaths on request		1	715
	Sahara one-piece top PP urinal			
	with small rubber collection bag			
	Paed	LM755109	1	8070
	with 5 small plastic collection bags			
	Paed	LM755110	1	8070
	with standard collection bag and connection tube			
	Standard	LM755120	1	8070
	with long collection bag and connection tube			
	Standard	LM755130	1	8070
	with five medium collection bags and connection tube			
	Standard	LM755140	1	8070
	with standard rubber bag and connection tube			
	Large	LM755150	1	8070
	with long rubber bag and connection tube			
	Large	LM755160	1	8070
	with five medium plastic bags and connection tube			
	Large	LM755170	1	8070

INCONTINENCE APPLIANCES

URINAL SYSTEMS

Manufacturer	Appliance	Order No.	Quantity	List Price p
DBT Medical Ltd	Peoplecare PP Male urinal:			
	PP flange 25mm child			
	Sheath size			
	13mm	LM844113	1	2620
	16mm	LM844116	1	2620
	19mm	LM844119	1	2620
	PP flange 29mm child			
	Sheath size			
	22mm	LM845122	1	2620
	25mm	LM845125	1	2620
	PP flange 32mm child			
	Sheath size			
	19mm	LM845219	1	2620
	22mm	LM845222	1	2620
	25mm	LM845225	1	2575
	PP flange 38mm adult			
	Sheath size			
	19mm	LM846319	1	2620
	22mm	LM846322	1	2620
	25mm	LM846325	1	2620
	29mm	LM846329	1	2620
	32mm	LM846332	1	2620
	PP flange 44mm adult			
	Sheath size			
	35mm	LM847435	1	2620
	38mm	LM847438	1	2620
	41mm	LM847441	1	2620
	PP Standard bag			
	Medium	LM881002	1	1352
	Large	LM881003	1	1677
	PP Curved Top			
	Small	LM874101	1	1020
	Meduim	LM874102	1	1020
	Large	LM874103	1	1020
	PP Straight Top			
	Small	LM875211	1	1020
	Meduim	LM875212	1	1020
	Large	LM875213	1	1020
	Ex-large	LM875214	1	1020
	Transverse rubber bag with tap for above urinal	LM881001	1	2769
	Double based PP Flange for above urinal	LM846350	1	2620
	Rubber pubic flange, adult, for above urinal	LM854229	1	3021
Ellis, Son & Paramore Ltd	Hallam Modular Urinals	NS200	1	3163
	Spare bag	NS200(a)	1	168
	Spare belt	NS200(b)	1	375
Hollister Ltd	Retracted Penis Pouch	9811	10	2783
	Retracted Penis Pouch with Flextend Skin Barrier	9873	10	2735

IXB

INCONTINENCE APPLIANCES

URINAL SYSTEMS

Manufacturer	Appliance		Order No.	Quantity	List Price p
Jade-Euro-Med Ltd (including products formerly listed under Coloplast Ltd & Mentor Medical Ltd)	Aquadry cones for use with pubic pressure flanges				
	Straight				
		Small	787140	1	1294
		Medium	787159	1	1294
		Large	787167	1	1294
	Curved				
		Small	787175	1	1294
		Medium	787183	1	1294
		Large	787191	1	1294
	Aquadry pubic pressure flange with rubber understraps				
	Child	12mm	787000	1	2993
		15mm	787019	1	2993
		18mm	787027	1	2993
		22mm	787035	1	2993
		25mm	787043	1	2993
	Adult	25mm	787078	1	3083
		29mm	787086	1	3083
		32mm	787094	1	3083
		35mm	787108	1	3083
		38mm	787116	1	3083
		41mm	787124	1	3083
		44mm	787132	1	3083
	Aquadry pubic pressure urinal 1 all-in-one appliance with pressure ring, tapered inner sleeve trimmed to fit and rubber understraps				
			470856	1	6260
	Aquadry pubic pressure urinal 2 all-in-one appliance with pressure ring, diaphragm and rubber straps				
		25mm	785709	1	6260
		32mm	785717	1	6260
		38mm	785725	1	6260
	Aquadry pubic pressure urinal 3 all-in-one appliance with pressure ring, diaphragm and scrotal support				
		25mm	785733	1	6260
		32mm	785741	1	6260
		38mm	785768	1	6260
	Aquadry rubber belt				
		61cm, 71cm, 91.5cm, 112cm	787205	1	361
	Aquadry urinal all-in-one appliance with inner sheath and rubber understraps				
		29mm	784001	1	6260
		32mm	784028	1	6260
		35mm	784036	1	6260
		38mm	784044	1	6260
		41mm	784052	1	6260
	Rubber leg bag connecting tube with female attachment for urinal				
			785776	1	315

INCONTINENCE APPLIANCES

URINAL SYSTEMS

Manufacturer	Appliance	Order No.	Quantity	List Price p
Jade-Euro-Med Ltd (including products formerly listed under Coloplast Ltd & Mentor Medical Ltd)	Male urinals - all fitted with taps			
	Day and night use urinal with diaphragm, Scrotal support and bag. STATE SIZE OF DIAPHRAGM	Fig 4A	1	5844
	Urinal with waistband, Scrotal support complete with inner sheath and bag	Fig 5	1	7112
	Adult male urinal with pressure ring, diaphragm, rubber understraps. STATE SIZE OF DIAPHRAGM	Fig 101	1	6323
	Day and night urinal with pressure ring, inner sheath, waistband and understraps. STATE SIZE OF SHEATH	Fig 104	1	6941
	Day and night urinal with sheath, waistbelt, understraps and plastic bag	Fig 105	1	6733
	Urinal with inner sheath, rubber understraps and plastic bag. STATE SIZE OF SHEATH	Fig 106	1	6239
	Day and night urinal, scrotal support and plastic bag	Fig 107	1	5995
	Day and night urinal to contain penis and scrotum, fitted with inner sheath and diaphragm complete with bag	Fig 111A	1	5873
	Male jockey appliance with bag. STATE WAIST SIZE	M200	1	6253
	Replacement belt for above. STATE WAIST SIZE	JB/200	1	1228
	Plastic bags	OLBWT(L)	5	1576
	Rubber bag	RB/M200	1	2626
+	Ring	SP/M200	1	102
	Stoke Mandeville replacement sheath (state size of sheath)	SMS	1	655
	Male PP urinal with 5 plastic bags (state size of sheath)	PP2	1	6681
	Spare parts for PP Urinals:			
	Flange with sheaths, state size	PP3	1	3317
	Cone - small straight	PP4	1	1315
	Cone - small curved	PP5	1	1315
	Cone - medium straight	PP6	1	1315
	Cone - medium curved	PP7	1	1315
	Cone - large straight	PP8	1	1315
	Cone - large curved	PP9	1	1315
	Cone - ex-large straight	PP10	1	1315
	Plastic bag small	OLBWT(S)	5	1576
	Plastic bag large	OLBWT(L)	5	1576
	Rubber bag with air vent for use with all Jade-Euro-Med urinals	PP13	1	2574

+to be deleted 1 June 2007

IXB

INCONTINENCE APPLIANCES

URINAL SYSTEMS

Manufacturer	Appliance	Order No.	Quantity	List Price p
Jade-Euro-Med Ltd (including products formerly listed under Coloplast Ltd & Mentor Medical Ltd)	Progress long life plastic urinal bags pk 10	M700	1	2805
	Progress long life plastic scrotal urinal bags pk 10	M800	1	2805
	Fridjohn urinal	M600	1	8385
	Y.B. Wet. A complete urinal system STATE SHEATH SIZE 25mm/29mm/32mm/36mm/41mm	M500	1	6805
	Essex appliance. A complete urinal system. STATE SHEATH SIZE 21mm/25mm/31mm/35mm/40mm	M400	1	5391
	1-piece belt, incorporating double based flange and bag	KM28	1	5685
	1-piece belt, with flange and 5 plastic bags	KM29	1	5685
	Male PP urinal, child, with integral flange Plastic bag: Curved cone Medium	WR013-01-R	1	6847
	Replacement PP flange with integral sheath for child pp urinals: Sheath 22mm Flange 25mm	WS025-22-L	1	3855
	Sheath 25mm Flange 32mm	WS032-25-K	1	3855
	Replacement curved rubber cone top for above urinals Small	WS130-01-S	1	1630
	Medium	WS130-03-W	1	1630
	Large	WS130-05-B	1	1630
	Replacement straight rubber cone top for above urinals Medium	WS135-03-T	1	1630
	Large	WS135-05-X	1	1630
	Ex-large	WS135-07-C	1	1630
	Replacement double-based PP flange child 32mm opening	WS160-32-V	1	3446
	adult 38mm opening	WS160-38-J	1	3446
	adult 44mm opening	WS160-44-D	1	3446
	Chailey male urinal, adolescent/adult with rubber bag	WP100-01-P	1	6462
	plastic bag	WP105-01-L	1	8185

INCONTINENCE APPLIANCES

URINAL SYSTEMS

Manufacturer	Appliance	Order No.	Quantity	List Price p
Jade-Euro-Med Ltd (including products formerly listed under Coloplast Ltd & Mentor Medical Ltd)	Spares for Chailey urinals 1 piece curved top with integral sheath and under-straps			
	child 22mm sheath	WS200-22-R	1	4312
	adult 22mm sheath	WS202-22-A	1	4312
	adult 25mm sheath	WS202-25-G	1	4312
	adult 29mm sheath	WS202-29-Q	1	4312
	adult 32mm sheath	WS202-32-D	1	4312
	adult 35mm sheath	WS202-35-K	1	4312
	adult 38mm sheath	WS202-38-R	1	4312
	adult 44mm sheath	WS202-44-L	1	4312
	- rubber belt			
	61cm	WS101-61-A	1	636
	66cm	WS101-91-26	1	636
	71cm	WS101-91-28	1	636
	76cm	WS101-91-30	1	636
	81cm	WS101-91-32	1	636
	86cm	WS101-91-34	1	636
	91cm	WS101-91-36	1	636
	97cm	WS101-91-38	1	636
	102cm	WS101-91-40	1	636
	107cm	WS101-91-42	1	636
	112cm	WS101-91-44	1	636
	117cm	WS101-91-46	1	636
	- rubber bags (suitable also for PP and	WS110-01-G	1	2051
	Chiron urinals)	WS110-05-Q	1	2810
	- plastic bags (suitable also for PP urinals & Chiron urinals)			
	wide neck	WS120-10-N	1	423
	adult	WS120-05-V	1	423
	child	WS120-01-M	1	423
	Male PP urinal, adult, with integral flange			
	rubber bag - various sizes	WP001-01-M	1	8002
		WP003-01-V	1	8002
		WP005-01-E	1	8002
	plastic bag - various sizes	WP011-01-S	1	7561
		WP013-01-B	1	7561
		WP015-01-K	1	7561
	Replacement PP flange for above 19mm	WS038-19-R	1	3855
	22mm	WS038-22-E	1	3855
	25mm	WS038-25-L	1	3855
	29mm	WS038-29-U	1	3855
	32mm	WS038-32-H	1	3855
	35mm	WS038-35-P	1	3855
	38mm	WS038-38-V	1	3855
	41mm	WS038-41-J	1	3855
	Male PP urinal, adult, with double-based flange			
	- rubber bag	WP031-01-D	1	8115
	- plastic bag - various sizes	WP035-01-V	1	7561
		WP041-01-J	1	7561

IXB

INCONTINENCE APPLIANCES

URINAL SYSTEMS

Manufacturer	Appliance		Order No.	Quantity	List Price p
Jade-Euro-Med	Replacement sheath for above urinals		WS160-01-J	10	148
Ltd (including	Rubber bag with vent tube for PP urinals				
products formerly	adult		WS140-05-G	1	3364
listed under	Rubber double bag, adult,		WS140-08-N	1	3602
Coloplast Ltd &	for PP urinals				
Mentor Medical	Stoke Mandeville sheath type urinal		WP110-01-U	1	7393
Ltd)	Stoke Mandeville double		WP113-01-H	1	9608
	rubber bag urinal				
	Replacement sheaths		WS160-02-L	10	443
	Replacement bag for WP113		WS140-07-L	1	3602
	Replacement sheath for WP113				
		22mm	WS162-22-B	1	1008
		25mm	WS162-25-H	1	1008
		29mm	WS162-29-R	1	1008
		32mm	WS162-32-E	1	1008
	Chiron male rubber urinal with		WP124-01-S	1	6653
	webbing belt				
	* Surrey model L/weight urinal				
	L- MK I	25mm	WP130-25-V	1	6018
		38mm	WP130-38-F	1	6018
	L - MK II	25mm	WP133-25-J	1	6018
		32mm	WP133-32-F	1	6018
		38mm	WP133-38-T	1	6018

* Replacement bags for the Surrey Urinal can be found on page 400

	Chiron male plastic urinal				
	(rubber sheaths)		WP145-01-H	1	3443
	Chiron geriatric urinal				
	(film type sheaths)		WP148-01-V	1	4999
	Replacement sheaths for WP145 & WP151				
		25mm	WS168-25-J	1	636
		29mm	WS168-29-S	1	636
	Replacement net suspensory		WS107-08-W	1	1495
	for WP107, WP129 & WP145				
	Transverse rubber bag &		WS145-01-U	1	3801
	stopcock (child)				
	Non allergic film type sheath		WS161-01-N	10	117
Manfred Sauer	URIbag pocket sized (when not in use)		URIbag	1	1323
UK Ltd (formerly	reusable urinal for men & urinary/ostomy				
Manfred Sauer	appliance users, 1.1 Litre capacity				
GmbH)	URIbag F pocket sized		URIbagF	1	1323
	(when not in use) reusable urinal for				
	females, 1.2 Litre capacity				
	URIfem female reusable bottle urinal		URIfem	1	1323
	(sterile up to 130°C) for women lying				
	down or in semi-sitting position in bed, 1				
	Litre capacity				

Manfred Sauer GmbH see Manfred Sauer UK Ltd

Mentor Medical Ltd see Jade-Euro-Med Ltd

INCONTINENCE APPLIANCES

URINAL SYSTEMS

Manufacturer	Appliance		Order No.	Quantity	List Price p
S G & P Payne	Male Incontinence Appliance with rubber belt				
	MK 1	- with combined rubber flange & understraps	0001	1	7137
	MK 2	- with rubber flange & fabric facepiece	0002	1	7674
	MK 3	- with combined rubber flange understraps and coned top	0003	1	6334
	Lightweight male Incontinence Appliance				
	MK 4	- with fabric facepiece & separate long flanged plastic bag with foam pad	0004	1	4524
	MK 5	- with fabric facepiece separate flange & long flanged plastic bag with material facepiece and belt	0005	1	6355
	MK 6	- with combined flange & understraps& long flanged plastic bag & rubber belt	0006	1	5573
	MK 7	- with flange material flange support reinforced coned top and plastic or rubber bag	0007	1	7996
	MK 8	- with flange material flange support long plastic bag	0008	1	6680
	MK 9	- with rubber flange & wide belt with scrotal support	0009	1	7996
	MK 10	- with flange support with wide belt & scrotal support separate flange & long flanged plastic bag	0010	1	6679
	MK 11	- with flange soft replaceable diaphragm material facepiece with belt and adjustable rubber understraps soft coned top plastic or rubber bag	0011	1	7996
	MK 12	- with flange soft replaceable diaphragm material facepiece with belt and adjustable rubber understraps long plastic bag	0012	1	6680
	Replacements for above appliances				
	Rubber flange with - feathered diaphragm (MK2,MK5,MK9,MK10)				
		Medium 32mm	0511	1	2067
		Large 38mm	0512	1	2067
		Ex-large 45mm	0513	1	2067
		and understrap (MK1,MK6)			
		Small 25mm	0501	1	3199
		Medium 32mm	0502	1	3199
		Large 38mm	0503	1	3199
		Ex-large 45mm	0504	1	3199
		Feathered diaphragm & combined reinforced top	0560	1	3629

IXB

INCONTINENCE APPLIANCES

URINAL SYSTEMS

Manufacturer	Appliance	Order No.	Quantity	List Price p
S G & P Payne	Rubber flange 38mm (MK11 MK12)	0516	1	2067
	Rubber flange 45mm (MK11, MK12)	0517	1	2067
	Soft replaceable rubber diaphragms (MK11, MK12)	0519	3	515
	Material facepiece with belt & loop (MK2,MK4,MK5)	0430	1	2396
	Reinforced cone top (MK1,MK2,MK9)			
	Small - to fit 25mm flange	0601	1	1390
	Medium - to fit any size flange	0602	1	1390
	Large - to fit any size flange	0603	1	1390
	Soft coned top (MK11)	0619	1	1390
	Plastic bag (MK1,MK2,MK3,MK7,MK9,MK11)	0801	1	349
	Rubber bag (MK1,MK2,MK3,MK7,MK9,MK11)	0901	1	2103
	Rubber belt (MK1, MK3, MK6)	0101	1	451
	Elastic belt (MK1,MK3,MK6)			
	Waist size 70cm	0201	1	954
	Waist size 75cm	0202	1	954
	Waist size 80cm	0203	1	954
	Waist size 85cm	0204	1	954
	Waist size 90cm	0205	1	954
	Waist size 95cm	0206	1	954
	Web belt (MK1,MK3,MK6)	0301	1	667
	Flange support with wide belt & scrotal support (MK9,MK10)			
	Small - Waist size 70/80cm	0420	1	2718
	Medium - Waist size 80/90cm	0421	1	2718
	Large - Waist size 90/100cm	0422	1	2718
	Material flange support (MK7, MK8)			
	70cm	0401	1	2718
	75cm	0402	1	2718
	80cm	0403	1	2718
	85cm	0404	1	2718
	90cm	0405	1	2718
	95cm	0406	1	2718
	100cm	0407	1	2718
	105cm	0408	1	2718
	110cm	0409	1	2718
	Night connector (MK1,MK2,MK3,MK7,MK9,MK11)	0701	1	451

INCONTINENCE APPLIANCES

URINAL SYSTEMS

Manufacturer	Appliance	Order No.	Quantity	List Price p
S G & P Payne	Long flanged plastic bag (MK5,MK6,MK8,MK10,MK12)			
	38mm - to fit 32/38mm flange	0811	1	472
	45mm - to fit 45mm flange	0812	1	472
	with foam pad (MK4)			
	38mm - to fit 32/38mm flange	0821	1	536
	45mm - to fit 45mm flange	0822	1	536
	Material facepiece with belt and adjustable rubber understraps (MK11, MK12)			
	Small	0414	1	2718
	Medium	0415	1	2718
	Large	0416	1	2718
	Material facepiece with support belt, loop and scrotal (MK2,MK4,MK5)	0441	1	2718
	Incontiaid Reuseable Urinal Bottle	1350	1	882
	Payne's Male Urine Director	0630	1	2554
	Payne's Female Urine Director	0631	1	2554
	PP Urinal Complete with rubber bag/plastic bag	0019	1	7137
	Pubic Pressure Flange			
	25mm with -			
	13mm sheath	0520	1	3199
	17mm sheath	0521	1	3199
	19mm sheath	0522	1	3199
	22mm sheath	0523	1	3199
	32mm with			
	22mm sheath	0524	1	3199
	25mm sheath	0525	1	3199
	38mm with			
	29mm sheath	0526	1	3199
	32mm sheath	0527	1	3199
	45mm with			
	35mm sheath	0528	1	3199
	38mm sheath	0529	1	3199
	42mm sheath	0530	1	3199
	Coned Top			
	Straight			
	Small for 25mm flange	0620	1	1390
	Medium for any size flange	0621	1	1390
	Large for any size flange	0622	1	1390
	Curved			
	Small for 25mm flange	0623	1	1390
	Medium for any size flange	0624	1	1390
	Large for any size flange	0625	1	1390

INCONTINENCE APPLIANCES

URINAL SYSTEMS

Manufacturer	Appliance	Order No.	Quantity	List Price p
S G & P Payne	Rubber bag with vent tube (MK1,MK2,MK3,MK7,MK9,MK11)	0910	1	2524
	Reinforced cone top with vent tube			
	Small	0610	1	1829
	Medium	0611	1	1829
	Large	0612	1	1829
	Stoke Mandeville condom urinal complete	0020	1	5890
	Spares for above:			
	Kipper bags	0920	1	3313
	Rubber tube & connector	0712	1	257
	Dry incontinence sheaths			
	plain end	1101	100	1714
	teated end	1106	100	1714
	Rubber tubing			
	latex 8mm	1203	per metre	530
	red 8mm	1204	per metre	530
	latex 10mm	1205	per metre	530
	red 10mm	1206	per metre	530
	Nylon connectors			
	GU	0711	1	150
	SM	0710	1	150
	GU Pattern Stoke Mandeville Condom Set	0021	1	6141
	As above with 1136ml bag	0022	1	7618
	Replacement parts for above urinals			
	Kipper bags - see Leg Bags			
	Nylon studs - GU	0711	1	150
	- SM	0710	1	150
	Nylon stud with latex tube	0712	1	257
	Adjustable web belt			
	Waist size up to 95cm	0304	1	703
	Waist size up to 115cm	0305	1	703
	Waist size up to 150cm	0306	1	703
	Male urinal for day and night use, air tube to bag, inner sheath and diaphragm to receiver, web belt and cotton suspensory bag	IU/9	1	5777
	Male urinal with long narrow bag, web belt and cotton suspensory bag	IU/365	1	6013
	Male urinal for day use, the receiver to contain the penis and scrotum, web waist band and tape understraps	IU/11	1	5518

INCONTINENCE APPLIANCES

URINAL SYSTEMS

Manufacturer	Appliance	Order No.	Quantity	List Price p
S G & P Payne	Male urinal for night use, similar to IU/11 but the receiver designed for use in bed	IU/12	1	5518
	Male urinal for day and night use, short rubber bag, detachable bag and night tube, web belt and cotton suspensory bag	IU/43	1	4599
	Replacement suspension bag - small, medium & large	IU/1458	1	581
Salts Healthcare	Male PP urinal			
	- rubber bag	ZL0001	1	5838
	- plastic bag (4)	ZL0001	1	5838
	Spare parts for above urinal			
	25mm flange			
	18mm sheath	ZL0053	1	2775
	32mm flange			
	25mm sheath	ZL0059	1	2775
	38mm flange			
	18mm sheath	ZL0060	1	2775
	22mm sheath	ZL0061	1	2775
	25mm sheath	ZL0062	1	2775
	29mm sheath	ZL0063	1	2775
	32mm sheath	ZL0064	1	2775
	44mm flange			
	35mm sheath	ZL0065	1	2775
	38mm sheath	ZL0066	1	2775
	Cone - small straight	ZL0100	1	1235
	small curved	ZL0101	1	1235
	medium straight	ZL0102	1	1235
	medium curved	ZL0103	1	1235
	large curved	ZL0105	1	1235
	ex-large straight	ZL0106	1	1235
	Pubic Pressure Flange Belt	ZL0034	1	2437
	- plastic bags			
	adult	ZL0152	4	1358
	- rubber bag			
	adult	ZL0155	1	1358
	child	ZL0154	1	1358
	transverse	ZL0153	1	1358
	- belt	ZL0010	1	413

IXB

INCONTINENCE APPLIANCES

URINAL SYSTEMS

Manufacturer	Appliance	Order No.	Quantity	List Price p
Ward Surgical	Jockey Male Urinal	WM27	1	7314
Appliance Co	Varsity Male Urinal	WM14	1	5646
	Day use, covered bag complete with belt suspensory and thigh strap	Fig 4	1	4671
	Male urinal Day and Night use covered bag air vent, belt suspensory	Fig 4A	1	4834
	Male urinal Day and Night use with short bag and belt	Fig 104	1	5004
	As above with covered bag	Fig 104a	1	5424
	As above with double chamber bag	Fig 104b	1	5638
	Male urinal Day and night use with long bag and belt	Fig 105	1	5004
	Paraplegic male urinal	Fig 110	1	6839
	Stoke Mandeville Pattern	WM18	1	6571
	Male PP urinal rubber bag	WM19	1	6123
	Stoke Mandeville spare sheaths - rubber	WM20	1	609
	Male PP urinal plastic bag (4)	WM21	1	5425
	Replacement for above			
	PP flange	WM22	1	2809
	PP cone	WM23	1	1110
	Rubber bag	WM24	1	1521
	Plastic bag	WM26	1	304
	Night use, covered bag complete with belt suspensory and thigh strap	Fig 5	1	5874
	Day and night use, covered bags, air vent complete with belt, suspensory and thigh strap	Fig 5a	1	5874
	Day and night use, long tube rubber bag with air vent, complete with belt and thigh strap	Fig 6	1	5333
	Male dribbling bag and tapes	Fig 9	1	2170
	Day and night use, short covered bag	Fig 101	1	5004
	Day and night use, short bag & belt	Fig 106	1	5004
	Male urinal - sheath and suspensory with short covered bag	WM56	1	5457
	Male urinal - sheath and suspensory with long covered bag	WM57	1	5457
	Night urinal with long tube	WM59	1	2637
	Stoke Mandeville sheath type urinal, with 30 rubber film sheaths, rubber bag and thigh strap and belt	WM49	1	5224
	Webbing Belt	WM102	1	924
	Elastic leg strap	WM103	10	528
	Net Suspensory	WM104	1	1215
	Spare rubber bag with vent	WM105	1	2639
	Spare Receiver	WM106	1	3800

INCONTINENCE APPLIANCES

MANUFACTURERS' ADDRESSES AND TELEPHONE NUMBERS
(INCONTINENCE APPLIANCES)

A1 Pharmaceuticals PLC, Unit 3 and 4 Bessemer Park, 250 Milkwood Road, Herne Hill, London SE24 0HG (0207 7387373)

Astra Tech Ltd, Stroud Water Business Park, Brunel Way, Stonehouse, Gloucester GL10 3SW (01453 791763)

B. Braun Medical Ltd, Thorncliffe Park, Sheffield, S35 2PW (0114 225 9000)

Bard Ltd, Forest House, Brighton Road, Crawley, West Sussex RH11 9BP (01293 527888)

Beambridge Medical, 46 Merrow Lane, Burpham, Guildford, Surrey GU4 7LQ (01483 827696/01483 571928)

Bio Diagnostics, Upton Industrial Estate, Rectory Road, Upton-upon-Severn, Worcestershire WR8 0LX (01684 592262)

Charles S Bullen (Stomacare) Ltd, 85/87 Kempston Street, Liverpool L3 8HE (0151 2076995)

Camp Ltd, Northgate House, Staple Gardens, Winchester, Hampshire SO23 8ST (01962 855248)

CliniMed Ltd, Cavell House, Knaves Beech Way, Loudwater, High Wycombe, Bucks, HP10 9QY (01628 850100)

CliniSupplies Ltd, Unit 9 Crystal Way, Elmgrove Road, Harrow, Middlesex, HA1 2HP (0208 8634168)

Coloplast Ltd, Peterborough Business Park, Peterborough PE2 6FX (01733 392000)

ConvaTec Ltd, Harrington House, Milton Road, Ickenham, Uxbridge, UB10 8PU (01895 628400)

Dansac Ltd, Victory House, Vision Park, Histon, Cambridge CB4 4ZR (01223 235100)

DBT Medical Ltd, 14 Eagle Industrial Estate, The Crofts, Witney, OX28 4DJ (01993 773673)

Ellis, Son & Paramore Ltd, Spring Street Works, Sheffield, S3 8PD (0114 2738921/221269)

Engineers & Doctors Ltd, Cornwallis House, Howard Chase, Basildon, Essex SS14 3BB (0800 1699189)

Flexicare Medical Ltd, Cynon Valley Business Park, Mountain Ash, Mid-Glamorgan, CF45 4ER (01443 474647)

GF Products, 3 Newnham Lane, Burwell, Cambridgeshire, CB5 0EA (01638 610028)

GP Supplies Ltd, Unit 1 behind AMC House, 12 Cumberland Avenue, Park Royal, London, NW10 7QL (0845 458 4040)

GTA (UK) Ltd, 34 Nottingham South Industrial Estate, Ruddington Lane, Wilford, Nottingham, NG11 7EP (0115 9815703)

Hollister Ltd, Rectory Court, 42 Broad Street, Wokingham, Berkshire, RG40 1AB (0118 989 5000) (Retail Pharmacy Order Line 0800 521392)

Hospital Management & Supplies Ltd, Salthouse Road, Brackmills, Northampton, NN4 OU4 (01604 704600)

Hunter Urology Ltd, 1 The Stable Yard, Woodhayes, Honiton, Devon, EX14 4TP (01404 44088)

Jade-Euro-Med Ltd, Unit 14, East Hanningfield Industrial Estate, Old Church Road, East Hanningfield, Chelmsford, Essex, CM3 8BG (01245 400413)

JBOL Ltd, 1 Folley Bridge, Oxford, OX1 4LB (01865 240572)

JLJ Healthcare Ltd, Number One 61 Whitehall Road, Halesowen, West Midlands, B63 3JS (0121 6023943)

L.IN.C Medical Systems Ltd, Loddington House, Main Street, Loddington, Leicestershire, LE7 9XE (01572 717515)

Malvern Medical Developments Ltd, Unit 10, Northbrook Close, Worcester, WR3 8BP (01905 731343)

Manfred Sauer GmbH see Manfred Sauer UK Ltd

INCONTINENCE APPLIANCES

MANUFACTURERS' ADDRESSES AND TELEPHONE NUMBERS (INCONTINENCE APPLIANCES)

Manfred Sauer UK Ltd, Unit 3 io Centre, Lodge Farm, Northampton NN5 7UW (0870 1904100)

Medasil (Surgical) Ltd, Medasil House, Hunslet Road, Leeds LS10 1AU (0113 2433491)

Mentor Medical Ltd, Building 10, Commerce Way, Lancing, West Sussex BN15 8TJ (01903 761122)

Neomedic Ltd: distributed by GP Supplies Ltd

North West Medical Supplies Ltd, Premier House, Southgate Way, Orton Southgate, Peterborough, PE2 6YG (01733 361336)

S G & P Payne, Percy House, Brook Street, Hyde, Cheshire SK14 2NS (0161 3678561)

Pennine Healthcare Ltd, City Gate, London Road, Derby DE24 8WY (01332 794880)

Rochester Medical Ltd, 10 Commerce Way, Lancing, West Sussex BN15 8TA (01903 875055)

Salts Healthcare Ltd, Richard Street, Aston, Birmingham, B7 4AA (0121 3332000)

Shiloh Healthcare Ltd: Lion Mill, Fitton Street, Royton, Oldham, OL2 5JX (0161 624 5641)

Teleflex Medical, Stirling Road, Cressex Business Park, High Wycombe, Buckinghamshire, HP12 3ST (01494 532761)

The Kendall Company (UK) Ltd see Tyco Healthcare

Tyco Healthcare, 154 Fareham Road, Gosport, Hampshire, PO13 0FN (01329 224000)

Universal Hospital Supplies, 313 Chase Road, London N14 6JA (0208 9206207)

Unomedical Ltd, Thornhill Road, North Moons Moat, Redditch, Worcestershire B98 9NL (01527 64222)

Ward Surgical Appliance Company Ltd, 57A Brightwell Avenue, Westcliffe-on-Sea, Essex, SS0 9EB (01702 354064)

STOMA APPLIANCES
(Colostomy, Ileostomy, Urostomy)

1.   Prescribers and suppliers should note that products not included in the list are not prescribable (See Part I Clause 2).

2.   Where the information is available, the **"Reference Capacity"** of a stoma bag will be given. This is intended to give a guide of comparison between different bag sizes, but *should not be taken to indicate actual usable capacity.* "Reference Capacity" shall be measured according to BS 7127:Part 101:1991, Appendix M, with the level of water set at the lower edge of the opening of wafer or flange.

3.   Only basic information has been provided and prescribers may on occasions wish to seek further information about certain products eg when assessing a patient for the first time. If so this is always available from the manufacturers (addresses and telephone numbers are given at the end of the entry). Information may also be sought from stoma nurses and community pharmacists.

4.   Where the prescriber has not specified the type of appliance or part thereof or accessory, the pharmacy or appliance contractor must endorse the prescription form stating the type supplied and submit the invoice if requested by the NHSBSA, Prescription Pricing Division.

IXC

STOMA APPLIANCES

ADHESIVE DISCS/RINGS/PADS/PLASTERS

Manufacturer	Appliance	Order No.	Quantity	List Price p
For a list of adhesive tapes prescribable under Drug Tariff see Part IXA				
C S Bullen Ltd	Double-sided Adhesive			
	Plaster Zinc Oxide			
	89mm x 89mm	UF 33	10	426
	102mm x 102mm	UF 34	10	526
	127mm x 127mm	UF 35	10	888
	Double Sided Adhesive			
	Plastic Acrylic Base			
	89mm x 89mm	UF 62	10	382
	102mm x 102mm	UF 63	10	491
	127mm x 127mm	UF 64	10	826
	Flange Retention Strips			
	102mm x 25mm	UF 440	100	381
	102mm x 51mm	UF 441	100	516
	Shelter Safe-Seal	UF7000	40	2150
CliniMed Ltd	HydroFrame Flange Extenders	WAF H33	20 (strips)	1266
Essentials Accessories				
Jade-Euro-Med Ltd	Kidney Seals - Adhesive Flange Retaining Strips			
(formerly Mentor	Small	WJ250-51-T	10	551
Medical Ltd)	Large	WJ250-75-J	10	551
	Double Sided - Adhesive Discs			
	76mm diam -			
	19mm opening	WJ002-19-R	10	520
	25mm opening	WJ002-25-L	10	520
	90mm diam -			
	32mm opening	WJ005-32-V	10	520
	38mm opening	WJ005-38-J	10	520
	Chiron Double-Sided Plasters			
	90mm square -			
	19mm opening	WJ010-19-N	10	706
	35mm opening	WJ010-35-L	10	706
	102mm square -			
	19mm opening	WJ011-19-S	10	811
	35mm opening	WJ011-35-Q	10	811
	127mm square -			
	19mm opening	WJ012-19-W	10	894
	35mm opening	WJ012-35-U	10	894
	150mm square -			
	19mm opening	WJ013-19-B	10	999
	102mm x 76mm -			
	19mm opening	WJ014-19-F	10	999
	102mm square -			
	25mm opening	WJ016-25-J	10	999
	125mm square -			
	25mm opening	WJ018-01-C	10	1096

STOMA APPLIANCES

ADHESIVE DISCS/RINGS/PADS/PLASTERS

Manufacturer	Appliance	Order No.	Quantity	List Price p
Mentor Medical Ltd	Carshalton Plasters Acrylic			
	25mm	48-530-40	10	553
	32mm	48-530-59	10	553
	38mm	48-530-67	10	553
	Carshalton Plasters Foam Ring			
	25mm	48-538-49	10	876
	32mm	48-538-57	10	876
	38mm	48-538-65	10	876
Mentor Medical Ltd also see Jade-Euro-Med Ltd				
OstoMart Ltd	OstoFix Flange Security Tape			
	2.5cm x 10cm	DGW1	100	396
	5cm x 10cm	DGW2	100	687
	OstoFix Forty Security Frames	DFW3	40	1850
Salts Healthcare	Transacryl Double Sided Plaster			
	25mm	833018	10	646
	32mm	833019	10	646
	38mm	833020	10	646
	Reliaseal Double-sided hypo-allergic adhesive disc			
	13mm round	906009	10	1962
	19mm round	906011	10	1962
	25mm round	906013	10	1962
	32mm round	906015	10	1962
	38mm round	906016	10	1962
	Secuplast Circular Plasters			
	32mm	SP32	10	1096
	38mm	SP38	10	1096
	45mm	SP45	10	1096
	57mm	SP57	10	1096
	70mm	SP70	10	1078
	Secuplast Hydro	SPH1	30	1150
T J Shannon Ltd	Easychange spare plasters with rings		5	655
	Rubber retaining ring	TJS 948h	5	662
	+ Double sided plasters	TJS 948a	25	1656
A H Shaw & Partners Ltd	Double Side plasters			
	128mm x 128mm hole cut to size	NSI 46	10	896
	102mm x 102mm hole cut to size	NSI 49	10	864
Ward Surgical Appliance Co	Double-Sided Plasters with opening	WM17	10	450
	Single-Sided Waterproof Plaster Strips			
	100mm x 25mm	WM17a	10	123
	100mm x 50mm	WM17b	10	185
Welland Medical Ltd	See CliniMed Ltd Essentials Accessories			

+to be deleted 1 June 2007

IXC

STOMA APPLIANCES

ADHESIVE PASTES, SPRAYS, SOLUTIONS

Manufacturer	Appliance	Order No.	Quantity	List Price p
Hollister Ltd	Medical Adhesive Aerosol	7730	90g	1609
Manfred Sauer UK Ltd (formerly Manfred Sauer GmbH)	* Original Skin Latex Adhesive in a 28g tube with a long pipette/nozzle applicator.	50.01	2	869
	* Pure Latex Skin Adhesive without any skin care components giving a stronger bond, in a 28g tube with a long pipette/nozzle applicator.	50.00	2	854
	* Lanolin Free Latex Skin Adhesive for people allergic to lanolin, in a 28g tube with a long pipette/nozzle applicator.	50.03	2	854
	* 50% reduction in skin care components, in a 28g tube with a long pipette/nozzle applicator.	50.05	2	854
	* 2% Resin giving a stronger bond than the original adhesive 50.01, in a 28g tube with a long pipette/nozzle applicator. Should only be tried after 50.01 is found to be too weak.	50.20	2	854
	* 12% Resin giving a stronger bond than the 2% resin adhesive 50.20, in a 28g tube with a long pipette/nozzle applicator. Should only be tried after 50.20 is found to be too weak.	50.22	2	854
	* Synthetic Skin Adhesive in a 28g tube with a long pipette/nozzle applicator.	50.36-2	2	1525
	* Synthetic Skin Adhesive in a 45ml bottle with brush in the lid	50.36	1	1525
Manfred Sauer GmbH see Manfred Sauer UK Ltd				
Salts Healthcare	Latex Adhesive Solution	833005	28ml	226

* Safe for direct application on the skin

STOMA APPLIANCES

ADHESIVE REMOVERS (SPRAYS, LIQUIDS, WIPES)

Manufacturer	Appliance	Order No.	Quantity	List Price p
CliniMed Ltd Essentials Accessories	Appeel No Sting Medical Adhesive Remover	3505	30 wipes	1470
		3500	50ml aerosol	887
	Clear Peel Adhesive Remover	3910	50ml	312
Coloplast Ltd	Comfeel Cleanser	4710	180ml bottle	1684
		4715	30 sachets	868
ConvaTec Ltd	ConvaCare Adhesive Remover Wipes	S208	100 wipes	1733
Hollister Ltd	Adhesive Remover	7731	76g	1372
	Universal Remover Wipes	7760	50	1306
Opus Healthcare Ltd	Lift medical Adhesive Remover	5500	30 sachets	870
		5501	100ml bottle	613
	Lift Plus Medical Adhesive Remover	5502	30 sachets	1420
		5503	50ml spray	865
	Ultra Cleanse	4400	30 sachets	853
		4401	200ml bottle	1656
OstoMart Ltd	OstoCLEAR	MRW1	30 sachets	856
		MRW2	100ml bottle	938
Pelican Healthcare	Citrus Fresh Adhesive Remover	133000	30 sachets	885
		133002	100ml	597
Salts Healthcare	Wipe Away Adhesive Remover	WA1	30 sachets	866

IXC

STOMA APPLIANCES

BAG CLOSURES
(Available separately from the bags)

Manufacturer	Appliance	Order No.	Quantity	List Price p
C S Bullen Ltd	Plastic Bag Clamp	400	10	650
	Soft Wire Ties	410	50	550
CliniMed Ltd	Soft-end Ties White	9760	30	284
CliniMed Ltd Essentials Accessories	Closure Clamps (Drainable Bags)	3750	1	117
Coloplast Ltd	Coloplast Clamp	9503	20	2064
ConvaTec Ltd	Clips (Beige) (1-pce pouch)	S207	10	332
	Soft Wire Ties	S205	50	574
	Curved Clip for Drainable Pouches	S202	10	588
Dansac Ltd	Opaque Soft Wire Ties	095-01	50	573
	Opaque Longer Soft Wire Ties	095-02	50	656
Hollister Ltd	Drainable Pouch Clamp Beige	8770	1	120
			10	1018
Mentor Medical Ltd	Closure Clips for Odourproof Bags	WN110-01-E	10	749
	Bag Clamp	32-285-17	10	969
Pelican Healthcare Ltd	Drainable Pouch Clips	130406	20	687
Salts Healthcare	Closure Clips	833044	5	215
	Drainable Pouch Clips	CL1	10	753

STOMA APPLIANCES

BAG COVERS

Note:
These stoma bag covers can be washed and reused many times. Cloth fabric ♦ types are more durable than those made of non-woven fabric ◊. Refer to the manufacturer's instructions.

Manufacturer	Appliance	Order No.	Quantity	List Price p
C S Bullen Ltd	♦ Night Bag Cover	UF57	1	857
	♦ Day Bag Cover	UF58	1	857
Coloplast Ltd	♦ Closed MC2000/MC2002			
	White	9011	5	2565
	Flesh	9021	5	2565
	♦ Open MC2000/MC2002			
	White	9012	5	2565
	Flesh	9022	5	2565
	♦ Mini Decorated Open MC2000			
	White	9013	5	2565
	Flesh	9023	5	2565
	♦ URO 2002 4260 White	9014	5	2565
	URO 2002 4240	9015	5	2565
	URO 2002 4241	9016	5	2565
	♦ ILEO B (Standard)	9003	5	2565
Cover Care	♦ Cover Care Pouch Covers			
	Mini 32/38mm pouches	L198	3	772
	45/57mm pouches	L199	3	772
	Large Urostomy pouches	L200	3	817
	Standard Drainable pouches	L201	3	817
	& urostomy pouches			
	Small 38/45 mm closed pouches	L203	3	817
	small drainable pouches,			
	combihesive closed pouches			
	Medium 57 & 70mm closed	L204	3	817
	pouches			
CUI (INT) Ltd	♦ Cuiwear Ostomy Support Underwear with in built pouch cover			
(formerly Cuiwear	Ladies	CF01-CF27	1	950
Ltd)		CF31-CF57	1	950
	Mens	CW01-CW15	1	950
		CN01-CN15	1	950
	♦ Cuiwear Urostomy Support Underwear with in built pouch cover with night			
	drainage			
	Ladies			
	Black	BS31-BS57	1	950
	White	BS01-BS27	1	950
Cuiwear Ltd see CUI (INT) Ltd				
Hi-Line Ltd	♦ Coversure Custom-made Covers			
	Appliance to be stated			
	White	Res C1	1	905
	Stone	Res C2	1	905
	White/Lace Front	Res C3	1	905
Impharm Nationwide	♦ Ostocovers (white or coloured)		3	698
Ltd				

STOMA APPLIANCES

BAG COVERS

Manufacturer	Appliance	Order No.	Quantity	List Price p
Jade-Euro-Med Ltd (formerly Mentor Medical Ltd)	♦ Cotton Bag Cover			
	Day Size	WN124-01-C	1	1219
	Night Size	WN125-04-N	1	1219
Mentor Medical Ltd	♦ Cotton Cover to fit Redifit Bags			
	25mm & 32mm opening	WN103-01-M	1	870
	38mm, 44mm & 51mm opening	WN103-04-T	1	870
	♦ Cotton Stomabag Covers			
	White	32-238-84	5	2736
	◊ "Symphony" Polythene Bag Cover	32-286-06	5	506
Mentor Medical Ltd also see Jade-Euro-Med Ltd				
Salts Healthcare	♦ Salts Cotton Bag Cover (appliance to be stated)	833029	1	420
	♦ Eakin Cotton Bag Covers Size of opening			
	Small	839030	1	488
		839031	1	488
	Large	839033	1	488
		839034	1	488
		839035	1	488
A H Shaw & Partners Ltd	♦ Day Bag Cover			
	Cotton	NSI 48	1	568
	Lycra	NSI 44	1	599
	♦ Night Bag Cover			
	Cotton	NSI 47	1	599
	Lycra	NSI 45	1	643
Ward Surgical Appliance Co	♦ White Linen Cover	15	1	652

STOMA APPLIANCES

BELTS

Manufacturer	Appliance	Order No.	Quantity	List Price p
B. Braun Medical	Almarys Twin Belt (support) 120mm for Two Piece System	31780	1	461
	Biotrol Waist Belt	F00780E	1	469
C S Bullen Ltd	38mm Elastic Belt with wire ring retainer			
	Small	UF 44	1	1035
	Medium	UF 45	1	1035
	Large	UF 46	1	1035
	25mm Elastic Belt with plastic retainer ring shield	UF 47	1	1095
	Waterproof Canvas retaining shield			
	Small	UF 48	1	1588
	Medium	UF 49	1	1588
	Large	UF 50	1	1588
	St Mark's Belt	UF551	1	4251
	Fitting windows in Stoma belt for use with Ileostomy bags or colostomy cups	UF 561	1	501
	Camilla Panty Girdle	BS210	1	1962
	Cloe Roll-on Girdle	BS225	1	1635
	Constance Panty Girdle	BS200	1	2593
J. Chawner Surgical Belts Ltd	Made to Measure Colostomy Belt with hole over stoma right and or left including steels; understraps, suspenders & zip as standard			
	made in Lycra	FC1	1	3130
Coloplast Ltd	Ileo Belt	0402	1	880
	K Flex Belt	0420	1	671
	Assura Seal Belt	0421	1	647
	Corsinel Made to measure support garments			
	Female 160010-160960		1	7837
	162010-162080		1	7837
	162340-162480		1	7837
	Male 170010-170480		1	7837
	172010-172040		1	7837
	172180-172240		1	7837
ConvaTec Ltd	System 2 Belt	S210	1	332

IXC

STOMA APPLIANCES

BELTS

Manufacturer	Appliance		Order No.	Quantity	List Price p
CoverCare	Male Support Belt				
	Waist Size:				
		Small 65-75cm	L100	1	2956
		Medium 77.5-87.5cm	L101	1	2956
		Large 90-100cm	L102	1	2956
		Ex- Large 102.5-112.5cm	L103	1	2956
	Provision for hole aperture		HOLE	1	566

(Patients who require a hole in belt should ensure belt fits correctly and with it on, ask stoma care nurse to mark central position of stoma with a cross (X); and return belt to supplier with sample of pouch used so that hole in belt can be customised to fit individual requirements).

Manufacturer	Appliance		Order No.	Quantity	List Price p
CUI (INT) Ltd	Fulcionel	Female	F301-F380	1	6950
(formerly		Male	M101-M140	1	6950
Cuiwear Ltd)					
Cuiwear Ltd see CUI (INT) Ltd					
Dansac Ltd	Dansac Belt & Plate Pack				
	1 adjustable elasticated belt with 5 plates				
	suitable for one and two piece appliances				
		50-63mm	09075-0000	1	4089
	Dansac Belt Pack				
	5 adjustable elasticated belts				
		50-63mm	09000-0000	5	4089
	Dansac Long Ostomy Belt				
		White 150cm	090-01	1	729
		Beige 100cm	090-02	1	729
		Beige 150cm	090-03	1	729
DBT Medical Ltd	Birkbeck Elastic Waistband & Shield				
		19mm	LM725219	5	4943
		38mm	LM725238	5	4943
		54mm	LM725254	5	4943
	Birkbeck Retaining ring - for use with above				
		19mm	LM725319	5	937
		38mm	LM725338	5	937
		54mm	LM725354	5	937
	Birkbeck Elastic Waist band		LM725100	5	3757
	White Sausage Belt		LM810004	per metre	845
Hi-Line Ltd	Breathable Stretch Unisex Ostomy Belt 21cm deep.				
	Sizes Small, Medium, Large, X Large, XX Large and XXX Large. With hole over stoma if required		Res 6	1	2957
	Breathable Stretch Unisex Ostomy Belt 13.5cm deep				
	Sizes Small, Medium, Large, X Large, XX Large and XXX Large. With hole over stoma if required		Res 6b	1	2396
	Lightweight Support Belt 13cm wide.				
	Small, Medium, Large, X Large, XX Large, XXX Large Hook & Eye or Velcro Fastening With hole over stoma		Res 3	1	2687

STOMA APPLIANCES

BELTS

Manufacturer	Appliance	Order No.	Quantity	List Price p
Hi-Line Ltd	Lightweight Support Belt (long) 21cm wide			
	Small, Medium, Large, X Large, XX Large,	Res 4	1	3118
	XXX Large Hook & Eye or Velcro Fastening			
	With hole over stoma			
	Ladies Ostomy belt including hole over stoma optional detachable suspenders*			
	*please indicate on order if required	Res 5	1	3719
	Medium control Ostomy Girdle/Pantie Brief including hole over stoma			
	With suspenders as required	Res 2	1	4191
	Ostomy Girdle/Pantie Brief including hole over stoma			
	With suspenders as required	Res 1	1	4264
	Seamless Two Way Stretch Unisex Colostomy Belt 26cm Deep			
	Small, Medium, Large, X Large, XX Large	Res 7	1	2219
	Seamless Two Way Stretch Unisex Colostomy Belt 27cm and above			
	Small, Medium, Large, X Large, XX Large	Res 8	1	2483
Hollister Ltd	Adapt Belt			
	66-109cm	7300	1	755
			10	6278
	74-124cm	7299	1	755
			10	6278
Jade-Euro-Med	Belt/double cotton face piece for St. Marks flange.			
Ltd (including	STATE HOLE SIZE	KM 22	1	1639
products	Belt/double cotton face piece with elastic fixing for St. Marks flange.			
formerly listed	STATE HOLE SIZE	KM 23	1	2138
under Mentor	Belt/double cotton face piece with tapes fixing for St. Marks flange.			
Medical Ltd)	STATE HOLE SIZE	KM 24	1	2161
	St Mark's Pattern Col. Belt			
	Male	KM 30	1	6263
	Female	KM 31	1	6263
	Ostomy Web and Elastic Belt with Button & Buckle			
	Fastening 25mm	KM 25	1	909
	Fastening 51mm	KM 26	1	1076
	Fastening 76mm	KM 27	1	1240
	Ostomy Girdle or Panti Brief, Hole over Stoma	KM 21	1	5306
	with or without Suspenders & or under-strap			
	(Range=KM2101 - KM2126)			
	Web & Elastic Belt			
	25mm wide			
	Small	WL002-25-01-S	1	1188
	Medium	WL002-25-02-U	1	1188
	Large	WL002-25-03-W	1	1188
	51mm wide			
	Lengths:			
	81cm	WL002-51-32-D	1	1385
	86cm	WL002-51-34-H	1	1385
	91cm	WL002-51-36-M	1	1385
	97cm	WL002-51-38-R	1	1385
	102cm	WL002-51-40-C	1	1385
	107cm	WL002-51-42-G	1	1385
	112cm	WL002-51-44-L	1	1385

IXC

STOMA APPLIANCES

BELTS

Manufacturer	Appliance	Order No.	Quantity	List Price p
Jade-Euro-Med	Short Web End and Buckle	WL005-25-P	1	802
Ltd (including	Web & Elastic Belt (25mm wide)			
products	61cm	WL008-25-24-U	1	1253
formerly listed	76cm	WL008-25-30-P	1	1253
under Mentor	81cm	WL008-25-32-T	1	1253
Medical Ltd)	91cm	WL008-25-36-C	1	1253
	Narrow Belt			
	Flange diam (38mm)			
	91cm	WL111-38-36-R	1	2471
	97cm	WL111-38-38-V	1	2471
	102cm	WL111-38-40-G	1	2471
	Web & Elastic Belt Child			
	25mm wide			
	71cm	WL129-25-28-J	1	999
	38mm wide			
	66cm	WL129-38-26-X	1	1391
	71cm	WL129-38-28-C	1	1391
	76cm	WL129-38-30-N	1	1391
	91cm	WL129-38-36-B	1	1391
	Elastic Non-Slip Belt			
	81cm	WL132-25-32-L	1	1391
	86cm	WL132-25-34-Q	1	1391
	97cm	WL132-25-38-Y	1	1391
	112cm	WL132-25-44-T	1	1391
	Non-slip belt			
	81cm	WL133-01-32-P	1	2037
	86cm	WL133-01-34-T	1	2037
	91cm	WL133-01-36-X	1	2037
	97cm	WL133-01-38-C	1	2037
	102cm	WL133-01-40-N	1	2037
Marlen USA	Adjustable Elastic Waist Belt	5004	1	270
Mentor Medical	Redifit Adjustable Belt			
Ltd	Small	WL123-01-H	1	999
	Medium	WL123-04-P	1	999
	Large	WL123-07-V	1	999
	Night Belt Two Way Stretch			
	Small	WL236-01-H	1	2785
	Medium	WL236-04-P	1	2785
	Large	WL236-07-V	1	2785
	Extra Large	WL236-09-A	1	2785
	Carshalton Belt			
	Medium	48-522-22	1	1053
	Large	48-524-19	1	1053
	Stoma Belt			
	Small - 43cm - 66cm	32-247-83	1	660
	Medium - 66cm x 109cm	32-248-80	1	648

Mentor Medical Ltd also see Jade-Euro-Med Ltd

STOMA APPLIANCES

BELTS

Manufacturer	Appliance	Order No.	Quantity	List Price p
Nu-Hope	Nu-Hope Support Belts			
Laboratories	(The standard opening is 60mm; the following alternative size and shape openings are			
(formerly	available by adding the appropriate suffix to the order code 50mm-E, 56mm-F, 63mm-G,			
Penlan Medical	68mm-A, 72mm-DC, 75mm-B, 80mm-C, Med Oval-H, Large Oval-J, Ex Large Oval-K)			
Ltd)	75mm wide			
	Small (70-78cm)	6400	1	3230
	Medium (80-88cm)	6401	1	3230
	Large (90-100cm)	6402	1	3230
	X-Large (103-115cm)	6403	1	3361
	XX-Large (118-130cm)	6404	1	3361
	100mm wide			
	Small (70-78cm)	6410	1	4024
	Medium (80-88cm)	6411	1	4024
	Large (90-100cm)	6412	1	4024
	X-Large (103-115cm)	6413	1	4188
	XX-Large (118-130cm)	6414	1	4188
	125mm wide			
	Small (70-78cm)	6420	1	4786
	Medium (80-88cm)	6421	1	4786
	Large (90-100cm)	6422	1	4786
	X-Large (103-115cm)	6423	1	4980
	XX-Large (118-130cm)	6424	1	4980
	150mm wide			
	Small (70-78cm)	6430	1	5545
	Medium (80-88cm)	6431	1	5545
	Large (90-100cm)	6432	1	5545
	X-Large (103-115cm)	6433	1	5769
	XX-Large (118-130cm)	6434	1	5769
	175mm wide (left)			
	Small (70-78cm)	6440	1	6396
	Medium (80-88cm)	6441	1	6396
	Large (90-100cm)	6442	1	6396
	X-Large (103-115cm)	6443	1	6650
	XX-Large (118-130cm)	6444	1	6650
	175mm wide (right)			
	Small (70-78cm)	6445	1	6396
	Medium (80-88cm)	6446	1	6396
	Large (90-100cm)	6447	1	6396
	X-Large (103-115cm)	6448	1	6650
	XX-Large (118-130cm)	6449	1	6650
	200mm wide (left)			
	Small (70-78cm)	6450	1	7258
	Medium (80-88cm)	6451	1	7258
	Large (90-100cm)	6452	1	7258
	X-Large (103-115cm)	6453	1	7552
	XX-Large (118-130cm)	6454	1	7552
	200mm wide (right)			
	Small (70-78cm)	6455	1	7258
	Medium (80-88cm)	6456	1	7258
	Large (90-100cm)	6457	1	7258
	X-Large (103-115cm)	6458	1	7552
	XX-Large (118-130cm)	6459	1	7552

IXC

STOMA APPLIANCES

BELTS

Manufacturer	Appliance	Order No.	Quantity	List Price p
Nu-Hope	225mm wide (left)			
Laboratories	Small (70-78cm)	6460	1	7420
(formerly	Medium (80-88cm)	6461	1	7420
Penlan Medical	Large (90-100cm)	6462	1	7420
Ltd)	X-Large (103-115cm)	6463	1	7565
	XX-Large (118-130cm)	6464	1	7565
	225mm wide (right)			
	Small (70-78cm)	6465	1	7420
	Medium (80-88cm)	6466	1	7420
	Large (90-100cm)	6467	1	7420
	X-Large (103-115cm)	6468	1	7565
	XX-Large (118-130cm)	6469	1	7565
	Prolapse Overbelt	P	1	1157
Oakmed Ltd	Made to Measure Ostomy Belt	B100	1	7679
	Made to Measure Pantie Girdle	P200	1	4981
	Made to Measure Ostomy Girdle	G300	1	4981
Omex Medical Ltd	Schacht Belt 91.5cm	780251	1	536
Orthotic Services Ltd	Made to Measure Ostomy Girdle in white - hole or panel over stoma as required; zips and suspenders as standard	OSL-012	1	3195
	(A measuring chart is available on application)			
OstoMart Ltd	Ostoshield (belt required)	Res50	1	667
	Ostoshield Belt Small/Medium only for use with Res 50 - Ostoshield	Res40	1	344
	Ostoshield Belt Large/Extra Large Only for use with Res 50 - Ostoshield	Res45	1	344
Pelican Healthcare Ltd	Pelican Adjustable Ostomy Belt	133006	1	721
Penlan Medical see Nu-Hope Laboratories				
E Sallis Ltd	Colostomy Belt for			
	Night use	14b	1	1178
		14c	1	614
	Day use	15a	1	3244
	Ostomy Girdle/Pantie Brief including hole over stoma, with suspenders as required			
	Made in elastane	Fit 15c	1	4109
	St Mark's Hospital Pattern			
	Colostomy Shield	17	1	1059

STOMA APPLIANCES

BELTS

Manufacturer	Appliance	Order No.	Quantity	List Price p
Salts Healthcare	Standard Adjustable Ostomy Belt			
	Beige 100cm	ABO1	1	737
	Eakin Stoma Support Belt with IsoFlex			
	20cm depth			
	Small (75-90cm)	839051	1	4669
	Medium (90-105cm)	839052	1	4669
	Large (105-120cm)	839053	1	4669
	X Large (120-135cm)	839054	1	4669
	26cm depth			
	Small (75-90cm)	839061	1	5188
	Medium (90-105cm)	839062	1	5188
	Large (105-120cm)	839063	1	5188
	X Large (120-135cm)	839064	1	5188
	25mm Single Elastic Belt with			
	2 loops:			
	Standard 89cm long	877002	1	389
	Ex-large 107cm long	877024	1	389
	25mm Single Elastic Belt with suspender ends	877007	1	456
	102mm Elastic Belt with waterproof panel	877008	1	1595
	With 4 loops & retaining ring	877009	1	2097
	25mm Button Belt	877011	1	389
	Button & Loop Belt	877012	1	389
	Baby Lycra Belt With Velcro Fastening			
	Standard 89cm long	877022	1	396
	Ex-large 107cm long	877023	1	396
	150mm Elastic Belt with Waterproof Panel	877017	1	1943
	Colostomy Belt	877018	1	7989
	Eakin Elasticated Belt			
	Small	839029	1	384
	Large	839036	1	384
	Comfizz Stoma Support Wear			
	Ladies Brief			
	Black Small/Medium	BRFBSM	1	1200
	Medium/Large	BRFBML	1	1200
	Large/X Large	BRFBLXL	1	1200
	White Small/Medium	BRFWSM	1	1200
	Medium/Large	BRFWML	1	1200
	Large/X Large	BRFWLXL	1	1200
	Unisex Boxer			
	Black Small/Medium	BOXBSM	1	1200
	Medium/Large	BOXBML	1	1200
	Large/X Large	BOXBLXL	1	1200
	White Small/Medium	BOXWSM	1	1200
	Medium/Large	BOXWML	1	1200
	Large/X Large	BOXWLXL	1	1200

IXC

SASH — Made to Measure 50mm polyester webbing Stoma Hernia Support Belt attached to plastic flange with hole over stoma

| | S1 | 1 | 3483 |

(Patients are required to complete an Order Form obtainable from Stoma Care Nurses or SASH (Address: Woodhouse, Woodside Road, Hockley, Essex, SS5 4RU Tel 01702 206 502) detailing waist size and enclosing a sample of pouch used so that the hole within the belt flange can be customised to fit individual requirements)

| T J Shannon Ltd | Elastic Belt (with button & buckle fastening) | TJS 962d | 1 | 494 |

STOMA APPLIANCES

BELTS

Manufacturer	Appliance	Order No.	Quantity	List Price p
A H Shaw & Partners Ltd	Colostomy Belt 102mm wide elastic web made to measure	NSI 10	1	1623
	102mm Ostomy Belt			
	With groin strap	NSI 10A	1	1856
	With lace fastenings	NSI 11	1	1973
	With wire spring	NSI 12	1	1817
	Double zip panel	NSI 36	1	941
	Colostomy Belt 152mm wide made to measure			
	With under-strap	NSI 13	1	2174
	With lace fastenings	NSI 14	1	2940
	Colostomy Belt 205mm wide made to measure			
	With under-strap	NSI 15	1	3121
	With lace fastenings	NSI 16	1	3726
	255mm Belt made to measure	NSI 17	1	3544
	With zip panel	NSI 18	1	4472
	306mm Belt made to measure	NSI 19	1	3894
	With zip panel	NSI 20	1	4743
	357mm Belt made to measure	NSI 21	1	3972
	With zip panel	NSI 22	1	4965
	Colostomy/Ileostomy Adjustable Belt			
	25mm wide	NSI 23	1	941
	102mm wide 3 sections	NSI 24	1	2381
	154mm wide 3 sections	NSI 25	1	3001
	Colostomy Night Belt in net or rayon, no hole, for use with dressing pad	NSI 32	1	1733
Ward Surgical Appliance Co	Day Colostomy Belt made to measure All sizes	23	1	4116
	Wide second stage rubberised ileostomy belt with 2 straps, and buttonholed ends for use with ileostomy boxes, or with celluloid hook ends for use with ileostomy bags	19	1	2415
	As above - with under-straps or suspenders	20	1	2715
	Fitting "windows" in belt for use with ileostomy bags or colostomy cups, or 4 stitched holes for studs of colostomy cups or shields	35	1	438
	Web and Elastic Belt with button and buckle fastening			
	25mm wide	WM 25	1	783
	51mm wide	WM 51	1	1010
	76mm wide	WM 75	1	1147
	Hookend Elastic Belt	WM 86	1	1093
Welland Medical Ltd	Welland Universal Belt System. 5 Universal belt rings with 1 adjustable elasticated belt			
	67mm belt ring	BLT067	1	3517
	73mm belt ring	BLT073	1	3458
	77mm belt ring	BLT077	1	3517
	82mm belt ring	BLT082	1	3517
	92mm belt ring	BLT092	1	3517
	98mm belt ring	BLT098	1	3458
	Universal Belt System Large (5 belt rings with 1 adjustable elasticated belt)			
	67mm belt rings	BLT167	1	3517
	73mm belt ring	BLT173	1	3458
	77mm belt rings	BLT177	1	3517
	82mm belt rings	BLT182	1	3517
	92mm belt rings	BLT192	1	3517
	98mm belt ring	BLT198	1	3458

STOMA APPLIANCES

COLOSTOMY BAGS

Manufacturer	Appliance		Order No.	Quantity	List Price p
B. Braun Medical	**Biotrol**				
	Colo S bag with skin protector adhesive				
	White	25mm	32-525	30	7282
		30mm	32-530	30	7282
		35mm	32-535	30	7282
		40mm	32-540	30	7282
		45mm	32-545	30	7282
		50mm	32-550	30	7282
		60mm	32-560	30	7282
	Elite bag with filter, skin protector adhesive, fabric backing				
	Beige	starter hole	36-810	30	7681
		25mm	36-825	30	7681
		30mm	36-830	30	7681
		35mm	36-835	30	7681
		40mm	36-840	30	7681
		45mm	36-845	30	7681
		50mm	36-850	30	7681
		60mm	36-860	30	7681
		70mm	36-870	30	7681
	Transparent	starter hole	30-810	30	7234
		25mm	30-825	30	7135
		30mm	30-830	30	7135
		35mm	30-835	30	7135
		40mm	30-840	30	7135
		45mm	30-845	30	7135
		50mm	30-850	30	7135
		60mm	30-860	30	7135
		70mm	30-870	30	7135
	White	starter hole	32-815	30	7681
		25mm	32-825	30	7681
		30mm	32-830	30	7681
		35mm	32-835	30	7681
		40mm	32-840	30	7681
		45mm	32-845	30	7681
		50mm	32-850	30	7681
		60mm	32-860	30	7681
		70mm	32-870	30	7681
	Elite Petite bag with filter, skin protector adhesive, fabric backing				
	Beige	starter hole	37-310	30	6529
		25mm	37-325	30	6529
		30mm	37-330	30	6529
		35mm	37-335	30	6529
		40mm	37-340	30	6529
		45mm	37-345	30	6529
	Mini S size (reference capacity : 75-69ml (see Note 2, page 257)) with filter, skin protector adhesive, fabric backing				
	Beige	25mm	33-025	30	6008
		30mm	33-030	30	6008
		35mm	33-035	30	6008
		40mm	33-040	30	6008

IXC

STOMA APPLIANCES

COLOSTOMY BAGS

Manufacturer	Appliance		Order No.	Quantity	List Price p
B. Braun Medical	**Biotrol**				
	Integrale bag with filter & skin protector adhesive				
	White	starter hole	32-415	30	7681
		25mm	32-425	30	7681
		30mm	32-430	30	7681
		35mm	32-435	30	7681
		40mm	32-440	30	7681
		45mm	32-445	30	7681
		50mm	32-450	30	7681
		60mm	32-460	30	7681
		70mm	32-470	30	7681
	Preference bag with filter, skin protector adhesive, fabric backing				
	Beige	starter hole	36-615	30	7305
		25mm	36-625	30	7305
		30mm	36-630	30	7305
		35mm	36-635	30	7305
		40mm	36-640	30	7305
		45mm	36-645	30	7305
		50mm	36-650	30	7305
		60mm	36-660	30	7305
	White	starter hole	32-610	30	7179
		25mm	32-625	30	7179
		30mm	32-630	30	7179
		35mm	32-635	30	7179
		40mm	32-640	30	7179
		45mm	32-645	30	7179
		50mm	32-650	30	7179
		60mm	32-660	30	7179
	Almarys bag with filter, Interface adhesive and all over soft non-woven cover				
	Transparent	starter hole	76-015	30	6620
	Beige	starter hole	76-115	30	6620
		25mm	76-025	30	6620
		30mm	76-030	30	6620
		35mm	76-035	30	6620
		40mm	76-040	30	6620
		45mm	76-045	30	6620
		50mm	76-050	30	6620
		60mm	76-060	30	6620
	Almarys Optima Closed bag with filter and all over soft non-woven cover				
	Transparent	starter hole 10mm	F018610E	30	6378
	Beige	starter hole 10mm	F008610E	30	6378
		25mm	F008625E	30	6378
		30mm	F008630E	30	6378
		35mm	F008635E	30	6378
		40mm	F008640E	30	6378
		45mm	F008645E	30	6378
		50mm	F008650E	30	6378
		60mm	F008660E	30	6378

STOMA APPLIANCES

COLOSTOMY BAGS

Manufacturer	Appliance		Order No.	Quantity	List Price p
B. Braun Medical	**Biotrol**				
	Almarys Optima Mini Closed bag with filter and all over soft non woven cover				
	Beige	20mm	F008920E	30	5643
		25mm	F008925E	30	5643
		30mm	F008930E	30	5643
		35mm	F008935E	30	5643
		40mm	F008940E	30	5643
	Almarys Preference Closed bag with filter, skin protector and microporous adhesive and all over soft non-woven cover				
	Transparent	starter hole 10mm	F018310E	30	6378
	Beige	starter hole 10mm	F008310E	30	6378
		25mm	F008325E	30	6378
		30mm	F008330E	30	6378
		35mm	F008335E	30	6378
		40mm	F008340E	30	6378
		45mm	F008345E	30	6378
		50mm	F008350E	30	6378
	Almarys Quiet Closed bag with filter and all over soft non-woven cover				
	Transparent	starter hole 10mm	F018110E	30	6378
	Beige	starter hole 10mm	F008110E	30	6378
		25mm	F008125E	30	6378
		30mm	F008130E	30	6378
		35mm	F008135E	30	6378
		40mm	F008140E	30	6378
		45mm	F008145E	30	6378
		50mm	F008150E	30	6378
		60mm	F008160E	30	6378
	Softima closed pouch with filter, skin protector and protective cover				
	Beige				
	Cut-to-fit	16-50mm	043016E	30	7470
		16-70mm	043070E	30	7470
	pre-cut	24mm	043024E	30	7470
		28mm	043028E	30	7470
		32mm	043032E	30	7470
		36mm	043036E	30	7470
		40mm	043040E	30	7470
		45mm	043045E	30	7470
	Transparent				
	cut-to-fit	16-50mm	043616E	30	7470
		16-70mm	043670E	30	7470
	Mini Beige				
	Cut-to-fit	16-50mm	043216E	30	7470

IXC

STOMA APPLIANCES

COLOSTOMY BAGS

Manufacturer	Appliance		Order No.	Quantity	List Price p
C S Bullen Ltd	**Shelter Closed Pouch** Bio dressing resin				
	Beige				
	cut-to-fit	13mm-80mm	2450/00	20	3690
	Clear				
	cut-to-fit	13mm-64mm	2250/00	20	3690
	pre-cut	19mm	2250/19	20	3690
		25mm	2250/25	20	3690
		32mm	2250/32	20	3690
		38mm	2250/38	20	3690
		44mm	2250/44	20	3690
		51mm	2250/51	20	3690
		58mm	2250/58	20	3690
		64mm	2250/64	20	3690
	Shelter Closed Pouch microporous adhesive				
	Beige				
	cut-to-fit	13mm-64mm	2240/00	20	2880
	pre-cut	19mm	2240/19	20	2880
		25mm	2240/25	20	2880
		32mm	2240/32	20	2880
		38mm	2240/38	20	2880
		44mm	2240/44	20	2880
		51mm	2240/51	20	2880
		58mm	2240/58	20	2880
		64mm	2240/64	20	2880
	Shelter Closed Pouch microporous adhesive, bio dressing resin				
	Clear				
	cut-to-fit	13mm-64mm	2245/00	20	3925
	pre-cut	19mm	2245/19	20	3925
		25mm	2245/25	20	3925
		32mm	2245/32	20	3925
		38mm	2245/38	20	3925
		44mm	2245/44	20	3925
		51mm	2245/51	20	3925
		58mm	2245/58	20	3925
		64mm	2245/64	20	3925

STOMA APPLIANCES

COLOSTOMY BAGS

Manufacturer	Appliance		Order No.	Quantity	List Price p
Coloplast Ltd	**Assura Inspire** Closed Bag with Integral Filter, Oval Adhesive and Soft Backing.				
	Midi Transparent				
	starter hole	20-65mm	12130	30	7476
	ready-cut	25mm	12134	30	7476
		30mm	12135	30	7476
		35mm	12136	30	7476
	Maxi Transparent				
	starter hole	20-75mm	12160	30	7476
	pre-cut	25mm	12164	30	7347
		30mm	12165	30	7347
		35mm	12166	30	7347
	Assura Inspire Closed Bag with Integral Filter, Oval Adhesive and Opaque Soft Cover Front and Back.				
	Midi Soft Cover				
	starter hole	20-65mm	12140	30	7476
	ready-cut	25mm	12144	30	7476
		30mm	12145	30	7476
		35mm	12146	30	7476
		40mm	12147	30	7476
		45mm	12148	30	7476
		50mm	12149	30	7476
	Maxi Soft Cover				
	starter hole	20-75mm	12170	30	7476
	pre-cut	25mm	12174	30	7347
		30mm	12175	30	7347
		35mm	12176	30	7347
	Assura Inspire Closed Bag with Integral Filter, Oval Adhesive and Soft Cover Front and Back.				
	Midi Design				
	starter hole	20-65mm	12150	30	7476
	ready-cut	25mm	12154	30	7476
		30mm	12155	30	7476
		35mm	12156	30	7476
		40mm	12157	30	7476
		45mm	12158	30	7476
		50mm	12159	30	7476
	Maxi Design				
	starter hole	20-75mm	12180	30	7476
	pre-cut	25mm	12184	30	7347
		30mm	12185	30	7347
		35mm	12186	30	7347
	Closed Bag with Integral Filter and Soft Cover front and back				
	Mini Soft Cover				
	starter hole	20-65mm	12110	30	5957
	Mini Design				
	starter hole	20-65mm	12120	30	5957
	Assura Closed Bag with Integral Filter and Soft Backing				
	Mini Opaque				
	starter hole	20mm	2421	30	5991
	ready-cut	25mm	2424	30	5991
		30mm	2425	30	5991
		35mm	2426	30	5991
		40mm	2427	30	5991

STOMA APPLIANCES

COLOSTOMY BAGS

Manufacturer	Appliance		Order No.	Quantity	List Price p
Coloplast Ltd	**Assura** Closed Bag with Integral Filter and Soft Backing				
	Midi Clear				
	starter hole	20mm	2471	30	7476
	ready-cut	25mm	2474	30	7476
		30mm	2475	30	7476
		35mm	2476	30	7476
		40mm	2477	30	7476
		45mm	2478	30	7476
		50mm	2479	30	7476
	Midi Opaque				
	starter hole	20mm	2461	30	7476
	ready-cut	25mm	2464	30	7476
		30mm	2465	30	7476
		35mm	2466	30	7476
		40mm	2467	30	7476
		45mm	2468	30	7476
		50mm	2469	30	7476
	Maxi Clear				
	starter hole	10-70mm	2482	30	7476
		20mm	2481	30	7476
	ready-cut	25mm	2484	30	7476
		30mm	2485	30	7476
		35mm	2486	30	7476
		40mm	2487	30	7476
		45mm	2488	30	7476
		50mm	2489	30	7476
	Maxi Opaque				
	starter hole	10-70mm	2512	30	7476
		20mm	2511	30	7476
	ready-cut	25mm	2514	30	7476
		30mm	2515	30	7476
		35mm	2516	30	7476
		40mm	2517	30	7476
	Paediatric Opaque				
	starter hole	10-35mm	2120	30	6516
	Closed Bag with Integral Filter and Opaque Soft Cover front and back				
	Mini				
	starter hole	20-55mm	12420	30	5985
	Midi				
	starter hole	20-55mm	12460	30	7476
	pre-cut	25mm	12464	30	7476
		30mm	12465	30	7476
		35mm	12466	30	7476
		40mm	12467	30	7476
		45mm	12468	30	7476
		50mm	12469	30	7476
	Maxi				
	starter hole	10-70mm	12580	30	7476
		20-55mm	12480	30	7476

STOMA APPLIANCES

COLOSTOMY BAGS

Manufacturer	Appliance	Order No.	Quantity	List Price p
Coloplast Ltd	**Assura Inspire 1 Piece** Closed Bags with Dual Filter			
	Midi Design - starter hole 20-65mm	14505	30	8054
	Soft cover - starter hole 20-65mm	14504	30	8054
	Maxi Design - starter hole 20-75mm	14508	30	8054
	Soft cover - starter hole 20-75mm	14507	30	8054
	Transparent - starter hole 20-75mm	14506	30	8054
	Assura Inspire Seal 1 Piece Integral Convexity Closed Bags with Integral Filter and Soft Backing			
	Important: This product with Integral convexity should only be used after prior assessment of suitability by an appropriate medical professional			
	Midi Transparent			
	starter hole 15-33mm	14092	10	2691
	15-43mm	14093	10	2691
	Maxi Transparent			
	starter hole 15-33mm	14002	10	2691
	15-43mm	14003	10	2691
	Assura Inspire Seal 1 Piece Integral Convexity Closed Bags with Integral Filter and Opaque Soft Cover Front and Back			
	Important: This product with Integral convexity should only be used after prior assessment of suitability by an appropriate medical professional			
	Midi Soft Cover			
	starter hole 15-33mm	14095	10	2691
	15-43mm	14096	10	2691
	Maxi Soft Cover			
	starter hole 15-33mm	14005	10	2691
	15-43mm	14006	10	2691
	Assura Seal Integral Convexity Closed Bags with Filter and Soft Backing			
	Important: This product with Integral Convexity should only be used after prior assessment of suitability by an appropriate medical professional			
	Midi Clear			
	21mm	12863	10	2447
	25mm	12864	10	2447
	28mm	12865	10	2447
	31mm	12866	10	2447
	35mm	12867	10	2447
	Midi Opaque			
	starter hole 15-33mm	12562	10	2447
	15-43mm	12563	10	2447
	Maxi Clear			
	21mm	12883	10	2447
	25mm	12884	10	2447
	28mm	12885	10	2447
	31mm	12886	10	2447
	35mm	12887	10	2447
	38mm	12888	10	2447
	Maxi Opaque			
	starter hole 15-33mm	12572	10	2447
	15-43mm	12573	10	2447
	Assura Inspire Soft Seal 1 piece Closed Bags with Shallow convexity			
	Important: This product with integral convexity should only be used after prior assessment of suitability by an appropriate medical professional			
	Midi Soft Cover			
	starter hole 15-33mm	14434	10	2747
	starter hole 15-43mm	14435	10	2747
	Midi Soft Cover 21mm	14451	10	2747
	25mm	14452	10	2747
	28mm	14453	10	2747
	31mm	14454	10	2747
	Maxi Soft Cover			
	starter hole 15-33mm	14444	10	2747
	starter hole 15-43mm	14445	10	2747
	Midi Transparent			
	starter hole 15-33mm	14431	10	2747

IXC

STOMA APPLIANCES

COLOSTOMY BAGS

Manufacturer	Appliance		Order No.	Quantity	List Price p
Coloplast Ltd	starter hole	15-43mm	14432	10	2747
	Maxi Transparent				
	starter hole	15-33mm	14441	10	2747
	starter hole	15-43mm	14442	10	2747
	Assura Conseal 1 Piece Plug				
	Important: This product should only be used after prior assessment of suitability by				
	an appropriate medical professional.				
	Length Size				
	35mm	stoma size 20-35mm	1435	10	2447
		stoma size 35-45mm	1485	10	2447
	45mm	stoma size 20-35mm	1445	10	2447
		stoma size 35-45mm	1495	10	2447
	MC2000				
	Clear	25mm	5625	30	8040
		30mm	5630	30	8040
		35mm	5635	30	8040
		40mm	5640	30	8040
		45mm	5645	30	8040
		50mm	5650	30	8040
		55mm	5655	30	8040
		60mm	5660	30	8040
	Opaque	25mm	5725	30	8040
		30mm	5730	30	8040
		35mm	5735	30	8040
		40mm	5740	30	8040
		45mm	5745	30	8040
		50mm	5750	30	8040
		55mm	5755	30	8040
		60mm	5760	30	8040
	PC3000				
	Clear	25mm	8725	30	7596
		30mm	8730	30	7596
		35mm	8735	30	7596
		40mm	8740	30	7596
		45mm	8745	30	7596
		50mm	8750	30	7596
	Opaque	25mm	8825	30	7596
		30mm	8830	30	7596
		35mm	8835	30	7596
		40mm	8840	30	7596
		45mm	8845	30	7596
		50mm	8850	30	7596
		55mm	8855	30	7596
	SenSura 1-piece Closed Bags				
	Mini Soft Cover				
	cut-to-fit	10-55/66mm	15620	30	8310
	Midi Soft Cover				
	cut-to-fit	10-55/66mm	15650	30	8310
	pre-cut	25mm	15652	30	8310
		30mm	15653	30	8310
		35mm	15654	30	8310
		40mm	15655	30	8310
		45mm	15656	30	8310
		50mm	15657	30	8310
	Midi Transparent				
	cut-to-fit	10-55/66mm	15640	30	8310
	Maxi Soft Cover				
	cut-to-fit	10-65/76mm	15680	30	8310
	pre-cut	25mm	15682	30	8310
		30mm	15683	30	8310
		35mm	15684	30	8310
	Maxi Transparent				
	cut-to-fit	10-65/76mm	15670	30	8310

STOMA APPLIANCES

COLOSTOMY BAGS

Manufacturer	Appliance		Order No.	Quantity	List Price p
ConvaTec Ltd	**Colodress Plus** (Stomahesive Wafer) Closed Pouches				
	Opaque starter hole				
		19mm	S861	30	7292
	pre-cut	25mm	S862	30	7292
		32mm	S863	30	7292
		38mm	S864	30	7292
		45mm	S865	30	7292
		50mm	S866	30	7292
		64mm	S867	30	7292
	Clear starter hole	19mm	S871	30	7292
	pre-cut	25mm	S872	30	7292
		32mm	S873	30	7292
		38mm	S874	30	7292
		45mm	S875	30	7292
		50mm	S876	30	7292
		64mm	S877	30	7292
	Mini	19mm	S901	30	6578
		25mm	S902	30	6578
		32mm	S903	30	6578
		38mm	S904	30	6578
		45mm	S905	30	6578
	Esteem Closed Pouches with Integral filter				
	Small - opaque				
	starter hole	20mm-60mm	S5001	30	6078
	pre-cut	25mm	S5002	30	6078
		30mm	S5003	30	6078
		35mm	S5011	30	5968
		40mm	S5004	30	6078
		50mm	S5005	30	6078
	Medium - clear				
	starter hole	20mm-80mm	S5006	30	6838
	pre-cut	25mm	S5007	30	6838
		30mm	S5008	30	6838
		35mm	S5012	30	6714
		40mm	S5009	30	6838
		50mm	S5010	30	6838
	Medium - opaque				
	starter hole	20mm-80mm	S5013	30	6838
	pre-cut	25mm	S5014	30	6838
		30mm	S5015	30	6838
		35mm	S5018	30	6714
		40mm	S5016	30	6838
		50mm	S5017	30	6838
	Large - clear				
	starter hole	20mm-80mm	S5020	30	6838
	Large - opaque				
	starter hole	20mm-80mm	S5027	30	6838
	pre-cut	25mm	S5028	30	6838
		30mm	S5029	30	6838
		35mm	S5034	30	6714
		40mm	S5030	30	6838
		50mm	S5031	30	6838
		60mm	S5032	30	6838
		70mm	S5033	30	6838

IXC

STOMA APPLIANCES

COLOSTOMY BAGS

Manufacturer	Appliance		Order No.	Quantity	List Price p
Dansac Ltd	**Dansac Light Convex**				
	Integral convexity closed bag with filter and soft cover front and back				
	Important: This product with integral convexity should only be used after prior assessment of suitability by an appropriate medical professional.				
	Opaque				
	starter hole	15-24mm	257-24	10	2369
		15-37mm	257-37	10	2369
		15-46mm	257-46	10	2369
	Opaque				
	pre-cut	20mm	257-20	10	2369
		25mm	257-25	10	2369
		30mm	257-30	10	2369
		35mm	257-35	10	2369
		40mm	257-40	10	2369
	Clear				
	starter hole	15-24mm	258-24	10	2369
		15-37mm	258-37	10	2369
		15-46mm	258-46	10	2369
	pre-cut	20mm	258-20	10	2369
		25mm	258-25	10	2369
		30mm	258-30	10	2369
		35mm	258-35	10	2369
		40mm	258-40	10	2369
		45mm	258-45	10	2369
	Unique				
	Opaque				
		starter hole	227-20	30	6796
		25mm	225-25	30	6796
		30mm	225-30	30	6796
		35mm	225-35	30	6796
		40mm	225-40	30	6796
		45mm	225-45	30	6796
		50mm	225-50	30	6796
		60mm	225-60	30	6796
	Clear				
		starter hole	228-20	30	6796
		25mm	226-25	30	6796
		30mm	226-30	30	6796
		35mm	226-35	30	6796
		40mm	226-40	30	6796
		45mm	226-45	30	6796
		50mm	226-50	30	6796
		60mm	226-60	30	6796
	Mini opaque (reference capacity: 220ml (see Note 2, page 257))				
	cut to fit	20-50mm	231-20	30	6378
	pre-cut	25mm	231-25	30	6378
		30mm	231-30	30	6378
		35mm	231-35	30	6378
		40mm	231-40	30	6378
	Oval Flange				
	Opaque - starter hole		223-15	30	6796
	Clear - starter hole		224-15	30	6796

STOMA APPLIANCES

COLOSTOMY BAGS

Manufacturer	Appliance		Order No.	Quantity	List Price p
Dansac Ltd	**Dansac Nova**				
	Opaque				
	starter hole	20-60mm	801-20	30	7302
	pre-cut	25mm	801-25	30	7302
		30mm	801-30	30	7302
		35mm	801-35	30	7302
		40mm	801-40	30	7302
		45mm	801-45	30	7302
		50mm	801-50	30	7302
	Clear				
	starter hole	20-60mm	802-20	30	7302
	pre-cut	25mm	802-25	30	7220
		30mm	802-30	30	7220
		35mm	802-35	30	7220
		40mm	802-40	30	7220
		45mm	802-45	30	7220
		50mm	802-50	30	7220
	Dansac Nova Mini				
	Opaque				
	starter hole	20-50mm	803-20	30	5974
	pre-cut	25mm	803-25	30	5974
		30mm	803-30	30	5974
		35mm	803-35	30	5974
		40mm	803-40	30	5974
	Dansac Nova 1 Maxi				
	Closed pouch with a skin protecting barrier				
	Clear				
	cut-to-fit	20-60mm	806-20	30	7242
	Opaque				
	cut-to-fit	20-60mm	805-20	30	7242
	Dansac Nova 1 X3 Closed				
	Clear				
	cut-to-fit	15-46mm	852-15	10	2600
	Opaque				
	cut-to-fit	15-46mm	851-15	10	2600
	pre-cut	20mm	851-20	10	2600
		25mm	851-25	10	2600
		30mm	851-30	10	2600
		35mm	851-35	10	2600
		40mm	851-40	10	2600

IXC

STOMA APPLIANCES

COLOSTOMY BAGS

Manufacturer	Appliance		Order No.	Quantity	List Price p
Dansac Ltd	**Dansac Nova 1 Convex** with integral 6mm convexity				
	Important: This product with integral convexity should only be used after assessment by a medical professional.				
	Opaque				
	cut-to-fit	15-24mm	831-24	10	2595
		15-37mm	831-37	10	2595
		15-46mm	831-46	10	2595
	pre-cut	20mm	831-20	10	2595
		25mm	831-25	10	2595
		30mm	831-30	10	2595
		35mm	831-35	10	2595
		40mm	831-40	10	2595
		45mm	831-45	10	2595
	Clear				
	cut-to-fit	15-24mm	832-24	10	2595
		15-37mm	832-37	10	2595
		15-46mm	832-46	10	2595
	Dansac Nova 1 Soft Convex with integral 5mm convexity				
	Important: This product with integral convexity should only be used after assessment by a medical professional				
	Opaque				
	pre-cut	20mm	871-20	10	2595
		25mm	871-25	10	2595
		30mm	871-30	10	2595
		35mm	871-35	10	2595
		40mm	871-40	10	2595
	Dansac NovaLife 1 Closed				
	Clear				
	cut-to-fit	20-45mm	808-20	30	7986
	Opaque				
	cut-to-fit	20-45mm	807-20	30	7986
		25-45mm	807-25	30	7986
		30-45mm	807-30	30	7986
		35-45mm	807-35	30	7986
		40-45mm	807-40	30	7986
	Unique Light				
	Closed pouch				
	Opaque-soft lining on both sides, tapered barrier and fully activated filter				
	cut-to-fit	20-60mm	255-20	30	6945
	pre-cut	25mm	255-25	30	6945
		30mm	255-30	30	6945
		35mm	255-35	30	6945
		40mm	255-40	30	6945
		45mm	255-45	30	6945
		50mm	255-50	30	6945
		60mm	255-60	30	6945

STOMA APPLIANCES

COLOSTOMY BAGS

Manufacturer	Appliance	Order No.	Quantity	List Price p
Hollister Ltd	**Compact**			
	Closed Pouch			
	Clear-with filter and white comfort backing on body-worn side			
	cut-to-fit13-64mm	3460	30	7272
	Beige-with filter and beige comfort backing on both sides			
	cut-to-fit 13-64mm	3470	30	7272
	pre-cut 25mm	3472	30	7272
	32mm	3478	30	7272
	38mm	3473	30	7272
	44mm	3479	30	7272
	51mm	3474	30	7272
	64mm	3475	30	7272
	Transparent - with filter and white comfort backing on body-worn side			
	cut-to-fit 13-64mm	3520	30	7272
	pre-cut 25mm	3522	30	7272
	32mm	3528	30	7272
	38mm	3523	30	7272
	44mm	3529	30	7272
	51mm	3524	30	7272
	64mm	3525	30	7272
	Karaya 5 seal without filter			
	Transparent			
	32mm	7168	30	6516
	38mm	7163	30	6516
	44mm	7169	30	6516
	51mm	7164	30	6516
	64mm	7165	30	6516
	76mm	7166	30	6516
	Karaya 5 seal with microporous adhesive and filter			
	Transparent			
	32mm	3328	30	7727
	38mm	3323	30	7727
	44mm	3329	30	7727
	51mm	3324	30	7727
	64mm	3325	30	7727
	76mm	3326	30	7727
	Microporous Adhesive only with filter			
	Transparent			
	25mm	3142	50	8291
	32mm	3148	50	8291
	38mm	3143	50	8291
	44mm	3149	50	8291
	51mm	3144	50	8291
	64mm	3145	50	8291
	Premium Bag with Karaya 5 seal microporous adhesive and filter			
	Transparent			
	32mm	3558	15	3898
	38mm	3553	15	3898
	44mm	3559	15	3898
	51mm	3554	15	3898
	64mm	3555	15	3898
	Impression "C" with convex wafer Beige with filter and beige Comfort backing on both sides			
	19mm	3490	10	2531
	22mm	3491	10	2531
	25mm	3492	10	2531
	29mm	3493	10	2531
	32mm	3494	10	2531
	35mm	3495	10	2531
	38mm	3496	10	2531
	41mm	3497	10	2531
	44mm	3498	10	2531
	51mm	3499	10	2531

STOMA APPLIANCES

COLOSTOMY BAGS

Manufacturer	Appliance	Order No.	Quantity	List Price p
Hollister Ltd	**Impression "C"** with convex wafer, Transparent front with filter and beige Comfort backing on body worn side			
	19mm	3590	10	2485
	22mm	3591	10	2485
	25mm	3592	10	2485
	29mm	3593	10	2485
	32mm	3594	10	2485
	35mm	3595	10	2485
	38mm	3596	10	2485
	41mm	3597	10	2485
	44mm	3598	10	2485
	51mm	3599	10	2485
	Moderma-Flex			
	Closed Pouch with skin-resting barrier, filter and beige comfort backing on bodyworn side. Transparent starter hole			
	15-55mm	22500	30	6748
	Closed pouch with skin-resting barrier, filter and beige comfort backing on both sides. Beige starter hole			
	15-55mm	22100	30	6748
	20mm	22120	30	6748
	25mm	22125	30	6748
	30mm	22130	30	6748
	35mm	22135	30	6748
	40mm	22140	30	6748
	45mm	22145	30	6748
	Maxi closed pouch with skin-resting barrier, anatomical shape with integral filter and beige comfort backing on bodyworn side. Beige - with comfort backing on both sides cut-to-fit			
	15-55mm	22300	30	7159
	pre-cut			
	25mm	22325	30	7159
	30mm	22330	30	7159
	35mm	22335	30	7159
	Transparent - with comfort backing on body side only			
	cut-to-fit 15-55mm	22400	30	7159
	Moderma Flex with Adapt conformable convex rings			
	Closed pouch, anatomical shape with integral filter. Flexible barrier plus Adapt conformable convex ring. Beige - with comfort backing on both sides			
	cut-to-fit 20-29mm + 20mm ring	22620	20	9024
	30-39mm + 30mm ring	22630	20	9024
	40-49mm + 40mm ring	22640	20	9024
	Transparent - with comfort backing on body side only			
	cut-to-fit 20-29mm + 20mm ring	22720	20	9024
	30-39mm + 30mm ring	22730	20	9024
	40-49mm + 40mm ring	22740	20	9024

STOMA APPLIANCES

COLOSTOMY BAGS

Manufacturer	Appliance	Order No.	Quantity	List Price p
Hollister Ltd	**Moderma Flex Convex**			
	Closed Pouch with integral convexity, anatomical shape, with integral filter			
	Maxi - Beige with comfort backing on both sides			
	cut-to-fit			
	15-38mm	22800	30	9300
	15-51mm	22801	30	9300
	pre-cut			
	20mm	22820	30	9300
	25mm	22825	30	9300
	30mm	22830	30	9300
	35mm	22835	30	9300
	Maxi - Transparent with comfort backing on body worn side			
	cut-to-fit			
	15-38mm	22900	30	9300
	15-51mm	22901	30	9300
	pre-cut			
	20mm	22920	30	9300
	25mm	22925	30	9300
	30mm	22930	30	9300
	35mm	22935	30	9300
Jade-Euro-Med Ltd	**Black Butyl** Screw-cap outlet			
	Day bag	KM 38	1	3146
	Night bag	KM 40	1	3669
	White Rubber Screw-cap outlet			
	Day bag	KM 44	1	1748
	Night bag	KM 46	1	2003
Marlen USA	**UltraLite** Closed Bag (formerly Ultra Closed Bag)			
	Opaque			
	Flat starter hole	801312	15	3033
	Transparent			
	Flat starter hole	861312	15	3033
	Flat pre-cut			
	Opaque			
	12mm	801412	15	3033
	16mm	801416	15	3033
	19mm	801419	15	3033
	22mm	801422	15	3033
	25mm	801425	15	3033
	29mm	801429	15	3033
	32mm	801432	15	3033
	34mm	801434	15	3033
	38mm	801438	15	3033
	41mm	801441	15	3033
	44mm	801444	15	3033
	48mm	801448	15	3033
	50mm	801450	15	3033
	54mm	801454	15	3033
	57mm	801457	15	3033
	60mm	801460	15	3033
	63mm	801463	15	3033
	67mm	801467	15	3033
	70mm	801470	15	3033
	73mm	801473	15	3033
	76mm	801476	15	3033
	Transparent			
	12mm	861412	15	3033
	16mm	861416	15	3033
	19mm	861419	15	3033
	22mm	861422	15	3033
	25mm	861425	15	3033
	29mm	861429	15	3033

IXC

STOMA APPLIANCES

COLOSTOMY BAGS

Manufacturer	Appliance	Order No.	Quantity	List Price p
Marlen USA	32mm	861432	15	3033
	34mm	861434	15	3033
	38mm	861438	15	3033
	41mm	861441	15	3033
	44mm	861444	15	3033
	48mm	861448	15	3033
	50mm	861450	15	3033
	54mm	861454	15	3033
	57mm	861457	15	3033
	60mm	861460	15	3033
	63mm	861463	15	3033
	67mm	861467	15	3033
	70mm	861470	15	3033
	73mm	861473	15	3033
	76mm	861476	15	3033
	Shallow Convex pre-cut			
	Opaque			
	12mm	801512	15	3033
	16mm	801516	15	3033
	19mm	801519	15	3033
	22mm	801522	15	3033
	25mm	801525	15	3033
	29mm	801529	15	3033
	32mm	801532	15	3033
	34mm	801534	15	3033
	38mm	801538	15	3033
	41mm	801541	15	3033
	44mm	801544	15	3033
	48mm	801548	15	3033
	50mm	801550	15	3033
	54mm	801554	15	3033
	57mm	801557	15	3033
	60mm	801560	15	3033
	63mm	801563	15	3033
	67mm	801567	15	3033
	70mm	801570	15	3033
	73mm	801573	15	3033
	76mm	801576	15	3033
	Transparent			
	12mm	861512	15	3033
	16mm	861516	15	3033
	19mm	861519	15	3033
	22mm	861522	15	3033
	25mm	861525	15	3033
	29mm	861529	15	3033
	32mm	861532	15	3033
	34mm	861534	15	3033
	38mm	861538	15	3033
	41mm	861541	15	3033
	44mm	861544	15	3033
	48mm	861548	15	3033
	50mm	861550	15	3033
	54mm	861554	15	3033
	57mm	861557	15	3033
	60mm	861560	15	3033
	63mm	861563	15	3033
	67mm	861567	15	3033
	70mm	861570	15	3033
	73mm	861573	15	3033
	76mm	861576	15	3033

STOMA APPLIANCES

COLOSTOMY BAGS

Manufacturer	Appliance	Order No.	Quantity	List Price p
Marlen USA	**Ultramax** Closed Bag			
	Opaque			
	Flat starter hole	83400	30	6900
	12mm	83412	30	6900
	16mm	83416	30	6900
	19mm	83419	30	6900
	22mm	83422	30	6900
	25mm	83425	30	6900
	29mm	83429	30	6900
	32mm	83432	30	6900
	34mm	83434	30	6900
	38mm	83438	30	6900
	41mm	83441	30	6900
	44mm	83444	30	6900
	50mm	83450	30	6900
	55mm	83455	30	6900
	Convex starter hole	83500	10	2451
	12mm	83512	10	2451
	16mm	83516	10	2451
	19mm	83519	10	2451
	22mm	83522	10	2451
	25mm	83525	10	2451
	29mm	83529	10	2451
	32mm	83532	10	2451
	34mm	83534	10	2451
	38mm	83538	10	2451
✖	41mm	83541	10	2451
✖	44mm	83544	10	2451
	Transparent			
	Flat starter hole	82400	30	6900
	12mm	82412	30	6900
	16mm	82416	30	6900
	19mm	82419	30	6900
	22mm	82422	30	6900
	25mm	82425	30	6900
	29mm	82429	30	6900
	32mm	82432	30	6900
	34mm	82434	30	6900
	38mm	82438	30	6900
	41mm	82441	30	6900
	44mm	82444	30	6900
	50mm	82450	30	6900
	55mm	82455	30	6900
	Convex starter hole	82500	10	2451
	12mm	82512	10	2451
	16mm	82516	10	2451
	19mm	82519	10	2451
	22mm	82522	10	2451
	25mm	82525	10	2451
	29mm	82529	10	2451
	32mm	82532	10	2451
	34mm	82534	10	2451
	38mm	82538	10	2451
✖	41mm	82541	10	2451
✖	44mm	82544	10	2451

✖**to be deleted 1 May 2007**

STOMA APPLIANCES

COLOSTOMY BAGS

Manufacturer	Appliance	Order No.	Quantity	List Price p
Mentor Medical Ltd	**Adhesive Stoma Bag**			
	25mm	32-232-80	90	14564
	32mm	32-233-88	90	14564
	38mm	32-234-85	90	14564
	With filter			
	25mm	32-242-87	90	16368
	32mm	32-243-84	90	16368
	38mm	32-244-81	90	16368
	44mm	32-241-04	90	16368
	51mm	32-245-89	90	16368
	64mm	32-246-86	90	16368
	Chiron			
	Disposable bags for 19mm stoma			
	305mm x 102mm	WD119-01-L	10	1143
	305mm x 127mm	WD119-02-N	10	1143
	Chironseal			
	Disposable bags for 22mm Stoma			
	305mm x 127mm	WD022-02-G	10	1287
	230mm x 127mm	WD022-03-J	10	1287
	305mm x 150mm	WD022-04-L	10	1287
	Disposable bags for 38mm Stoma			
	305mm x 102mm	WD038-01-L	10	1287
	305mm x 127mm	WD038-02-N	10	1287
	230mm x 127mm	WD038-03-Q	10	1287
	305mm x 150mm	WD038-04-S	10	1287
	Reinforced Disposable bags Sealed			
	at both ends	WD525-01-A	10	1715
		WD538-02-V	10	1715
	Spout outlet bag PVC	WD600-10-A	10	3527
	EC1 Range			
	Beige			
	starter hole 15-64mm	32-330-06	30	7822
	fixed size - 25mm	32-330-14	30	7822
	fixed size - 32mm	32-330-22	30	7822
	fixed size - 38mm	32-330-30	30	7822
	fixed size - 44mm	32-330-49	30	7822
	fixed size - 51mm	32-330-57	30	7822
	fixed size - 64mm	32-330-65	30	7822
	Clear			
	starter hole 15-64mm	32-334-05	30	7822
	fixed size - 25mm	32-334-13	30	7822
	fixed size - 32mm	32-334-21	30	7822
	fixed size - 38mm	32-334-48	30	7822
	fixed size - 44mm	32-334-56	30	7822
	fixed size - 51mm	32-334-80	30	7822
	fixed size - 64mm	32-334-99	30	7822

STOMA APPLIANCES

COLOSTOMY BAGS

Manufacturer	Appliance	Order No.	Quantity	List Price p
Mentor Medical Ltd	**Mirage** Closed Pouches			
	Beige			
	starter hole 19-44mm	32-510-10	30	6610
	starter hole 19-64mm	32-510-15	30	6610
	25mm	32-510-25	30	6610
	32mm	32-510-32	30	6610
	38mm	32-510-38	30	6610
	44mm	32-510-44	30	6610
	51mm	32-510-51	30	6610
	64mm	32-510-64	30	6610
	Large Outline cut 19-90mm	32-510-90	10	2388
	Clear			
	starter hole 19-44mm	32-515-10	30	6610
	starter hole 19-64mm	32-515-15	30	6610
	25mm	32-515-25	30	6610
	32mm	32-515-32	30	6610
	38mm	32-515-38	30	6610
	44mm	32-515-44	30	6610
	51mm	32-515-51	30	6610
	64mm	32-515-64	30	6610
	Large Outline cut 19-90mm	32-515-90	10	2388
	Mirage Flushable Soft-backed Closed Pouches			
	Beige			
	starter hole 19-44mm	32-610-19	30	7153
	25mm	32-610-25	30	7153
	32mm	32-610-32	30	7153
	38mm	32-610-38	30	7153
	44mm	32-610-44	30	7153
	51mm	32-610-51	30	7153
	Clear			
	starter hole 19-44mm	32-615-19	30	7153
	25mm	32-615-25	30	7153
	32mm	32-615-32	30	7153
	38mm	32-615-38	30	7153
	44mm	32-615-44	30	7153
	51mm	32-615-51	30	7153
	Omni 1-piece closed bag			
	Beige			
	starter hole 15-44mm	32-311-86	30	7935
	fixed size 25mm	32-311-00	30	7935
	fixed size 32mm	32-311-19	30	7935
	fixed size 38mm	32-311-27	30	7935
	fixed size 44mm	32-311-35	30	7935
	fixed size 51mm	32-311-43	30	7935
	Redifit			
	Continuation bags with Karaya			
	32mm	WA009-32-N	20	8293
	44mm	WA009-44-V	20	8293
	64mm	WA009-64-C	20	8293

IXC

STOMA APPLIANCES

COLOSTOMY BAGS

Manufacturer	Appliance	Order No.	Quantity	List Price p
Mentor Medical Ltd	**Symphony** 'WC Disposable' Closed bag			
	Beige			
	starter hole 15-44mm	32-336-18	30	8184
	fixed size 25mm	32-336-26	30	8184
	fixed size 32mm	32-336-34	30	8184
	fixed size 38mm	32-336-42	30	8184
	fixed size 44mm	32-336-50	30	8184
	fixed size 51mm	32-336-69	30	8184
	Clear			
	fixed size 25mm	32-335-10	30	8184
	fixed size 32mm	32-335-29	30	8184
	fixed size 38mm	32-335-37	30	8184
	fixed size 44mm	32-335-45	30	8184
	fixed size 51mm	32-335-53	30	8184
	Symphony Classic Soft-backed "WC Disposable" Closed Bag			
	Beige			
	starter hole 15-51mm	32-340-15	30	8184
	fixed size 25mm	32-340-25	30	8184
	fixed size 32mm	32-340-32	30	8184
	fixed size 38mm	32-340-38	30	8184
	fixed size 44mm	32-340-44	30	8184
	fixed size 51mm	32-340-51	30	8184
Oakmed Ltd	**Option** - Mini Pouch with Soft Covering to one side			
	cut-to-fit 10mm-50mm			
	Clear	0910K	30	5644
	Opaque	1010K	30	5644
	Option - Colostomy with Soft Covering to one side			
	Clear			
	starter hole			
	20mm	0120K	30	6234
	25mm	0125K	30	6234
	30mm	0130K	30	6234
	35mm	0135K	30	6234
	40mm	0140K	30	6234
	45mm	0145K	30	6234
	50mm	0150K	30	6234
	55mm	0155K	30	6234
	60mm	0160K	30	6234
	Opaque			
	starter hole			
	20mm	0220K	30	6234
	25mm	0225K	30	6234
	30mm	0230K	30	6234
	35mm	0235K	30	6234
	40mm	0240K	30	6234
	45mm	0245K	30	6234
	50mm	0250K	30	6234
	55mm	0255K	30	6234
	60mm	0260K	30	6234

STOMA APPLIANCES

COLOSTOMY BAGS

Manufacturer	Appliance	Order No.	Quantity	List Price p
Oakmed Ltd	**Option** - Colostomy Plus with Soft Covering to one side			
	Clear starter hole			
	20mm	0520K	30	6384
	25mm	0525K	30	6384
	30mm	0530K	30	6384
	35mm	0535K	30	6384
	40mm	0540K	30	6384
	45mm	0545K	30	6384
	50mm	0550K	30	6384
	55mm	0555K	30	6384
	60mm	0560K	30	6384
	Opaque starter hole			
	20mm	0620K	30	6384
	25mm	0625K	30	6384
	30mm	0630K	30	6384
	35mm	0635K	30	6384
	40mm	0640K	30	6384
	45mm	0645K	30	6384
	50mm	0650K	30	6384
	55mm	0655K	30	6384
	60mm	0660K	30	6384
	Option - Mini Pouch with Filter and Soft Covering to both sides			
	Opaque			
	cut-to-fit 10mm - 50mm	1110K	30	5751
	Option - Colostomy with Filter and Soft Covering to both sides			
	Opaque starter hole			
	20mm	0320K	30	6503
	25mm	0325K	30	6503
	30mm	0330K	30	6503
	35mm	0335K	30	6503
	40mm	0340K	30	6503
	45mm	0345K	30	6503
	50mm	0350K	30	6503
	55mm	0355K	30	6503
	60mm	0360K	30	6503
	Option - Colostomy Plus with Filter and Soft Covering to both sides			
	Opaque starter hole			
	20mm	0420K	30	6661
	25mm	0425K	30	6661
	30mm	0430K	30	6661
	35mm	0435K	30	6661
	40mm	0440K	30	6661
	45mm	0445K	30	6661
	50mm	0450K	30	6661
	55mm	0455K	30	6661
	60mm	0460K	30	6661
	Option - Colostomy Maxi with Filter and Soft Covering to one side			
	Clear			
	cut-to-fit 20mm-100mm	0720K	30	7058
	Option - Colostomy Maxi with Filter and Soft Covering to both sides			
	Opaque			
	cut-to-fit 20mm-100mm	0820K	30	7202
	Option - Colostomy Maxi with Filter and Soft Covering to both sides without window			
	Opaque			
	cut-to-fit 20mm-100mm	0820KWW	30	7076

STOMA APPLIANCES

COLOSTOMY BAGS

Manufacturer	Appliance	Order No.	Quantity	List Price p
Oakmed Ltd	**Option** - Colostomy Microskin			
	Opaque starter hole			
	20mm	M-0320K	30	7251
	25mm	M-0325K	30	7251
	30mm	M-0330K	30	7251
	35mm	M-0335K	30	7251
	40mm	M-0340K	30	7251
	45mm	M-0345K	30	7251
	50mm	M-0350K	30	7251
	55mm	M-0355K	30	7251
	60mm	M-0360K	30	7251
	Option - Colostomy Plus Microskin			
	Opaque starter hole			
	20mm	M-0420K	30	7353
	25mm	M-0425K	30	7353
	30mm	M-0430K	30	7353
	35mm	M-0435K	30	7353
	40mm	M-0440K	30	7353
	45mm	M-0445K	30	7353
	50mm	M-0450K	30	7353
	55mm	M-0455K	30	7353
	60mm	M-0460K	30	7353
	Option - Colostomy Maxi with Filter and Soft Covering to both sides			
	Opaque			
	cut-to-fit 20mm-100mm	0820K	30	7202
	Option - Colostomy Maxi with Filter and Soft Covering to both sides without window			
	Opaque			
	cut-to-fit 20mm-100mm	0820KWW	30	7076
	Option - Colostomy Microskin			
	Opaque starter hole			
	20mm	M-0320K	30	7251
	25mm	M-0325K	30	7251
	30mm	M-0330K	30	7251
	35mm	M-0335K	30	7251
	40mm	M-0340K	30	7251
	45mm	M-0345K	30	7251
	50mm	M-0350K	30	7251
	55mm	M-0355K	30	7251
	60mm	M-0360K	30	7251
	Option - Colostomy Plus Microskin			
	Opaque starter hole			
	20mm	M-0420K	30	7353
	25mm	M-0425K	30	7353
	30mm	M-0430K	30	7353
	35mm	M-0435K	30	7353
	40mm	M-0440K	30	7353
	45mm	M-0445K	30	7353
	50mm	M-0450K	30	7353
	55mm	M-0455K	30	7353
	60mm	M-0460K	30	7353

STOMA APPLIANCES

COLOSTOMY BAGS

Manufacturer	Appliance	Order No.	Quantity	List Price p
Oakmed Ltd	**Option Alginate** Mini Pouch			
	Opaque			
	starter hole 20mm	A-1110K	30	8077
	Option Alginate Colostomy pouch			
	Opaque			
	starter hole			
	20mm	A-0320K	30	8077
	25mm	A-0325K	30	8077
	30mm	A-0330K	30	8077
	35mm	A-0335K	30	8077
	40mm	A-0340K	30	8077
	45mm	A-0345K	30	8077
	50mm	A-0350K	30	8077
	55mm	A-0355K	30	8077
	60mm	A-0360K	30	8077
	Option Alginate Colostomy Plus			
	Opaque			
	starter hole			
	20mm	A-0420K	30	8077
	25mm	A-0425K	30	8077
	30mm	A-0430K	30	8077
	35mm	A-0435K	30	8077
	40mm	A-0440K	30	8077
	45mm	A-0445K	30	8077
	50mm	A-0450K	30	8077
	55mm	A-0455K	30	8077
	60mm	A-0460K	30	8077
Omex Medical Ltd	Schacht Colostomy Pouches	785474	100	3426
Peak Medical	**Colomate** Closed 1 piece pouch Beige non-woven front and back and high capacity filter			
	Small			
	starter hole 10mm	CSB110	30	6500
	Medium			
	starter hole 13mm	CMB113	30	7900
	pre-cut 25mm	CMB125	30	7900
	28mm	CMB128	30	7900
	32mm	CMB132	30	7900
	35mm	CMB135	30	7900
	38mm	CMB138	30	7900
	45mm	CMB145	30	7900
	52mm	CMB152	30	7900

IXC

STOMA APPLIANCES

COLOSTOMY BAGS

Manufacturer	Appliance		Order No.	Quantity	List Price p
Peak Medical	Large				
	starter hole	13mm	CLB113	30	7900
	pre-cut	25mm	CLB125	30	7900
		28mm	CLB128	30	7900
		32mm	CLB132	30	7900
		35mm	CLB135	30	7900
		38mm	CLB138	30	7900
		45mm	CLB145	30	7900
		52mm	CLB152	30	7900

Colomate Closed 1 piece pouch in transparent with high capacity filter

	Small				
	starter hole	10mm	CST110	30	6500

Colomate Closed 1 piece pouch transparent with beige needle-pin overlap and high capacity filter

	Large				
	starter hole	13mm	CLT113	30	7900
	pre-cut	25mm	CLT125	30	7900
		28mm	CLT128	30	7900
		32mm	CLT132	30	7900
		35mm	CLT135	30	7900
		38mm	CLT138	30	7900
		45mm	CLT145	30	7900
		52mm	CLT152	30	7900

Colomate Closed 1 piece pouch, oval 60mm x 90mm hydrocolloid barrier, transparent with beige needle-pin overlap and high capacity filter

	Large				
	starter hole	10mm	CLTO110	30	7900

Colomate Closed Anatomical 1 piece pouch Beige non-woven front and back and high capacity filter

	Medium/Large				
	starter hole	13mm	CMLB113	30	7900
	pre-cut	25mm	CMLB125	30	7900
		28mm	CMLB128	30	7900
		32mm	CMLB132	30	7900
		35mm	CMLB135	30	7900
		38mm	CMLB138	30	7900
		45mm	CMLB145	30	7900
		52mm	CMLB152	30	7900

STOMA APPLIANCES

COLOSTOMY BAGS

Manufacturer	Appliance	Order No.	Quantity	List Price p
Pelican Healthcare Ltd	**Pelican Select**			
	with skin protector,fabric both sides, filter			
	Closed pouches			
	Clear			
	cut-to-fit 20-65mm	100700	30	7220
	pre-cut 27mm	101727	30	7220
	34mm	101734	30	7220
	41mm	101741	30	7220
	48mm	101748	30	7220
	55mm	101755	30	7220
	Opaque			
	cut-to-fit 20-65mm	100720	30	7220
	pre-cut 27mm	100727	30	7220
	34mm	100734	30	7220
	41mm	100741	30	7220
	48mm	100748	30	7220
	55mm	100755	30	7220
	Mini Closed Pouches			
	Clear cut-to-fit			
	20-65mm	100600	30	6056
	Opaque cut-to-fit			
	20-65mm	100620	30	6056
	Pelican Select Afresh Closed Pouch with skin protector, fabric on both sides, split fabric backing for viewing/positioning and filter.			
	Opaque - Standard shape			
	cut-to-fit 20-65mm	102120	30	7111
	pre-cut 22.5mm	102122	30	7111
	25mm	102125	30	7111
	27.5mm	102127	30	7111
	30mm	102130	30	7111
	32.5mm	102132	30	7111
	35mm	102135	30	7111
	37.5mm	102137	30	7111
	40mm	102140	30	7111
	45mm	102145	30	7111
	50mm	102150	30	7111
	55mm	102155	30	7111
	Clear - Standard shape			
	cut-to-fit 20-65mm	102220	30	7111
	pre-cut 22.5mm	102222	30	7111
	25mm	102225	30	7111
	27.5mm	102227	30	7111
	30mm	102230	30	7111
	32.5mm	102232	30	7111
	35mm	102235	30	7111
	37.5mm	102237	30	7111
	40mm	102240	30	7111
	45mm	102245	30	7111
	50mm	102250	30	7111
	55mm	102255	30	7111

IXC

STOMA APPLIANCES

COLOSTOMY BAGS

Manufacturer	Appliance	Order No.	Quantity	List Price p
Pelican Healthcare Ltd	Opaque - Mini shape			
	cut-to-fit 20-65mm	102320	30	7111
	pre-cut 22.5mm	102322	30	7111
	25mm	102325	30	7111
	27.5mm	102327	30	7111
	30mm	102330	30	7111
	32.5mm	102332	30	7111
	35mm	102335	30	7111
	37.5mm	102337	30	7111
	40mm	102340	30	7111
	45mm	102345	30	7111
	50mm	102350	30	7111
	55mm	102355	30	7111
	Clear - Mini shape			
	cut-to-fit 20-65mm	102300	30	7111
	Opaque - Maxi shape			
	cut-to-fit 20-65mm	102420	30	7191
	Clear - Maxi shape			
	cut-to-fit 20-65mm	102400	30	7191

Pelican Select Closed Convex Pouch - integral convexity with filter and split fabric backing
Important: This product with integral convexity should only be used after prior assessment of suitability by an appropriate medical professional.

	Appliance	Order No.	Quantity	List Price p
	Opaque - Standard			
	cut-to-fit 12-40mm	103312	10	2733
	pre-cut 20mm	103320	10	2733
	22.5mm	103322	10	2733
	25mm	103325	10	2733
	27.5mm	103327	10	2733
	30mm	103330	10	2733
	32.5mm	103332	10	2733
	35mm	103335	10	2733
	37.5mm	103337	10	2733
	40mm	103340	10	2733
	Clear - Standard			
	cut-to-fit 12-40mm	103412	10	2733
	pre-cut 20mm	103420	10	2733
	22.5mm	103422	10	2733
	25mm	103425	10	2733
	27.5mm	103427	10	2733
	30mm	103430	10	2733
	32.5mm	103432	10	2733
	35mm	103435	10	2733
	37.5mm	103437	10	2733
	40mm	103440	10	2733

STOMA APPLIANCES

COLOSTOMY BAGS

Manufacturer	Appliance	Order No.	Quantity	List Price p
Pelican Healthcare Ltd	Opaque - Maxi			
	cut-to-fit 2-40mm	103512	10	2733
	pre-cut 20mm	103520	10	2733
	22.5mm	103522	10	2733
	25mm	103525	10	2733
	27.5mm	103527	10	2733
	30mm	103530	10	2733
	32.5mm	103532	10	2733
	35mm	103535	10	2733
	37.5mm	103537	10	2733
	40mm	103540	10	2733
	Opaque - Mini			
	cut-to-fit 12-40mm	103112	10	2733
	Clear - Maxi			
	cut-to-fit 12-40mm	103612	10	2733
ProSys International Ltd	**Independence** - 1 piece closed pouch with integral filter, soft covering both sides and viewing curtain			
	starter hole			
	20mm	PR100-20	30	7475
Salts Healthcare	**Cohflex - with filter**			
	Closed			
	starter hole (10-60mm)			
	Flesh/Flesh	515410	30	6775
	Flesh/Clear	515420	30	6775
	pre-cut Flesh/Flesh			
	25mm	515425	30	6775
	30mm	515430	30	6775
	35mm	515435	30	6775
	40mm	515440	30	6775
	45mm	515445	30	6775
	50mm	515450	30	6775
	Coloset			
	Closed bag			
	Small starter	713656	30	1181
	Confidence			
	Closed pouches			
	Opaque			
	starter hole			
	13mm	C13	30	6852
	pre-cut			
	25mm	C25	30	6852
	32mm	C32	30	6852
	38mm	C38	30	6852
	45mm	C45	30	6852
	52mm	C52	30	6852
	Mini Closed pouches			
	starter hole			
	13mm	CM13	30	5398
	Closed pouches - transparent/overlap film			
	Standard			
	starter hole			
	13mm	CT13	30	6560

STOMA APPLIANCES

COLOSTOMY BAGS

Manufacturer	Appliance	Order No.	Quantity	List Price p
Salts Healthcare	Closed pouches - transparent/no overlap			
	Standard			
	starter hole			
	13mm	CTT13	30	6560
	Closed pouches-transparent/overlap film			
	pre-cut			
	25mm	CT25	30	6758
	32mm	CT32	30	6758
	38mm	CT38	30	6758
	Closed pouches-transparent/overlap film			
	Large			
	starter hole			
	13mm	CLT13	30	6642
	Closed pouches - transparent/no overlap			
	Large			
	starter hole			
	13mm	CLTT13	30	6642

Confidence Comfort closed pouches - Opaque film/beige overlap comfort backing on both sides. Hypoallergenic hydrocolloid, protected filter, anatomical shape.

	Standard			
	starter hole			
	13mm	CFO13	30	7750
	Large			
	starter hole			
	13mm	CFLO13	30	7750

Confidence Comfort closed pouches - Transparent film. Comfort backing on body side. Hypoallergenic hydrocolloid, protected filter, anatomical shape.

	Standard			
	starter hole			
	13mm	CFT13	30	7750
	Large			
	starter hole			
	13mm	CFLT13	30	7750

Confidence Comfort closed pouches - Transparent film/beige overlap comfort backing on both sides. Hypoallergenic hydrocolloid, protected filter, anatomical shape.

	Standard			
	starter hole			
	13mm	CF13	30	7901
	pre-cut			
	25mm	CF25	30	7901
	32mm	CF32	30	7901
	35mm	CF35	30	7901
	38mm	CF38	30	7901
	41mm	CF41	30	7901
	Large			
	starter hole			
	13mm	CFL13	30	7901
	pre-cut			
	25mm	CFL25	30	7901
	32mm	CFL32	30	7901
	35mm	CFL35	30	7901
	38mm	CFL38	30	7901
	41mm	CFL41	30	7901

Confidence Gold
with hypoallergenic hydrocolloid and soft beige comfort backing on both sides, filter

	Closed Pouches			
	Opaque			
	starter hole			
	13mm	CNW13	30	6734

STOMA APPLIANCES

COLOSTOMY BAGS

Manufacturer	Appliance	Order No.	Quantity	List Price p
Salts Healthcare	pre-cut			
	25mm	CNW25	30	6734
	32mm	CNW32	30	6734
	35mm	CNW35	30	6734
	38mm	CNW38	30	6734
	Mini Closed Pouches			
	starter hole			
	13mm	CMNW13	30	5306
	Closed Pouches - Transparent			
	Film/Beige Overlap Comfort Backing			
	Standard			
	starter hole			
	13mm	CTNW13	30	6447
	pre-cut 25mm	CTNW25	30	6642
	32mm	CTNW32	30	6642
	35mm	CTNW35	30	6642
	38mm	CTNW38	30	6642
	45mm	CTNW45	30	6642
	52mm	CTNW52	30	6642
	Large			
	starter hole			
	13mm	CLTNW13	30	6642

Confidence Gold Convex
1 piece integral convexity with hypoallergenic hydrocolloid and soft beige comfort backing on both sides, filter.
Important: This product with integral convexity should only be used after assessment by a medical professional.
Closed Pouches Transparent
Film/Beige Overlap Comfort Backing
Standard
starter hole

	13-25mm	CC13-25	10	2599
	13-38mm	CC13-38	10	2599
	13-52mm	CC13-52	10	2599
pre-cut	21mm	CC21	10	2599
	25mm	CC25	10	2599
	28mm	CC28	10	2599
	32mm	CC32	10	2599
	35mm	CC35	10	2599
	38mm	CC38	10	2599
	41mm	CC41	10	2599
	45mm	CC45	10	2599

Eakin
Closed bag
Clear

	32mm	839130	20	5009
	45mm	839131	20	5009
	64mm	839132	20	5009

Simplicity 1 - with filter
Closed
starter hole (10mm-60mm)

	White/White	511310	30	7951
	White/Clear	511311	30	7951
pre-cut				
	White/White			
	30mm	511330	30	7951
	40mm	511340	30	7951
	50mm	511350	30	7951
	60mm	511360	30	7951

STOMA APPLIANCES

COLOSTOMY BAGS

Manufacturer	Appliance	Order No.	Quantity	List Price p
Salts Healthcare	**Simplicity 1 Anatomical**			
	Closed			
	Opaque - starter hole	541310	30	7538
	30mm	541330	30	7538
	40mm	541340	30	7538
	50mm	541350	30	7538
T J Shannon Ltd	Night bags	TJS 948e	1	2813
	Day bags	TJS 948f	1	2458
	Disposable bags	TJS 948g	100	1218
	Day bags tap outlet	TJS 948j	1	2813
	Night bags tap outlet	TJS 948k	1	3067
	Bags with elastic necks		50	2456
	Disposable bags and plaster sealed both ends		12	672
A H Shaw & Partners Ltd	Hainsworth bags with body mould adhesive hole size 25mm, 32mm, 38mm, and 51mm	NSI 63	20	4861
	Hainsworth bags with Healwell adhesive hole size 25mm, 32mm, 38mm, and 51mm	NSI 39	20	2552
	Stick on bags with plasters	NSI 62	10	967
	Shaw double seal			
	280mm x 154mm	NSI 64	100	1163
	Colostomy bags			
	350mm x 204mm	NSI 65	100	1272
Ward Surgical Appliance Co				
	Colostomy Disposable bags, sealed both ends			
	30.5cm x 102mm with			
	102mm x 76mm plasters	WM 15	10	887
	30.5cm x 127mm with			
	102mm x 102mm plasters	WM 16	10	887
	Rubber colostomy bag with mount outlet	WM 12	1	1531
Welland Medical Ltd	**Curvex** closed pouches with soft flexible flange, all over soft cover and filter			
	Beige			
	25mm plateau starter hole	CCS 513	10	2407
	32mm plateau starter hole	CCM 513	10	2407
	32mm plateau 25mm pre-cut	CCM 525	10	2407
	32mm plateau 32mm pre-cut	CCM 532	10	2407
	43mm plateau starter hole	CCL 513	10	2407
	43mm plateau 32mm pre-cut	CCL 532	10	2407
	43mm plateau 38mm pre-cut	CCL 538	10	2407
	Clear			
	25mm plateau starter hole	CCS 713	10	2407
	32mm plateau starter hole	CCM 713	10	2407
	43mm plateau starter hole	CCL 713	10	2407

STOMA APPLIANCES

COLOSTOMY BAGS

Manufacturer	Appliance		Order No.	Quantity	List Price p
Welland Medical Ltd	**Silhouette** Standard Length Closed Pouches				
	Beige				
		10mm	SCS 510	30	6626
		25mm	SCS 525	30	6626
		29mm	SCS 529	30	6626
		32mm	SCS 532	30	6626
		35mm	SCS 535	30	6626
		38mm	SCS 538	30	6626
		44mm	SCS 544	30	6626
		51mm	SCS 551	30	6626
		60mm	SCS 560	30	6626
	Clear				
		10mm	SCS 710	30	6626
		25mm	SCS 725	30	6626
		29mm	SCS 729	30	6626
		32mm	SCS 732	30	6626
		35mm	SCS 735	30	6626
		38mm	SCS 738	30	6626
		44mm	SCS 744	30	6626
		51mm	SCS 751	30	6626
		60mm	SCS 760	30	6626
	Silhouette Vogue Shorter Length Closed Pouches				
	Beige	10mm	SCV 510	30	5878
		25mm	SCV 525	30	5878
		29mm	SCV 529	30	5878
		32mm	SCV 532	30	5878
		35mm	SCV 535	30	5878
		38mm	SCV 538	30	5878
		44mm	SCV 544	30	5878
		51mm	SCV 551	30	5878
	Vogue Mini Bags				
	Beige	starter hole 10mm	VOG 910	30	6126
		25mm	VOG 925	30	6126
		29mm	VOG 929	30	6126
		32mm	VOG 932	30	6126
		35mm	VOG 935	30	6126
		38mm	VOG 938	30	6126
		44mm	VOG 944	30	6126
		51mm	VOG 951	30	6126
	Welland Colostomy Bags with soft backing				
	Beige	starter hole 10mm	FSC 910	30	6908
		25mm	FSC 925	30	6908
		29mm	FSC 929	30	6908
		32mm	FSC 932	30	6908
		35mm	FSC 935	30	6908
		38mm	FSC 938	30	6908
		44mm	FSC 944	30	6908
		51mm	FSC 951	30	6908
		60mm	FSC 960	30	6908
	Clear	starter hole 10mm	FSC 710	30	6908
		25mm	FSC 725	30	6908
		29mm	FSC 729	30	6908
		32mm	FSC 732	30	6908
		35mm	FSC 735	30	6908
		38mm	FSC 738	30	6908
		44mm	FSC 744	30	6908
		51mm	FSC 751	30	6908
		60mm	FSC 760	30	6908

IXC

STOMA APPLIANCES

COLOSTOMY BAGS

Manufacturer	Appliance	Order No.	Quantity	List Price p
Welland Medical Ltd	**Welland FreeStyle** Colostomy Pouches (incorporating Dual-Carb Filter)			
	Closed pouch with clear odour barrier film on flange side, opaque odour barrier film on filter side. Both sides covered with beige polyethylene soft back.			
	Medium 13mm starter hole (cuts to 60mm)			
		FMC 513	30	7079
	pre-cut			
	25mm	FMC 525	30	6944
	29mm	FMC 529	30	6944
	32mm	FMC 532	30	6944
	35mm	FMC 535	30	6944
	38mm	FMC 538	30	6944
	44mm	FMC 544	30	6944
	Large 13mm starter hole (cuts to 60mm)			
		FLC 513	30	7079
	pre-cut			
	25mm	FLC 525	30	7079
	29mm	FLC 529	30	7079
	32mm	FLC 532	30	7079
	35mm	FLC 535	30	6944
	38mm	FLC 538	30	7079
	44mm	FLC 544	30	7079
	Closed pouch with clear odour barrier film on both sides and a white polyethylene soft back layer on the flange side.			
	Medium 13mm starter hole (cuts to 60mm)			
		FMC 713	30	7079
	Large 13mm starter hole (cuts to 60mm)			
		FLC 713	30	7079
	pre-cut			
	25mm	FLC 725	30	6944
	29mm	FLC 729	30	6944
	32mm	FLC 732	30	6944
	35mm	FLC 735	30	6944
	38mm	FLC 738	30	6944
	44mm	FLC 744	30	6944
	Closed pouch with integral convexity with soft backing			
	Beige soft backing to both sides			
	Medium 13mm starter hole (cuts to 35mm)			
		NCM 513	10	2666
	pre-cut			
	25mm	NCM 525	10	2666
	29mm	NCM 529	10	2666
	32mm	NCM 532	10	2666
	35mm	NCM 535	10	2666
	Large 13mm starter hole (cuts to 48mm)			
		NCL 513	10	2666
	pre-cut			
	35mm	NCL 535	10	2666
	38mm	NCL 538	10	2666
	44mm	NCL 544	10	2666
	Clear with white soft backing on flange side			
	Medium 13mm starter hole (cuts to 35mm)			
		NCM 713	10	2666
	Large 13mm starter hole (cuts to 48mm)			
		NCL 713	10	2666

STOMA APPLIANCES

COLOSTOMY BAGS

Manufacturer	Appliance	Order No.	Quantity	List Price p
Welland Medical Ltd	**Welland FreeStyle Flushable** Colostomy Pouches (incorporating Dual-Carb Filter)			
	Seam welded closed pouch with softback layer on both sides, a hydrocolloid wafer and an inner collection pouch which is toilet disposable			
	Medium			
	19mm	FFM 519	30	8256
	25mm	FFM 525	30	8256
	29mm	FFM 529	30	8256
	32mm	FFM 532	30	8256
	35mm	FFM 535	30	8256
	38mm	FFM 538	30	8256
	44mm	FFM 544	30	8256
	Large			
	19mm	FFL 519	30	8256
	25mm	FFL 525	30	8256
	29mm	FFL 529	30	8256
	32mm	FFL 532	30	8256
	35mm	FFL 535	30	8256
	38mm	FFL 538	30	8256
	44mm	FFL 544	30	8256
	Welland FreeStyle Oval Colostomy Pouches with soft backing			
	Beige			
	starter hole 13mm	FCV 513	30	7053
	Clear			
	starter hole 13mm	FCV 713	30	7053
	Welland Impact Colostomy Bags with Toilet disposable liner and soft backing			
	Mini			
	Beige 19mm	IMP 219	30	5845
	25mm	IMP 225	30	5845
	29mm	IMP 229	30	5845
	32mm	IMP 232	30	5845
	35mm	IMP 235	30	5845
	38mm	IMP 238	30	5845
	44mm	IMP 244	30	5845
	51mm	IMP 251	30	5845
	Standard			
	Beige 19mm	IMP 919	30	7113
	25mm	IMP 925	30	7113
	29mm	IMP 929	30	7113
	32mm	IMP 932	30	7113
	35mm	IMP 935	30	7113
	38mm	IMP 938	30	7113
	44mm	IMP 944	30	7113
	51mm	IMP 951	30	7113
	Maxi			
	Beige 19mm	IMP 319	30	7113
	25mm	IMP 325	30	7113
	29mm	IMP 329	30	7113
	32mm	IMP 332	30	7113
	35mm	IMP 335	30	7113
	38mm	IMP 338	30	7113
	44mm	IMP 344	30	7113
	51mm	IMP 351	30	7113
	Welland Ovation Closed Pouch with oval skin protector.			
	Clear			
	starter hole 10mm	FCO 710	30	7143
	Beige			
	starter hole 10mm	FCO 910	30	7143

IXC

STOMA APPLIANCES

COLOSTOMY SETS

Manufacturer	Appliance	Order No.	Quantity	List Price p
Jade-Euro-Med Ltd (formerly Mentor Medical Ltd)	Chiron Appliances Adhesive model with spout bag			
	MK I	WE001-38-W	1	7905
	MK III	WE007-38-X	1	7905
Mentor Medical Ltd see Jade-Euro-Med Ltd				
Omex Medical Ltd	Schacht Odourproof Colostomy Appliance	785466	1	2955
T J Shannon Ltd	Easychange Colostomy Appliance 27mm, 40mm, 57mm		1	492
	Colostomy Outfit	TJS 948A	1	8301
	Colostomy Outfit	TJS 948NA	1	8038
	Colostomy Outfit	TJS 948T	1	4401
	Adhesive Appliance	TJS 948B	1	5360
A H Shaw & Partners Ltd	Complete Colostomy outfit comprising of a 102mm wide elastic web belt with groin-strap 660mm, 715mm etc. to 107cm, 1 Colostomy facepiece (flange), 100 Colostomy bags 280mm x 154mm	NSI 6	1	4504
	Complete Colostomy outfit comprising of an adjustable 102mm wide elastic web belt with groin-strap 660mm, 715mm etc. to 107cm, 1 Colostomy facepiece, 100 Colostomy bags 280mm x 154mm	NSI 8	1	4919

STOMA APPLIANCES

DEODORANTS

Manufacturer	Appliance	Order No.	Quantity	List Price p
Anglo Venture 2000 Ltd	Friends Ostomy Deodorant Spray			
	Cinnamon	012345	75ml	355
	Victorian Rose	012346	75ml	355
	Lemon	012347	75ml	355
C S Bullen Ltd	Shelter Deodorant	520	125ml	321
	Shelter Deodorant Sachet	530	50	975
CliniMed Ltd Essentials Accessories	LiMone Ostomy Deodorant Spray	3905	50ml	482
Coloplast Ltd	Coloplast OAD	1523	36ml	463
Dansac Ltd	Nodor S	080-00	50ml	420
		080-01	250ml	859
Ecolab	Atmocol Pocket Spray	785911	25ml	209
Hollister Ltd	Adapt Lubricating Deodorant	78500	236ml	897
	Adapt Lubricating Deodorant Sachet	78501	50	1274
Loxley Products	Day-drop	LL04	7.5ml	109
		LL05	15ml	181
		LL06	30ml	309
	Lemon Day-drop	LL07	7.5ml	109
		LL08	15ml	181
	Lemon Day-drop Spray	LL010	50ml	345
Mentor Medical Ltd	Chironair Odour Control Liquid	WN003-01-F	110ml	662
Opus Healthcare	NaturCare (pump spray)	1100	50ml	390
	NaturCare Fragrant (pump spray)	1101	50ml	390
	NaturCare Zest (pump spray)	1102	50ml	390
	NaturCare Breeze (pump spray)	1103	50ml	390
	NaturCare (aerosol spray)	1100A	50ml	469
	NaturCare Fragrant (aerosol spray)	1101A	50ml	469
	NaturCare Zest (aerosol spray)	1102A	50ml	469
	NaturCare Breeze (aerosol spray)	1103A	50ml	469
OstoMart	OstoMIST Odour Neutralising Spray			
	Blackberry	BDW1	100ml	755
		BDW2	50ml	387
	Grapefruit	DWR1	100ml	755
		DWR2	50ml	387
	Apple	DPA1	100ml	755
		DPA2	50ml	387
	OstoZYME Odour Neutralising Lubricating Gel sachets	TCB3	30 x 8ml	1750
Pelican Healthcare Ltd	Dor Pouch Deodorant	130103	7ml	217
	Citrus Fresh Pouch Deodorant Spray	2200	50ml	403

STOMA APPLIANCES

DEODORANTS

Manufacturer	Appliance	Order No.	Quantity	List Price p
Salts Healthcare	Noroma	833021	28ml	269
		833056	227ml	877
	Fresh Aire	FA1	50ml	382
T J Shannon	Colostomy Plus		7ml	298
A H Shaw & Partners Ltd	Forest Breeze	NSI 61	14ml	385
UCI Healthcare Ltd	Auricare Faecal Odour Eliminator	ACD125	125ml	907
		ACD60	60ml	427

DISCHARGE SOLIDIFYING AGENTS

Manufacturer	Appliance	Order No.	Quantity	List Price p
B.Braun Medical	Ileo Gel Tablets	005010	30	916
C S Bullen Ltd	Absorbian Core (only for use with Absorbian drainable pouch)	UFAS04	20	1500
	Absorbian Sachet	UFAS-01	30	750
	Absorbian Sachet Plus	UFAS-02	30	750
	Absorbian Wand	UFAS-03	60	1500
CliniMed Ltd Essentials Accessories	Morform Sachet	3837	60	1835
Oakmed Ltd	Gel-X Capsules		140	1453
	Gel-X Tablets		140	1425
Opus Healthcare Ltd	AbsorbaGel	9900	150	4500
OstoMart	OstoSORB 3g sachets	PFW5	30	918
ProSys International Ltd	ProSys Absorbent Strips	P100AS	100	950

FILTERS/BRIDGES

Manufacturer	Appliance	Order No.	Quantity	List Price p
B. Braun Medical	Biotrol Flatus Filters	35-500	50	1335
Coloplast Ltd	Filtrodor Filters	0509	50	2200
Cuxson Gerrard	Flatus Patches T33 3.8cm x 3.8cm	FLA 830	50	360
Hollister Ltd	Replacement Filter elements for series 366 drainable bags	7766	20	337
			100	1654
Mentor Medical Ltd	Doublesure Flatus Filter (pack)	WJ130-11-N	10	399
	Stoma Bridge	32-298-07	20	358
	Spare filters for Beta & Omni range	32-297-34	20	842
	Spare filters for Mirage drainable pouches	32-560-20	20	461
Opus Healthcare Ltd	ClearWay Stoma Bridge	7700	30	966
	ClearWay Stoma Bridge Mini	8800	30	968
Salts Healthcare	Metal Bridges- for use with other disposable bags	833053	30	1546

STOMA APPLIANCES

FLANGES

Manufacturer	Appliance	Order No.	Quantity	List Price p
C S Bullen Ltd	Lenbul			
	25mm diameter 51mm base	UF 24	1	934
	38mm diameter 76mm base	UF 25	1	1421
	51mm diameter 102mm base	UF 26	1	1658
DBT Medical Ltd	St Mark's Flanges made in two Rubbers with Hard Centre			
	22mm int diam, 16mm deep, 76mm base	LM 841101	2	3720
	32mm int diam, 16mm deep, 76mm base	LM 841103	2	3720
	32mm int diam, 10mm deep, 76mm base	LM 841104	2	3720
	38mm int diam, 16mm deep, 76mm base	LM 841105	2	3720
	38mm int diam, 10mm deep, 76mm base	LM 841106	2	3720
	44mm int diam, 16mm deep, 102mm base	LM 841107	2	3720
	25mm int diam, 13mm deep, 76mm base	LM 841110	2	3720
	51mm int diam, 16mm deep, 102mm base	LM 841109	2	3720
	St Mark's Flanges made in Soft Honey Coloured Rubber			
	25mm int diam, 13mm deep, 51mm base	LM 842101	2	2170
	32mm int diam, 16mm deep, 76mm base	LM 842103	2	2170
	32mm int diam, 10mm deep, 76mm base	LM 842104	2	2170
	38mm int diam, 16mm deep, 76mm base	LM 842105	2	2170
	38mm int diam, 10mm deep, 76mm base	LM 842106	2	2170
	44mm int diam, 16mm deep, 102mm base	LM 842107	2	2170
	51mm int diam, 16mm deep, 102mm base	LM 842109	2	2170
	25mm int diam, 13mm deep, 76mm base	LM 842111	2	2170
	Any of the above Flanges are available with a Diaphragm, or Cowl, or Dressing Retainer at the extra cost of:			330

IXC

STOMA APPLIANCES

FLANGES

Manufacturer	Appliance	Order No.	Quantity	List Price p
DBT Medical Ltd	St Mark's Flanges, Black Firm Rubber			
	22mm int diam, 13mm deep, 51mm base	LM 843101	2	2483
	32mm int diam, 16mm deep, 76mm base	LM 843103	2	2483
	32mm int diam, 10mm deep, 76mm base	LM 843104	2	2483
	38mm int diam, 16mm deep, 76mm base	LM 843105	2	2483
	38mm int diam, 10mm deep, 76mm base	LM 843106	2	2483
	44mm int diam, 16mm deep, 102mm base	LM 843107	2	2483
	51mm int diam, 16mm deep, 102mm base	LM 843109	2	2483
	Birkbeck Flanges, White Rubber			
	20mm int diam, 16mm deep, 75mm base	LM 722019	2	2483
	38mm int diam, 16mm deep, 90mm base	LM 722038	2	2483
Jade-Euro-Med Ltd (including products formerly listed under Mentor Medical Ltd)	Colostomy flange St Mark's pattern, state size	KM54	1	1485
	Colostomy flange St Mark's pattern with diaphragm, state size	KM55	1	1485
	Chiron Flanges, 38mm int diam,			
	10mm deep	WK102-38-K	1	1856
	32mm 16mm deep	WK104-32-F	1	1856
	38mm 16mm deep	WK104-38-T	1	1856
	Rubber Flange			
	38mm int diam, 16mm deep	WK108-38-L	1	1856
	St Mark's Pattern Flanges			
	25mm diam, 13mm deep			
	51mm base	WK111-25-B	1	1581
	76mm base	WK113-25-K	1	1581
	32mm diam, 10mm deep			
	76mm base	WK115-32-Q	1	1581
	32mm diam, 16mm deep			
	76mm base	WK117-32-Y	1	1581
	38mm diam, 10mm deep			
	76mm base	WK119-38-V	1	1581
	38mm diam, 16mm deep			
	76mm base	WK121-38-R	1	1581
	44mm diam, 16mm deep	WK123-44-U	1	1581
	102mm base			
	51mm diam, 16mm deep	WK125-51-A	1	1581
	102mm base			
	38mm with dressing retainer	WK126-01-N	1	1997
	38mm with 16mm canopy	WK126-02-Q	1	1997

STOMA APPLIANCES

FLANGES

Manufacturer	Appliance	Order No.	Quantity	List Price p
Jade-Euro-Med Ltd (including products formerly listed under Mentor Medical Ltd)	Flanges all Blue Rubber			
	25mm int diam, 13mm deep, 51mm base	WK132-25-R	1	1680
	38mm int diam, 10mm deep, 76mm base	WK135-38-P	1	1680
	Flanges Blue and Brown			
	25mm int diam, 13mm deep, 76mm base	WK141-25-S	1	2437
	38mm int diam, 10mm deep, 76mm base	WK144-38-Q	1	2437
	38mm int diam, 16mm deep, 76mm base	WK147-38-D	1	2437
	Rubber Flanges, double base hole 38mm int diam	WK160-38-J	1	2460
Mentor Medical Ltd	Redifit belt flange			
	25mm	WL124-01-25	1	75
	32mm	WL124-01-32	1	75
	38mm	WL124-01-38	1	75
	44mm	WL124-01-44	1	75
	51mm	WL124-01-51	1	75
	64mm	WL124-01-64	1	75
	75mm	WL124-01-75	1	75

Mentor Medical Ltd also see Jade-Euro-Med Ltd

Omex Medical Ltd	Schacht Colo Flanges and Locking Rings	784583	1	540
	Schacht Ileo Flanges and Locking Rings	784575	1	540
Salts Healthcare	Latex Foam Diaphragm with Rigid Face Piece Flanges 38mm	811002	1	4660
	Latex Sheath for use with 811002 Flanges	811003	1	775
	SF1 Soft Rubber Flanges 25mm	822001	1	821
	SF4 Soft Rubber Flange 38mm	822004	1	834
	SF5 Semi-Rigid Flange 38mm	822005	1	1429
	SF6 Semi-Rigid Hard Rubber Flange 38mm	822006	1	953
A H Shaw & Partners Ltd	Rubber Adhesive Flange	NSI 1	1	681
	Rubber Non-Stick Flange	NSI 2	1	824
	Colostomy facepiece rubber-foam face, hole diameter 45mm, 65mm, 77mm	NSI 9	1	1246
Ward Surgical Appliance Co	Plastic/Rubber airfilled Flange	WM 88	1	1784
	St Mark's standard flange	WM 100	1	1174
	St Mark's flange with diaphragm	WM 101	1	1435

IXC

STOMA APPLIANCES

ILEOSTOMY (DRAINABLE) BAGS

Manufacturer	Appliance		Order No.	Quantity	List Price p
B. Braun Medical	**Biotrol**				
	Elite bag with skin protector adhesive and fabric backing				
	Beige	starter hole	38-810	30	7860
		20mm	38-820	30	7860
		25mm	38-825	30	7860
		30mm	38-830	30	7860
		35mm	38-835	30	7860
		40mm	38-840	30	7860
		45mm	38-845	30	7860
		50mm	38-850	30	7860
		60mm	38-860	30	7860
		70mm	38-870	30	7860
	Transparent	starter hole	31-810	30	7415
		20mm	31-820	30	7280
		25mm	31-825	30	7280
		30mm	31-830	30	7280
		35mm	31-835	30	7280
		40mm	31-840	30	7280
		45mm	31-845	30	7280
		50mm	31-850	30	7280
		60mm	31-860	30	7280
		70mm	31-870	30	7280
	White	starter hole	34-815	30	7860
		20mm	34-820	30	7860
		25mm	34-825	30	7860
		30mm	34-830	30	7860
		35mm	34-835	30	7860
		40mm	34-840	30	7860
		45mm	34-845	30	7860
		50mm	34-850	30	7860
		60mm	34-860	30	7860
		70mm	34-870	30	7860
	Elite Petite bag with skin protector adhesive and fabric backing				
	Beige	starter hole	37-710	30	6744
		25mm	37-725	30	6744
		30mm	37-730	30	6744
		35mm	37-735	30	6744
		40mm	37-740	30	6744
		45mm	37-745	30	6744
	Ileo S Bag with skin protector				
	White	starter hole	32-715	30	7860
		20mm	32-720	30	7860
		25mm	32-725	30	7860
		30mm	32-730	30	7860
		35mm	32-735	30	7860
		40mm	32-740	30	7860
		45mm	32-745	30	7860
		50mm	32-750	30	7860
		60mm	32-760	30	7860
		70mm	32-770	30	7860
	Post-op Bag				
	Transparent	Small	32-210	30	8190
		Large	32-215	30	11503

STOMA APPLIANCES

ILEOSTOMY (DRAINABLE) BAGS

Manufacturer	Appliance		Order No.	Quantity	List Price p
B.Braun Medical	Preference Bag with skin protector, microporous adhesive and fabric backing				
	Beige	starter hole	34-615	30	7860
		20mm	34-620	30	7860
		25mm	34-625	30	7860
		30mm	34-630	30	7860
		35mm	34-635	30	7860
		40mm	34-640	30	7860
		45mm	34-645	30	7860
		50mm	34-650	30	7860
		60mm	34-660	30	7860
	Almarys Optima Drainable bag with all over soft non-woven cover				
	Transparent	starter hole	F018710E	30	6845
	Beige	starter hole	F008710E	30	6845
		25mm	F008725E	30	6845
		30mm	F008730E	30	6845
		35mm	F008735E	30	6845
		40mm	F008740E	30	6845
		45mm	F008745E	30	6845
		50mm	F008750E	30	6845
		60mm	F008760E	30	6845
	Almarys Optima Mini Drainable bag with all over soft non woven cover				
	Beige	20mm	F008820E	30	6367
		25mm	F008825E	30	6367
		30mm	F008830E	30	6367
		35mm	F008835E	30	6245
		40mm	F008840E	30	6367
	Almarys Optima Drainable bag with filter and soft cover				
	Transparent	starter hole 10mm	F019510E	30	6728
	Beige	starter hole 10mm	F009510E	30	6728
		25mm	F009525E	30	6728
		30mm	F009530E	30	6728
		35mm	F009535E	30	6728
		40mm	F009540E	30	6728
		45mm	F009545E	30	6728
		50mm	F009550E	30	6728
		60mm	F009560E	30	6728
	Softima drainable pouch with filter, skin protector, protective cover and "Flow Control" soft outlet				
	Beige				
	cut-to-fit	16-60mm	043716E	30	8612
	pre-cut	24mm	043724E	30	8612
		28mm	043728E	30	8612
		32mm	043732E	30	8612
		36mm	043736E	30	8612
		40mm	043740E	30	8612
		45mm	043745E	30	8612
	Transparent				
	cut-to-fit	16-60mm	043816E	30	8612

IXC

STOMA APPLIANCES

ILEOSTOMY (DRAINABLE) BAGS

Manufacturer	Appliance		Order No.	Quantity	List Price p
C S Bullen Ltd	**Absorbian** drainable pouch - 2 Openings with Bio-dressing resin, microporous adhesive and skin barrier				
	Clear				
	cut-to-fit	13mm-80mm	UFAS05	15	3190
	Lenbul				
	With screw outlet				
		Day Bag	F5	1	1321
		Night Bag	F6	1	1455
	Shelter Drainable Pouch				
	Extra Large Opaque				
	cut-to-fit	13-80mm	3600/00	15	2440
	Bio dressing, resin				
	Beige				
	cut-to-fit	13mm-64mm	3250/00	15	2540
		13mm-80mm	3450/00	15	2555
	pre-cut	19mm	3250/19	15	2540
		25mm	3250/25	15	2540
		32mm	3250/32	15	2540
		38mm	3250/38	15	2540
		44mm	3250/44	15	2540
		51mm	3250/51	15	2540
		58mm	3250/58	15	2540
		64mm	3250/64	15	2540
	Clear Infant				
	cut-to-fit	8mm-51mm	3350/00	15	2540
	Newborn				
	cut-to-fit	8mm-25mm	3550/00	15	2540
	Microporous adhesive, bio dressing resin				
	Beige				
	cut-to-fit	13mm-64mm	3245/00	15	2440
		13mm-80mm	3445/00	15	2795
	pre-cut	19mm	3245/19	15	2440
		25mm	3245/25	15	2440
		32mm	3245/32	15	2440
		38mm	3245/38	15	2440
		44mm	3245/44	15	2440
		51mm	3245/51	15	2440
		58mm	3245/58	15	2440
		64mm	3245/64	15	2440
	Pouch with 2 openings Microporous adhesive, bio dressing resin				
	Beige				
	cut-to-fit	13mm-64mm	4102/00	15	2780
	pre-cut	19mm	4102/19	15	2780
		25mm	4102/25	15	2780
		32mm	4102/32	15	2780
		38mm	4102/38	15	2780
		44mm	4102/44	15	2780
		51mm	4102/51	15	2780
		57mm	4102/57	15	2780
		64mm	4102/64	15	2780
	Shelter Drainable Pouch Microporous adhesive				
	Clear				
	cut-to-fit	13-64mm	3200/00	15	2780
	pre-cut	19mm	3200/19	15	2780
		25mm	3200/25	15	2780
		32mm	3200/32	15	2780
		38mm	3200/38	15	2780
		44mm	3200/44	15	2780
		51mm	3200/51	15	2780
		58mm	3200/58	15	2780
		64mm	3200/64	15	2780

STOMA APPLIANCES

ILEOSTOMY (DRAINABLE) BAGS

Manufacturer	Appliance		Order No.	Quantity	List Price p
C S Bullen Ltd	**Shelter Soft and Secure**				
	Bio dressing resin, skin barrier and integral closure				
	cut-to-fit	13mm-64mm	SS3250/00	15	3530
		13mm-80mm	SS3450/00	15	3545
	pre-cut	19mm	SS3250/19	15	3530
		25mm	SS3250/25	15	3530
		32mm	SS3250/32	15	3530
		38mm	SS3250/38	15	3530
		44mm	SS3250/44	15	3530
		51mm	SS3250/51	15	3530
		58mm	SS3250/58	15	3530
		64mm	SS3250/64	15	3530
	Microporous adhesive, bio dressing resin, skin barrier and integral closure				
	cut-to-fit	13mm-64mm	SS3245/00	15	3430
		13mm-80mm	SS3445/00	15	3785
	pre-cut	19mm	SS3245/19	15	3430
		25mm	SS3245/25	15	3430
		32mm	SS3245/32	15	3430
		38mm	SS3245/38	15	3430
		44mm	SS3245/44	15	3430
		51mm	SS3245/51	15	3430
		58mm	SS3245/58	15	3430
		64mm	SS3245/64	15	3430
	Extra large capacity				
	cut-to-fit	13mm-80mm	SS3600/00	15	3430
	Microporous adhesive, skin barrier and integral closure				
	cut-to-fit	13-64mm	SS3200/00	15	3770
	pre-cut	19mm	SS3200/19	15	3770
		25mm	SS3200/25	15	3770
		32mm	SS3200/32	15	3770
		38mm	SS3200/38	15	3770
		44mm	SS3200/44	15	3770
		51mm	SS3200/51	15	3770
		58mm	SS3200/58	15	3770
		64mm	SS3200/64	15	3770
Coloplast Ltd	**Assura Inspire** Drainable Bag with Hide-Away Outlet and Integral Dual Filter				
	Mini Soft Cover				
	cut-to-fit	12-55mm	14801	30	9122
	Midi Transparent				
	cut-to-fit	12-55mm	14803	30	9122
	Midi Soft Cover				
	cut-to-fit	12-55mm	14804	30	9122
	Midi Design				
	cut-to-fit	12-55mm	14805	30	9122
	Maxi Transparent				
	cut-to-fit	12-70mm	14806	30	9122
	Maxi Soft Cover				
	cut-to-fit	12-70mm	14807	30	9122
	Maxi Design				
	cut-to-fit	12-70mm	14808	30	9122

IXC

STOMA APPLIANCES

ILEOSTOMY (DRAINABLE) BAGS

Manufacturer	Appliance		Order No.	Quantity	List Price p
Coloplast Ltd	**Assura Inspire** Drainable Bag with Integral Filter and Soft Backing				
	Mini Transparent				
	starter hole	10-55mm	13300	30	7563
	Midi Transparent				
	starter hole	10-55mm	13330	30	7563
	pre-cut	25mm	13334	30	7431
		30mm	13335	30	7431
		35mm	13336	30	7431
	Maxi Transparent				
	starter hole	10-70mm	13360	30	7563
	pre-cut	25mm	13364	30	7431
		30mm	13365	30	7431
		35mm	13366	30	7431
	Inspire Drainable Bag with Integral Filter and Opaque Soft Cover Front and Back				
	Mini Soft Cover				
	starter hole	10-55mm	13310	30	7563
	Midi Soft Cover				
	starter hole	10-55mm	13340	30	7563
	ready cut	25mm	13344	30	7563
		30mm	13345	30	7563
		35mm	13346	30	7563
	Maxi Soft Cover				
	starter hole	10-70mm	13370	30	7563
	pre-cut	25mm	13374	30	7431
		30mm	13375	30	7431
		35mm	13376	30	7431
	Inspire Drainable Bag with Integral Filter and Soft Cover Front and Back				
	Mini Design				
	starter hole	10-55mm	13320	30	7563
	Midi Design				
	starter hole	10-55mm	13350	30	7563
	pre-cut	25mm	13354	30	7431
		30mm	13355	30	7431
		35mm	13356	30	7431
	Maxi Design				
	starter hole	10-70mm	13380	30	7563
	pre-cut	25mm	13384	30	7431
		30mm	13385	30	7431
		35mm	13386	30	7431
	Assura Drainable Bag with soft backing				
	Mini Opaque				
	starter hole	10mm	2400	30	7563
	Midi Clear				
	starter hole	10mm	2450	30	7563
		25mm	2454	30	7563
		30mm	2455	30	7563
		35mm	2456	30	7563
		40mm	2457	30	7563
	Midi Opaque				
	starter hole	10mm	2440	30	7563
		25mm	2444	30	7563
		30mm	2445	30	7563
		35mm	2446	30	7563
		40mm	2447	30	7563

STOMA APPLIANCES

ILEOSTOMY (DRAINABLE) BAGS

Manufacturer	Appliance		Order No.	Quantity	List Price p
Coloplast Ltd	Maxi Clear				
	starter hole	10mm	2490	30	7563
		25mm	2494	30	7563
		30mm	2495	30	7563
		35mm	2496	30	7563
		40mm	2497	30	7563
	Maxi Opaque				
	starter hole	10mm	2520	30	7563
		25mm	2524	30	7563
		30mm	2525	30	7563
		35mm	2526	30	7563
		40mm	2527	30	7563

Drainable Bag with Integral Filter and Soft Cover Front and Back.

	Paediatric Clear				
	starter hole	10-35mm	2115	30	6540
	Paediatric Opaque				
	starter hole	10-35mm	2110	30	6540
	Large Post-Op for high output Clear				
	starter hole	10-70mm	12805	10	2884

Drainable Bag with opaque Soft Cover front and back

	Mini				
	starter hole	10-55mm	12400	30	7563
	Midi				
	starter hole	10-55mm	12440	30	7563
	pre-cut	25mm	12444	30	7563
		30mm	12445	30	7563
		35mm	12446	30	7563
		40mm	12447	30	7563
	Maxi				
	starter hole	10-70mm	12490	30	7563

Assura Seal Integral Convexity Drainable Bags with Soft Backing
Important:This product with Integral Convexity should only be used after prior assessment of suitability by an appropriate medical professional.

	Maxi Clear	21mm	12953	10	2612
		25mm	12954	10	2612
		28mm	12955	10	2612
		31mm	12956	10	2612
		35mm	12957	10	2612
		38mm	12958	10	2612
		41mm	12959	10	2612
	Maxi Opaque				
	starter hole	15-33mm	12582	10	2612
		15-43mm	12583	10	2612
	Maxi Opaque	18mm	12962	10	2612
		21mm	12963	10	2612
		25mm	12964	10	2612
		28mm	12965	10	2612
		31mm	12966	10	2612
		35mm	12967	10	2612
		38mm	12968	10	2612
		41mm	12969	10	2612

IXC

STOMA APPLIANCES

ILEOSTOMY (DRAINABLE) BAGS

Manufacturer	Appliance	Order No.	Quantity	List Price p
Coloplast Ltd	**Assura Inspire Seal** Integral Convexity Drainable Bags with integral filter and Soft Backing with Hide-away outlet.			
	Important: This product with Integral Convexity should only be used after prior assessment of suitability by an appropriate medical professional.			
	Maxi Transparent			
	starter hole 15-33mm	14102	10	2805
	15-43mm	14103	10	2805
	pre-cut 21mm	14163	10	2805
	pre-cut 25mm	14164	10	2805
	pre-cut 28mm	14165	10	2805
	pre-cut 31mm	14166	10	2805
	Assura Inspire Seal Integral Convexity Drainable Bags with integral filter, opaque Soft Cover Front and Back with Hide-away outlet.			
	Important: This product with Integral Convexity should only be used after prior assessment of suitability by an appropriate medical professional.			
	Midi Soft Cover			
	starter hole 15-33mm	14195	10	2805
	15-43mm	14196	10	2805
	Maxi Soft Cover			
	starter hole 15-33mm	14105	10	2805
	15-43mm	14106	10	2805
	pre-cut 21mm	14173	10	2805
	pre-cut 25mm	14174	10	2805
	pre-cut 28mm	14175	10	2805
	pre-cut 31mm	14176	10	2805
	Maxi Design			
	starter hole 15-33mm	14108	10	2774
	15-43mm	14109	10	2772
	Assura Inspire Drainable Bag with Integral Filter, opaque Soft Cover Front and Back with Hide-away outlet			
	Mini Opaque			
	starter hole 12-55mm	13810	30	8590
	Midi Opaque			
	starter hole 12-55mm	13840	30	8590
	pre-cut 25mm	13844	30	8590
	pre-cut 30mm	13845	30	8590
	pre-cut 35mm	13846	30	8590
	Maxi Opaque			
	starter hole 12-70mm	13870	30	8590
	pre-cut 25mm	13874	30	8590
	pre-cut 30mm	13875	30	8590
	pre-cut 35mm	13876	30	8590
	Assura Inspire Drainable Bag with Integral Filter, Soft Backing with Hide-away outlet			
	Midi Transparent			
	starter hole 12-55mm	13830	30	8590
	Maxi Transparent			
	starter hole 12-70mm	13860	30	8590

STOMA APPLIANCES

ILEOSTOMY (DRAINABLE) BAGS

Manufacturer	Appliance		Order No.	Quantity	List Price p
Coloplast Ltd	**Assura** Inspire Drainable Bag with Integral Filter, opaque design Soft Cover Front and Back with Hide-away outlet				
	Midi Design				
	starter hole	12-55mm	13850	30	8590
	Maxi Design				
	starter hole	12-70mm	13880	30	8494
	Assura Inspire Soft Seal Drainable bags with Hide-Away outlet				
	Important: This product with Integral Convexity should only be used after prior assessment of suitability by an appropriate medical professional.				
	Midi Soft Cover				
	starter hole	15-33mm	14404	10	4088
		15-43mm	14405	10	4088
	Maxi Soft Cover				
	starter hole	15-33mm	14414	10	4088
		15-43mm	14415	10	4088
	Maxi Soft Cover				
	pre-cut	21mm	14421	10	4088
		25mm	14422	10	4088
		28mm	14423	10	4088
		31mm	14424	10	4088
	Maxi Design				
	starter hole	15-33mm	14417	10	4088
		15-43mm	14418	10	4088
	Maxi Transparent				
	starter hole	15-33mm	14411	10	4088
		15-43mm	14412	10	4088
	✖ **Ileo B**				
	Clear	22mm	0401	100	19320
	Decorated White				
		20mm	0405	100	19320
	Mini Decorated White				
		20mm	0404	100	19200
	MC 2000				
	Clear	20mm	5920	30	8520
		25mm	5925	30	8520
		30mm	5930	30	8520
		35mm	5935	30	8520
		40mm	5940	30	8520
		45mm	5945	30	8520
		50mm	5950	30	8520
		55mm	5955	30	8520
		60mm	5960	30	8520
	Opaque	25mm	6325	30	8520
		30mm	6330	30	8520
		35mm	6335	30	8520
		40mm	6340	30	8520
		45mm	6345	30	8520
	Large Open Adjustable				
		10mm-80mm	6100	30	8520
	Mini Opaque	20mm	5820	30	8040
		25mm	5825	30	8040
		30mm	5830	30	8040
		35mm	5835	30	8040
		40mm	5840	30	8040

✖**to be deleted 1 May 2007**

IXC

STOMA APPLIANCES

ILEOSTOMY (DRAINABLE) BAGS

Manufacturer	Appliance		Order No.	Quantity	List Price p
Coloplast Ltd	**PC 3000**				
	Clear	20mm	8520	30	7782
		25mm	8525	30	7782
		30mm	8530	30	7782
		35mm	8535	30	7782
		40mm	8540	30	7782
		45mm	8545	30	7782
		50mm	8550	30	7782
	Opaque	20mm	8620	30	7782
		25mm	8625	30	7782
		30mm	8630	30	7782
		35mm	8635	30	7782
		40mm	8640	30	7782
	Mini starter hole				
		15mm	8980	30	7047
		20mm	8981	30	7047
		30mm	8983	30	7047
	SenSura 1-piece Drainable Bags with Hide-away outlet				
	Mini Soft Cover				
	cut-to-fit	10-55/66mm	15720	30	9330
	Midi Soft Cover				
	cut-to-fit	10-55/66mm	15760	30	9330
	pre-cut	25mm	15762	30	9330
		30mm	15763	30	9330
		35mm	15764	30	9330
	Midi Split Soft Cover				
	cut-to-fit	10-55/66mm	15761	30	9330
	Midi Transparent				
	cut-to-fit	10-55/66mm	15740	30	9330
	Maxi Soft Cover				
	cut-to-fit	10-65/76mm	15780	30	9330
	pre-cut	25mm	15782	30	9330
		30mm	15783	30	9330
		35mm	15784	30	9330
	Maxi Split Soft Cover				
	cut-to-fit	10-65/76mm	15781	30	9330
	Maxi Transparent				
	cut-to-fit	10-65/76mm	15770	30	9330
ConvaTec Ltd	**Esteem** Drainable Pouches with Integral Filter and InvisiClose Outlet				
	Medium - Opaque				
	cut-to-fit	20-70mm	S5079	30	8508
	pre-cut	25mm	S5080	30	8508
		30mm	S5081	30	8508
		35mm	S5082	30	8508
		40mm	S5083	30	8508
		50mm	S5084	30	8508
	Small - Opaque				
	cut-to-fit	20-50mm	S5072	30	8508
	pre-cut	25mm	S5073	30	8508
		30mm	S5074	30	8508
		35mm	S5075	30	8508
		40mm	S5076	30	8508
		50mm	S5077	30	8508
	Medium - Transparent				
	cut-to-fit	20-70mm	S5078	30	8508
	Small - Transparent				
	cut-to-fit	20-50mm	S5071	30	8508

STOMA APPLIANCES

ILEOSTOMY (DRAINABLE) BAGS

Manufacturer	Appliance		Order No.	Quantity	List Price p
ConvaTec Ltd	**Esteem** Drainable Pouches with Integral Filter				
	Small - clear				
	starter hole	20mm	S5040	10	2142
	Small - opaque				
	starter hole	20mm	S5041	10	2142
	pre-cut	25mm	S5042	10	2142
		30mm	S5043	10	2142
		35mm	S5046	10	2106
		40mm	S5044	10	2142
		50mm	S5045	10	2142
	Medium - clear				
	starter hole	20mm	S5047	10	2381
	Medium - opaque				
	starter hole	20mm	S5048	10	2381
	pre-cut	25mm	S5049	10	2381
		30mm	S5050	10	2381
		35mm	S5054	10	2339
		40mm	S5051	10	2381
		50mm	S5052	10	2381
		60mm	S5053	10	2381
	Large - clear				
	starter hole	20mm	S5055	10	2381
	pre-cut	25mm	S5056	10	2381
		30mm	S5057	10	2381
		35mm	S5069	10	2339
		40mm	S5058	10	2381
		50mm	S5059	10	2381
		60mm	S5060	10	2381
		70mm	S5061	10	2381
	Large - opaque				
	starter hole	20mm	S5062	10	2381
	pre-cut	25mm	S5063	10	2381
		30mm	S5064	10	2381
		35mm	S5070	10	2339
		40mm	S5065	10	2381
		50mm	S5066	10	2381
		60mm	S5067	10	2381
		70mm	S5068	10	2381
	Esteem Drainable Pouches No Filter and InvisiClose Outlet				
	Paediatric Extra Small - Transparent				
	cut-to-fit	0-23mm	S5090	10	2700
	Esteem One-Piece Convex Drainable Pouch with InvisiClose Outlet, Flexible Hydrocolloid Collar, Filter and 2-sided Flocking				
	Opaque				
	pre-cut	19mm	S5151	10	4282
		22mm	S5152	10	4282
		25mm	S5153	10	4282
		28mm	S5154	10	4282
		32mm	S5155	10	4282
		35mm	S5156	10	4282
		38mm	S5157	10	4282
		45mm	S5158	10	4282
		50mm	S5159	10	4282

IXC

STOMA APPLIANCES

ILEOSTOMY (DRAINABLE) BAGS

Manufacturer	Appliance		Order No.	Quantity	List Price p
ConvaTec Ltd	**Esteem** One-Piece Convex Drainable Pouch with InvisiClose Outlet, Flexible Hydrocolloid Collar, Filter and 1-sided Flocking				
	Transparent				
	pre-cut	19mm	S5161	10	4282
		22mm	S5162	10	4282
		25mm	S5163	10	4282
		28mm	S5164	10	4282
		32mm	S5165	10	4282
		35mm	S5166	10	4282
		38mm	S5167	10	4282
		45mm	S5168	10	4282
		50mm	S5169	10	4282
	Ileodress Pouches				
	Small Size				
	Opaque	19mm starter hole	S851	10	2509
		25mm starter hole	S852	10	2509
		32mm starter hole	S853	10	2509
		38mm starter hole	S855	10	2509
		45mm starter hole	S856	10	2509
		50mm starter hole	S857	10	2509
		64mm starter hole	S860	10	2509
	Standard Size				
	Clear	19mm starter hole	S841	10	2538
		38mm precut	S845	10	2538
		45mm precut	S846	10	2538
		50mm precut	S847	10	2538
		64mm precut	S850	10	2538
	Standard Size				
	Opaque	19mm starter hole	S831	10	2538
		25mm precut	S832	10	2538
		32mm precut	S833	10	2538
		38mm precut	S835	10	2538
		45mm precut	S836	10	2538
		50mm precut	S837	10	2538
		64mm precut	S840	10	2538
	Ileodress Plus				
	- with modified Stomahesive wafer, perforated plastic backing and beige clip pouches				
	Standard Size				
	Clear	19mm starter hole	S420	10	2538
		38mm pre-cut	S423	10	2538
		45mm pre-cut	S424	10	2538
		50mm pre-cut	S425	10	2538
		64mm pre-cut	S426	10	2538
	Opaque	19mm starter hole	S411	10	2538
		25mm pre-cut	S412	10	2538
		32mm pre-cut	S413	10	2538
		38mm pre-cut	S414	10	2538
		45mm pre-cut	S415	10	2538
		50mm pre-cut	S416	10	2538
		64mm pre-cut	S417	10	2538
	Small Size				
	Opaque	19mm starter hole	S430	10	2241
		25mm	S431	10	2241
		32mm	S432	10	2241
		38mm	S433	10	2241
		45mm	S434	10	2241
		50mm	S436	10	2241
	Little-Ones				
	Mini Size	8mm starter hole	S880	15	3492
	Stomadress Pouches				
	Clear	8mm starter hole	S439	10	2468

STOMA APPLIANCES

ILEOSTOMY (DRAINABLE) BAGS

Manufacturer	Appliance		Order No.	Quantity	List Price p
Dansac Ltd	**Invent** Drainable with filter, soft spunlace material on both sides anatomically shaped				
	Opaque				
	cut-to-fit	15-60mm	339-15	30	7249
	pre-cut	20mm	339-20	30	7249
		25mm	339-25	30	7249
		30mm	339-30	30	7249
		35mm	339-35	30	7249
		40mm	339-40	30	7249
		45mm	339-45	30	7249
		50mm	339-50	30	7249
	InVent Mini Drainable with filter, soft spunlace material on both sides, anatomically shaped				
	Opaque				
	cut-to-fit	15-50mm	335-15	30	7267
		25mm	335-25	30	7267
		30mm	335-30	30	7267
		35mm	335-35	30	7267
	InVent Symmetrical Drainable with filter, soft spunlace cover front and back (opaque) and back only (clear), symmetrically shaped				
	Clear				
	cut-to-fit	15-60mm	338-15	30	7117
	pre-cut	25mm diam	338-25	30	7117
		30mm diam	338-30	30	7117
		35mm diam	338-35	30	7117
	Opaque				
	cut-to-fit	15-60mm	337-15	30	7117
		25mm diam	337-25	30	7117
		30mm diam	337-30	30	7117
		35mm diam	337-35	30	7117
		40mm diam	337-40	30	7117
		45mm diam	337-45	30	7117
	Dansac InVent Convex Integral convexity drainable bag with filter, soft spunlace cover front and back, anatomically shaped Important: This product with integral convexity should only be used after prior assessment of suitability by an appropriate medical professional				
	Opaque				
	starter hole	15-24mm	341-24	10	2546
		15-37mm	341-37	10	2546
		15-46mm	341-46	10	2546
	Opaque				
	pre-cut				
		25mm	341-25	10	2546
		30mm	341-30	10	2546
		35mm	341-35	10	2546

STOMA APPLIANCES

ILEOSTOMY (DRAINABLE) BAGS

Manufacturer	Appliance	Order No.	Quantity	List Price p
Dansac Ltd	**Dansac InVent Symm Convex**			

Integral convexity drainable bag with filter, soft spunlace cover front and back (opaque) and back only (clear) symmetrically shaped
Important: This product with integral convexity should only be used after prior assessment of suitability by an appropriate medical professional

		Order No.	Quantity	List Price p
Opaque				
starter hole	15-24mm	343-24	10	2546
	15-37mm	343-37	10	2546
	15-46mm	343-46	10	2546
Opaque				
pre-cut	25mm	343-25	10	2546
	30mm	343-30	10	2546
	35mm	343-35	10	2546
Clear				
starter hole	15-24mm	344-24	10	2546
	15-37mm	344-37	10	2546
	15-46mm	344-46	10	2546
Clear				
pre-cut	20mm	344-20	10	2546
	25mm	344-25	10	2546
	30mm	344-30	10	2546

Dansac Nova 1 Convex EasiFold Drainable with integral 6mm convexity.
Important: This product with integral convexity should only be used after assessment by a medical professional

		Order No.	Quantity	List Price p
Opaque				
cut-to-fit	15-24mm	841-24	10	3868
	15-37mm	841-37	10	3868
	15-46mm	841-46	10	3868
pre-cut	20mm	841-20	10	3868
	25mm	841-25	10	3868
	30mm	841-30	10	3868
	35mm	841-35	10	3868
Clear				
cut-to-fit	15-24mm	842-24	10	3868
	15-37mm	842-37	10	3868
	15-46mm	842-46	10	3868

Dansac Nova 1 Soft Convex EasiFold Drainable with 5mm integral convexity
Important: This product with integral convexity should only be used after assessment by a medical professional

		Order No.	Quantity	List Price p
Opaque				
pre-cut	20mm	881-20	10	3868
	25mm	881-25	10	3868
	30mm	881-30	10	3868
	35mm	881-35	10	3868
Clear				
pre-cut	25mm	882-25	10	3868
	30mm	882-30	10	3868
	35mm	882-35	10	3868

Dansac Nova 1 Soft Convex High Output with 5mm integral convexity, drainable bag with twin filters, soft covers and soft-tap closure
Important: This product with integral convexity should only be used after prior assessment of suitability by an appropriate medical professional.

		Order No.	Quantity	List Price p
Clear				
pre-cut	25mm	820-25	10	3080
	30mm	820-30	10	3080
	35mm	820-35	10	3080

STOMA APPLIANCES

ILEOSTOMY (DRAINABLE) BAGS

Manufacturer	Appliance		Order No.	Quantity	List Price p
Dansac Ltd	**Dansac Nova 1 Drainable**				
	With twin filter and water repellent soft covers includes increased outlet.				
	Anatomical				
	Opaque				
	cut-to-fit	15-60mm	811-15	30	7223
	Clear				
	Cut-to-fit	15-60mm	812-15	30	7223
	Symmetrical				
	Opaque				
	cut-to-fit	15-60mm	813-15	30	7223
		25-60mm	813-25	30	7223
		30-60mm	813-30	30	7223
		35-60mm	813-35	30	7223
		40-60mm	813-40	30	7223
	Clear				
	cut-to-fit	15-60mm	814-15	30	7223
	Dansac Nova 1 Drainable Infant.				
	One piece drainable ostomy pouch with flange opening				
	Clear				
	cut-to-fit	0-40mm	818-00	30	6916
	cut-to-fit	10-40mm	818-10	30	6916
	Dansac Nova 1 Drainable with EasiFold closure.				
	With Twin filter and water repellent soft covers				
	Symmetrical				
	Opaque				
	cut-to-fit	15-60mm	823-15	30	8335
		20-60mm	823-20	30	8335
		25-60mm	823-25	30	8335
		30-60mm	823-30	30	8335
		35-60mm	823-35	30	8335
		40-60mm	823-40	30	8335
		45-60mm	823-45	30	8335
	Clear				
	cut-to-fit	15-60mm	824-15	30	8346
	Dansac Nova 1 Mini EasiFold Drainable bag. Twin filter and soft covers front and back. Plus Integrated Closure System.				
	Clear				
	cut-to-fit	15-50mm	826-15	30	8350
	Opaque				
	cut-to-fit	15-50mm	825-15	30	8350
	Dansac Nova 1 Maxi EasiFold				
	Drainable bag, twin filter and soft covers front and back, plus integrated closure system				
	Opaque				
	cut-to-fit	15-90mm	815-15	10	2787
	Clear				
	cut-to-fit	15-90mm	816-15	10	2787

STOMA APPLIANCES

ILEOSTOMY (DRAINABLE) BAGS

Manufacturer	Appliance		Order No.	Quantity	List Price p
Dansac Ltd	**Dansac Nova 1 EasiFold X3 Drainable**				
	Clear				
	cut-to-fit	15-46mm	862-15	10	3874
	Opaque				
	cut-to-fit	15-46mm	861-15	10	3874
	pre-cut	18mm	861-18	10	3874
		20mm	861-20	10	3874
		23mm	861-23	10	3874
		25mm	861-25	10	3874
		28mm	861-28	10	3874
		30mm	861-30	10	3874
		32mm	861-32	10	3874
		35mm	861-35	10	3874
	Unique				
	Maxi Clear				
	cut-to-fit	10mm-90mm	324-10	10	2512
	Opaque	starter hole	321-15	30	7014
		20mm	319-20	30	7014
		25mm	319-25	30	7014
		30mm	319-30	30	7014
		35mm	319-35	30	7014
		40mm	319-40	30	7014
		45mm	319-45	30	7014
		50mm	319-50	30	7014
		60mm	319-60	30	7014
	Clear	starter hole	322-15	30	7014
		25mm	320-25	30	7014
		30mm	320-30	30	7014
		35mm	320-35	30	7014
		40mm	320-40	30	7014
	Mini opaque (reference capacity: 250ml (see Note 2, page 257))				
	cut-to-fit	15mm-50mm	315-15	30	6910
	pre-cut				
		25mm	315-25	30	6910
		30mm	315-30	30	6910
	Mini clear (reference capacity: 250ml (see Note 2, page 257))				
	cut-to-fit	15mm-50mm	316-15	30	6770
	Oval flange				
		Opaque starter hole	317-15	30	7014
		Clear starter hole	318-15	30	7014

STOMA APPLIANCES

ILEOSTOMY (DRAINABLE) BAGS

Manufacturer	Appliance	Order No.	Quantity	List Price p
DBT Medical	Birkbeck			
	with Screwcap outlet			
	Black Rubber			
	Day Bag			
	19mm	LM 723225	1	2960
	38mm	LM 723230	1	2960
	54mm	LM 723235	1	2960
	Night Bag			
	19mm	LM 723275	1	3385
	38mm	LM 723280	1	3385
	54mm	LM 723295	1	3385
	Disposable Plastic Bag	LM 724000	100	1725
	Pink Rubber			
	Day Bag			
	19mm	LM 724225	1	2960
	38mm	LM 724230	1	2960
	54mm	LM 724235	1	2960
	Night Bag			
	19mm	LM 724275	1	3385
	38mm	LM 724280	1	3385
	54mm	LM 724295	1	3385
	White Rubber			
	with Screwcap outlet			
	Day Bag			
	38mm	LM 882111	1	1326
	44mm	LM 882112	1	1326
	51mm	LM 882113	1	1326
	with air vent			
	38mm	LM 882114	1	1586
	on body side			
	38mm	LM 882115	1	1431
	Child's			
	Day Bag			
	19mm	LM 882101	1	1278
	25mm	LM 882102	1	1278
	28mm	LM 882103	1	1278
	Night Bag			
	19mm	LM 882121	1	1563
	25mm	LM 882122	1	1563
	28mm	LM 882123	1	1563
Hollister Ltd	**Compact** Drainable Pouch			
	Clear-with beige comfort backing on body-worn side			
	cut-to-fit 13-64mm	3250	10	2545
	Beige-with beige comfort backing on both sides			
	cut-to-fit 13-64mm	3251	10	2545
	25mm	3252	10	2545
	32mm	3258	10	2545
	38mm	3253	10	2545
	Mini-Drainable Pouch Beige-with beige comfort backing on both sides			
	cut-to-fit 13-51mm	3241	10	2328

IXC

STOMA APPLIANCES

ILEOSTOMY (DRAINABLE) BAGS

Manufacturer	Appliance	Order No.	Quantity	List Price p
Hollister Ltd	**Karaya 5 seal**			
	with microporous adhesive			
	229mm Length			
	32mm	3138	30	8536
	38mm	3133	30	8536
	44mm	3139	30	8536
	51mm	3134	30	8536
	30.5cm Length			
	Opaque 25mm	3112	30	8301
	32mm	3118	30	8301
	38mm	3113	30	8301
	44mm	3119	30	8301
	51mm	3114	30	8301
	64mm	3115	30	8301
	30.5cm Length			
	Transparent			
	25mm	3222	30	8536
	32mm	3228	30	8536
	38mm	3223	30	8536
	44mm	3229	30	8536
	51mm	3224	30	8536
	64mm	3225	30	8536
	76mm	3226	30	8536
	41cm Length			
	Transparent			
	32mm	3278	30	8536
	38mm	3273	30	8536
	44mm	3279	30	8536
	51mm	3274	30	8536
	64mm	3275	30	8536
	76mm	3276	30	8536
	with microporous adhesive and quiet film			
	Transparent			
	32mm	3608	15	4188
	38mm	3603	15	4188
	44mm	3609	15	4188
	51mm	3604	15	4188
	64mm	3605	15	4188
	76mm	3606	15	4188
	Premium			
	with integral filter holder and twenty replacement filters			
	25mm	3662	15	4568
	32mm	3668	15	4568
	38mm	3663	15	4568
	44mm	3669	15	4568
	51mm	3664	15	4568
	64mm	3665	15	4568
	Impression with Convex wafer			
	Transparent			
	19mm	3610	10	2750
	22mm	3611	10	2750
	25mm	3612	10	2750
	29mm	3613	10	2750
	32mm	3614	10	2750
	35mm	3615	10	2750
	38mm	3616	10	2750
	41mm	3617	10	2750
	44mm	3618	10	2750

STOMA APPLIANCES

ILEOSTOMY (DRAINABLE) BAGS

Manufacturer	Appliance	Order No.	Quantity	List Price p
Hollister Ltd	**Impression "C"** with convex wafer			
	Beige with beige Comfort backing on both sides			
	19mm	3260	10	2640
	22mm	3261	10	2640
	25mm	3262	10	2640
	29mm	3263	10	2640
	32mm	3264	10	2640
	35mm	3265	10	2640
	38mm	3266	10	2640
	41mm	3267	10	2640
	51mm	3269	10	2640
	Transparent with beige Comfort backing on body worn side			
	19mm	3280	10	2592
	22mm	3281	10	2592
	25mm	3282	10	2592
	29mm	3283	10	2592
	32mm	3284	10	2592
	35mm	3285	10	2592
	38mm	3286	10	2592
	41mm	3287	10	2592
	Moderma - Flex			
	Drainable Pouch with skin resting barrier, filter, transparent front. Anatomical shape.			
	Beige comfort backing on body worn side.			
	starter hole			
	15-55mm	26500	30	7433
	Drainable Pouch with skin-resting barrier, filter. Anatomical shape.			
	Beige comfort backing on both sides.			
	starter hole			
	15-55mm	26200	30	7433
	20mm	26220	30	7433
	25mm	26225	30	7433
	30mm	26230	30	7433
	35mm	26235	30	7433
	40mm	26240	30	7433
	Mini Drainable Pouch with skin resting barrier, filter.			
	Beige comfort backing on both sides.			
	starter hole			
	15-55mm	26100	30	7433
	20mm	26120	30	7433
	25mm	26125	30	7433
	30mm	26130	30	7433
	35mm	26135	30	7433
	40mm	26140	30	7433
	Moderma - Flex with Adapt conformable convex rings			
	Drainable pouch, with integral filter. Lock and Roll closure system with flexible barrier plus Adapt conformable convex ring.			
	Midi - Beige with comfort backing on both sizes, anatomical shape			
	cut-to-fit 20-29mm + 20mm ring	28620	20	10186
	30-39mm + 30mm ring	28630	20	10186
	40-49mm + 40mm ring	28640	20	10186
	Midi - Transparent with comfort backing on body side only, anatomical shape.			
	cut-to-fit 20-29mm + 20mm ring	28720	20	10186
	30-39mm + 30mm ring	28730	20	10186
	40-49mm + 40mm ring	28740	20	10186
	Maxi - Beige with comfort backing on both sides, symmetrical shape			
	cut-to-fit 20-29mm + 20mm ring	28820	20	10186
	30-39mm + 30mm ring	28830	20	10186
	40-49mm + 40mm ring	28840	20	10186
	Maxi - Transparent with comfort backing on body side only, symmetrical shape.			
	cut-to-fit 20-29mm + 20mm ring	28920	20	10186
	30-39mm + 30mm ring	28930	20	10186
	40-49mm + 40mm ring	28940	20	10186

IXC

STOMA APPLIANCES

ILEOSTOMY (DRAINABLE) BAGS

Manufacturer	Appliance		Order No.	Quantity	List Price p
Hollister Ltd	**Moderma Flex with Lock n Roll Closure**				
	Mini Drainable Pouch, symmetrical shape with integral filter and lock and roll closure system				
	Beige comfort backing on both sides				
	cut-to-fit	15-55mm	28100	30	7350
		20mm	28120	30	7350
		25mm	28125	30	7350
		30mm	28130	30	7350
		35mm	28135	30	7350
		40mm	28140	30	7350
	Drainable Pouch, anatomical shape, flexible barrier plus integral filter and Lock and Roll closure system.				
	Midi - Beige with comfort backing on both sides				
	cut-to-fit	15-55mm	28200	30	8339
		20mm	28220	30	8339
		25mm	28225	30	8339
		30mm	28230	30	8339
		35mm	28235	30	8339
		40mm	28240	30	8339
	Midi - Transparent with comfort backing on body side only				
	cut-to-fit	15-55mm	28500	30	8339
	Drainable Pouch, symmetrical shape, flexible barrier plus integral filter and Lock and Roll closure system				
	Maxi - Beige with comfort backing on both sides				
	cut-to-fit	15-55mm	28300	30	8492
		20mm	28320	30	8492
		25mm	28325	30	8492
		30mm	28330	30	8492
		35mm	28335	30	8492
		40mm	28340	30	8492
	Maxi - Transparent with comfort backing on body side only				
	cut-to-fit	15-55mm	28400	30	8492
	Moderma Flex Convex				
	Drainable pouch with integral convexity, symmetrical shape, integral filter and Lock 'n' Roll closure system				
	Maxi - Beige with comfort backing on both sides				
	cut-to-fit	15-38mm	26800	30	10950
		15-51mm	26801	30	10950
	pre-cut	20mm	26820	30	10950
		25mm	26825	30	10950
		30mm	26830	30	10950
		35mm	26835	30	10950
	Maxi - Transparent with comfort backing on body worn side				
	cut-to-fit	15-38mm	26900	30	10950
		15-51mm	26901	30	10950
	pre-cut	20mm	26920	30	10950
		25mm	26925	30	10950
		30mm	26930	30	10950
		35mm	26935	30	10950

STOMA APPLIANCES

ILEOSTOMY (DRAINABLE) BAGS

Manufacturer	Appliance		Order No.	Quantity	List Price p
Jade-Euro-Med Ltd	**Black Butyl**				
(including products	Spout outlet				
formerly listed under		Day Bag	KM 42	1	3322
Mentor Medical Ltd)		Night Bag	KM 43	1	3322
	+ White Rubber				
	Spout outlet				
		Day Bag	KM 48	1	1571
		Night Bag	KM 49	1	1571
	Chiron				
	Black Butyl Screw Cap Outlet				
	Day Bag	38mm	WF005-38-W	1	3732
		44mm	WF005-44-R	1	3732
	Night Bag	38mm	WF025-38-H	1	4479
		44mm	WF025-44-C	1	4479
	Latex Rubber Screw cap outlet				
	Day Bag	38mm	WF003-38-N	1	1896
	Night Bag	38mm	WF023-38-Y	1	2509
	White Rubber Screw cap outlet				
	Day Bag	38mm	WF001-38-E	1	2149
		44mm	WF001-44-Y	1	2149
		51mm	WF001-51-V	1	2149
	Night Bag	38mm	WF021-38-Q	1	2509
	Screw cap outlet on body side				
	Day Bag	38mm	WF002-38-J	1	2149
	Night Bag	38mm	WF031-01-V	1	2053
	Children's Bag	38mm	WF011-38-K	1	1696
Marlen USA	**UltraLite** Ileostomy Bag (formerly UltraLite Small Bag)				
	Opaque starter hole Flat pre-cut		501312	15	3396
		12mm	501412	15	3396
		16mm	501416	15	3396
		19mm	501419	15	3396
		22mm	501422	15	3396
		25mm	501425	15	3396
		29mm	501429	15	3396
		32mm	501432	15	3396
		34mm	501434	15	3396
		38mm	501438	15	3396
		41mm	501441	15	3396
		44mm	501444	15	3396
		48mm	501448	15	3396
		50mm	501450	15	3396
		54mm	501454	15	3396
		57mm	501457	15	3396
		60mm	501460	15	3396
		63mm	501463	15	3396
		67mm	501467	15	3396
		70mm	501470	15	3396
		73mm	501473	15	3396
		76mm	501476	15	3396

IXC

+to be deleted 1 June 2007

STOMA APPLIANCES

ILEOSTOMY (DRAINABLE) BAGS

Manufacturer	Appliance		Order No.	Quantity	List Price p
Marlen USA	Shallow Convex Flange pre-cut				
	Opaque	12mm	501512	15	3475
		16mm	501516	15	3475
		19mm	501519	15	3475
		22mm	501522	15	3475
		25mm	501525	15	3475
		29mm	501529	15	3475
		32mm	501532	15	3475
		34mm	501534	15	3475
		38mm	501538	15	3475
		41mm	501541	15	3475
		44mm	501544	15	3475
		48mm	501548	15	3475
		50mm	501550	15	3475
		54mm	501554	15	3475
		57mm	501557	15	3475
		60mm	501560	15	3475
		63mm	501563	15	3475
		67mm	501567	15	3475
		70mm	501570	15	3475
		73mm	501573	15	3475
		76mm	501576	15	3475
	UltraMax				
	Opaque				
		Flat starter hole	53400	30	7018
		12mm	53412	30	7018
		16mm	53416	30	7018
		19mm	53419	30	7018
		22mm	53422	30	7018
		25mm	53425	30	7018
		29mm	53429	30	7018
		32mm	53432	30	7018
		34mm	53434	30	7018
		38mm	53438	30	7018
		41mm	53441	30	7018
		44mm	53444	30	7018
		50mm	53450	30	7018
		55mm	53455	30	7018
		Convex starter hole	53500	10	2620
		12mm	53512	10	2620
		16mm	53516	10	2620
		19mm	53519	10	2620
		22mm	53522	10	2620
		25mm	53525	10	2620
		29mm	53529	10	2620
		32mm	53532	10	2620
		34mm	53534	10	2620
		38mm	53538	10	2620
	✖	41mm	53541	10	2620
	✖	44mm	53544	10	2620

STOMA APPLIANCES

ILEOSTOMY (DRAINABLE) BAGS

Manufacturer	Appliance		Order No.	Quantity	List Price p
Marlen USA	Transparent				
		Flat starter hole	52400	30	7018
		12mm	52412	30	7018
		16mm	52416	30	7018
		19mm	52419	30	7018
		22mm	52422	30	7018
		25mm	52425	30	7018
		29mm	52429	30	7018
		32mm	52432	30	7018
		34mm	52434	30	7018
		38mm	52438	30	7018
		41mm	52441	30	7018
		44mm	52444	30	7018
		50mm	52450	30	7018
		55mm	52455	30	7018
		Convex starter hole	52500	10	2620
		12mm	52512	10	2620
		16mm	52516	10	2620
		19mm	52519	10	2620
		22mm	52522	10	2620
		25mm	52525	10	2620
		29mm	52529	10	2620
		32mm	52532	10	2620
		34mm	52534	10	2620
		38mm	52538	10	2620
	✖	41mm	52541	10	2620
	✖	44mm	52544	10	2620
Mentor Medical Ltd	**Adhesive Stoma Bag**				
		19mm	32-250-89	60	10647
		25mm	32-251-86	60	10647
		32mm	32-252-83	60	10647
		38mm	32-253-80	60	10647
		51mm	32-254-88	60	10647
	Cavendish				
	Clear PVC Bag	25mm	WD650-25-R	10	3609
		32mm	WD650-32-N	10	3609
		38mm	WD650-38-B	10	3609
		32mm	WC010-32-U	10	3587
		38mm	WC010-38-H	10	3587
		32mm	WC013-32-H	10	4321
		38mm	WC013-38-V	10	4321
	EC1 Range				
		10-64mm	32-331-62	30	8195
		19mm	32-331-03	30	8195
		25mm	32-331-11	30	8195
		32mm	32-331-38	30	8195
		38mm	32-331-46	30	8195
		44mm	32-331-54	30	8195
	Mini	(Clear)	32-333-08	30	8195
		(Opaque)	32-333-16	30	8195

✖to be deleted 1 May 2007

IXC

STOMA APPLIANCES

ILEOSTOMY (DRAINABLE) BAGS

Manufacturer	Appliance		Order No.	Quantity	List Price p
Mentor Medical Ltd	Post Op				
	Large outline	10-90mm	32-338-12	30	11960
	Small outline	10-64mm	32-338-04	30	8452
	Mirage Drainable Pouches				
	Beige	starter hole 19-44mm	32-520-10	30	7094
		25mm	32-520-25	30	7094
		32mm	32-520-32	30	7094
		38mm	32-520-38	30	7094
		44mm	32-520-44	30	7094
		51mm	32-520-51	30	7094
		Large Outline cut 19-90mm			
			32-520-90	10	2471
	Clear	starter hole 19-44mm	32-525-10	30	7094
		starter hole 19-64mm	32-525-15	30	7094
		25mm	32-525-25	30	7094
		32mm	32-525-32	30	7094
		38mm	32-525-38	30	7094
		44mm	32-525-44	30	7094
		51mm	32-525-51	30	7094
		Large Outline cut 19-90mm			
			32-525-90	10	2470
	Omni-1-Piece				
	with flatus filter and 20 replacement filters				
	Beige	starter hole 10-44mm	32-299-55	20	5458
		25mm	32-299-12	20	5458
		32mm	32-299-20	20	5458
		38mm	32-299-39	20	5458
		44mm	32-299-47	20	5458
	Clear	starter hole 10-44mm	32-318-79	20	5458
	Redifit with Karaya				
	Clear Medium				
		25mm	WA027-25-T	20	8016
		44mm	WA027-44-X	20	8016
	Opaque Medium				
		25mm	WA018-25-S	20	8016
		32mm	WA018-32-P	20	8016
		38mm	WA018-38-C	20	8016
		44mm	WA018-44-W	20	8016
		51mm	WA018-51-T	20	8016
	Small				
		25mm	WA020-25-N	20	8016
		32mm	WA020-32-K	20	8016
		38mm	WA020-38-X	20	8016

Mentor Medical Ltd also see Jade-Euro-Med Ltd

STOMA APPLIANCES

ILEOSTOMY (DRAINABLE) BAGS

Manufacturer	Appliance		Order No.	Quantity	List Price p
Oakmed Ltd	**Option** - Mini Ileostomy with Soft Covering to one side				
	cut-to-fit 10mm-50mm				
	Clear		2410K	30	5978
	Opaque		2510K	30	5978
	Option - Ileostomy with Soft Covering to one side				
	Clear				
	starter hole	20mm	2020K	30	6384
		25mm	2025K	30	6384
		30mm	2030K	30	6384
		35mm	2035K	30	6384
		40mm	2040K	30	6384
		45mm	2045K	30	6384
		50mm	2050K	30	6384
		55mm	2055K	30	6384
		60mm	2060K	30	6384
	Opaque				
	starter hole	20mm	2120K	30	6384
		25mm	2125K	30	6384
		30mm	2130K	30	6384
		35mm	2135K	30	6384
		40mm	2140K	30	6384
		45mm	2145K	30	6384
		50mm	2150K	30	6384
		55mm	2155K	30	6384
		60mm	2160K	30	6384
	Option - Ileostomy Alginate with Velcro Fastening				
	Opaque				
	starter hole	20mm	AV-4120K	30	8447
		25mm	AV-4125K	30	8447
		30mm	AV-4130K	30	8447
		35mm	AV-4135K	30	8447
		40mm	AV-4140K	30	8447
		45mm	AV-4145K	30	8447
		50mm	AV-4150K	30	8447
		55mm	AV-4155K	30	8447
		60mm	AV-4160K	30	8447
	Option - Ileostomy Midi with Filter and Soft Covering to one side				
	Clear				
	starter hole	20mm	3220k	30	6341
		25mm	3225k	30	6341
		30mm	3230k	30	6341
		35mm	3235k	30	6341
		40mm	3240k	30	6341
		45mm	3245k	30	6341
		50mm	3250k	30	6341
		55mm	3255k	30	6341
		60mm	3260k	30	6341
	Opaque				
	starter hole	20mm	3320k	30	6341
		25mm	3325k	30	6341
		30mm	3330k	30	6341
		35mm	3335k	30	6341
		40mm	3340k	30	6341
		45mm	3345k	30	6341
		50mm	3350k	30	6341
		55mm	3355k	30	6341
		60mm	3360k	30	6341

STOMA APPLIANCES

ILEOSTOMY (DRAINABLE) BAGS

Manufacturer	Appliance		Order No.	Quantity	List Price p
Oakmed Ltd	**Option** - Ileostomy with Filter and Soft Covering to one side				
	Clear				
	starter hole	20mm	3020k	30	6704
		25mm	3025k	30	6704
		30mm	3030k	30	6704
		35mm	3035k	30	6704
		40mm	3040k	30	6704
		45mm	3045k	30	6704
		50mm	3050k	30	6704
		55mm	3055k	30	6704
		60mm	3060k	30	6704
	Opaque				
	starter hole	20mm	3120k	30	6704
		25mm	3125k	30	6704
		30mm	3130k	30	6704
		35mm	3135k	30	6704
		40mm	3140k	30	6704
		45mm	3145k	30	6704
		50mm	3150k	30	6704
		55mm	3155k	30	6704
		60mm	3160k	30	6704
	Option - Mini Ileostomy with Soft Cover to Both Sides				
	Opaque				
	starter hole				
	cut-to-fit	10mm-50mm	2610K	30	6193
	Option - Ileostomy Midi with Filter and Soft Covering to both sides				
	Opaque				
	starter hole	20mm	4320k	30	6647
		25mm	4325k	30	6647
		30mm	4330k	30	6647
		35mm	4335k	30	6647
		40mm	4340k	30	6647
		45mm	4345k	30	6647
		50mm	4350k	30	6647
		55mm	4355k	30	6647
		60mm	4360k	30	6647
	Option - Ileostomy with Filter and Soft Covering to both sides				
	Opaque				
	starter hole	20mm	4120k	30	7002
		25mm	4125k	30	7002
		30mm	4130k	30	7002
		35mm	4135k	30	7002
		40mm	4140k	30	7002
		45mm	4145k	30	7002
		50mm	4150k	30	7002
		55mm	4155k	30	7002
		60mm	4160k	30	7002

STOMA APPLIANCES

ILEOSTOMY (DRAINABLE) BAGS

Manufacturer	Appliance		Order No.	Quantity	List Price p
Oakmed Ltd	**Option** - Ileostomy Microskin with Velcro Fastening				
	Opaque				
	starter hole	20mm	MV-4120K	30	8447
		25mm	MV-4125K	30	8447
		30mm	MV-4130K	30	8447
		35mm	MV-4135K	30	8447
		40mm	MV-4140K	30	8447
		45mm	MV-4145K	30	8447
		50mm	MV-4150K	30	8447
		55mm	MV-4155K	30	8447
		60mm	MV-4160K	30	8447
	Option - Ileostomy with Velcro Fastening				
	Opaque				
	starter hole	20mm	V-4120K	30	8447
		25mm	V-4125K	30	8447
		30mm	V-4130K	30	8447
		35mm	V-4135K	30	8447
		40mm	V-4140K	30	8447
		45mm	V-4145K	30	8447
		50mm	V-4150K	30	8447
		55mm	V-4155K	30	8447
		60mm	V-4160K	30	8447
	Option - Ileostomy Microskin with window, Filter and Soft Covering to both sides				
	Opaque				
	starter hole	20mm	M-4120K	30	8103
		25mm	M-4125K	30	8103
		30mm	M-4130K	30	8103
		35mm	M-4135K	30	8103
		40mm	M-4140K	30	8103
		45mm	M-4145K	30	8103
		50mm	M-4150K	30	8103
		55mm	M-4155K	30	8103
		60mm	M-4160K	30	8103
	Option - Ileostomy Midi Microskin				
	Opaque				
	starter hole	20mm	M-4320K	30	7818
		25mm	M-4325K	30	7818
		30mm	M-4330K	30	7818
		35mm	M-4335K	30	7818
		40mm	M-4340K	30	7818
		45mm	M-4345K	30	7818
		50mm	M-4350K	30	7818
		55mm	M-4355K	30	7818
		60mm	M-4360K	30	7818
	Option - Ileo Microskin Mini				
	Opaque				
	cut-to-fit 13mm-50mm		M-2610K	30	7008
	Option Ileo Oval - Ileostomy pouch with filter and soft covering to one side, MacKintosh liners				
	Clear				
	cut-to-fit	20mm-80mm	6020k	20	6953

STOMA APPLIANCES

ILEOSTOMY (DRAINABLE) BAGS

Manufacturer	Appliance		Order No.	Quantity	List Price p
Omex Medical Ltd	Schacht		470511	50	2100
Pelican Healthcare Ltd	**Pelican Pouch** - with Skin Protector, Adhesive, Comfort Backing, Paediatric/Neonatal Pouch				
		7mm-40mm	120705	30	7523
	Pelican Select Drainable Pouch with skin protector, fabric both sides Clear				
	cut-to-fit	20mm-65mm	110620	30	7342
	Opaque cut-to-fit	20mm-65mm	110720	30	7325
	Pelican Select Paediatric Pouch - with skin protector, plain fabric both sides Clear				
	cut-to-fit	10mm-50mm	101600	30	6567
	Opaque cut-to-fit	10mm-50mm	101602	30	6567
	Paediatric Pouch - with skin protector, fabric both sides with printed motif Clear				
	cut-to-fit	10mm-50mm	101601	30	6567
	Opaque cut-to-fit	10mm-50mm	101603	30	6567
	Paediatric Pouch - with filter, skin protector, fabric both sides with printed motif Clear				
	cut-to-fit	10mm-50mm	101608	30	6891
	Neonatal Pouch - Plain split fabric front and back Clear				
	cut-to-fit	10mm-50mm	101604	30	6345
	Neonatal Pouch - Split fabric front and back with printed motif Clear				
	cut-to-fit	10mm-50mm	101605	30	6345
	Pelican Select Drainable DuoVent - with two filters, easy access outlet, skin protector, fabric both sides Clear - Standard				
	cut-to-fit	15mm-65mm	110215	30	7235
	Opaque - Standard cut-to-fit	15-65mm	110315	30	7235
	Clear - Mini cut-to-fit	15-65mm	111200	30	7012
	Opaque - Mini cut-to-fit	15-65mm	111215	30	7012

ILEOSTOMY (DRAINABLE) BAGS

Manufacturer	Appliance		Order No.	Quantity	List Price p
Pelican Healthcare Ltd	**Pelican Select Afresh** - Drainable Pouch with Clipless System & Integral Filter				
	Opaque Maxi				
	pre-cut	20mm	112520	30	7925
		25mm	112525	30	7925
		27.5mm	112527	30	7925
		30mm	112530	30	7925
		32.5mm	112532	30	7925
		35mm	112535	30	7925
		37.5mm	112537	30	7925
		40mm	112540	30	7925
		45mm	112545	30	7925
		50mm	112550	30	7925
		55mm	112555	30	7925
	Clear Maxi				
	pre-cut	20mm	112620	30	7925
		25mm	112625	30	7925
		27.5mm	112627	30	7925
		30mm	112630	30	7971
		32.5mm	112632	30	7925
		35mm	112635	30	7925
		37.5mm	112637	30	7925
		40mm	112640	30	7925
		45mm	112645	30	7925
		50mm	112650	30	7925
		55mm	112655	30	7925
	Pelican Select Afresh - Drainable Pouch with filter				
	Opaque Maxi				
	cut-to-fit	15-65mm	112515	30	7925
	Clear Maxi				
	cut-to-fit	15-65mm	112615	30	7925
	Opaque Standard				
	cut-to-fit	15-65mm	112115	30	7925
	pre-cut	20mm	112120	30	7925
		25mm	112125	30	7925
		27.5mm	112127	30	7925
		30mm	112130	30	7925
		32.5mm	112132	30	7925
		35mm	112135	30	7925
		37.5mm	112137	30	7925
		40mm	112140	30	7925
		45mm	112145	30	7925
		50mm	112150	30	7925
		55mm	112155	30	7925

IXC

STOMA APPLIANCES

ILEOSTOMY (DRAINABLE) BAGS

Manufacturer	Appliance		Order No.	Quantity	List Price p
Pelican Healthcare Ltd	**Pelican Select Afresh** - Drainable Pouch with filter				
	Clear Standard				
	cut-to-fit	15-65mm	112215	30	7925
	pre-cut	20mm	112220	30	7925
		25mm	112225	30	7925
		27.5mm	112227	30	7925
		30mm	112230	30	7925
		32.5mm	112232	30	7925
		35mm	112235	30	7925
		37.5mm	112237	30	7925
		40mm	112240	30	7925
		45mm	112245	30	7925
		50mm	112250	30	7925
		55mm	112255	30	7925
	Opaque Mini				
	cut-to-fit	15-65mm	112315	30	7925
	pre-cut	20mm	112320	30	7925
		25mm	112325	30	7925
		27.5mm	112327	30	7925
		30mm	112330	30	7925
		32.5mm	112332	30	7925
		35mm	112335	30	7925
		37.5mm	112337	30	7925
		40mm	112340	30	7925
		45mm	112345	30	7925
		50mm	112350	30	7925
		55mm	112355	30	7925
	Clear Mini				
	cut-to-fit	15-65mm	112415	30	7925

Pelican Select Afresh

Paediatric Pouch-with filter, skin protector, fabric, printed motif and clipless outlet
Clear

	cut-to-fit	10-50mm	112701	30	8015

Paediatric Pouch-with filter, skin protector, fabric and clipless outlet
Opaque

	cut-to-fit	10-50mm	112702	30	8015

Neonatal Pouch-with filter, skin protector, fabric, printed motif and clipless outlet
Clear

	cut-to-fit	0-40mm	112703	30	8015

Neonatal Pouch-with filter, skin protector, fabric and clipless outlet
Opaque

	cut-to-fit	0-40mm	112704	30	8015

STOMA APPLIANCES

ILEOSTOMY (DRAINABLE) BAGS

Manufacturer	Appliance	Order No.	Quantity	List Price p
Pelican Healthcare Ltd	**Pelican Select Drainable Convex Pouch** - integral convexity with filter, split fabric backing and clipless outlet			
	Important: This product with integral convexity should only be used after prior assessment of suitability by an appropriate medical professional.			
	Opaque - Standard			
	cut-to-fit 12-40mm	113312	10	4023
	20mm	113320	10	4023
	22.5mm	113322	10	4023
	25mm	113325	10	4023
	27.5mm	113327	10	4023
	30mm	113330	10	4023
	32.5mm	113332	10	4023
	35mm	113335	10	4023
	37.5mm	113337	10	4023
	40mm	113340	10	4023
	Clear - Standard			
	cut-to-fit 12-40mm	113412	10	4023
	20mm	113420	10	4023
	22.5mm	113422	10	4023
	25mm	113425	10	4023
	27.5mm	113427	10	4023
	30mm	113430	10	4023
	32.5mm	113432	10	4023
	35mm	113435	10	4023
	37.5mm	113437	10	4023
	40mm	113440	10	4023
	Opaque - Maxi			
	cut-to-fit 12-40mm	113512	10	4023
	20mm	113520	10	4023
	22.5mm	113522	10	4023
	25mm	113525	10	4023
	27.5mm	113527	10	4023
	30mm	113530	10	4023
	32.5mm	113532	10	4023
	35mm	113535	10	4023
	37.5mm	113537	10	4023
	40mm	113540	10	4023
	Opaque - Mini			
	cut-to-fit 12-40mm	113112	10	4023
	Clear - Mini			
	cut-to-fit 12-40mm	113212	10	4023
	Clear - Maxi			
	cut-to-fit 12-40mm	113612	10	4023
ProSys International Ltd	**Independence** - 1 piece drainable pouch with integral filter, soft covering to both sides, viewing curtain and Ezefold outlet			
	starter hole 20mm	PR200-20	30	8495

IXC

STOMA APPLIANCES

ILEOSTOMY (DRAINABLE) BAGS

Manufacturer	Appliance	Order No.	Quantity	List Price p
Salts Healthcare	**Cohflex**			
	Drainable			
	starter hole 10-60mm			
	Flesh/Flesh	514410	30	7272
	Flesh/Clear	514420	30	7272
	pre-cut			
	Flesh/Flesh			
	25mm	514425	30	7272
	30mm	514430	30	7272
	35mm	514435	30	7272
	40mm	514440	30	7272
	45mm	514445	30	7272
	Paediatric			
	10mm starter	632310	30	6444
	Paediatric (Flesh)			
	10mm starter	632410	30	6439
	Confidence Drainable pouches			
	Small			
	starter hole			
	13mm	DS13	30	5307
	Confidence			
	Drainable pouches - transparent/overlap film			
	Standard starter hole			
	13mm	DT13	30	6370
	Drainable pouches - transparent/no overlap			
	Standard starter hole			
	13mm	DTT13	30	6370
	Drainable pouches - transparent /overlap film			
	Large starter hole			
	13mm	DLT13	30	6652
	Drainable pouches - transparent/no overlap			
	Large starter hole			
	13mm	DLTT13	30	6652
	Confidence Comfort Drainable			
	Drainable pouches with an easy clean integral closure. Hypoallergenic hydrocolloid, integral filter and soft beige cover.			
	Large Opaque starter hole			
	13-65mm	CFDL13	30	8450
	Large Transparent starter hole			
	13-70mm	CFDLT13	30	8450
	Large with oval wafer starter hole			
	13mm	DLTO13	30	8600
	Standard Opaque starter hole			
	13-65mm	CFD13	30	8450
	pre-cut			
	25mm	CFD25	30	8450
	32mm	CFD32	30	8450
	35mm	CFD35	30	8450
	38mm	CFD38	30	8450
	45mm	CFD45	30	8450
	Standard Transparent/overlap starter hole			
	13-65mm	CFDT13	30	8450
	Small Opaque starter hole			
	13-65mm	CFDS13	30	8450

STOMA APPLIANCES

ILEOSTOMY (DRAINABLE) BAGS

Manufacturer	Appliance	Order No.	Quantity	List Price p
Salts Healthcare	**Confidence Gold**			
	with hypoallergenic hydrocolloid and soft beige comfort backing on both sides			
	Drainable Pouches			
	Opaque starter hole			
	13mm	DNW13	30	6538
	Small Drainable Pouches			
	starter hole			
	13mm	DSNW13	30	5216
	Drainable Pouches - Transparent Film/Beige			
	Overlap Comfort Backing			
	Standard			
	starter hole			
	13mm	DTNW13	30	6260
	Large starter hole			
	13mm	DLTNW13	30	6538
	Confidence Gold Soft and Secure			
	Drainable pouches with an easy clean, soft and secure integral closure.			
	Hypoallergenic hydrocolloid, transparent overlap, beige comfort backing on both			
	sides, filter			
	Standard			
	starter hole			
	13mm	SST13	30	8337
	pre-cut			
	25mm	SST25	30	8337
	32mm	SST32	30	8337
	35mm	SST35	30	8337
	38mm	SST38	30	8337
	45mm	SST45	30	8337
	Confidence Gold Convex			
	1 Piece integral convexity with hypoallergenic hydrocolloid and soft beige comfort			
	backing on both sides, filter.			
	Important: This product with integral convexity should only be used after			
	assessment by a medical professional.			
	Drainable Pouches			
	Transparent film/beige overlap comfort backing			
	Standard			
	starter hole			
	13-25mm	CD13-25	10	2694
	13-38mm	CD13-38	10	2694
	13-52mm	CD13-52	10	2694
	pre-cut 21mm	CD21	10	2694
	25mm	CD25	10	2694
	28mm	CD28	10	2694
	32mm	CD32	10	2694
	35mm	CD35	10	2694
	38mm	CD38	10	2694
	41mm	CD41	10	2694
	45mm	CD45	10	2694

IXC

STOMA APPLIANCES

ILEOSTOMY (DRAINABLE) BAGS

Manufacturer	Appliance	Order No.	Quantity	List Price p
Salts Healthcare	**Confidence Gold Convex Soft and Secure**			
	Drainable pouches with 1 piece integral Convexity with an easy clean soft and secure closure. Hypoallergenic Hydrocolloid, transparent overlap, soft beige comfort backing on both sides, filter.			
	Important: This product with integral convexity should only be used after assessment by a medical professional.			
	Standard			
	starter hole			
	13-25mm	SSCT1325	10	4017
	13-38mm	SSCT1338	10	4017
	13-52mm	SSCT1352	10	4017
	pre-cut			
	21mm	SSCT21	10	4017
	25mm	SSCT25	10	4017
	28mm	SSCT28	10	4017
	32mm	SSCT32	10	4017
	35mm	SSCT35	10	4017
	38mm	SSCT38	10	4017
	41mm	SSCT41	10	4017
	45mm	SSCT45	10	4017
	Confidence Gold with Filter			
	With hypoallergenic hydrocolloid and soft beige comfort backing on both sides, filter			
	Drainable Pouches - Opaque			
	starter hole			
	13mm	GDF13	30	6759
	Small starter hole			
	13mm	GDSF13	30	6759
	Drainable Pouches - Transparent Film/Beige, Overlap comfort backing			
	Standard			
	starter hole			
	13mm	GDTF13	30	6759
	Eakin			
	Clear			
	Large			
	32mm	839120	20	5787
	45mm	839121	20	5787
	64mm	839122	20	5787
	Small			
	32mm	839110	20	5787
	45mm	839111	20	5787
	64mm	839112	20	5787
	Koenig Rutzen All Rubber Black Screw Outlet			
	Large			
	25mm	161125	1	3578
	29mm	161129	1	3578
	32mm	161132	1	3578
	35mm	161135	1	3578
	38mm	161138	1	3578
	44mm	161144	1	3578
	51mm	161151	1	3578
	Small			
	25mm	161225	1	3578
	32mm	161232	1	3578
	38mm	161238	1	3578
	Special	161099	1	3717

STOMA APPLIANCES

ILEOSTOMY (DRAINABLE) BAGS

Manufacturer	Appliance	Order No.	Quantity	List Price p
Salts Healthcare	Spout Outlet			
	Large			
	25mm	171125	1	2676
	29mm	171129	1	2676
	32mm	171132	1	2676
	38mm	171138	1	2676
	44mm	171144	1	2676
	51mm	171151	1	2676
	Small			
	25mm	171225	1	2676
	32mm	171232	1	2676
	38mm	171238	1	2676
	Special	171099	1	2775
	Koenig Rutzen with metal bridge, screw outlet			
	Large			
	25mm	165125	1	4801
	32mm	165132	1	4801
	38mm	165138	1	4801
	44mm	165144	1	4801
	Small			
	25mm	165225	1	4756
	32mm	165232	1	4756
	38mm	165238	1	4756
	Special	165099	1	4986
	with metal bridge, spout outlet			
	Large			
	32mm	175132	1	3467
	38mm	175138	1	3467
	with reinforced rubber plate, black, screw outlet			
	Large			
	25mm	163125	1	4801
	32mm	163132	1	4801
	38mm	163138	1	4801
	Small			
	25mm	163225	1	4801
	32mm	163232	1	4801
	Special	163099	1	4829
	Koenig Rutzen with reinforced rubber plate, black, spout outlet			
	Large			
	25mm	173125	1	3597
	32mm	173132	1	3597
	38mm	173138	1	3597
	Small			
	25mm	173225	1	3597
	32mm	173232	1	3597
	38mm	173238	1	3597
	with plate and metal bridge, screw outlet			
	Large			
	25mm	168125	1	5595
	32mm	168132	1	5595
	38mm	168138	1	5595
	44mm	168144	1	5595
	51mm	168151	1	5595

IXC

STOMA APPLIANCES

ILEOSTOMY (DRAINABLE) BAGS

Manufacturer	Appliance	Order No.	Quantity	List Price p
Salts Healthcare	Small			
	25mm	168225	1	5595
	32mm	168232	1	5595
	38mm	168238	1	5595
	Special	168099	1	5809
	Spout Outlet			
	Large			
	32mm	178132	1	4430
	38mm	178138	1	4430
	Light White			
	Opaque			
	Large			
	25mm	273125	30	5704
	32mm	273132	30	5704
	38mm	273138	30	5704
	Medium			
	25mm	273325	30	5704
	32mm	273332	30	5704
	38mm	273338	30	5704
	Small			
	32mm	273232	30	5704
	Adhesive Bag			
	Opaque			
	Large			
	25mm	274125	30	6456
	32mm	274132	30	6456
	38mm	274138	30	6456
	44mm	274144	30	6456
	Medium			
	25mm	274325	30	6456
	32mm	274332	30	6456
	38mm	274338	30	6456
	Small			
	25mm	274225	30	6456
	32mm	274232	30	6456
	38mm	274238	30	6456
	Simplicity 1			
	Drainable			
	starter hole (10mm-60mm)			
	White/White	510310	30	8293
	White/Clear	510311	30	8293
	pre-cut			
	White/White			
	30mm	510330	30	8293
	40mm	510340	30	8293
	50mm	510350	30	8293
	60mm	510360	30	8293
	Simplicity 1 Anatomical			
	Clear - starter hole	540311	30	8083
	Opaque - starter hole	540310	30	8083
	30mm	540330	30	8083
	40mm	540340	30	8083
	50mm	540350	30	8083
	60mm	540360	30	8083

STOMA APPLIANCES

ILEOSTOMY (DRAINABLE) BAGS

Manufacturer	Appliance	Order No.	Quantity	List Price p
A H Shaw & Partner Ltd	**Black Rubber Day Bag**			
	(with screw cap)			
	22mm	NSI 66	1	2733
	29mm		1	2733
	38mm		1	2733
	Black Rubber Night Bag			
	(with screw cap)			
	22mm	NSI 67	1	2895
	29mm		1	2895
	38mm		1	2895
Ward Surgical Appliance Co	**Black Rubber**			
	(with screw outlet)			
	19mm, 35mm or 54mm			
	Day Size	WM 08	1	1849
	Night Size	WM 09	1	1932
	White Rubber			
	with screw outlet			
	Day Size	WM 01	1	1264
	Night Size	WM 02	1	1421
	with spout outlet			
	Day Size	WM 03	1	1264
	Night Size	WM 04	1	1421
	with tap outlet			
	Day Size	WM 05	1	1851
	Night Size	WM 06	1	2052
	with flange attached	WM 99	1	2795
	Donald Rose registered design rubber bags with celluloid collars, solid, flat or fluid rims.	9	1	1977
	New improved rubber bag only, complete with collar.	12	1	2146
	Extra tap outlet and skirt (also extra for Donald Rose RD bag)	13	1	252
	Shaped rubber night bag with long vertical spring vulcanite screw outlet	18	1	1967
Welland Medical Ltd	**Curvex** drainable pouches with soft flexible flange, all-over soft cover, Integral Closure and Dual-Carb Filter			
	Maxi size, beige double sided softback			
	25mm plateau starter hole	CDS 513	10	3977
	32mm plateau starter hole	CDM 513	10	3977
	32mm plateau 25mm pre-cut	CDM 525	10	3977
	32mm plateau 32mm pre-cut	CDM 532	10	3977
	43mm plateau starter hole	CDL 513	10	3977
	43mm plateau 32mm pre-cut	CDL 532	10	3977
	43mm plateau 38mm pre-cut	CDL 538	10	3977
	Maxi size, clear front			
	25mm plateau starter hole	CDS 713	10	3977
	32mm plateau starter hole	CDM 713	10	3977
	43mm plateau starter hole	CDL 713	10	3977

IXC

STOMA APPLIANCES

ILEOSTOMY (DRAINABLE) BAGS

Manufacturer	Appliance	Order No.	Quantity	List Price p
Welland Medical Ltd	**Curvex** drainable pouches with soft flexible flange, all-over soft cover and filter			
	Beige			
	25mm plateau starter hole	CFS 513	10	2516
	32mm plateau starter hole	CFM 513	10	2516
	43mm plateau starter hole	CFL 513	10	2516
	Curvex drainable pouches with soft flexible flange, soft cover and filter			
	Clear			
	25mm plateau starter hole	CFS 713	10	2516
	32mm plateau starter hole	CFM 713	10	2516
	43mm plateau starter hole	CFL 713	10	2516
	FreeStyle drainable pouches with hydrocolloid wafer, protected Dual-Carb charcoal-based filter and integral closure			
	Beige double-sided softback large bags			
	13mm starterhole			
	(cut to 60mm)	FLD 513	30	8485
	25mm	FLD 525	30	8485
	29mm	FLD 529	30	8485
	32mm	FLD 532	30	8485
	35mm	FLD 535	30	8485
	38mm	FLD 538	30	8485
	44mm	FLD 544	30	8485
	White softback on body side large bags			
	13mm starter hole			
	(cut to 60mm)	FLD 713	30	8187
	Beige double-sided softback medium anatomical bags			
	13mm starter hole			
	(cut to 60mm)	FMD 513	30	8485
	25mm	FMD 525	30	8485
	29mm	FMD 529	30	8485
	32mm	FMD 532	30	8485
	35mm	FMD 535	30	8485
	38mm	FMD 538	30	8485
	44mm	FMD 544	30	8485
	FreeStyle Drainable Pouch with integral convexity with soft backing and Dual Carb Filter and Integral closure			
	Beige soft backing to both sides			
	Medium			
	13mm starter hole			
	(cut to 35mm)	NDM 513	10	3977
	25mm	NDM 525	10	3977
	29mm	NDM 529	10	3977
	32mm	NDM 532	10	3977
	35mm	NDM 535	10	3977
	Large			
	13mm starter hole			
	(cut to 48mm)	NDL 513	10	3977
	35mm	NDL 535	10	3977
	38mm	NDL 538	10	3977
	44mm	NDL 544	10	3977
	Clear with soft backing on flange side			
	Medium			
	13mm starter hole			
	(cut to 35mm)	NDM 713	10	3977
	Large			
	13mm starter hole			
	(cut to 48mm)	NDL 713	10	3977

STOMA APPLIANCES

ILEOSTOMY (DRAINABLE) BAGS

Manufacturer	Appliance	Order No.	Quantity	List Price p
Welland Medical Ltd	**Silhouette Plus** Drainable Pouches with filter			
	Beige			
	19mm	SDF 519	30	7135
	25mm	SDF 525	30	7135
	29mm	SDF 529	30	7135
	32mm	SDF 532	30	7135
	35mm	SDF 535	30	7135
	38mm	SDF 538	30	7135
	44mm	SDF 544	30	7135
	51mm	SDF 551	30	7135
	Clear			
	19mm	SDF 719	30	7135
	25mm	SDF 725	30	7135
	29mm	SDF 729	30	7135
	32mm	SDF 732	30	7135
	35mm	SDF 735	30	7135
	38mm	SDF 738	30	7135
	44mm	SDF 744	30	7135
	51mm	SDF 751	30	7135
	Standard Length Drainable Bags with soft backing			
	Beige			
	starter hole 19mm	FSI 919	30	7162
	25mm	FSI 925	30	7162
	29mm	FSI 929	30	7162
	32mm	FSI 932	30	7162
	35mm	FSI 935	30	7162
	38mm	FSI 938	30	7162
	44mm	FSI 944	30	7162
	51mm	FSI 951	30	7162
	Clear			
	starter hole 19mm	FSI 719	30	7162
	25mm	FSI 725	30	7162
	29mm	FSI 729	30	7162
	32mm	FSI 732	30	7162
	35mm	FSI 735	30	7162
	38mm	FSI 738	30	7162
	44mm	FSI 744	30	7162
	51mm	FSI 751	30	7162
	Welland Ovation Drainable Pouch with oval skin protector			
	Beige starter hole 10mm	FSI 910	30	7541
	Clear starter hole 10mm	FSI 710	30	7541
	Welland Ovation Drainable Pouch with large vertical oval skin protector			
	Clear starter hole 10mm	FVI 710	10	2471
	Large Post-Op Drainable Bag with Softbacking			
	Clear starter hole 10mm	FSP 700	30	7382
	Beige starter hole 10mm	FSP 900	30	7382
	Welland Ovation Mini Drainable Pouch with oval skin protector			
	Clear starter hole 10mm	FSM 710	30	6600
	Welland Ovation Mini Drainable with vertical skin protector			
	Clear starter hole 10mm	FVM 710	10	2162

IXC

STOMA APPLIANCES

ILEOSTOMY SETS

Manufacturer	Appliance	Order No.	Quantity	List Price p
DBT Medical Ltd	**Birkbeck**			
	Appliance "A"			
	19mm	LM 720119	1	10334
	38mm	LM 720138	1	10334
	54mm	LM 720154	1	10334
	Appliance "B"			
	19mm	LM 720519	1	6669
	38mm	LM 720538	1	6669
	54mm	LM 720554	1	6669
Ward Surgical Appliance Co	Donald Rose Ileostomy Appliance			
	First Stage	1	1	4838
	Second Stage	8	1	4786
	New Improved	11	1	5079

STOMA APPLIANCES

IRRIGATION/WASH - OUT APPLIANCES - (Replacement Parts)
(SLEEVES/DRAINS/BAGS/CONES/LUBRICATION)
NB. Complete Appliances are not prescribable

Manufacturer	Appliance	Order No.	Quantity	List Price p
Astra Tech Ltd	Medena Ileostomy Catheter	M8730	5	503
B. Braun Medical	Biotrol Irrigation			
	Sleeves	F05066E	50	4305
	Cone	F05062E	1	298
Coloplast Ltd	Disposable Sleeve	1540	30	3813
	Disposable Sleeve	1560	30	3813
	Colotip	1110	1	723
	Irrigator Bag	1511	1	1369
Dansac Ltd	Irri-Drain with Ring Holder for Silicone Ring	950-20	20	2526
	Silicone Ring	09547-0000	1	507
	Irri-Drain Adhesive	950-35	20	2463
	Water Container	95200-0000	1	1976
	Clamp	95210-0000	1	855
	Cone	95205-0000	1	1269
	Brush	95220-0000	1	215
	Tube	95215-0000	1	151
Hollister Ltd	Stoma Cone/Irrigator Kit	7718	1	2242
	Irrigator Drain	7724	20	3093
	Replacement Cones	7723	10	7954
			1	972
	Stoma Lubricant	7740	1	550
Medicina Ltd	Medicina Caecostomy and ACE Washout sets			
	For Caecostomy Button	AS01	1	880
	For Caecostomy Tube or ACE Catheter	AS02	1	880
	Ace Stopper	AP8/15-AP14/100	1	1400
	Ace Dressing			
	Standard	SD01	30	2700
	Key Hole	KD08-KD18	30	4800
Oakmed Ltd	Option Connect 2 Irrigation Sleeve	JH990	30	3741
	Oakmed Option PEG	PEG 50-3	30	4800
		PEG 50-7	30	4800
		PEG 75-10	30	4800
		PEG 75-15	30	4800
Ward Surgical Appliance Co	Belt	WM 79	1	838

STOMA APPLIANCES

PRESSURE PLATES/SHIELDS

Manufacturer	Appliance	Order No.	Quantity	List Price p
Coloplast Ltd	Supporting Plate	1120	1	689
ConvaTec Ltd	Combihesive Natura			
	Convex Inserts (for use with Combihesive Natura flanges)			
	38mm (25mm internal dia)	S7624	5	150
	45mm (32mm internal dia)	S7626	5	150
	45mm (35mm internal dia)	S7627	5	150
	57mm (41mm internal dia)	S7629	5	150
Jade-Euro-Med Ltd (formerly Mentor Medical Ltd)	Surrey Model Plastic Pressure Plate			
	32mm diam	WK001-32-L	1	836
	Standard Plastic Pressure Plates to use with Lightweight Bag attached Flange			
	25mm int diameter	WK004-25-C	1	836
	38mm int diameter	WK004-38-M	1	836
	Stainless Wire Pressure Frames, Hook and Lug			
	To fit			
	32mm Flange	WK012-32-V	1	1019
	38mm Flange	WK012-38-J	1	1019
	44mm Flange	WK012-44-D	1	1019
	51mm Flange	WK012-51-A	1	1019
Mentor Medical Ltd see Jade-Euro-Med Ltd				
OstoMart Ltd	Ostoshield (without belt)	Res50	1	667
	Ostoshield Belt Small/Medium 45cm/85cm	Res40	1	344
	Ostoshield Belt Large/Extra Large 66cm/124cm	Res45	1	344

STOMA APPLIANCES

PRESSURE PLATES/SHIELDS

Manufacturer	Appliance	Order No.	Quantity	List Price p
Salts Healthcare	Plastic Retaining Shield			
	Single	833008	1	363
	SS Wire Retaining Ring			
	Medium	833011	1	346
	Plastic Retaining Shield			
	Large	833030	1	444
	Light White Anti-Sag Ring			
	For Belt use	833038	1	164
	For Velcro Belt Fastening	833086	1	187
	Light White Stabilising Ring	833039	1	144
	Convex Plate for Light White Bag			
	32mm	833046	5	1568
	44mm	833048	5	1568
	Pressure Plate for Simplicity, Kombo & Solo			
	50mm	833059	1	226
	60mm	833060	1	226
	Pressure Plate Kombo			
	50mm	833090	1	214
	60mm	833091	1	214
	Second Nature			
	Convex Inserts (for use with Second Nature Adhesive Flanges)			
	38mm (19mm internal dia)	CI3819	5	142
	38mm (22mm internal dia)	CI3822	5	142
	38mm (25mm internal dia)	CI3825	5	142
	45mm (29mm internal dia)	CI4529	5	142
	45mm (32mm internal dia)	CI4532	5	142
	45mm (35mm internal dia)	CI4535	5	142
	57mm (38mm internal dia)	CI5738	5	142
	57mm (41mm internal dia)	CI5741	5	142
T J Shannon	Facepiece	TJS 948b	1	837
Ward Surgical Appliance Co				
	Celluloid Colostomy Cup			
	With sponge or solid rim, Small, Medium or Large	WM10	1	3683
	With Sponge Rubber or Solid Rim, Belt Fitting	WM11	1	4201
	St Mark's Shields (celluloid)			
	4 studs	WM13	1	800

IXC

STOMA APPLIANCES

SKIN FILLERS AND PROTECTIVES
(Barrier Creams, Pastes, Aerosols, Lotions, Powders, Gels and Wipes)

Manufacturer	Appliance	Order No.	Quantity	List Price p
3M Health Care Ltd	3M Cavilon Durable Barrier Cream			
	2g sachet	3392S	20	758
		3391E	28g	400
		3392E	92g	815
	3M Cavilon No Sting Barrier Film			
	Pump Spray (Sterilised)	3346P	28ml	667
	Foam Applicators (Sterile) (1ml)	3343P	5	498
	(3ml)	3345P	5	799
	Stoma Wipe	3344E	30	2340
C S Bullen Ltd	Balspray Aerosol	UF95	1	712
	Karaya Gum Powder	UF65	70g	473
CliniMed Ltd	CliniShield Wipes	3800	50	1365
Essentials	LBF No Sting Barrier Film (Sterile)	3820	30 sachets	2377
Accessories	Ostagel Skin Cleanser bottle	8801	100ml	272
	sachets 1.5ml	8802	30	870
Coloplast Ltd	Coloplast Strip Paste	2655	10 strips	751
	Comfeel Barrier Cream	4720	60g	463
	Comfeel Protective Film			
	Sachets	4735	30	1059
	Applicator	4731	1	502
	Conveen Prep	62042	54	1004
	Ostomy Powder	1907	25g	228
ConvaTec Ltd	ConvaCare Protective Barrier Wipes	S209	100 wipes	1733
	Orabase Paste see Part IXA page 200			
	Orahesive Powder	S106	25g	233
	Stomahesive Paste	S105	60g	761
Dansac Ltd	Soft Paste	77550-0	50g	347
Hollister Ltd	Adapt Barrier Strips (6g strip)	79400	10 strips	743
	Adapt Paste	79300	57g	357
	Karaya Paste	7910	128g	812
	Karaya Powder	7905	71g	936
	Premium Powder	7906	1	248
	Skin Gel Protective Dressing Wipes	7917	50	1337
Manfred Sauer UK	Preventox Skin Protecting Film	50.50	50	869
Ltd (formerly	Individually Packed Wipes			
Manfred Sauer	Preventox Skin Protecting Film with	50.58	50ml	713
GmbH)	Roll-on applicator			

Manfred Sauer GmbH see Manfred Sauer UK Ltd

STOMA APPLIANCES

SKIN FILLERS AND PROTECTIVES (Barrier Creams, Pastes, Aerosols, Lotions, Powders, Gels and Wipes)

Manufacturer	Appliance	Order No.	Quantity	List Price p
MedLogic Global Ltd	SuperSkin Liquid Barrier Film			
	(0.7g)	SS0009	10	814
	(2g)	SS0010	10	1323
Mentor Medical Ltd	Chiron Barrier Cream	WM102-01-A	52g	554
	Karaya Powder	WM083-01-R	100g	803
	Derma-gard Skin Wipes	32-291-06	50	1622
Opus Healthcare Ltd	LaVera Barrier Cream	3300	30 sachets	1119
	SkinSafe Non Sting Protective Film	6600	50 sachets	3571
	SkinSafe Non Sting Protective Film Spray	6601	50ml	1150
OstoMart Ltd	OstoCLENZ No rinse Skin Cleansing Gel	LGS2	100ml	267
	(sachets 2ml)	LGS3	30	1140
	OstoGuard Barrier Cream	RMC1	60g	460
	(sachets 2g)	RMC2	20	761
	OstoGuard No sting protective skin barrier film			
	(3ml sachet)	RMC3	30	1950
	(30ml dab on bottle)	RMC4	bottle	600
	OstoSEAL Protective Powder	ABP1	25g	228
S G & P Payne	Payne's Barrier Cream	1320	50g	407
Pelican Healthcare Ltd	Pelican Paste	130101	100g	758
	Pelican Ultra Barrier Cream	130105	50ml	451
	Pelican Protect	133004	30	2360
	Pelican Strip Paste	130400	30	2209
Salts Healthcare	Stoma Paste	SP60	60g	360
	Karaya Powder 4oz Puffer Pack	833004	1	508
	Ostomy Cleaning Soap (Saltair Soap)	833007	110ml	305
	Peri-Prep Wipes	840001	50	1650
Teleflex Medical	Rusch Translet Barrier Wipes	732730	30	616
Welland Medical Ltd	See CliniMed Ltd Essential Accessories			

IXC

STOMA APPLIANCES

SKIN PROTECTORS
(Wafers, Blankets, Foam Pads, Washers)

Manufacturer	Appliance	Order No.	Quantity	List Price p
B. Braun Medical	Biotrol Skin Protectors			
	10cm x 10cm	32-075	10	1881
	10cm diam	32-076	10	1881
C S Bullen Ltd	Karaya Gum Washers in tins			
	51mm diameter			
	Regular			
	51mm x 22mm opening	UF601	10	1285
	51mm x 29mm opening	UF602	10	1285
	Extra Hard			
	51mm x 22mm opening	UF6601	10	1285
	51mm x 29mm opening	UF6602	10	1285
	64mm diameter			
	Regular			
	64mm x 32mm opening	UF603	10	1490
	Extra Hard			
	64mm x 32mm opening	UF6603	10	1490
	76mm diameter			
	Regular			
	76mm x 22mm opening	UF 604	10	1709
	76mm x 29mm opening	UF 605	10	1709
	76mm x 38mm opening	UF 606	10	1709
	76mm x 51mm opening	UF 607	10	1709
	Extra Hard			
	76mm x 22mm opening	UF 6604	10	1709
	76mm x 29mm opening	UF 6605	10	1709
	76mm x 38mm opening	UF 6606	10	1709
	76mm x 51mm opening	UF 6607	10	1709
CliniMed Ltd	Hyperseal Washers			
Essentials	Small	HWA 300	20	2400
Accessories	Large	HWA 350	5	1000

STOMA APPLIANCES

SKIN PROTECTORS (Wafers, Blankets, Foam Pads, Washers)

Manufacturer	Appliance	Order No.	Quantity	List Price p
Coloplast Ltd	Coloplast Protective Sheets Non Sterile			
	10cm x 10cm	3210	10	2349
	15cm x 15cm	3215	5	2781
	20cm x 20cm	3220	5	5060
	Coloplast Protective Rings			
	10mm	2310	30	4077
	15mm	2315	30	4077
	20mm	2320	30	4077
	25mm	2325	30	4077
	30mm	2330	30	4077
	40mm	2340	30	4077
	50mm	2350	30	4077
ConvaTec Ltd	Stomahesive Wafers			
	100mm x 100mm	S100	5	1147
	200mm x 200mm	S101	3	2811
	Varihesive Wafers			
	100mm x 100mm	S108	5	1003
Dansac Ltd	Dansac GX-tra Seals			
	Washers			
	20mm (50mm outer diameter)	725-20/30	30	4081
	30mm (60mm outer diameter)	725-30/30	30	4081
	40mm (70mm outer diameter)	725-40/30	30	4081
	50mm (80mm outer diameter)	725-50/30	30	4081
Hollister Ltd	Adapt Barrier Rings			
	48mm	7805	10	1690
	98mm	7806	10	2130
	Adapt Conformable Rings			
	17-26mm	79520	10	1700
	27-36mm	79530	10	1700
	37-46mm	79540	10	1700
	Hollister Skin Barrier			
	102mm x 102mm	7700	5	1160
	203mm x 203mm	7701	4	3650
Jade-Euro-Med Ltd (formerly Mentor Medical Ltd)	White Foam Pads			
	76mm diam			
	25mm opening	WJ275-25-A	5	546
	29mm opening	WJ275-29-J	5	746
	32mm opening	WJ275-32-W	5	746
	38mm opening	WJ275-38-K	5	746
	90mm diam			
	32mm opening	WJ290-32-L	5	746
	38mm opening	WJ290-38-Y	5	746

IXC

STOMA APPLIANCES

SKIN PROTECTORS (Wafers, Blankets, Foam Pads, Washers)

Manufacturer	Appliance	Order No.	Quantity	List Price p
Mentor Medical Ltd	Karaya Washers to fit (Redifit) Bag			
	25mm	WM080-25-T	10	1610
	32mm	WM080-32-Q	10	1610
	38mm	WM080-38-D	10	1610
	51mm	WM080-51-U	10	1610
	Downs Adhesive Karaya Gum Washers			
	22mm centre opening 51mm base	WM051-23-C	10	1306
	29mm centre opening 51mm base	WM051-28-N	10	1306
	22mm centre opening 70mm base	WM070-23-J	10	1610
	29mm centre opening 70mm base	WM070-28-U	10	1610
	Karaya Rings			
	19mm	32-263-87	20	2932
	25mm	32-264-84	20	2932
	32mm	32-265-81	20	2932
	38mm	32-266-89	20	2932
	Seel-a-Peel Squares			
	100mm sq	32-292-03	20	4521
	150mm sq	32-292-11	5	2783
	Rings			
	19mm	32-293-00	20	2682
	25mm	32-293-19	20	2682
	32mm	32-293-27	20	2682
	38mm	32-293-35	20	2682
	44mm	32-293-43	20	2682
Mentor Medical Ltd also see Jade-Euro-Med Ltd				
Oakmed Ltd	Option Seals Rings			
	20mm	WM-100	10	1801
Omex Medical Ltd	Schacht Foam Rings			
	Colostomy	784885	10	752
	Ileostomy	784893	10	752
Peak Medical	Varimate hydrocolloid double-sided adhesive wedges			
	Small	VMW60	60	2800
	Large	VMW40	40	2800
Pelican Healthcare Ltd	Pelican Skin Proctector			
	100mm x 100mm	130320	10	2197
	Pelican Superseal Washers			
	20mm	130325	32	4546
	30mm	130326	32	4546

STOMA APPLIANCES

SKIN PROTECTORS (Wafers, Blankets, Foam Pads, Washers)

Manufacturer	Appliance	Order No.	Quantity	List Price p
Salts Healthcare	Salts Saltair Twin Pack			
	Small	833001	1	1066
	Large	833002	1	1491
	Salts Small Karaya Washers	833003	10	871
	Foam Seals as in small twin pack	833031	10	217
	Salts Large Karaya Washers	833084	10	1419
	Foam Seals as in large twin pack	833085	10	217
	Cohesive Slims			
	Small 48mm	839005	30	5394
	Cohesive Washers			
	Small 48mm	839002	20	3666
	Large 98mm	839001	10	2448
	Protective Wafer			
	10cm x 10cm	PW1010	10	2237
	15cm x 15cm	PW1515	5	2400
SASH	SoftPads	SP101	8	1210
T J Shannon Ltd	Kaygee Washers			
	64mm base			
	(29mm or 22mm hole)		10	733
	70mm base			
	(35mm or 22mm hole)		10	733
A H Shaw & Partners Ltd	Shaw Healwell Squares hole sizes 25mm, 32mm and 38mm	NSI 53	12	1189
	Body Mould Squares hole sizes 25mm, 32mm and 38mm	NSI 56	5	1254
	Washers hole sizes 25mm, 32mm	NSI 59	10	1149
	Rings hole sizes 25mm, 32mm and 38mm	NSI 55	5	1149
	Shaw Healwell Rings hole sizes 25mm, 32mm and 38mm	NSI 52	21	1028
Welland Medical Ltd	See CliniMed Ltd Essentials Accessories			

IXC

STOMA APPLIANCES

STOMA CAPS/DRESSINGS

Manufacturer	Appliance	Order No.	Quantity	List Price p
B. Braun Medical	Biotrol Petite	F00015E	30	3564
	15-35mm (starter hole)	F00011E	30	3564
C S Bullen Ltd	Shelter Stomacap			
	Microporous adhesive			
	cut-to-fit			
	13mm-64mm	1240/00	15	1495
	pre-cut			
	19mm	1240/19	15	1495
	25mm	1240/25	15	1495
	32mm	1240/32	15	1495
	38mm	1240/38	15	1495
	44mm	1240/44	15	1495
	51mm	1240/51	15	1495
	58mm	1240/58	15	1495
	64mm	1240/64	15	1495
	Mini Stomacap			
	cut-to-fit			
	10mm-32mm	1740/00	50	4500
	Microporous adhesive, bio dressing resin			
	cut-to-fit			
	13mm-64mm	1245/00	15	1795
	pre-cut			
	19mm	1245/19	15	1795
	25mm	1245/25	15	1795
	32mm	1245/32	15	1795
	38mm	1245/38	15	1795
	44mm	1245/44	15	1795
	51mm	1245/51	15	1795
	58mm	1245/58	15	1795
	64mm	1245/64	15	1795
Coloplast Ltd	Colocap	1014	100	12970
	Assura Minicap Opaque 20mm starter hole	2501	30	3867
ConvaTec Ltd	Colodress Plus Stoma Cap 19mm starter hole	S821	30	3749
Dansac Ltd	Dansac Nova Mini Caps (Opaque)			
	cut-to-fit			
	20-50mm	829-20	30	3757
	pre-cut			
	25mm	829-25	30	3757
	30mm	829-30	30	3757
	40mm	829-40	30	3757
	50mm	829-50	30	3757
	Dansac Unique Mini Cap (Opaque)			
	cut-to-fit			
	20-50mm	229-20	30	3764
	pre-cut			
	30mm	229-30	30	3764
	40mm	229-40	30	3764
	50mm	229-50	30	3764
Hollister Ltd	Hollister Stoma Cap			
	51mm	3184	30	3765
	76mm	3186	30	3765

STOMA APPLIANCES

STOMA CAPS/DRESSINGS

Manufacturer	Appliance	Order No.	Quantity	List Price p
Mentor Medical Ltd	Leisure Pouch	32-287-11	20	2639
Oakmed Ltd	Option Stoma Cap	1320K	50	5444
	Option Stoma Cap with Soft Covering and Filter Opaque for:-			
	cut-to-fit 20mm - 50mm	1420K	50	5912
	50mm flange	1750K	30	3221
	Option Stoma Cap Mini with Soft Covering Opaque for:-			
	cut-to-fit 20mm - 40mm	1120K	50	5810
	Option Stoma Cap with Soft Covering Opaque for:-			
	cut-to-fit 20mm - 50mm	1520K	50	5810
Peak Medical	Colomate Mini Stoma Cap 1-piece beige high capacity filter cut-to-fit			
	starter hole 20mm	CCB120	30	3800
	pre-cut 35mm	CCB135	30	3800
Pelican Healthcare	Pelican Select Minuet 10-40mm (starter hole)	102380	30	3787
	Pelican Select Minuet Plus Stoma Cap			
	10-55mm (starter hole)	102382	30	3787
Salts Healthcare	Confidence Gold Stomacap with Filter starter hole			
	13mm	SCG13	30	3408
	Confidence Stomacap with Filter starter hole			
	13mm	SC13	30	3467
	Second Nature Stoma Cap with filter			
	32mm	2SC32	30	3228
	38mm	2SC38	30	3228
	45mm	2SC45	30	3228
	57mm	2SC57	30	3228
Ward Surgical Appliance Co	Two zip fasteners fitted to colostomy belt	36	1	795
	Waterproof front, fitted to colostomy belt	37	1	656
	Donald Rose rubber ileo/colostomy bath belt with internal chamber for dressings, with stud fastenings for adjustment	51	1	1970
	Woven understraps with buttonhold ends	21	1 pair	304

TUBING

Manufacturer	Appliance	Order No.	Quantity	List Price p
Hollister Ltd	Premium Urostomy drain tube adaptor	7331	10	2231
Salts Healthcare	Salts Night Tube Adaptor	833043	2	110
	Urostomy Night Drainage Adaptor	NDA6	6	1223
Ward Surgical Appliance Co				
	Metal Spring Tubing Clip	48	1	221

IXC

STOMA APPLIANCES

TWO PIECE OSTOMY SYSTEMS

Manufacturer	Appliance	Order No.	Quantity	List Price p
B. Braun Medical	**Almarys Twin +**			
	Base Plate			
	40mm (15-35mm)	036240E	10	2961
	50mm (15-45mm)	036250E	10	2961
	60mm (15-55mm)	036260E	10	2961
	80mm (15-75mm)	036280E	10	2961
	Convex Base Plate			
	Important: This product with integral convexity should only be used after prior assessment of suitability by an appropriate medical professional.			
	40mm/17mm	036342E	5	1534
	40mm/20mm	036343E	5	1534
	50mm/24mm	036351E	5	1534
	50mm/27mm	036352E	5	1534
	50mm/30mm	036353E	5	1534
	50mm/17-30mm	036355E	5	1534
	60mm/34mm	036361E	5	1534
	60mm/37mm	036362E	5	1534
	60mm/40mm	036363E	5	1534
	60mm/17-40mm	036365E	5	1534
	80mm/17-60mm	036385E	5	1534
	Closed Pouch with filter and protective cover			
	Beige 40mm	037240E	30	4254
	50mm	037250E	30	4254
	60mm	037260E	30	4254
	80mm	037280E	30	4254
	Transparent			
	40mm	037340E	30	4254
	50mm	037350E	30	4254
	60mm	037360E	30	4254
	80mm	037380E	30	4254
	Drainable pouch with filter, protective cover and "Flow Control" soft outlet			
	Beige 40mm	038840E	30	4461
	50mm	038850E	30	4461
	60mm	038860E	30	4461
	Transparent			
	40mm	038740E	30	4461
	50mm	038750E	30	4461
	60mm	038760E	30	4461
	High Flow Drainable collection pouch			
	Beige 50mm	039850E	30	11392
	60mm	039860E	30	11392
	Transparent			
	80mm	039880E	30	11392
	Biotrol LockRing 2			
	Flange			
	35mm	22-135	5	1412
	50mm	22-150	5	1412
	75mm	22-175	5	1412

STOMA APPLIANCES

TWO PIECE OSTOMY SYSTEMS

Manufacturer	Appliance			Order No.	Quantity	List Price p
B. Braun Medical	Hydrocolloid Flange					
			35mm	24-235	5	1385
			50mm	24-250	5	1385
			62mm	24-262	5	1385
			75mm	24-275	5	1385
	Closed Bag					
		Beige	35mm	22-835	30	3458
			50mm	22-850	30	3458
			62mm	22-862	30	3458
			75mm	22-875	30	3458
		White	35mm	22-335	30	3518
			50mm	22-350	30	3518
		Transparent				
			75mm	22-375	30	3518
	Drainable Bag					
		Beige	35mm	22-535	30	3458
			50mm	22-550	30	3458
			62mm	22-562	30	3458
			75mm	22-575	30	3458
		White	35mm	22-435	30	3518
			50mm	22-450	30	3518
		Transparent				
			75mm	22-475	30	3518
	Biotrol					
	Paediatric					
	Closed Bag					
	Beige					
			35mm	23-435	30	3084
	Urostomy Bag					
	Transparent					
		Baby	35mm	23-835	10	2600
		Child	35mm	23-935	10	2600
	Urostomy Bag					
	Transparent					
			35mm	22-635	10	2646
			50mm	22-650	10	2646
			75mm	22-775	10	2646
	Softima Key					
	Flexible Base Plate					
			40mm	63040E	10	3623
			50mm	63050E	10	3623
			60mm	63060E	10	3623
			80mm	63080E	10	3623

STOMA APPLIANCES

TWO PIECE OSTOMY SYSTEMS

Manufacturer	Appliance	Order No.	Quantity	List Price p
B. Braun Medical	Drainable Pouch with Filter and Flow Control			
	Beige 40mm	63340E	30	4824
	50mm	63350E	30	4824
	60mm	63360E	30	4824
	Transparent			
	40mm	63440E	30	4824
	50mm	63450E	30	4824
	60mm	63460E	30	4824
	Closed Pouch with Filter			
	Beige 40mm	63140E	30	4884
	50mm	63150E	30	4884
	60mm	63160E	30	4884
	80mm	63180E	30	4884
	Transparent			
	40mm	63240E	30	4884
	50mm	63250E	30	4884
	60mm	63260E	30	4884
	80mm	63280E	30	4884
C S Bullen Ltd	**Shelter**			
	Flexible Plate Microporous adhesive and Bio dressing resin			
	38mm	745/38	5	1125
	45mm	745/45	5	1125
	57mm	745/57	5	1125
	Rigid Plate Bio dressing resin			
	38mm	750/38	5	1105
	45mm	750/45	5	1105
	57mm	750/57	5	1105
	Closed Pouch			
	38mm	2700/38	10	1026
	45mm	2700/45	10	1026
	57mm	2700/57	10	1026
	Drainable Pouch			
	38mm	3700/38	10	1026
	45mm	3700/45	10	1026
	57mm	3700/57	10	1026
	Stoma Cap			
	38mm	1700/38	10	885
	45mm	1700/45	10	885
	57mm	1700/57	10	885
	Drainable Pouch Extra Large			
	38mm	4700/38	10	1231
	45mm	4700/45	10	1231
	57mm	4700/57	10	1231
	70mm	4700/70	10	1231

STOMA APPLIANCES

TWO PIECE OSTOMY SYSTEMS

Manufacturer	Appliance	Order No.	Quantity	List Price p
Coloplast Ltd	**Assura** Base Plates with 10mm starter hole:			
	40mm for 15-35mm stoma	13141	5	1598
	50mm for 15-45mm stoma	13151	5	1598
	60mm for 15-55mm stoma	13161	5	1598
	Convex inserts for use with the above - see "Pressure Plates"			
	Assura Base Plates 40mm for paediatric bags	2180	5	1621
	Assura Extra			
	Base Plates			
	40mm flange	2831	5	1921
	50mm flange	2832	5	1921
	60mm flange	2833	5	1921
	Assura Seal Extra			
	Base Plates with integral deep convexity			
	40mm flange starter hole 15-23mm	14243	5	1921
	50mm flange starter hole 15-33mm	14246	5	1921
	60mm flange starter hole 15-43mm	14249	5	1921
	Assura Seal Integral Convexity Baseplates			
	Important: This product with Integral Convexity should only be used after prior assessment of suitability by an appropriate medical professional.			
	40mm flange for 15mm pre-cut	12721	5	1522
	40mm flange for 18mm pre-cut	12722	5	1522
	40mm flange for 21mm pre-cut	12723	5	1522
	50mm flange starter hole 15mm	12717	5	1522
	50mm flange for 25mm pre-cut	12724	5	1522
	50mm flange for 28mm pre-cut	12725	5	1522
	50mm flange for 31mm pre-cut	12726	5	1522
	60mm flange starter hole 15-43mm	12718	5	1522
	60mm flange for 35mm pre-cut	12727	5	1522
	60mm flange for 38mm pre-cut	12728	5	1522
	60mm flange for 41mm pre-cut	12729	5	1522
	Assura Soft Seal Baseplates with shallow convexity			
	Important: This product with integral convexity should only be used after prior assessment of suitability by an appropriate medical professional			
	40mm flange starter hole 15-23mm	14261	5	1708
	40mm flange 18mm pre-cut	14271	5	1708
	40mm flange 21mm pre-cut	14272	5	1708
	50mm flange starter hole 15-33mm	14262	5	1708
	50mm flange 25mm pre-cut	14273	5	1708
	50mm flange 28mm pre-cut	14274	5	1708
	50mm flange 31mm pre-cut	14275	5	1708
	60mm flange starter hole 15-43mm	14263	5	1708
	60mm flange 35mm pre-cut	14276	5	1708
	60mm flange 38mm pre-cut	14277	5	1708
	60mm flange 41mm pre-cut	14278	5	1708

IXC

STOMA APPLIANCES

TWO PIECE OSTOMY SYSTEMS

Manufacturer	Appliance	Order No.	Quantity	List Price p
Coloplast Ltd	**Assura** Soft Seal Extra Baseplate			
	Important: This product with integral convexity should only be used after prior			
	assessment of suitability by an appropriate medical professional.			
	40mm flange starter hole 15-23mm	14281	5	1884
	50mm flange starter hole 15-33mm	14282	5	1884
	60mm flange starter hole 15-43mm	14283	5	1884
	40mm flange pre-cut 18mm	14291	5	1884
	40mm flange pre-cut 21mm	14292	5	1884
	50mm flange pre-cut 25mm	14293	5	1884
	50mm flange pre-cut 28mm	14294	5	1884
	50mm flange pre-cut 31mm	14295	5	1884
	60mm flange pre-cut 35mm	14296	5	1884
	60mm flange pre-cut 38mm	14297	5	1884
	60mm flange pre-cut 41mm	14298	5	1884
	Assura Closed Bags:			
	Paediatric Opaque			
	40mm	2160	30	3078
	Mini Opaque			
	40mm	2724	30	3390
	50mm	2725	30	3390
	Midi Clear			
	40mm	2774	30	4125
	50mm	2775	30	4125
	60mm	2776	30	4125
	Midi Opaque			
	40mm	2764	30	4125
	50mm	2765	30	4125
	60mm	2766	30	4125
	Maxi Clear			
	40mm	2784	30	4125
	50mm	2785	30	4125
	60mm	2786	30	4125
	Maxi Opaque			
	40mm	2814	30	4125
	50mm	2815	30	4125
	60mm	2816	30	4125
	Minicap Opaque			
	40mm	2804	30	3300
	50mm	2805	30	3300
	Assura Uro Minicap 2 piece			
	Opaque with 40mm coupling	2807	30	13779
	Opaque with 50mm coupling	2808	30	13731
	Assura Drainable Bags			
	Paediatric Opaque			
	40mm	2150	30	3567
	Midi Clear			
	40mm	2754	30	4125
	50mm	2755	30	4125
	60mm	2756	30	4125
	Midi Opaque			
	40mm	2744	30	4125
	50mm	2745	30	4125
	60mm	2746	30	4125

STOMA APPLIANCES

TWO PIECE OSTOMY SYSTEMS

Manufacturer	Appliance	Order No.	Quantity	List Price p
Coloplast Ltd	Maxi Clear			
	40mm	2794	30	4125
	50mm	2795	30	4125
	60mm	2796	30	4125
	Maxi Opaque			
	40mm	2824	30	4125
	50mm	2825	30	4125
	60mm	2826	30	4125
	Closed Bag with Integral Filter and Opaque Soft Cover front and back			
	Midi			
	40mm	12461	30	4125
	50mm	12462	30	4125
	60mm	12463	30	4125
	Maxi			
	40mm	12481	30	4125
	50mm	12482	30	4125
	60mm	12483	30	4125
	Drainable Bag with Opaque Soft Cover front and back			
	Midi			
	40mm	12441	30	4125
	50mm	12442	30	4125
	60mm	12443	30	4125
	Assura Urostomy Bag (include 4 drain tube adaptors per pack)			
	Midi Clear with soft backing on body-worn side			
	40mm	2854	30	8238
	50mm	2855	30	8238
	Maxi Clear with soft backing on body-worn side			
	40mm	2874	30	8238
	50mm	2875	30	8238
	60mm	2876	30	8238
	Paediatric Clear with soft backing on body-worn side			
	40mm	2175	30	8238
	Maxi Opaque with soft backing on body-worn side			
	40mm	2864	30	8238
	50mm	2865	30	8238
	60mm	2866	30	8238
	Paediatric Opaque with soft backing on body-worn side			
	40mm	2170	30	8238
	Assura Inspire			
	Closed Bag with integral filter and soft backing			
	Midi Transparent			
	40mm	12344	30	4182
	50mm	12345	30	4182
	60mm	12346	30	4182
	Maxi Transparent			
	40mm	12374	30	4182
	50mm	12375	30	4182
	60mm	12376	30	4182
	Closed Bag with integral filter and opaque soft cover front and back			
	Midi Soft Cover			
	40mm	12354	30	4182
	50mm	12355	30	4182
	60mm	12356	30	4182

IXC

STOMA APPLIANCES

TWO PIECE OSTOMY SYSTEMS

Manufacturer	Appliance	Order No.	Quantity	List Price p
Coloplast Ltd	Maxi Soft Cover			
	40mm	12384	30	4182
	50mm	12385	30	4182
	60mm	12386	30	4182
	Closed Bag with integral filter and soft cover front and back			
	Midi Design			
	40mm	12364	30	4182
	50mm	12365	30	4182
	60mm	12366	30	4182
	Maxi Design			
	40mm	12394	30	4182
	50mm	12395	30	4182
	60mm	12396	30	4182
	Drainable Bag with integral filter and soft backing			
	Midi Transparent			
	40mm	13444	30	4182
	50mm	13445	30	4182
	60mm	13446	30	4182
	Maxi Transparent			
	40mm	13474	30	4182
	50mm	13475	30	4182
	60mm	13476	30	4182
	Drainable Bag with integral filter and opaque soft cover front and back			
	Midi Soft Cover			
	40mm	13454	30	4182
	50mm	13455	30	4182
	60mm	13456	30	4182
	Maxi Soft Cover			
	40mm	13484	30	4182
	50mm	13485	30	4182
	60mm	13486	30	4182
	Drainable Bag with integral filter and soft cover front and back			
	Midi Design			
	40mm	13464	30	4182
	50mm	13465	30	4182
	60mm	13466	30	4182
	Maxi Design			
	40mm	13494	30	4185
	50mm	13495	30	4182
	60mm	13496	30	4182
	Assura Inspire with Hide-away outlet			
	Drainable Bag with integral filter and soft backing with Hide-away outlet.			
	Midi Transparent			
	40mm	13944	30	4437
	50mm	13945	30	4437
	60mm	13946	30	4437
	Maxi Transparent			
	40mm	13974	30	4437
	50mm	13975	30	4437
	60mm	13976	30	4437

STOMA APPLIANCES

TWO PIECE OSTOMY SYSTEMS

Manufacturer	Appliance	Order No.	Quantity	List Price p
Coloplast Ltd	Drainable Bag with integral filter, opaque soft cover front and back with Hide-away outlet.			
	Mini Soft Cover			
	40mm	13924	30	4437
	50mm	13925	30	4437
	60mm	13926	30	4437
	Midi Soft Cover			
	40mm	13954	30	4437
	50mm	13955	30	4437
	60mm	13956	30	4437
	Maxi Soft Cover			
	40mm	13984	30	4437
	50mm	13985	30	4437
	60mm	13986	30	4437
	Drainable Bag with integral filter, opaque design soft cover front and back with Hide-away outlet.			
	Midi Design			
	40mm	13964	30	4437
	50mm	13965	30	4437
	60mm	13966	30	4437
	Assura Multichamber Urostomy Bag			
	Midi Transparent			
	40mm	14217	30	8238
	50mm	14218	30	8238
	60mm	14219	30	8238
	Maxi Transparent			
	40mm	14227	30	8238
	50mm	14228	30	8238
	60mm	14229	30	8238
	Midi White			
	40mm	14214	30	8238
	50mm	14215	30	8238
	60mm	14216	30	8238
	Maxi White			
	40mm	14224	30	8238
	50mm	14225	30	8238
	60mm	14226	30	8238

IXC

STOMA APPLIANCES

TWO PIECE OSTOMY SYSTEMS

Manufacturer	Appliance	Order No.	Quantity	List Price p
Coloplast Ltd	**Easiflex** Baseplate			
	35mm flange, starter hole 10-33mm	14301	10	3694
	50mm flange, starter hole 10-48mm	14302	10	3694
	70mm flange, starter hole 10-68mm	14303	10	3694
	90mm flange, starter hole 15-88mm	14309	5	1815
	Extra 35mm flange, starter hole 10-33mm	14304	10	3694
	Extra 50mm flange, starter hole 10-48mm	14305	10	3694
	Extra 70mm flange, starter hole 10-68mm	14306	10	3694
	35mm flange, pre-cut 18mm	14381	10	3694
	35mm flange, pre-cut 21mm	14382	10	3694
	35mm flange, pre-cut 25mm	14383	10	3694
	35mm flange, pre-cut 28mm	14384	10	3694
	50mm flange, pre-cut 25mm	14385	10	3694
	50mm flange, pre-cut 28mm	14386	10	3694
	50mm flange, pre-cut 31mm	14387	10	3694
	50mm flange, pre-cut 35mm	14388	10	3694
	50mm flange, pre-cut 41mm	14389	10	3694
	Extra 35mm flange, pre-cut 18mm	14391	10	3694
	Extra 35mm flange, pre-cut 21mm	14392	10	3694
	Extra 35mm flange, pre-cut 25mm	14393	10	3694
	Extra 35mm flange, pre-cut 28mm	14394	10	3694
	Extra 50mm flange, pre-cut 25mm	14395	10	3694
	Extra 50mm flange, pre-cut 28mm	14396	10	3694
	Extra 50mm flange, pre-cut 31mm	14397	10	3694
	Extra 50mm flange, pre-cut 35mm	14398	10	3694
	Extra 50mm flange, pre-cut 41mm	14399	10	3694
	Paediatric			
	17mm flange, starter hole 0-15mm	14307	10	3629
	27mm flange, starter hole 0-25mm	14308	10	3629
	Easiflex Closed Bags with Dual Filter			
	Mini Soft Cover			
	35mm	14471	30	4980
	50mm	14472	30	4980
	Mini Design			
	35mm	14473	30	4980
	50mm	14474	30	4980
	Midi Transparent			
	35mm	14461	30	4980
	50mm	14462	30	4980
	Midi Soft Cover			
	35mm	14464	30	4980
	50mm	14465	30	4980
	50mm Custom Peel	14466	30	4980
	Midi Design			
	35mm	14467	30	4980
	50mm	14468	30	4980
	50mm Custom Peel	14469	30	4980
	Maxi Transparent			
	35mm	14481	30	4980
	50mm	14482	30	4980
	50mm Custom Peel	14483	30	4980
	70mm	14478	30	4980

STOMA APPLIANCES

TWO PIECE OSTOMY SYSTEMS

Manufacturer	Appliance	Order No.	Quantity	List Price p
Coloplast Ltd	Maxi Soft Cover			
	35mm	14484	30	4980
	50mm	14485	30	4980
	50mm Custom Peel	14486	30	4980
	70mm	14479	30	4980
	Maxi Design			
	35mm	14487	30	4980
	50mm	14488	30	4980
	50mm Custom Peel	14489	30	4980
	Extra Large Transparent			
	70mm	14476	30	4980
	Extra Large Soft Cover			
	70mm	14477	30	4980
	Easiflex Drainable Bags with Hide-Away Outlet			
	Midi Transparent			
	35mm	14341	30	4917
	50mm	14342	30	4917
	Midi Soft Cover			
	35mm	14346	30	4917
	50rnm	14347	30	4917
	50mm Custom Peel	14348	30	4917
	Midi design			
	35mm	14351	30	4917
	50mm	14352	30	4917
	50mm Custom Peel	14353	30	4917
	Maxi Transparent			
	35mm	14356	30	4917
	50mm	14357	30	4917
	50mm Custom Peel	14358	30	4917
	70mm	14344	30	4917
	Maxi Soft Cover			
	35mm	14361	30	4917
	50mm	14362	30	4917
	50mm Custom Peel	14363	30	4917
	70mm	14349	30	4917
	Maxi Design			
	35mm	14366	30	4917
	50mm	14367	30	4917
	50mm Custom Peel	14368	30	4917
	Extra Large Transparent			
	70mm	14359	30	4917
	Extra Large Soft Cover			
	70mm	14364	30	4917
	Mini Soft Cover			
	35mm	14376	30	4824
	50mm	14377	30	4824
	Paediatric Transparent			
	17mm	14681	30	4917
	27mm	14682	30	4917
	Paediatric Design			
	17mm	14691	30	4917
	27mm	14692	30	4917
	XXL Transparent			
	90mm	14378	30	4917
	XXL Soft Cover			
	90mm	14379	30	4917

STOMA APPLIANCES

TWO PIECE OSTOMY SYSTEMS

Manufacturer	Appliance	Order No.	Quantity	List Price p
Coloplast Ltd	**Easiflex Soft Seal** baseplate			
	Important: This product with integral convexity should only be used after prior assessment of suitability by an appropiate medical professional.			
	35mm flange, starter hole 15-23mm	14401	5	1886
	50mm flange, starter hole 15-33mm	14402	5	1886
	50mm flange, starter hole 15-43mm	14403	5	1886
	35mm flange, pre-cut 18mm	14641	5	1886
	35mm flange, pre-cut 21mm	14642	5	1886
	50mm flange, pre-cut 25mm	14643	5	1886
	50mm flange, pre-cut 28mm	14644	5	1886
	50mm flange, pre-cut 31mm	14645	5	1886
	50mm flange, pre-cut 35mm	14646	5	1886
	50mm flange, pre-cut 38mm	14647	5	1886
	50mm flange, pre-cut 41mm	14648	5	1886
	Easiflex Soft Seal Extra baseplate			
	35mm flange, starter hole 15-23mm	14601	5	2075
	50mm flange, starter hole 15-33mm	14602	5	2075
	50mm flange, starter hole 15-43mm	14603	5	2075
	MC 2002			
	Base Plates			
	40mm flanges 15mm stoma	6742	5	1677
	40mm flanges 25mm stoma	6743	5	1677
	60mm flanges 35mm stoma	6764	5	1677
	60mm flanges 45mm stoma	6765	5	1677
	Closed Pouches			
	Clear			
	40mm	6641	30	4542
	60mm	6661	30	4542
	Opaque			
	40mm	6642	30	4542
	60mm	6662	30	4542
	Open Pouches			
	Clear - 40mm	6541	30	5013
	60mm	6561	30	5013
	Opaque - 40mm	6542	30	5013
	60mm	6562	30	5013
	Belt Plates			
	40mm	4270	1	68
	60mm	4271	1	68
	URO2002			
	Base Plates			
	40mm flange	4245	5	1720
	60mm flange	4265	5	1720
	Bags			
	40mm Large	4240	20	6660
	Small	4241	20	6660
	60mm Large	4260	20	6660
	Conseal			
	Base Plates			
	40mm	1200	5	1607
	50mm	1250	5	1607
	Colostomy Plug			
	40 x 35mm	1235	10	1464
	40 x 45mm	1245	10	1464
	50 x 35mm	1285	10	1464
	50 x 45mm	1295	10	1464
	Closed Bag			
	40mm	1210	30	4344
	50mm	1260	30	4344

STOMA APPLIANCES

TWO PIECE OSTOMY SYSTEMS

Manufacturer	Appliance	Order No.	Quantity	List Price p
ConvaTec Ltd	**Combihesive Natura**			
	Durahesive Convex flange with Flexible Collar. Mouldable			
	Important: This product with integral convexity should only be used after prior			
	assessment of suitability by an appropriate medical professional.			
	13-22mm (for 45mm pouches)	S7304	10	3185
	22-33mm (for 45mm pouches)	S7305	10	3185
	33-45mm (for 57mm pouches)	S7306	10	3185
	Durahesive with Convex-IT Flange			
	Important: This product with deep convexity should only be used after prior			
	assessment of suitability by an appropriate medical professional.			
	13mm/45mm	S7325	5	1587
	16mm/45mm	S7326	5	1587
	19mm/45mm	S7327	5	1587
	22mm/45mm	S7328	5	1587
	25mm/45mm	S7329	5	1587
	28mm/45mm	S7330	5	1587
	32mm/45mm	S7331	5	1587
	35mm/45mm	S7332	5	1587
	38mm/57mm	S7335	5	1587
	41mm/57mm	S7336	5	1587
	45mm/57mm	S7337	5	1587
	50mm/57mm	S7338	5	1587
	Flexible Flange with Micropore Surround (Oval)			
	32mm	S7244	5	1558
	38mm	S7245	5	1558
	45mm	S7246	5	1558
	57mm	S7247	5	1558
	70mm	S7248	5	1558
	Flexible Flange with Micropore Surround (Square)			
	Wafer size 100mm x 100mm			
	32mm	S7238	10	2956
	38mm	S7239	10	2956
	45mm	S7240	10	2956
	Wafer size 127mm x 127mm			
	57mm	S7241	10	2956
	70mm	S7242	10	2956
	Stomahesive Flange			
	32mm	S7294	10	2728
	38mm	S7295	10	2728
	45mm	S7296	10	2728
	57mm	S7297	10	2728
	70mm	S7298	10	2728
	100mm	S7299B	5	1364
	Stomahesive Flexible Flange			
	32mm	S7340	10	2947
	38mm	S7341	10	2947
	45mm	S7342	10	2947
	57mm	S7343	10	2947
	70mm	S7344	10	2947
	Flange Cap with Filter			
	Opaque			
	38mm	S7250	25	2577
	45mm	S7251	25	2577
	57mm	S7252	25	2577

IXC

STOMA APPLIANCES

TWO PIECE OSTOMY SYSTEMS

Manufacturer	Appliance	Order No.	Quantity	List Price p
ConvaTec Ltd	**Combihesive Natura**			
	Closed Pouch with filter			
	Standard Size - Opaque			
	32mm	S7254	30	3769
	38mm	S7255	30	3769
	45mm	S7256	30	3769
	57mm	S7257	30	3769
	70mm	S7258	30	3769
	Midi Size - Opaque			
	32mm	S7290F	20	2219
	38mm	S7291F	20	2219
	45mm	S7292F	20	2219
	57mm	S7293F	20	2219
	Closed pouch no filter			
	Standard size - Opaque			
	32mm	S7215	30	3543
	38mm	S7216	30	3543
	45mm	S7217	30	3543
	57mm	S7218	30	3543
	70mm	S7219	30	3543
	Mini size - Opaque			
	32mm	S7290	20	2066
	38mm	S7291	20	2066
	45mm	S7292	20	2066
	57mm	S7293	20	2066
	Convex inserts for use with above - see Pressure Plates			
	Drainable Pouch			
	Standard Size - Opaque			
	32mm	S7269	10	1248
	38mm	S7270	10	1248
	45mm	S7271	10	1248
	57mm	S7272	10	1248
	70mm	S7273	10	1248
	Small Size - Opaque			
	32mm	S7279	10	1248
	38mm	S7280	10	1248
	45mm	S7281	10	1248
	57mm	S7282	10	1248
	70mm	S7283	10	1248
	Standard Size - Clear			
	32mm	S7228	10	1248
	38mm	S7229	10	1248
	45mm	S7230	10	1248
	57mm	S7231	10	1248
	70mm	S7232	10	1248
	100mm	S7233	10	2214
	Drainable Pouch with Filter			
	Standard Size - Opaque one sided for:-			
	32mm flange	S7411	10	1248
	38mm flange	S7412	10	1248
	45mm flange	S7413	10	1248
	57mm flange	S7414	10	1248
	70mm flange	S7415	10	1248
	Standard Size - Opaque for:-			
	32mm flange	S7400	10	1224
	38mm flange	S7401	10	1224
	45mm flange	S7402	10	1224
	57mm flange	S7403	10	1224
	70mm flange	S7404	10	1224

STOMA APPLIANCES

TWO PIECE OSTOMY SYSTEMS

Manufacturer	Appliance	Order No.	Quantity	List Price p
ConvaTec Ltd	**Combihesive Natura**			
	Small Size - Opaque for:-			
	32mm flange	S7406	10	1224
	38mm flange	S7407	10	1224
	45mm flange	S7408	10	1224
	57mm flange	S7409	10	1224
	70mm flange	S7410	10	1224
	Stomahesive Flange with Flexible Hydrocolloid Collar			
	32mm	S7201	10	3254
	38mm	S7202	10	3254
	45mm	S7203	10	3254
	57mm	S7204	10	3254
	70mm	S7205	10	3254
	Urostomy Pouch with Improved Accuseal Tap			
	Standard Size - Clear for:-			
	32mm flange	S7380	10	2733
	38mm flange	S7381	10	2733
	45mm flange	S7382	10	2733
	57mm flange	S7383	10	2733
	70mm flange	S7384	10	2733
	Urostomy Pouch with Improved Accuseal Tap			
	Standard Size - Opaque for:-			
	32mm flange	S7370	10	2733
	38mm flange	S7371	10	2733
	45mm flange	S7372	10	2733
	57mm flange	S7373	10	2733
	Small Size - Opaque for:-			
	32mm flange	S7390	10	2733
	38mm flange	S7391	10	2733
	45mm flange	S7392	10	2733
	57mm flange	S7393	10	2733
	Urostomy Pouch with Standard Tap			
	Standard Size - Clear for:-			
	32mm flange	S7350	10	2668
	38mm flange	S7351	10	2668
	45mm flange	S7352	10	2668
	57mm flange	S7353	10	2668
	70mm flange	S7354	10	2889
	100mm flange	S7355	10	4011
	Small Size - Clear for:-			
	32mm flange	S7360	10	2668
	38mm flange	S7361	10	2668
	45mm flange	S7362	10	2668
	57mm flange	S7363	10	2668
	Combihesive Natura Drainable Pouches with InvisiClose Outlet, Integral Filter and 2-sided Flocking			
	Standard - Opaque			
	pre-cut			
	32mm	S7431F	30	4384
	38mm	S7432F	30	4384
	45mm	S7433F	30	4384
	57mm	S7434F	30	4384
	70mm	S7435F	30	4384
	Small - Opaque			
	pre-cut			
	32mm	S7436F	30	4384
	38mm	S7437F	30	4384
	45mm	S7438F	30	4384
	57mm	S7439F	30	4384
	70mm	S7440F	30	4384

IXC

STOMA APPLIANCES

TWO PIECE OSTOMY SYSTEMS

Manufacturer	Appliance	Order No.	Quantity	List Price p
ConvaTec Ltd	**Combihesive Natura** Drainable Pouches with InvisiClose Outlet, Integral Filter and 1-sided Flocking			
	Standard - Opaque pre-cut			
	32mm	S7447F	30	4384
	38mm	S7448F	30	4384
	45mm	S7449F	30	4384
	57mm	S7450F	30	4384
	70mm	S7451F	30	4384
	Combihesive Natura Drainable Pouches with InvisiClose Outlet, 1-sided Flocking			
	Standard - Clear pre-cut			
	32mm	S7441N	30	4384
	38mm	S7442N	30	4384
	45mm	S7443N	30	4384
	57mm	S7444N	30	4384
	70mm	S7445N	30	4384
	Combihesive Natura Little Ones			
	Stomahesive Wafer with Flexible Collar			
	32mm (75mm x 75mm)	S7811	5	1559
	45mm (100mm x 100mm)	S7812	5	1559
	Closed Pouch			
	32mm	S7891	20	2091
	45mm	S7892	20	2091
	Drainable Pouch			
	32mm	S7880	10	1225
	45mm	S7881	10	1225
	Urostomy Pouch			
	32mm	S7850	10	2670
	Combihesive Natura High Output			
	Drainable Pouch with Filter Opaque for:-			
	45mm	S7467	5	1998
	57mm	S7468	5	1998
	70mm	S7469	5	1998
	Consecura Low Profile			
	Locking flange with Micropore surround			
	35mm	S601LP	5	1446
	45mm	S602LP	5	1446
	57mm	S603LP	5	1446
	70mm	S604LP	5	1446
	Stomahesive Locking Flange			
	35mm	S590LP	5	1446
	45mm	S591LP	5	1446
	57mm	S592LP	5	1446
	70mm	S593LP	5	1446
	100mm	S594LP	5	3195
	Closed Pouch with Filter Standard Size			
	Opaque for:			
	35mm flange	S616LP	30	3635
	45mm flange	S617LP	30	3635
	57mm flange	S618LP	30	3635
	70mm flange	S619LP	30	3635
	Clear for:-			
	35mm flange	S630LP	30	3635
	45mm flange	S631LP	30	3635
	57mm flange	S632LP	30	3635
	70mm flange	S633LP	30	3635

STOMA APPLIANCES

TWO PIECE OSTOMY SYSTEMS

Manufacturer	Appliance	Order No.	Quantity	List Price p
ConvaTec Ltd	Drainable Pouch Standard Size			
	Opaque for:-			
	35mm flange	S606LP	10	1204
	45mm flange	S607LP	10	1204
	57mm flange	S608LP	10	1204
	70mm flange	S609LP	10	1204
	Clear for:-			
	35mm flange	S611LP	10	1204
	45mm flange	S612LP	10	1204
	57mm flange	S613LP	10	1204
	70mm flange	S614LP	10	1204
	100mm flange	S615LP	10	2063
	Urostomy Pouch with Accuseal Tap Standard Size -			
	Clear for:-			
	35mm flange	S640LP	10	2625
	45mm flange	S641LP	10	2625
	57mm flange	S642LP	10	2625
	Opaque for:-			
	35mm flange	S655LP	10	2625
	45mm flange	S656LP	10	2625
	57mm flange	S657LP	10	2625
	70mm flange	S658LP	10	2625
	Urostomy Pouch with Fold-up Tap Standard Size -			
	Clear for:-			
	35mm flange	S635LP	10	2625
	45mm flange	S636LP	10	2625
	57mm flange	S637LP	10	2625
	Esteem Synergy			
	Durahesive Convex Skin Barrier with Flexible Collar Mouldable			
	13-22mm (for 13-35mm pouches)	S1180	10	3762
	22-33mm (for 13-48mm pouches)	S1181	10	3762
	33-45mm (for 13-61mm pouches)	S1182	10	3762
	Stomahesive Skin Barrier			
	cut-to-fit			
	13-35mm	S1130	10	3220
	13-48mm	S1131	10	3220
	13-61mm	S1132	10	3220
	13-89mm	S1133	10	3220
	Paediatric - Extra Small			
	0-23mm	S1171	5	1745
	Paediatric			
	4.8-31mm	S1172	5	1745
	Stomahesive Skin Barrier with Flexible Collar			
	cut-to-fit			
	13-35mm	S1100	10	3489
	13-48mm	S1101	10	3489
	13-61mm	S1102	10	3489
	pre-cut			
	19mm	S1142	10	3486
	25mm	S1144	10	3486
	32mm	S1146	10	3486
	35mm	S1147	10	3486
	38mm	S1148	10	3486
	45mm	S1150	10	3486
	Stomahesive Skin Barrier with Flexible Hydrocolloid Collar			
	cut-to-fit			
	13-35mm	S1190	10	3762
	13-48mm	S1191	10	3762
	13-61mm	S1192	10	3762
	Paediatric			
	4.8-31mm	S1173	5	1855

IXC

STOMA APPLIANCES

TWO PIECE OSTOMY SYSTEMS

Manufacturer	Appliance	Order No.	Quantity	List Price p
ConvaTec Ltd	Closed Pouch with Filter (2-sided Comfort Backing)			
	Opaque - Standard (22.8cm) for:-			
	13-35mm barrier	S1062F	30	4472
	13-48mm barrier	S1063F	30	4472
	13-61mm barrier	S1064F	30	4472
	Opaque - Small (19.8cm) for:-			
	13-35mm barrier	S1053F	30	4192
	13-48mm barrier	S1054F	30	4192
	13-61mm barrier	S1055F	30	4192
	Closed Pouch with Filter (1-sided Comfort Backing)			
	Transparent - Standard (22.8cm) for:-			
	13-35mm barrier	S1050F	30	4472
	13-48mm barrier	S1051F	30	4472
	13-61mm barrier	S1052F	30	4472
	Transparent - Small (19.8cm) for:-			
	13-35mm barrier	S1056F	30	4192
	13-48mm barrier	S1057F	30	4192
	13-61mm barrier	S1058F	30	4192
	Closed Pouch with Filter			
	Transparent - Paediatric for:-			
	4.8-31mm barriers	S1272F	10	1660
	Opaque - Paediatric for:-			
	4.8-31mm barriers	S1274F	10	1660
	Closed Pouch without Filter (2-sided Comfort Backing)			
	Opaque - Standard (22.8cm) for:-			
	13-35mm barrier	S1058N	30	4192
	13-48mm barrier	S1056N	30	4192
	13-61mm barrier	S1057N	30	4192
	Opaque - Small (19.8cm) for:-			
	13-35mm barrier	S1053N	30	3627
	13-48mm barrier	S1054N	30	3627
	13-61mm barrier	S1055N	30	3627
	Closed Pouch without Filter (1-sided Comfort Backing)			
	Opaque - Mini (16.3cm) for:-			
	13-35mm barrier	S1060N	20	2422
	13-48mm barrier	S1061N	20	2422
	Drainable Pouch with InvisiClose outlet and Filter (2-sided Comfort Backing)			
	Opaque - Standard - Right (30.8cm) for:-			
	13-35mm barrier	S1210F	30	5010
	13-48mm barrier	S1211F	30	5010
	13-61mm barrier	S1212F	30	5010
	Opaque - Small - Right (27.6cm) for:-			
	13-35mm barrier	S1230F	30	5010
	13-48mm barrier	S1231F	30	5010
	Drainable Pouch with Filter (2-sided Comfort Backing)			
	Opaque - Standard - Right (30.4cm) for:-			
	13-35mm barrier	S1020F	10	1493
	13-48mm barrier	S1021F	10	1493
	13-61mm barrier	S1022F	10	1493
	Opaque - Small - Right (26.5cm) for:-			
	13-35mm barrier	S1040F	10	1493
	13-48mm barrier	S1041F	10	1493
	Drainable Pouch with InvisiClose outlet and Filter (1-sided Comfort Backing)			
	Transparent - Standard - Right (30.8cm) for:-			
	13-35mm barrier	S1220F	30	5010
	13-48mm barrier	S1221F	30	5010
	13-61mm barrier	S1222F	30	5010
	Opaque - Standard - Left (30.8cm) for:-			
	13-35mm barrier	S1215F	30	5010
	13-48mm barrier	S1216F	30	5010
	13-61mm barrier	S1217F	30	5010

STOMA APPLIANCES

TWO PIECE OSTOMY SYSTEMS

Manufacturer	Appliance	Order No.	Quantity	List Price p
ConvaTec Ltd	Drainable Pouch with Filter (1-sided Comfort Backing)			
	Transparent - Standard - Right (30.4cm) for:-			
	13-35mm barrier	S1005F	10	1493
	13-48mm barrier	S1006F	10	1493
	13-61mm barrier	S1007F	10	1493
	Transparent - Standard - Left (30.4cm) for:-			
	13-35mm barrier	S1001F	10	1493
	13-48mm barrier	S1002F	10	1493
	13-61mm barrier	S1003F	10	1493
	Drainable Pouch with InvisiClose outlet and filter			
	Opaque - Paediatric for:-			
	4.8-31mm barriers	S1273F	10	1670
	Transparent - Paediatric for:-			
	4.8-31mm barriers	S1275F	10	1670
	Drainable Pouch with InvisiClose outlet and no Filter (2-sided Comfort Backing)			
	Opaque - Small - Right (27.6cm) for:-			
	13-35mm barrier	S1235N	10	1616
	13-48mm barrier	S1236N	10	1616
	Drainable Pouch with InvisiClose outlet and no filter			
	Transparent - Paediatric Extra Small for:-			
	0-23mm barrier	S1271	10	1650
	Drainable Pouch no Filter (2-sided Comfort Backing)			
	Opaque - Standard - Right (30.4cm) for:-			
	13-35mm barrier	S1020N	10	1444
	13-48mm barrier	S1021N	10	1444
	13-61mm barrier	S1022N	10	1444
	Opaque - Small - Right (26.5cm) for:-			
	13-35mm barrier	S1040N	10	1444
	13-48mm barrier	S1041N	10	1444
	Opaque - Standard - Left (30.4cm) for:-			
	13-35mm barrier	S1025N	10	1444
	13-48mm barrier	S1026N	10	1444
	13-61mm barrier	S1027N	10	1444
	Opaque - Small - Left (26.5cm) for:-			
	13-35mm barrier	S1045N	10	1444
	13-48mm barrier	S1046N	10	1444
	Drainable Pouch no Filter (1-sided Comfort Backing)			
	Transparent - Extra Large - Straight (35.2cm) for:-			
	13-89mm barrier	S1009N	10	2985
	Urostomy pouch with Accuseal Tap (includes 2 drain tube adapters per pack) and 1-sided comfort backing (For use with Esteem Synergy Durahesive Convex skin barrier)			
	Standard - Opaque for:-			
	13-35mm barrier	S1080	10	3568
	13-48mm barrier	S1081	10	3568
	13-61mm barrier	S1082	10	3568
	Small - Opaque for:-			
	13-35mm barrier	S1090	10	3568
	13-48mm barrier	S1091	10	3568
	Standard - Transparent for:-			
	13-35mm barrier	S1085	10	3568
	13-48mm barrier	S1086	10	3568
	13-61mm barrier	S1087	10	3568
	Small - Transparent for:-			
	13-35mm barrier	S1075	10	3568
	13-48mm barrier	S1076	10	3568

IXC

STOMA APPLIANCES

TWO PIECE OSTOMY SYSTEMS

Manufacturer	Appliance	Order No.	Quantity	List Price p
Dansac Ltd	**Dansac Nova 2 High Output** Drainable pouch with twin filter and soft covers, plus a tap closure system			
	Opaque			
	55mm flange	1207-55	10	2650
	70mm flange	1207-70	10	2650
	Clear			
	55mm flange	1208-55	10	2650
	70mm flange	1208-70	10	2650
	Dansac Nova 2 Mini Closed pouch			
	Opaque			
	36mm Flange	1203-36	30	3273
	43mm Flange	1203-43	30	3273
	55mm Flange	1203-55	30	3273
	Dansac Nova 2 Mini EasiFold Drainable pouch			
	Opaque			
	36mm Flange	1219-36	10	1448
	43mm Flange	1219-43	10	1448
	55mm Flange	1219-55	10	1448
	Clear			
	36mm Flange	1220-36	10	1448
	43mm Flange	1220-43	10	1448
	55mm Flange	1220-55	10	1448
	Dansac Nova 2 Easifold Large Two-piece large drainable pouch with filter and EasiFold closure			
	Opaque			
	55mm flange	1221-55	10	1420
	70mm flange	1221-70	10	1420
	Clear			
	55mm flange	1222-55	10	1420
	70mm flange	1222-70	10	1420
	Nova 2 Convex Flange			
	Important: this product with deep convexity should only be used after prior assessment of suitability by an appropriate medical professional.			
	36mm Flange			
	cut-to-fit 15-23mm	1536-15	5	1526
	pre-cut 20mm	1536-20	5	1526
	pre-cut 23mm	1536-23	5	1526
	43mm Flange			
	cut-to-fit 15-30mm	1543-15	5	1526
	pre-cut 25mm	1543-25	5	1526
	pre-cut 30mm	1543-30	5	1526
	55mm Flange			
	cut-to-fit 15-42mm	1555-15	5	1526
	pre-cut 35mm	1555-35	5	1526
	pre-cut 40mm	1555-40	5	1526
	Nova 2 Easifold Drainable Pouches			
	Opaque Symmetrical			
	36mm Flange	1215-36	10	1420
	43mm Flange	1215-43	10	1420
	55mm Flange	1215-55	10	1420
	70mm Flange	1215-70	10	1420
	Clear Symmetrical			
	36mm Flange	1216-36	10	1420
	43mm Flange	1216-43	10	1420
	55mm Flange	1216-55	10	1420
	70mm Flange	1216-70	10	1420
	Nova 2 X3			
	43mm Flange (3mm depth)			
	cut-to-fit (15-30mm)	1343-15	5	1526
	pre-cut 25mm	1343-25	5	1526

STOMA APPLIANCES

TWO PIECE OSTOMY SYSTEMS

Manufacturer	Appliance	Order No.	Quantity	List Price p
Dansac Ltd	**55mm Flange** (3mm depth)			
	cut-to-fit (15-42mm)	1355-15	5	1526
	pre-cut 32mm	1355-32	5	1526
	pre-cut 35mm	1355-35	5	1526
	Nova 2 Soft Convex Flange			
	43mm Flange (5mm depth)			
	pre-cut 18mm	1443-18	5	1526
	pre-cut 21mm	1443-21	5	1526
	pre-cut 25mm	1443-25	5	1526
	pre-cut 28mm	1443-28	5	1526
	55mm Flange (5mm depth)			
	pre-cut 32mm	1455-32	5	1526
	pre-cut 35mm	1455-35	5	1526
	pre-cut 38mm	1455-38	5	1526
	Nova 2 Flange			
	36mm Flange			
	starter hole 12-28mm	1136-12	5	1470
	starter hole 15-28mm	1136-15	5	1497
	pre-cut 20mm	1136-20	5	1497
	pre-cut 25mm	1136-25	5	1497
	43mm Flange			
	starter hole 15-35mm	1143-15	5	1497
	pre-cut 25mm	1143-25	5	1497
	pre-cut 30mm	1143-30	5	1497
	55mm Flange			
	starter hole 15-47mm	1155-15	5	1497
	pre-cut 35mm	1155-35	5	1497
	pre-cut 40mm	1155-40	5	1497
	70mm Flange			
	starter hole 15-60mm	1170-15	5	1497
	pre-cut 45mm	1170-45	5	1497
	pre-cut 50mm	1170-50	5	1497
	Nova 2 Closed Pouches including water repellent soft fabric cover and twin filter technology			
	Opaque			
	36mm Flange	1201-36	30	3778
	43mm Flange	1201-43	30	3778
	55mm Flange	1201-55	30	3778
	70mm Flange	1201-70	30	3778
	Clear			
	36mm Flange	1202-36	30	3778
	43mm Flange	1202-43	30	3778
	55mm Flange	1202-55	30	3778
	70mm Flange	1202-70	30	3778
	Nova 2 Drainable Pouches including filtration system and water repellent soft fabric covers			
	Opaque			
	43mm Flange	1213-43	10	1256
	55mm Flange	1213-55	10	1256
	Nova 2 Sym Drainable Pouches including filtration system and water repellent soft fabric covers			
	Opaque			
	43mm Flange	1211-43	10	1256
	55mm Flange	1211-55	10	1256
	Clear			
	36mm Flange	1212-36	10	1256
	43mm Flange	1212-43	10	1256
	55mm Flange	1212-55	10	1256
	70mm Flange	1212-70	10	1256

IXC

STOMA APPLIANCES

TWO PIECE OSTOMY SYSTEMS

Manufacturer	Appliance	Order No.	Quantity	List Price p
Dansac Ltd	**Nova 2 Urostomy pouch**			
	Opaque			
	36mm Flange	1217-36	10	2683
	43mm Flange	1217-43	10	2683
	55mm Flange	1217-55	10	2683
	Clear			
	36mm Flange	1218-36	10	2683
	43mm Flange	1218-43	10	2683
	55mm Flange	1218-55	10	2683
	Unique 2 Flexi Flange			
	36mm Flange (100mm x 100mm)			
	starter hole (15-28mm)	536-15	5	1541
	pre-cut 25mm	536-25	5	1541
	43mm Flange (100mm x 100mm)			
	starter hole (15-35mm)	543-15	5	1541
	pre-cut 30mm	543-30	5	1541
	55mm Flange (100mm x 100mm)			
	starter hole (15-47mm)	555-15	5	1541
	pre-cut 35mm	555-35	5	1541
	pre-cut 40mm	555-40	5	1541
	80mm Flange (125mm x 125mm)			
	starter hole (15-70mm)	580-15	5	1572
	Unique 2 S Flange			
	36mm Flange (100mm x 100mm)			
	starter hole (15-28mm)	436-15	5	1487
	pre-cut 20mm	436-20	5	1487
	pre-cut 25mm	436-25	5	1487
	43mm Flange (100mm x 100mm)			
	starter hole (15-35mm)	443-15	5	1487
	pre-cut 30mm	443-30	5	1487
	55mm Flange (100mm x 100mm)			
	starter hole (15-47mm)	455-15	5	1487
	pre-cut 35mm	455-35	5	1487
	80mm Flange (125mm x 125mm)			
	starter hole (15-70mm)	480-15	5	1489
	Unique 2 Convex Flange			
	Important: This product with deep convexity should only be used after prior assessment of suitability by an appropriate medical professional.			
	36mm Flange (100mm x 100mm)			
	starter hole (15-25mm)	736-15	5	1544
	pre-cut 20mm	736-20	5	1544
	pre-cut 25mm	736-25	5	1544
	43mm Flange (100mm x 100mm)			
	starter hole (15-32mm)	743-15	5	1544
	pre-cut 25mm	743-25	5	1544
	pre-cut 30mm	743-30	5	1544
	55mm Flange (115mm x 115mm)			
	starter hole (15-44mm)	755-15	5	1544
	pre-cut 35mm	755-35	5	1544
	Urostomy Drainable Pouch			
	(includes 1 Dansac Drain Tube Adaptor and 3 caps)			
	Opaque with spunlace backing for:			
	36mm Flange	401-36	10	2674
	43mm Flange	401-43	10	2674
	55mm Flange	401-55	10	2674
	Clear with spunlace backing for:			
	36mm Flange	402-36	10	2674
	43mm Flange	402-43	10	2674
	55mm Flange	402-55	10	2674

STOMA APPLIANCES

TWO PIECE OSTOMY SYSTEMS

Manufacturer	Appliance	Order No.	Quantity	List Price p
Dansac Ltd	**Unique 2 Closed Pouch**			
	Opaque with spunlace cover next to skin for:			
	36mm Flange	501-36	30	3766
	43mm Flange	501-43	30	3766
	55mm Flange	501-55	30	3766
	80mm Flange	501-80	30	3766
	Clear with spunlace cover next to skin for:			
	36mm Flange	502-36	30	3766
	43mm Flange	502-43	30	3766
	55mm Flange	502-55	30	3766
	80mm flange	502-80	30	3766
	Unique 2 Plus Closed Pouch			
	Opaque with spunlace cover front and back for:			
	36mm Flange	505-36	30	3757
	43mm Flange	505-43	30	3757
	55mm Flange	505-55	30	3757
	80mm Flange	505-80	30	3757
	Unique 2 Mini Closed Pouch			
	Opaque with spunlace cover front and back for:			
	36mm Flange	503-36	30	3190
	43mm Flange	503-43	30	3190
	55mm Flange	503-55	30	3190
	Unique 2 MiniCap			
	Opaque for:			
	43mm Flange	507-43	30	3347
	55mm Flange	507-55	30	3347
	Unique 2 Drainable Regular			
	Opaque with spunlace cover next to skin for:			
	36mm Flange	511-36	10	1245
	43mm Flange	511-43	10	1245
	55mm Flange	511-55	10	1245
	80mm Flange	511-80	10	1245
	Clear with spunlace cover next to skin for:			
	55mm Flange	512-55	10	1245
	80mm Flange	512-80	10	1245
	Unique 2 Drainable Large			
	Opaque with spunlace cover next to skin for:			
	36mm Flange	521-36	10	1245
	43mm Flange	521-43	10	1245
	55mm Flange	521-55	10	1245
	80mm Flange	521-80	10	1245
	Clear with spunlace cover next to skin for:			
	36mm Flange	522-36	10	1245
	43mm Flange	522-43	10	1245
	55mm Flange	522-55	10	1245
	80mm Flange	522-80	10	1245
	InVent 2 - Drainable with filter, soft spunlace backing on both sides, anatomically shaped			
	Opaque			
	36mm Flange	513-36	10	1224
	43mm Flange	513-43	10	1224
	55mm Flange	513-55	10	1224
	InVent 2 Mini Drainable with filter, soft spun lace material on both sides, anatomically shaped			
	Opaque			
	36mm Flange	519-36	10	1227
	43mm Flange	519-43	10	1227

IXC

STOMA APPLIANCES

TWO PIECE OSTOMY SYSTEMS

Manufacturer	Appliance	Order No.	Quantity	List Price p
Dansac Ltd	**InVent 2 Sym - Drainable Symmetrical pouch with filter,** soft spunlace backing, symmetrically shaped			
	Opaque			
	36mm Flange	515-36	10	1245
	43mm Flange	515-43	10	1245
	55mm Flange	515-55	10	1245
	Clear			
	55mm Flange	516-55	10	1245
	80mm Flange	518-80	10	1245
Hollister Ltd	**Conform 2**			
	Fixed Flange			
	35mm flange 13-30mm stoma	23100	5	1472
	35mm flange 20mm stoma	23120	5	1472
	35mm flange 25mm stoma	23125	5	1472
	35mm flange 30mm stoma	23130	5	1472
	45mm flange 30mm stoma	24130	5	1472
	45mm flange 13-40mm stoma	24100	5	1472
	55mm flange 13-50mm stoma	25100	5	1472
	55mm flange 45mm stoma	25145	5	1472
	70mm flange 13-65mm stoma	27100	5	1472
	Flex Wear Flange			
	35mm fixed flange 20mm	33120	5	1447
	35mm fixed flange 25mm	33125	5	1447
	35mm fixed flange 30mm	33130	5	1447
	45mm fixed flange 13-40mm	34100	5	1447
	45mm fixed flange 35mm	34135	5	1447
	45mm fixed flange 40mm	34140	5	1447
	55mm fixed flange 13-40mm	35200	5	1447
	Floating Flange			
	45mm flange 13-30mm stoma	24200	5	1472
	55mm flange 13-40mm stoma	25200	5	1472
	70mm flange 13-55mm stoma	27200	5	1472
	Flex Wear Floating Flange - Adhesive Border			
	Flat Barrier			
	cut-to-fit			
	45mm flange, 13-30mm	34500	5	1550
	55mm flange, 13-40mm	35500	5	1550
	70mm flange, 13-55mm	37500	5	1550
	pre-cut			
	45mm flange, 20mm	34520	5	1550
	45mm flange, 25mm	34525	5	1550
	45mm flange, 30mm	34530	5	1550
	55mm flange, 35mm	35535	5	1550
	55mm flange, 40mm	35540	5	1550
	Convex Barrier			
	cut-to-fit			
	45mm flange, 13-25mm	34600	5	1630
	55mm flange, 13-38mm	35600	5	1630
	70mm flange, 13-51mm	37600	5	1630
	pre-cut			
	45mm flange, 22mm	34622	5	1630
	45mm flange, 25mm	34625	5	1630
	55mm flange, 29mm	35629	5	1630
	55mm flange, 32mm	35632	5	1630
	Convex-Floating Flange			
	45mm flange 13-25mm stoma	24300	5	1580
	45mm flange 22mm stoma	24322	5	1580
	45mm flange 25mm stoma	24325	5	1580
	55mm flange 13-38mm stoma	25300	5	1580
	55mm flange 29mm stoma	25329	5	1580
	55mm flange 32mm stoma	25332	5	1580
	70mm flange 15-51mm stoma	27300	5	1580

STOMA APPLIANCES

TWO PIECE OSTOMY SYSTEMS

Manufacturer	Appliance	Order No.	Quantity	List Price p
Hollister Ltd	Closed Pouch			
	With beige comfort backing			
	45mm	24400	30	3568
	55mm	25400	30	3568
	70mm	27400	30	3568
	transparent front, beige comfort backing on body worn side			
	45mm	24500	30	3568
	55mm	25500	30	3568
	70mm	27500	30	3568
	Conform 2			
	Drainable Pouch			
	Transparent			
	45mm	24600	10	1201
	55mm	25600	10	1201
	70mm	27600	10	1201
	Drainable Pouch with Filter - anatomical shape			
	Beige			
	35mm	23720	30	3740
	45mm	24720	30	3740
	55mm	25720	30	3740
	Transparent			
	35mm	23820	30	3740
	45mm	24820	30	3740
	55mm	25820	30	3740
	Beige with comfort backing on both sides			
	45mm	24420	30	4046
	55mm	25420	30	4046
	70mm	27420	30	4046
	Mini Drainable Pouch with Filter, Beige			
	35mm	23710	30	3740
	45mm	24710	30	3740
	55mm	25710	30	3740
	Urostomy Pouches			
	Beige			
	35mm	23730	10	2648
	45mm	24730	10	2648
	55mm	25730	10	2648
	Transparent			
	35mm	23830	10	2648
	45mm	24830	10	2648
	55mm	25830	10	2648
	Conform 2 with Lock'n'Roll Closure			
	Drainable Pouch, anatomical shape with integral filter and Lock and Roll closure system			
	Midi - Beige with comfort backing on both sides			
	35mm	23750	30	4305
	45mm	24750	30	4305
	55mm	25750	30	4305
	Midi - Transparent with comfort backing on body side only			
	35mm	23850	30	4305
	45mm	24850	30	4305
	55mm	25850	30	4305
	Drainable Pouch, symmetrical shape with integral filter and Lock and Roll closure system			
	Mini - Beige with comfort backing on both sides			
	35mm	23743	30	3750
	45mm	24743	30	3750
	55mm	25743	30	3750
	Maxi - Beige with comfort backing on both sides			
	35mm	23760	30	4384
	45mm	24760	30	4384
	55mm	25760	30	4384
	70mm	27760	30	4384

IXC

STOMA APPLIANCES

TWO PIECE OSTOMY SYSTEMS

Manufacturer	Appliance	Order No.	Quantity	List Price p
Hollister Ltd	Maxi - Transparent with comfort backing on body side only			
	35mm	23860	30	4384
	45mm	24860	30	4384
	55mm	25860	30	4384
	70mm	27860	30	4384
	Tandem Range			
	Floating Flange - Barrier and adhesive			
	cut-to-fit			
	25mm	3727	5	1475
	32mm	3722	5	1475
	44mm	3723	5	1475
	57mm	3724	5	1475
	89mm	3726	5	1530
	pre-cut			
	19mm	3747	5	1475
	25mm	3742	5	1475
	32mm	3748	5	1475
	38mm	3743	5	1475
	44mm	3749	5	1475
	Floating Flange - Barrier only			
	cut-to-fit			
	25mm	3767	5	1475
	32mm	3762	5	1475
	44mm	3763	5	1475
	57mm	3764	5	1475
	89mm	3766	5	1530
	Tandem Range - Impression CPL			
	Convex Flange			
	Convex Flange			
	pre-cut			
	13mm	3730	5	1579
	16mm	3731	5	1579
	19mm	3732	5	1579
	22mm	3733	5	1579
	25mm	3734	5	1579
	29mm	3735	5	1579
	32mm	3736	5	1579
	35mm	3737	5	1579
	38mm	3738	5	1579
	41mm	3739	5	1579
	44mm	37310	5	1579
	51mm	37311	5	1579
	Convex Flange - Barrier only			
	pre-cut			
	13mm	3780	5	1579
	16mm	3781	5	1579
	19mm	3782	5	1579
	22mm	3783	5	1579
	25mm	3784	5	1579
	29mm	3785	5	1579
	32mm	3786	5	1579
	35mm	3787	5	1579
	38mm	3788	5	1579

STOMA APPLIANCES

TWO PIECE OSTOMY SYSTEMS

Manufacturer	Appliance	Order No.	Quantity	List Price p
Hollister Ltd	**Tandem Range - Impression CPL Pouches**			
	cut-to-fit			
	Up to 25mm	3794	5	1579
	Up to 38mm	3798	5	1579
	Up to 51mm	37911	5	1579
	Closed Pouch			
	Beige - with filter and comfort backing on both sides			
	44mm	3342	30	3636
	57mm	3343	30	3636
	70mm	3344	30	3636
	Drainable Pouch			
	Transparent - with comfort backing on body-worn side only			
	38mm	3807	10	1224
	44mm	3802	10	1224
	57mm	3803	10	1224
	70mm	3804	10	1224
	102mm	3806	10	2353
	Beige - with comfort backing on both sides			
	38mm	3817	10	1224
	44mm	3812	10	1224
	57mm	3813	10	1224
	70mm	3814	10	1224
	Urostomy Pouch			
	Transparent - with comfort backing on the body-worn side			
	38mm	3907	10	2695
	44mm	3902	10	2695
	57mm	3903	10	2695
	70mm	3904	10	2695
Mentor Medical Ltd	Beta 2 Piece kit	32-294-08	1	6018
	Beta 2 Piece spare bags	32-294-16	90	16570
Oakmed Ltd	**Option Connect 2**			
	Option Connect 2 Skin Wafer			
	cut-to-fit			
	15mm-45mm	JH0015	10	3318
	pre-cut			
	20mm	JH0020	10	3318
	25mm	JH0025	10	3318
	30mm	JH0030	10	3318
	35mm	JH0035	10	3318
	40mm	JH0040	10	3318
	45mm	JH0045	10	3318
	Colostomy with Filter and Soft Covering to both sides			
	To fit up to 45mm Stoma	JH600	30	4139
	Colostomy with Filter and Soft Covering to both sides includes a window			
	To fit up to 45mm Stoma	JH610	30	4139
	Colostomy with Filter and Soft Covering to one side Clear			
	To fit up to 45mm Stoma	JH620	30	4139

IXC

STOMA APPLIANCES

TWO PIECE OSTOMY SYSTEMS

Manufacturer	Appliance	Order No.	Quantity	List Price p
Oakmed Ltd	Colostomy Mini with Filter and Soft Covering to both sides			
	To fit up to 45mm Stoma	JH500	30	4016
	Colostomy Mini with Filter and Soft Covering to both sides includes a window			
	To fit up to 45mm Stoma	JH510	30	4016
	Colostomy Mini with Filter and Soft Covering to one side Clear			
	To fit up to 45mm Stoma	JH520	30	4016
	Colostomy Plus with Filter and Soft Covering to both sides			
	To fit up to 45mm Stoma	JH700	30	4275
	Colostomy Plus with Filter and Soft Covering to both sides includes a window			
	To fit up to 45mm Stoma	JH710	30	4275
	Colostomy Plus with Filter and Soft Covering to one side			
	Clear To fit up to 45mm Stoma	JH720	30	4275
	Ileostomy with Filter and Soft Covering to both sides			
	To fit up to 45mm Stoma	JH300	30	4597
	Ileostomy with Filter and Soft Covering to both sides includes a window			
	To fit up to 45mm Stoma	JH310	30	4597
	Ileostomy with Filter and Soft Covering to one side			
	Clear To fit up to 45mm Stoma	JH320	30	4597
	Ileostomy Midi with Filter and Soft Covering to both sides			
	To fit up to 45mm Stoma	JH200	30	4564
	Ileostomy Midi with Filter and Soft Covering to both sides includes a window			
	To fit up to 45mm Stoma	JH210	30	4564
	Ileostomy Midi with Filter and Soft Covering to one side Clear			
	To fit up to 45mm Stoma	JH220	30	4564
	Ileostomy Mini with Filter and Soft Covering to both sides			
	To fit up to 45mm Stoma	JH100	30	4285
	Ileostomy Mini with Filter and Soft Covering to both sides includes a window			
	To fit up to 45mm Stoma	JH110	30	4285
	Ileostomy Mini with Filter and Soft Covering to one side Clear			
	To fit up to 45mm Stoma	JH120	30	4285
	Stoma Cap Soft Cover with Filter	JH900	30	4139
	Option Connect 2 Skin Wafer	JH0090 Oval	10	9313
	cut-to-fit 20mm-90mm			

Option Connect 2 PL
Ileostomy

Opaque 20mm-90mm	JHPL90	20	10062

Option Connect 2 Alginate Skin Wafer
cut-to-fit

	Order No.	Quantity	List Price p
15mm - 45mm	AJH0015	10	3690
pre-cut			
20mm	AJH0020	10	3690
25mm	AJH0025	10	3690
30mm	AJH0030	10	3690
35mm	AJH0035	10	3690
40mm	AJH0040	10	3690
45mm	AJH0045	10	3690

STOMA APPLIANCES

TWO PIECE OSTOMY SYSTEMS

Manufacturer	Appliance	Order No.	Quantity	List Price p
Oakmed Ltd	**Option Connect 2 Microskin Skin Wafer**			
	cut-to-fit			
	15mm - 45mm	MJH0015	10	3690
	pre-cut			
	20mm	MJH0020	10	3690
	25mm	MJH0025	10	3690
	30mm	MJH0030	10	3690
	35mm	MJH0035	10	3690
	40mm	MJH0040	10	3690
	45mm	MJH0045	10	3690
	Option Connect 2 Ileo with Velcro Fastening			
	To fit upto 45mm stoma	VJH310	30	4828
	Option Range			
	Option Flange			
	50mm	F500K	5	1409
	70mm	F700K	5	1409
	Colostomy with Filter and Soft Covering to both sides Opaque for:-			
	50mm flange	CA50K	30	3543
	Colostomy Plus with Filter and Soft Covering to one side Clear for:-			
	70mm flange	CD70K	30	3558
	Colostomy Plus with Filter and Soft Covering to both sides Opaque for:-			
	70mm flange	CC70K	30	3600
	Colostomy Plus with Soft Covering to both sides Opaque for:-			
	50mm flange	CH50K	30	3538
	Ileostomy Midi with Filter and Soft Covering to one side Clear for:-			
	50mm flange	IG50K	30	3558
	70mm flange	IG70K	30	3558
	Ileostomy with filter and Soft Covering to one side Clear for:-			
	50mm flange	IB50K	30	3558
	70mm flange	IB70K	30	3558
	Ileostomy Midi with Filter and Soft Covering to both sides Opaque for:-			
	50mm flange	ID50K	30	3579
	70mm flange	ID70K	30	3579
	Ileostomy with Filter and Soft Covering to both sides Opaque for:-			
	50mm flange	IA50K	30	3579
	70mm flange	IA70K	30	3579
Peak Medical	**Combimate** 2-piece Standard Flange			
	38mm flange			
	starter hole 13mm	FH3813	5	1495
	pre-cut 22mm	FH3822	5	1495
	pre-cut 25mm	FH3825	5	1495
	pre-cut 28mm	FH3828	5	1495
	45mm flange			
	starter hole 13mm	FH4513	5	1495
	pre-cut 22mm	FH4522	5	1495
	pre-cut 25mm	FH4525	5	1495
	pre-cut 28mm	FH4528	5	1495
	pre-cut 32mm	FH4532	5	1495
	pre-cut 35mm	FH4535	5	1495
	57mm flange			
	starter hole 13mm	FH5713	5	1495
	pre-cut 32mm	FH5732	5	1495
	pre-cut 35mm	FH5735	5	1495
	pre-cut 38mm	FH5738	5	1495
	70mm flange			
	starter hole 13mm	FH7013	5	1495

STOMA APPLIANCES

TWO PIECE OSTOMY SYSTEMS

Manufacturer	Appliance	Order No.	Quantity	List Price p
Peak Medical	**Combimate** Closed pouch, Beige non-woven both sides, high capacity filter			
	Small			
	38mm flange	CSB238	30	4000
	45mm flange	CSB245	30	4000
	Medium			
	38mm flange	CMB238	30	4000
	45mm flange	CMB245	30	4000
	57mm flange	CMB257	30	4000
	Large			
	38mm flange	CLB238	30	4000
	45mm flange	CLB245	30	4000
	57mm flange	CLB257	30	4000
	70mm flange	CLB270	30	4000
	Combimate Closed pouch, Beige non-woven backing, semi-transparent, with needle-pin overlap, high capacity filter			
	Large			
	45mm flange	CLT245	30	4000
	57mm flange	CLT257	30	4000
	70mm flange	CLT270	30	4000
	Combimate Anatomical Closed pouch, Beige non-woven both sides, high capacity filter			
	Medium/Large			
	38mm flange	CMLB238	30	4000
	45mm flange	CMLB245	30	4000
	57mm flange	CMLB257	30	4000
	70mm flange	CMLB270	30	4000
	Combimate Advance flange with non-woven layer			
	38mm flange, 13mm starter hole	FA3813	5	1800
	45mm flange, 13mm starter hole	FA4513	5	1800
	57mm flange, 13mm starter hole	FA5713	5	1800
	70mm flange, 13mm starter hole	FA7013	5	1800
	Combimate Colocap 2-piece stoma cap with high capacity filter			
	38mm flange	CCB238	30	3347
	45mm flange	CCB245	30	3347
	57mm flange	CCB257	30	3347
	Combimate Softflex 2-piece Flange			
	38mm flange			
	starter hole 13mm	FFB3813	5	1800
	pre-cut 22mm	FFB3822	5	1800
	pre-cut 25mm	FFB3825	5	1800
	pre-cut 28mm	FFB3828	5	1800
	45mm flange			
	starter hole 13mm	FFB4513	5	1800
	pre-cut 22mm	FFB4522	5	1800
	pre-cut 25mm	FFB4525	5	1800
	pre-cut 28mm	FFB4528	5	1800
	pre-cut 32mm	FFB4532	5	1800
	pre-cut 35mm	FFB4535	5	1800
	57mm flange			
	starter hole 13mm	FFB5713	5	1800
	pre-cut 32mm	FFB5732	5	1800
	pre-cut 35mm	FFB5735	5	1800
	pre-cut 38mm	FFB5738	5	1800
	70mm flange			
	starter hole 13mm	FFB7013	5	1800

STOMA APPLIANCES

TWO PIECE OSTOMY SYSTEMS

Manufacturer	Appliance	Order No.	Quantity	List Price p
Peak Medical	**Combimate Supersoft** flange			
	38mm flange			
	13mm starter hole	FSS3813	5	1800
	pre-cut 22mm	FSS3822	5	1800
	pre-cut 25mm	FSS3825	5	1800
	pre-cut 28mm	FSS3828	5	1800
	45mm flange			
	13mm starter hole	FSS4513	5	1800
	pre-cut 22mm	FSS4522	5	1800
	pre-cut 25mm	FSS4525	5	1800
	pre-cut 28mm	FSS4528	5	1800
	pre-cut 32mm	FSS4532	5	1800
	pre-cut 35mm	FSS4535	5	1800
	57mm flange			
	13mm starter hole	FSS5713	5	1800
	pre-cut 32mm	FSS5732	5	1800
	pre-cut 35mm	FSS5735	5	1800
	pre-cut 38mm	FSS5738	5	1800
	70mm flange			
	13mm starter hole	FSS7013	5	1800

Combimate Supersoft flange with shallow convexity
Important: This product with integral convexity should only be used after prior assessment of suitability by an appropriate medical professional.

		Order No.	Quantity	List Price p
	38mm flange			
	13mm starter hole	FC3813	3	1250
	pre-cut 16mm	FC3816	3	1250
	pre-cut 19mm	FC3819	3	1250
	45mm flange			
	13mm starter hole	FC4513	3	1250
	pre-cut 22mm	FC4522	3	1250
	pre-cut 25mm	FC4525	3	1250
	pre-cut 28mm	FC4528	3	1250
	57mm flange			
	13mm starter hole	FC5713	3	1250
	pre-cut 32mm	FC5732	3	1250
	pre-cut 35mm	FC5735	3	1250
	pre-cut 38mm	FC5738	3	1250
	pre-cut 41mm	FC5741	3	1250
	70mm flange			
	13mm starter hole	FC7013	3	1250

Combimate Supersoft flange with deep convexity
Important: This product with integral convexity should only be used after prior assessment of suitability by an appropriate medical professional.

		Order No.	Quantity	List Price p
	45mm flange			
	13mm starter hole	FXC4513	3	1250
	pre-cut 19mm	FXC4519	3	1250
	pre-cut 22mm	FXC4522	3	1250
	57mm flange			
	13mm starter hole	FXC5713	3	1250
	pre-cut 25mm	FXC5725	3	1250
	pre-cut 28mm	FXC5728	3	1250
	pre-cut 32mm	FXC5732	3	1250
	70 mm flange			
	13mm starter hole	FXC7013	3	1250
	pre-cut 32mm	FXC7032	3	1250
	pre-cut 35mm	FXC7035	3	1250
	pre-cut 39mm	FXC7039	3	1250
	pre-cut 44mm	FXC7044	3	1250

IXC

STOMA APPLIANCES

TWO PIECE OSTOMY SYSTEMS

Manufacturer	Appliance	Order No.	Quantity	List Price p
Salts Healthcare	**Black Rubber Bag** (for use with flange)			
	Screw outlet			
	Large	362129	1	3539
	Small	362229	1	3539
	Special	362099	1	3676
	Spout outlet			
	Large	372129	1	2472
	Small	372229	1	2472
	White Rubber Bag (for use with flange)			
	Screw outlet			
	Small	461229	1	1178
	Second Nature Wafer 110 x 100mm			
	32mm flange	2FL32	5	1299
	38mm flange	2FL38	5	1299
	45mm flange	2FL45	5	1299
	Wafer 134 x 124m			
	57mm flange	2FL57	5	1299
	Wafer 151 x 140mm			
	70mm flange	2FL70	10	2932
	Convex inserts for use with above - see "Pressure Plates"			
	Second Nature Closed Pouches			
	Opaque for:			
	32mm Flange	2C32	30	3789
	38mm Flange	2C38	30	3789
	45mm Flange	2C45	30	3789
	57mm Flange	2C57	30	3789
	Transparent/overlap film for:			
	45mm Flange	2CT45	30	3789
	57mm Flange	2CT57	30	3789
	Large 70mm Flange	2CLT70	30	3724
	Transparent/no overlap			
	Large 70mm Flange	2CLTT70	30	3724
	Second Nature Drainable Pouches			
	Opaque for:			
	32mm Flange	2D32	30	3725
	38mm Flange	2D38	30	3725
	45mm Flange	2D45	30	3725
	57mm Flange	2D57	30	3725
	Transparent/overlap film for:			
	45mm Flange	2DT45	30	3725
	57mm Flange	2DT57	30	3725
	Transparent/overlap film			
	Large 70mm Flange	2DLT70	30	3660
	Transparent/no overlap			
	Large 70mm Flange	2DLTT70	30	3660
	Second Nature Mini Closed Pouches			
	Opaque for:			
	32mm Flange	2CM32	30	3157
	38mm Flange	2CM38	30	3157
	45mm Flange	2CM45	30	3157
	57mm Flange	2CM57	30	3157
	Second Nature Mini Drainable Pouches			
	Opaque for:			
	32mm Flange	2DM32	30	3619
	38mm Flange	2DM38	30	3619
	45mm Flange	2DM45	30	3619
	57mm Flange	2DM57	30	3619

STOMA APPLIANCES

TWO PIECE OSTOMY SYSTEMS

Manufacturer	Appliance	Order No.	Quantity	List Price p
Salts Healthcare	**Second Nature** Urostomy Pouch -			
	transparent/overlap (includes 2 drain tube connectors per pack)			
	32mm Flange	2U32	10	2639
	38mm Flange	2U38	10	2639
	45mm Flange	2U45	10	2639
	57mm Flange	2U57	10	2639
	Secuplast Circular Plasters see Adhesive Discs/Rings/Pads/Plasters			
	Secu-Ring to fit:			
	32mm Flange	SR32	10	1154
	38mm Flange	SR38	10	1154
	45mm Flange	SR45	10	1154
	57mm Flange	SR57	10	1154
	70mm Flange	SR70	10	1133
Welland Medical Ltd	**FreeStyle** closed pouches with dual carb filter			
	Midi size with beige softback front			
	45mm	F2C445	30	4880
	55mm	F2C455	30	4880
	Midi size with clear front			
	45mm	F2C645	30	4880
	55mm	F2C655	30	4880
	Maxi size with beige softback front			
	45mm	F2C545	30	4880
	55mm	F2C555	30	4880
	Maxi size with clear front			
	45mm	F2C745	30	4880
	55mm	F2C755	30	4880
	FreeStyle two piece drainable pouches with integral closure and dual carb filter			
	Midi Size and beige softback front			
	45mm	F2D445	30	4810
	55mm	F2D455	30	4810
	Midi Size and clear front			
	45mm	F2D645	30	4810
	55mm	F2D655	30	4810
	Maxi Size and beige softback front			
	45mm	F2D545	30	4810
	55mm	F2D555	30	4810
	Maxi Size and clear front			
	45mm	F2D745	30	4810
	55mm	F2D755	30	4810
	FreeStyle			
	45mm flange			
	13mm starter hole	F2F413	5	1806
	pre-cut 25mm	F2F425	5	1806
	pre-cut 29mm	F2F429	5	1806
	pre-cut 32mm	F2F432	5	1806
	pre-cut 35mm	F2F435	5	1806
	pre-cut 38mm	F2F438	5	1806
	55mm flange			
	13mm starter hole	F2F513	5	1806
	pre-cut 38mm	F2F538	5	1806
	pre-cut 44mm	F2F544	5	1806

IXC

STOMA APPLIANCES

TWO PIECE OSTOMY SYSTEMS

Manufacturer	Appliance	Order No.	Quantity	List Price p
Welland Medical Ltd	**Silhouette 2** closed pouch with soft backing and filter			
	Beige			
	45mm	UNC545	30	3481
	60mm	UNC560	30	3481
	Silhouette 2 drainable pouch with soft backing and filter			
	Beige			
	45mm	UNF545	30	3535
	60mm	UNF560	30	3535
	Silhouette 2 urostomy pouch with soft backing and tap			
	Beige			
	45mm	UNU945	10	2589
	Clear			
	45mm	UNU745	10	2589
	60mm	UNU760	10	2536
	Silhouette 2 urostomy hydrocolloid flange			
	45mm Flange starter hole	UUU413	5	1292
	60mm Flange starter hole	UUU613	5	1264
	Silhouette 2 hydrocolloid flange			
	45mm Flange			
	starter hole	UNH410	5	1305
	pre-cut 25mm	UNH425	5	1305
	pre-cut 32mm	UNH432	5	1305
	pre-cut 38mm	UNH438	5	1305
	60mm Flange			
	starter hole	UNH610	5	1305
	pre-cut 32mm	UNH632	5	1305
	pre-cut 44mm	UNH644	5	1305
	pre-cut 51mm	UNH651	5	1305
	pre-cut 57mm	UNH657	5	1305
	Silhouette 2 dual adhesive flange			
	45mm Flange			
	starter hole	UNB410	5	1305
	pre-cut 25mm	UNB425	5	1305
	pre-cut 32mm	UNB432	5	1305
	pre-cut 38mm	UNB438	5	1305
	60mm Flange			
	starter hole	UNB610	5	1305
	pre-cut 32mm	UNB632	5	1305
	pre-cut 44mm	UNB644	5	1305
	pre-cut 51mm	UNB651	5	1305
	pre-cut 57mm	UNB657	5	1305

STOMA APPLIANCES

UROSTOMY BAGS

Manufacturer	Appliance	Order No.	Quantity	List Price p
B. Braun Medical	**Softima Uro Silk** 1 piece urostomy pouch			
	Beige			
	cut-to-fit 12-55mm	043914E	30	14700
	Transparent			
	cut-to-fit 12-55mm	043913E	30	14700
C S Bullen Ltd	**Lenbul**			
	Bag with tap			
	Day	U5	1	1536
	Night	U6	1	1754
	Bag with large opening			
	Day	U7	1	1594
	Night	U8	1	1821
Coloplast Ltd	**Assura** (include 4 drain tube adaptors per pack)			
	Urostomy Bag with Soft Backing			
	Midi Clear with soft backing on body-worn side			
	cut-to-fit 10-55mm	2550	30	13779
	Midi Eu with soft backing on body-worn side			
	cut-to-fit 10-55mm	2540	30	13779
	Maxi Clear with soft backing on body-worn side			
	cut-to-fit 10-55mm	2570	30	13779
	Maxi Opaque with soft backing on body-worn side			
	cut-to-fit 10-55mm	2560	30	13779
	Paediatric Clear with soft backing on body-worn side			
	cut-to-fit 10-35mm	2135	30	13779
	Paediatric Opaque with soft backing on body-worn side			
	cut-to-fit 10-35mm	2130	30	13779
	Assura Seal Integral Convexity Urostomy Bag			
	Maxi Clear			
	15mm	12991	10	4471
	18mm	12992	10	4471
	21mm	12993	10	4471
	25mm	12994	10	4471
	28mm	12995	10	4471
	31mm	12996	10	4471
	Maxi Transparent			
	starter hole			
	15-33mm	12595	10	4471
	15-43mm	12596	10	4471
	pre-cut			
	35mm	12997	10	4471
	Assura Soft Seal Multichamber One piece			
	Important: This product with integral convexity should only be used after prior assessment of suitability by an appropriate medical professional.			
	Maxi Transparent			
	15-33mm	14716	10	5600
	15-43mm	14717	10	5600
	Maxi White			
	15-33mm	14712	10	5600
	15-43mm	14713	10	5600

IXC

STOMA APPLIANCES

UROSTOMY BAGS

Manufacturer	Appliance	Order No.	Quantity	List Price p
Coloplast Ltd	**Assura** Multichamber One Piece			
	Urostomy Bag with Soft Backing			
	Midi Transparent			
	cut-to-fit 10-55mm	14212	30	17087
	Maxi Transparent			
	cut-to-fit 10-55mm	14222	30	17087
	Midi White			
	cut-to-fit 10-55mm	14211	30	17087
	Maxi White			
	cut-to-fit 10-55mm	14221	30	17087
ConvaTec Ltd	**Esteem** Urostomy pouch with Fold-Up Tap (includes 2 drain tube adapters per pack)			
	Standard - Opaque			
	cut-to-fit			
	13-45mm	S5140	10	4982
	pre-cut			
	20mm	S5141	10	4982
	25mm	S5142	10	4982
	30mm	S5143	10	4982
	35mm	S5144	10	4982
	Small -Opaque			
	cut-to-fit			
	13-45mm	S5120	10	4982
	pre-cut			
	20mm	S5121	10	4982
	25mm	S5122	10	4982
	30mm	S5123	10	4982
	35mm	S5124	10	4982
	Standard-Transparent			
	cut-to-fit			
	13-45mm	S5130	10	5074
	pre-cut			
	20mm	S5131	10	5074
	25mm	S5132	10	5074
	30mm	S5133	10	5074
	35mm	S5134	10	5074
	Small-Transparent			
	cut-to-fit			
	13-45mm	S5110	10	5074
	pre-cut			
	20mm	S5111	10	5074
	25mm	S5112	10	5074
	30mm	S5113	10	5074
	35mm	S5114	10	5074
	Urodress			
	19mm	S896	10	5074
	25mm	S897	10	5074
	32mm	S898	10	5074
	38mm	S899	10	5074
	45mm	S900	10	5074
	Urodress Deep Convex Urostomy Pouch			
	Clear Standard			
	16mm	S910	5	2233
	19mm	S911	5	2233
	22mm	S912	5	2233
	25mm	S913	5	2233
	28mm	S914	5	2233
	32mm	S915	5	2233
	35mm	S916	5	2233
	38mm	S917	5	2233

STOMA APPLIANCES

UROSTOMY BAGS

Manufacturer	Appliance	Order No.	Quantity	List Price p
Dansac Ltd	**Dansac Nova 1** Convex Urostomy pouch with 6mm convex depth			
	Clear			
	cut-to-fit			
	15-24mm	894-24	10	5200
	15-37mm	894-37	10	5200
	15-46mm	894-46	10	5200
	pre-cut			
	20mm	894-20	10	5200
	25mm	894-25	10	5200
	30mm	894-30	10	5200
	Nova 1 Urostomy pouch with 3mm soft convexity			
	Clear			
	pre-cut			
	15mm	892-15	10	5065
	20mm	892-20	10	5065
	25mm	892-25	10	5065
	30mm	892-30	10	5065
	Opaque			
	cut-to-fit			
	12-46mm	891-12	10	5057
	pre-cut			
	15mm	891-15	10	5057
	20mm	891-20	10	5057
	25mm	891-25	10	5057
	30mm	891-30	10	5057
	Transparent			
	cut-to-fit			
	12-46mm	892-12	10	5057
DBT Medical Ltd	Birkbeck Black Rubber			
	Day Bag			
	19mm	LM 723125	1	3385
	Pink Rubber			
	Day Bag			
	19mm	LM 724125	1	3385
	Night Bag			
	19mm	LM 724175	1	3693
	White Rubber Glasgow Bag			
	Small tap	LM 884230	1	2246
	Large tap	LM 884232	1	2246
	White Rubber Transverse			
	Bag Right			
	Small	LM 884104	1	2246
	Medium	LM 884105	1	2246
	Large	LM 884106	1	2246
	White Rubber Transverse			
	Bag Left			
	Small	LM 884114	1	2246
	Medium	LM 884115	1	2246
	Large	LM 884116	1	2246

IXC

STOMA APPLIANCES

UROSTOMY BAGS

Manufacturer	Appliance	Order No.	Quantity	List Price p
Hollister Ltd	**Compact** Urostomy Pouch (All include 1 drain tube per pack)			
	Transparent-with beige comfort backing on body-worn side			
	cut-to-fit			
	13-64mm	1401	10	5040
	pre-cut			
	13mm	1440	10	5040
	16mm	1441	10	5040
	19mm	1447	10	5040
	25mm	1442	10	5040
	32mm	1448	10	5040
	38mm	1443	10	5040
	44mm	1449	10	5040
	First Choice Urostomy Pouch			
	Urostomy Pouch with microporous II adhesive and synthetic skin barrier			
	cut-to-fit			
	13-64mm	1460	10	5170
	Lo-Profile			
	With Microporous II Adhesive and Karaya 5 Seal			
	Gasket Size:			
	25mm	1432	10	5695
	32mm	1438	10	5695
	38mm	1433	10	5695
	44mm	1439	10	5695
	51mm	1434	10	5695
	Impression			
	With Convex wafer (transparent)			
	16mm	1481	10	5270
	19mm	1482	10	5270
	22mm	1483	10	5270
	25mm	1484	10	5270
	29mm	1485	10	5270
	32mm	1486	10	5270
	35mm	1487	10	5270
	38mm	1488	10	5270
	44mm	1489	10	5270
	Impression "C" with convex wafer Transparent with beige comfort backing on body-worn side			
	13mm	1450	10	4605
	16mm	1451	10	4605
	19mm	1452	10	4605
	22mm	1453	10	4605
	25mm	1454	10	4605
	29mm	1455	10	4605
	32mm	1456	10	4605
	35mm	1457	10	4605
	38mm	1458	10	4605
	44mm	1459	10	4605
	51mm	14510	10	4605

STOMA APPLIANCES

UROSTOMY BAGS

Manufacturer	Appliance	Order No.	Quantity	List Price p
Hollister Ltd	**Moderma Flex**			
	Beige			
	15-55mm	29100	10	4829
	20mm	29120	10	4829
	25mm	29125	10	4829
	30mm	29130	10	4829
	35mm	29135	10	4829
	Transparent			
	15-55mm	29500	10	4829
	Moderma Flex with Adapt conformable convex rings			
	Urostomy pouch with flexible barrier plus Adapt conformable convex ring			
	Beige - with comfort backing on both sides			
	cut-to-fit			
	20-29mm + 20mm ring	29820	20	14180
	30-39mm + 30mm ring	29830	20	14180
	40-49mm + 40mm ring	29840	20	14180
	Transparent - with comfort backing on body side only			
	cut-to-fit			
	20-29mm + 20mm ring	29920	20	14180
	30-39mm + 30mm ring	29930	20	14180
	40-49mm + 40mm ring	29940	20	14180
	Moderma Flex Convex			
	Midi urostomy pouch with integral convexity, symmetrical shape			
	Beige with comfort backing on both sides			
	cut-to-fit			
	15-25mm	29200	10	4950
	15-38mm	29201	10	4950
	pre-cut			
	20mm	29220	10	4950
	25mm	29225	10	4950
	30mm	29230	10	4950
	35mm	29235	10	4950
	Transparent with comfort backing on body worn side			
	cut-to-fit			
	15-25mm	29300	10	4950
	15-38mm	29301	10	4950
	pre-cut			
	20mm	29320	10	4950
	25mm	29325	10	4950
	30mm	29330	10	4950
	35mm	29335	10	4950

IXC

STOMA APPLIANCES

UROSTOMY BAGS

Manufacturer	Appliance	Order No.	Quantity	List Price p
Jade-Euro-Med Ltd	White rubber urostomy bags			
(including products	Night bag tap outlet	KM 47	1	2003
formerly listed under	Day bag tap outlet	KM 45	1	1748
Mentor Medical Ltd)				
	Chiron			
	Black Rubber Day Bag 22mm	WF205-22-T	1	4074
	Latex Rubber Day Bag 38mm	WF203-38-B	1	2823
	Latex Rubber Night Bag 38mm	WF213-38-G	1	3092
	White Rubber Day Bag 38mm	WF201-38-S	1	2823
	White Rubber Night Bag 38mm	WF211-38-X	1	3201
	White Rubber Night Bag 44mm	WF211-44-S	1	3201
	White Rubber Night Bag 51mm	WF211-51-P	1	3201
	Mitcham			
	Maxi			
	adhesive			
	25mm	WH119-25-G	10	4639
	non-adhesive			
	25mm	WH009-25-U	10	3788
	38mm	WH009-38-E	10	3788
	Mini			
	non-adhesive			
	25mm	WH005-25-C	10	3788
	32mm	WH005-32-Y	10	3788
	Standard			
	adhesive			
	25mm	WH111-25-W	10	4639
	38mm	WH111-38-G	10	4639
	non-adhesive			
	19mm	WH002-19-U	10	3788
	25mm	WH002-25-P	10	3788
	32mm	WH002-32-L	10	3788
	38mm	WH002-38-Y	10	3788
*	With Foam Pads			
	*Replacement Bags for Surrey Urinal on page 248			
	non-adhesive			
	25mm	WH012-25-U	1	638
	32mm	WH012-32-R	1	638
	38mm	WH012-38-E	1	638

STOMA APPLIANCES

UROSTOMY BAGS

Manufacturer	Appliance	Order No.	Quantity	List Price p
Marlen USA	**UltraLite** (formerly Ultra)			
	Transparent			
	starter hole			
	12mm	761312	10	4132
	Flat pre-cut			
	12mm	761412	10	4132
	16mm	761416	10	4132
	19mm	761419	10	4132
	22mm	761422	10	4132
	25mm	761425	10	4132
	29mm	761429	10	4132
	32mm	761432	10	4132
	34mm	761434	10	4132
	38mm	761438	10	4132
	41mm	761441	10	4132
	44mm	761444	10	4132
	48mm	761448	10	4132
	50mm	761450	10	4132
	54mm	761454	10	4132
	57mm	761457	10	4132
	60mm	761460	10	4132
	63mm	761463	10	4132
	67mm	761467	10	4132
	70mm	761470	10	4132
	73mm	761473	10	4132
	76mm	761476	10	4132
	Shallow Convex pre-cut			
	12mm	761512	10	4132
	16mm	761516	10	4132
	19mm	761519	10	4132
	22mm	761522	10	4132
	25mm	761525	10	4132
	29mm	761529	10	4132
	32mm	761532	10	4132
	34mm	761534	10	4132
	38mm	761538	10	4132
	41mm	761541	10	4132
	44mm	761544	10	4132
	48mm	761548	10	4132
	50mm	761550	10	4132
	54mm	761554	10	4132
	57mm	761557	10	4132
	60mm	761560	10	4132
	63mm	761563	10	4132
	67mm	761567	10	4132
	70mm	761570	10	4132
	73mm	761573	10	4132
	76mm	761576	10	4132

IXC

STOMA APPLIANCES

UROSTOMY BAGS

Manufacturer	Appliance	Order No.	Quantity	List Price p
Marlen USA	**Ultramax**			
	Transparent			
	Flat starter hole	72400	10	4660
	12mm	72412	10	4660
	16mm	72416	10	4660
	19mm	72419	10	4660
	22mm	72422	10	4660
	25mm	72425	10	4660
	29mm	72429	10	4660
	32mm	72432	10	4660
	34mm	72434	10	4660
	38mm	72438	10	4660
	41mm	72441	10	4660
	44mm	72444	10	4660
	50mm	72450	10	4660
	55mm	72455	10	4660
	Convex starter hole	72500	10	4660
	12mm	72512	10	4660
	16mm	72516	10	4660
	19mm	72519	10	4660
	22mm	72522	10	4660
	25mm	72525	10	4660
	29mm	72529	10	4660
	32mm	72532	10	4660
	34mm	72534	10	4660
	38mm	72538	10	4660
	✖ 41mm	72541	10	4660
	✖ 44mm	72544	10	4660
Mentor Medical Ltd	**Carshalton**			
	with acrylic adhesive			
	25mm	48-534-58	10	2276
	32mm	48-534-66	10	2276
	38mm	48-534-74	10	2276
	Triangular			
	25mm	48-532-37	10	2276
	32mm	48-532-45	10	2276
	Rediflow			
	adhesive			
	25mm	WG001-25-C	20	6816
	32mm	WG001-32-Y	20	6816
	38mm	WG001-38-M	20	6816

Mentor Medical Ltd also see Jade-Euro-Med Ltd

✖to be deleted 1 May 2007

STOMA APPLIANCES

UROSTOMY BAGS

Manufacturer	Appliance		Order No.	Quantity	List Price p
Nu-Hope Laboratories (formerly Penlan Medical Ltd)	**Nu-Hope** Urostomy Pouch Flat				
	Standard				
	pre-cut	13mm	8254	10	4833
		16mm	8255	10	4833
		19mm	8256	10	4833
		22mm	8257	10	4833
		25mm	8258	10	4833
		28mm	8259	10	4833
		31mm	8260	10	4833
		34mm	8261	10	4833
		38mm	8262	10	4833
		41mm	8263	10	4833
		44mm	8264	10	4833
		50mm	8266	10	4833
		56mm	8268	10	5008
		63mm	8270	10	5008
		69mm	8272	10	5008
		75mm	8274	10	5008
	Large				
	pre-cut	13mm	8254-L	10	4622
		16mm	8255-L	10	4622
		19mm	8256-L	10	4622
		22mm	8257-L	10	4622
		25mm	8258-L	10	4622
		28mm	8259-L	10	4622
		31mm	8260-L	10	4622
		34mm	8261-L	10	4622
		38mm	8262-L	10	4622
	Regular Convexity Standard				
	pre-cut	13mm	8254-C	10	5283
		16mm	8255-C	10	5283
		19mm	8256-C	10	5283
		22mm	8257-C	10	5283
		25mm	8258-C	10	5283
		28mm	8259-C	10	5283
		31mm	8260-C	10	5283
		34mm	8261-C	10	5283
		38mm	8262-C	10	5283
	Large				
	pre-cut	13mm	8254-LC	10	5447
		16mm	8255-LC	10	5447
		19mm	8256-LC	10	5447
		22mm	8257-LC	10	5447
		25mm	8258-LC	10	5447
		28mm	8259-LC	10	5447
		31mm	8260-LC	10	5447
		34mm	8261-LC	10	5447
		38mm	8262-LC	10	5447
	Deep Convexity Standard				
	pre-cut	13mm	8254-DC	10	5523
		16mm	8255-DC	10	5523
		19mm	8256-DC	10	5523
		22mm	8257-DC	10	5523
		25mm	8258-DC	10	5523
		28mm	8259-DC	10	5523
		31mm	8260-DC	10	5523
		34mm	8261-DC	10	5523
		38mm	8262-DC	10	5523

IXC

STOMA APPLIANCES

UROSTOMY BAGS

Manufacturer	Appliance		Order No.	Quantity	List Price p
Nu-Hope Laboratories	Large				
(formerly Penlan	pre-cut	13mm	8254-L-DC	10	5695
Medical Ltd)		16mm	8255-L-DC	10	5695
		19mm	8256-L-DC	10	5695
		22mm	8257-L-DC	10	5695
		25mm	8258-L-DC	10	5695
		28mm	8259-L-DC	10	5695
		31mm	8260-L-DC	10	5695
		34mm	8261-L-DC	10	5695
		38mm	8262-L-DC	10	5695
Oakmed Ltd	**Option** Urostomy with soft covering to both sides with window				
	cut-to-fit	13-50mm	GC1300	20	8713
	pre-cut	16mm	GC1600	20	8713
		19mm	GC1900	20	8713
		22mm	GC2200	20	8713
		25mm	GC2500	20	8713
		32mm	GC3200	20	8713
		38mm	GC3800	20	8713
	Option Urostomy Microskin with soft covering to both sides				
	Opaque				
	cut-to-fit	13-50mm	MJ1300	20	8727
	pre-cut	16mm	MJ1600	20	8727
		19mm	MJ1900	20	8727
		22mm	MJ2200	20	8727
		25mm	MJ2500	20	8727
		32mm	MJ3200	20	8727
		38mm	MJ3800	20	8727
	Option Urostomy Mini Microskin				
	Opaque				
	cut-to-fit	13mm-40mm	TC1300	20	8574
Peak Medical	**Uromate** 1 piece urostomy pouch, semi-transparent, beige non-woven backing and needle-pin overlap, non-return valve, soft bottom outlet tap				
	Medium				
		13mm starter hole	UMT113B	20	9900
	pre-cut				
		16mm	UMT116B	20	9900
		19mm	UMT119B	20	9900
		22mm	UMT122B	20	9900
		25mm	UMT125B	20	9900
		28mm	UMT128B	20	9900
		32mm	UMT132B	20	9900
	Large				
		13mm starter hole	ULT113B	20	9900
	pre-cut				
		16mm	ULT116B	20	9900
		19mm	ULT119B	20	9900
		22mm	ULT122B	20	9900
		25mm	ULT125B	20	9900
		28mm	ULT128B	20	9900
		32mm	ULT132B	20	9900
		35mm	ULT135B	20	9900
		38mm	ULT138B	20	9900
	Uromate 1 piece urostomy or fistula pouch, semi-transparent, beige non-woven, non-return valve, soft bottom outlet tap				
		10mm starter hole	UXST110	20	9900

STOMA APPLIANCES

UROSTOMY BAGS

Manufacturer	Appliance		Order No.	Quantity	List Price p
Pelican Healthcare Ltd	**Pelican Select** Urostomy Pouch with soft covering to both sides				
	cut-to-fit	15mm-65mm	114215	30	14564
	pre-cut	20mm	114220	30	14564
		25mm	114225	30	14564
		27.5mm	114227	30	14564
		30mm	114230	30	14564
		32.5mm	114232	30	14564
		35mm	114235	30	14564
		37.5mm	114237	30	14564
		40mm	114240	30	14564
		45mm	114245	30	14564
		50mm	114250	30	14564
		55mm	114255	30	14564
	Mini				
	cut-to-fit	15mm-65mm	114415	30	14564
	Maxi				
	cut-to-fit	15mm-65mm	114615	30	14564
	Pelican Select Convex Urostomy Pouch with soft convexity				
	Important: This product with integral convexity should only be used after prior assessment of suitability by an appropriate medical professional.				
	cut-to-fit	12mm-40mm	115412	10	5006
	pre-cut	20mm	115420	10	5006
		22.5mm	115422	10	5006
		25mm	115425	10	5006
		27.5mm	115427	10	5006
		30mm	115430	10	5006
		32.5mm	115432	10	5006
		35mm	115435	10	5006
		37.5mm	115437	10	5006
		40mm	115440	10	5006
	Mini				
	cut-to-fit	12mm-40mm	115212	10	5006
	Maxi				
	cut-to-fit	12mm-40mm	115612	10	5006
	Pelican Select Paediatric Urostomy Pouch with clear medical film, split fabric backing and teddy print				
	cut-to-fit	10mm-50mm	112706	30	14564
Penlan Medical see Nu-Hope Laboratories					
Salts Healthcare	**Confidence** Urostomy Pouch transparent/overlap film (includes 2 drain tube connectors per pack)				
	starter hole				
		13mm	U13	10	4304
	pre-cut				
		25mm	U25	10	4304
		32mm	U32	10	4304
		38mm	U38	10	4304
	Confidence Gold				
	Urostomy Pouch with hypoallergenic hydrocolloid and transparent film/soft beige overlap comfort backing on both sides. (Includes 2 drain tube connectors per pack)				
	Standard				
	starter hole				
		13mm	UNW13	10	4451
	pre-cut				
		25mm	UNW25	10	4451
		32mm	UNW32	10	4451
		38mm	UNW38	10	4451
		45mm	UNW45	10	4451

IXC

STOMA APPLIANCES

UROSTOMY BAGS

Manufacturer	Appliance	Order No.	Quantity	List Price p
Salts Healthcare	Urostomy Pouch with hypoallergenic hydrocolloid and transparent film/soft beige overlap comfort backing on both sides. (Includes 2 drain tube connectors per pack)			
	Small			
	starter hole			
	13mm	USNW13	10	4451
	Confidence Gold Convex Urostomy Pouch			
	1 Piece integral convexity with hypoallergenic hydrocolloid and transparent film/beige overlap comfort backing on both sides. (Includes 2 drain tube connectors per pack)			
	Important:This product with Integral Convexity should only be used after prior assessment of suitability by an appropriate medical professional.			
	starter hole			
	13-25mm	CU1325	10	4669
	13-38mm	CU1338	10	4669
	13-52mm	CU1352	10	4669
	pre-cut			
	21mm	CU21	10	4669
	25mm	CU25	10	4669
	28mm	CU28	10	4669
	32mm	CU32	10	4669
	35mm	CU35	10	4669
	38mm	CU38	10	4669
	Koenig Rutzen			
	All Rubber Black with Tap outlet and N-R valve			
	Large			
	25mm	181125	1	4620
	32mm	181132	1	4620
	Medium			
	25mm	181325	1	4620
	32mm	181332	1	4620
	38mm	181338	1	4620
	with metal bridge, tap outlet and N-R valve			
	Large			
	38mm	185138	1	5402
	Medium			
	32mm	185332	1	5402
	All Rubber White Tap outlet			
	Large			
	32mm	281132	1	1913
	MB with Bridge, Tap outlet and N-R valve			
	Large			
	25mm	188125	1	6486
	32mm	188132	1	6486
	38mm	188138	1	6486
	Light White			
	Opaque			
	Large			
	25mm	294125	20	9552
	32mm	294132	20	9552
	38mm	294138	20	9552
	Adhesive Bag			
	Clear			
	Large			
	25mm	299125	20	9988
	32mm	299132	20	9988
	38mm	299138	20	9988

STOMA APPLIANCES

UROSTOMY BAGS

Manufacturer	Appliance	Order No.	Quantity	List Price p
Salts Healthcare	with Realistic Washer			
	Clear			
	Large			
	25mm	293125	20	12549
	32mm	293132	20	12549
	38mm	293138	20	12549
	Opaque			
	Large			
	25mm	292125	20	12525
	32mm	292132	20	12525
	38mm	292138	20	12525
Ward Surgical Appliance Co				
	Ureterostomy Bag			
	tap outlet, 19mm, 35mm or 54mm opening			
	Night Size	WM 47	1	2019
	Day Size	WM 48	1	1891
Welland Medical Ltd	**Curvex Uro**			
	Urostomy pouch with flexible convex flange and soft backing			
	Clear			
	25mm plateau, cut-to-fit	CUS713	10	4728
	32mm plateau, cut-to-fit	CUM713	10	4728
	43mm plateau, cut-to-fit	CUL713	10	4728
	Beige			
	25mm plateau, cut-to-fit	CUS913	10	4728
	32mm plateau, cut-to-fit	CUM913	10	4728
	43mm plateau, cut-to-fit	CUL913	10	4728
	Silhouette URO			
	Urostomy pouch with soft backing			
	Clear			
	13mm	SUR 713	10	4427
	16mm	SUR 716	10	4427
	19mm	SUR 719	10	4427
	22mm	SUR 722	10	4427
	25mm	SUR 725	10	4427
	32mm	SUR 732	10	4427
	38mm	SUR 738	10	4427
	Beige			
	13mm	SUR 913	10	4427
	16mm	SUR 916	10	4427
	19mm	SUR 919	10	4427
	22mm	SUR 922	10	4427
	25mm	SUR 925	10	4427
	32mm	SUR 932	10	4427
	38mm	SUR 938	10	4427

IXC

STOMA APPLIANCES

MANUFACTURERS' ADDRESSES AND TELEPHONE NUMBERS (STOMA APPLIANCES)

3M Health Care Ltd, 3M House, Morley Street, Loughborough, Leics, LE11 1EP (01509 611611)

Anglo Venture 2000 Ltd, The Mill, Hatfield Health, Bishop's Stortford, Herts, CM22 7DL (01279 730733)

Astra Tech Ltd, Stroud Water Business Park, Brunel Way, Stonehouse, Gloucestershire GL10 3SW (01453 791763)

B. Braun Medical, Thorncliffe Park, Sheffield, S35 2PW (0114 225 9000)

Charles S Bullen (Stomacare) Ltd, 85/87 Kempston Street, Liverpool, L3 8HE (0151 2076995)

J. Chawner Surgical Belts Ltd, Tudor Business Centre, Marsden Road, Redditch, B98 7AY (01527 62200)

CliniMed Ltd, Cavell House, Knaves Beech Way, Loudwater, High Wycombe, Bucks, HP10 9QY (01628 850100)

Coloplast Ltd, Peterborough Business Park, Peterborough, PE2 6FX (01733 392000)

ConvaTec Ltd, Harrington House, Milton Road, Ickenham, Uxbridge, UB10 8PU (01895 628400)

Cover Care, Trent House, Meadowbank Way, Eastwood, Nottingham, NG16 3SB (01773 536816)

CUI (INT) Ltd, 16 Dublin Street, Balbriggan, County Dublin, Ireland (00353 1 8414788)

Cuiwear Ltd see CUI (INT) Ltd

Cuxson Gerrard & Company Ltd, 125 Broadwell Road, Oldbury, Warley, West Midlands, B69 4BF (0121 5447117)

Dansac Ltd, Victory House, Vision Park, Histon, Cambridge CB4 4ZR (01223 235100)

DBT Medical Ltd, 14 Eagle Industrial Estate, The Crofts, Witney, OX28 4DJ (01993 773673)

Ecolab, Lotherton Way, Garforth, Leeds LS25 2JY (0113 2320066)

Hi-Line Ltd, 1 The Carlton Business Centre, Carlton, Nottingham, NG4 3AA (0115 9403080)

Hollister Ltd, Rectory Court, 42 Broad Street, Wokingham, Berkshire, RG40 1AB (0118 989 5000) (Retail Pharmacy Order Line 0800 521392)

Impharm Nationwide Ltd, PWS Building, Nelson Street, Bolton, BL3 2JW (01204 371155)

Jade-Euro-Med Ltd, Unit 14, East Hanningfield Industrial Estate, Old Church Road, East Hanningfield, Chelmsford, Essex CM3 8BG (01245 400413)

Loxley Products: Unit 8, South Lincolnshire Enterprise Agency, Station Road East, Grantham, Lincolnshire, NG31 6HX (01476 560194)

Manfred Sauer GmbH see Manfred Sauer UK Ltd

Manfred Sauer UK Ltd, Unit 3, io Centre, Lodge Farm, Northampton NN5 7UW (0870 1904100)

Marlen USA products: distributed by Marlen Healthcare Ltd, Shell Buildings, Maltmill Lane, Blackheath, Halesowen, West Midlands (0121 7082077)

Medicina Ltd, Unit 1 Adlington Business Village, Huyton Road, Adlington, PR7 4JH (01257 482200)

Medlogic Global Ltd, Western Wood Way, Language Science Park, Plympton, Plymouth, Devon, PL7 5BG (01752 209955)

Mentor Medical Ltd, Building 10, Commerce Way, Lancing, West Sussex BN15 8TJ (01903 761122)

STOMA APPLIANCES

MANUFACTURERS' ADDRESSES AND TELEPHONE NUMBERS (STOMA APPLIANCES)

Nu-Hope Laboratories: distributed by Penlan Medical Ltd, 2 New Row, Deeping St James, Lincolnshire, PE6 8NA (0784 1838036)

Oakmed Ltd, 54 Adams Avenue, Northampton, NN1 4LJ (01604 239250)

Omex Medical Ltd, Opal Drive, Foxmilne, Milton Keynes, MK15 0DG (01908 258285)

Opus Healthcare, PO Box 8204, Ardleigh, Colchester, CO7 7WH (01206 230741)

Orthotic Services Ltd, Heartlands House, 19 Cato Street, The Heartlands, Birmingham, B7 4TS (0121 3596323)

OstoMart Ltd, 1 The Carlton Business Centre, Carlton, Nottingham, NG4 3AA (0115 9403080)

S G & P Payne, Percy House, Brook Street, Hyde, Cheshire, SK14 2NS (0161 3678561)

Peak Medical, Holywell House Annexe, Holywell Street, Chesterfield, Derbyshire, S41 7SH (01246 209329)

Pelican Healthcare Ltd, Cardiff Business Park, Cardiff, CF14 5WF (02920 747787)

ProSys International Ltd, 60 Cottenham Park Road, Wimbledon, London, SW20 0TB (02089 447585)

E Sallis Ltd, Vernon Works, Waterford Street, Old Basford, Nottingham, NG6 0DH (0115 9787841/2)

Salts Healthcare Ltd, Richard Street, Aston, Birmingham, B7 4AA (0121 3332000)

SASH, Woodhouse, Woodside Road, Hockley, Essex, SS5 4RU (01702 206502)

T J Shannon Ltd, 59 Bradford Street, Bolton, BL2 1HT (01204 521789)

A H Shaw and Partners Ltd, Manor Road, Ossett, West Yorkshire, WF5 0LF (01924 273474)

Teleflex Medical, Stirling Road, Cressex Business Park, High Wycombe, Buckinghamshire, HP12 3ST (01494 532761)

UCI Healthcare Ltd, Unit 8, Southill, Cornbury Park,Charlbury, Oxon OX7 3EW (0160 8811815)

Ward Surgical Appliance Company Ltd, 57A Brightwell Avenue, Westcliffe-on-Sea, Essex SSO 9EB (01702 354064)

Welland Medical Ltd Products: distributed by CliniMed Ltd, Cavell House, Knaves Beech Way, Loudwater, High Wycombe, Bucks. HP10 9QY (01628 850100)

IXC

This Page is Intentionally Blank

CHEMICAL REAGENTS

APPROVED LIST OF CHEMICAL REAGENTS

The only chemical reagents which may be supplied as part of the pharmaceutical services are those listed in Part IXR of the Tariff.

The price listed in respect of a chemical reagent specified in the following list is the basic price on which payment will be calculated pursuant to Part II, Clause 6A for the dispensing of that chemical reagent.

The Notes to Part IX shall also apply to Part IXR when 'chemical reagent(s)' shall be substituted for 'appliance(s)'.

Chemical reagents are listed in the order; detection strips (urine), and detection strips (blood).

All quantities within this section are those of the manufacturer's original pack and are special containers (see Drug Tariff Part II, Clause 10B)

	Chemical Reagent	Quantity	Basic Price P
1.	**DETECTION STRIPS, URINE**		
	(Supplied with an instruction sheet, analysis record and colour chart)		
1.1	**Detection Strips, urine for Glycosuria**		
1.1.1	**Clinistix**	50	325
1.1.2	**Diabur Test 5000**	50	269
1.1.3	**Diastix**	50	276
1.1.4	**Medi-Test Glucose**	50	226
1.2	**Detection Strips, urine for Ketonuria** *(Acetonuria)*		
1.2.1	**Ketostix**	50	292
1.2.2	**Ketur Test**	50	258
1.3	**Detection Strips, urine for Proteinuria**		
1.3.1	**Albustix**	50	402
1.3.2	**Medi Test Protein 2**	50	316
2.	**DETECTION STRIPS, BLOOD FOR GLUCOSE**		
	(Supplied with an instruction sheet, analysis record and colour chart)		
	Meters for use with Blood Glucose Testing Strips or Discs are not available on prescription		
2.1	**Colorimetric Strips - visually readable**		
2.1.1	**Glucoflex-R**	50	1423
2.1.2	**Hypoguard Supreme**	50	1200
2.2	**Biosensor Strips - to be read only with the appropriate meter**		
2.2.1	**Advantage Plus**	50	1419
2.2.2	**Ascensia Microfill**	50	1417
2.2.3	**Aviva**	50	1393
2.2.4	**Freestyle**	50	1406
2.2.5	**GlucoMen Sensors**	50	1315
2.2.6	**GlucoMen Visio**	50	1397

IXR

CHEMICAL REAGENTS

APPROVED LIST OF CHEMICAL REAGENTS

		Chemical Reagent		Quantity	Basic Price P
	2.2.7	Medisense G2		50	1315
	2.2.8	Medisense Optium Plus		50	1397
	2.2.9	Medisense SoftSense		50	1396
*	2.2.10	Microdot		50	1296
	2.2.11	On-Call Plus		50	705
	2.2.12	One Touch Ultra		50	1397
	2.2.13	PocketScan		50	1365
	2.2.14	Sensocard		50	1567
	2.2.15	TrueTrack System		50	1370

2.3 Biosensor Discs - to be read only with the appropriate meter

2.3.1	Ascensia Autodisc test sensor discs		5 discs of 10 strips each	1406

2.4 Colorimetric Strips - to be read only with the appropriate meter

2.4.1	Active		50	1419
2.4.2	BM-Accutest		50	1376
2.4.3	Compact	3 drums of 17 strips each		1431
2.4.4	One Touch		50	1382
2.4.5	Prestige Smart System		50	1396

3. DETECTION STRIPS, BLOOD FOR KETONES (Beta-Hydroxybuterate)
    - to be read only with the appropriate meter

3.1	Optium ß-Ketone Test Strips	70784-35	10	1880

4. DETECTION STRIPS, BLOOD FOR DETERMINATION OF INTERNATIONAL NORMALISED RATIO (INR)
    - to be read only with the appropriate meter

4.1	CoaguChek PT	1937634	12	3167
		1937642	48	12383
4.2	CoaguChek XS PT	04625358	24	6334
		04625315	48	12383
4.3	HemoSense INRatio	0100071	12	3053
		0100139	48	11935
4.4	ProTime 3 cuvettes	49006000	6	1554
		49005000	25	6325

*The manufacturer of this product does not provide additional free patient support services

HOME OXYGEN THERAPY SERVICE

1.   HOME OXYGEN

1.1   Clinical best practice guidelines advise that oxygen therapy should be provided for patients in the home only after careful evaluation and never on a placebo basis. Oxygen may be supplied depending on the type of therapy required by a patient - for example, short burst (or intermittent) or long term therapy. The British Thoracic Society has issued updated clinical best practice guidelines for the assessment and provision of oxygen therapy. See the BTS website at www.brit-thoracic.org.uk

1.2   Extracts from the guidelines are included below.

Home Oxygen Service Arrangements from 1 February 2006

1.3   On 7 June 2005, the Department of Health and the Welsh Assembly Government announced the award of contracts to four companies for the delivery of an integrated (cylinder, concentrator, liquid) home oxygen service in England and Wales, which starts on **1 February 2006**. These four companies will meet all home oxygen needs in 10 oxygen service regions in England and one in Wales. Contact details for each supplier providing the service in each oxygen service region in England and in Wales are included at section 9. There is a free phone arrangement.

Home Oxygen Order Form (HOOF)

1.4   The supplier will provide the home oxygen service ordered by clinical staff on a Home Oxygen Order Form (HOOF) - **not Form FP10 or WP10 in Wales.** This form can be obtained by downloading it from

www.primarycarecontracting.nhs.uk or

http://howis.wales.nhs.uk/sites3/docopen.cfm?orgid=521&ID=60627

or supplies of printed forms are available from local NHS stores.

Ordering Home Oxygen Services

1.5   From 1 February 2006, other registered health care professionals, as well as GPs, may order home oxygen services for delivery direct to patients at home. Clinical staff should indicate the service(s) required on the form, together with details of the patient's oxygen flow rate and hours of use. Where a patient is awaiting referral for clinical assessment, advice is that a flow rate of 2l/min might be specified when ordering home oxygen. On assessment, the clinical specialist team will determine whether a patient's flow rate and hours of use require adjustment.

1.6   Services that may be ordered include:

- Emergency Oxygen Therapy
- Short Burst Oxygen Therapy
- Long Term Oxygen Therapy
- Ambulatory Oxygen Therapy

1.7   The supplier will provide the equipment that best meets the clinical needs of the patient as indicated on the HOOF. The supplier is also responsible for arrangements for the payment of patient's electricity costs associated with use of equipment supplied.

1.8   Clinicians should order a **service** (as above) and are not required to specify the provision of certain oxygen equipment. However, clinical staff may wish to discuss with the supplier, as appropriate, where it is felt that a patient has particular needs (for example, where a patient has a disability and uses a wheelchair or in relation to the special needs of a child or infant requiring home oxygen therapy). The supplier will need to be aware of these needs when deciding which equipment to supply to an individual patient. Clinical staff may also include details of any particular patient need on the HOOF.

1.9   These services, including advice to clinical staff, patients and their carers on the use of oxygen equipment supplied, are available on a 24 hour, 7 day a week basis. There is a free phone arrangement.

HOME OXYGEN THERAPY SERVICE

1.10   Details of the service specification, including requirements to support the discharge of patients from hospital and the response times for the delivery of each service, are available on the websites listed at paragraph 1.4.

2.   EMERGENCY HOME OXYGEN SERVICE

2.1   Where a clinician decides that a patient requires oxygen at home as soon as possible, the supplier may be requested to deliver this to the patient's home within four hours. Home oxygen may be ordered on an emergency basis for a minimum period of three days. This period should allow clinicians sufficient time to review a patient's needs and to place an order for another oxygen therapy service (for example, short burst oxygen where there is intermittent need for oxygen).

2.2   An order for emergency oxygen will continue to be met on this basis until the supplier receives a revised order for another oxygen therapy service from a clinician. If a revised order is not received after the initial three day period has elapsed, the supplier will continue to provide oxygen on an emergency basis for a subsequent three day period and the per diem cost for this three day service will continue to apply.

2.3   It is inappropriate to order home oxygen on an emergency basis where a patient or carer has forgotten to order supplies - particularly if the patient has access to a back up cylinder to meet his/her immediate needs. Each oxygen service supplier operates a 24 hour, 7 day a week helpline and patients and carers may be directed to their local free phone service.

3.   SHORT BURST THERAPY (INTERMITTENT THERAPY)

3.1   Short burst oxygen therapy refers to the intermittent use of supplemental oxygen at home usually for periods of about 10 to 20 minutes at a time to relieve dyspnoea. Traditionally, short burst oxygen therapy is used

- for pre-oxygenation before exercise
- for breathlessness during recovery from exercise
- for control of breathlessness at rest
- in palliative care
- after an exacerbation of Chronic Obstructive Pulmonary Disease (COPD) to bridge the time to full long term oxygen therapy (LTOT) assessment.

3.2   The British Thoracic Society (BTS) clinical guidelines recognise that further research is needed to support firm recommendations in relation to short burst oxygen therapy but advise that, where episodic breathlessness is not relieved by other treatments, short burst oxygen therapy should be considered for patients with the following conditions:

- severe COPD
- interstitial lung disease
- heart failure
- palliative care

3.3   Whilst the guidelines recognise that there is no specific methodology to support the clinical assessment of short burst oxygen therapy, it is recommended that other causes of breathlessness may need to be excluded or, as appropriate, the patient may need to be assessed for long term oxygen therapy (LTOT). In addition, the guidelines recommend that short burst oxygen therapy should only continue to be ordered for a patient where an improvement in breathlessness and/or exercise tolerance can be documented.

HOME OXYGEN THERAPY SERVICE

4.   LONG TERM OXYGEN THERAPY (LTOT)

4.1   Long term oxygen therapy is the provision of oxygen for a prolonged period of usually 15 hours or more a day (including at night). Once started, LTOT is likely to be life long.

4.2   The British Thoracic Society clinical guidelines draw attention to patients with the following conditions who may benefit from the provision of LTOT:

- Chronic obstructive pulmonary disease
- Severe chronic asthma
- Interstitial lung disease
- Cystic fibrosis
- Bronchiectasis
- Pulmonary vascular disease
- Primary pulmonary hypertension
- Pulmonary malignancy
- Chronic heart failure

4.3   The guidelines suggest that patients for whom there is clear evidence of the value of LTOT will be those with chronic obstructive airways disease, chronic hypoxaemia and oedema. The guidelines recommend that respiratory care specialist staff, with access to respiratory function services, should assess all these patients.

4.4   The BTS guidelines also draw attention to the benefit of LTOT for other groups of patients. For example, the provision of home oxygen therapy for palliation of dyspnoea in pulmonary malignancy and other causes of disabling dyspnoea due to terminal disease.

5.   AMBULATORY OXYGEN

5.1   Ambulatory oxygen refers to the provision of oxygen therapy during exercise and activities of daily living. Ambulatory oxygen therapy may be ordered for patients on LTOT who are mobile and need to or can leave the home on a regular basis. The BTS clinical guidelines indicate that ambulatory oxygen therapy might be considered for patients with the following conditions

- Chronic obstructive pulmonary disease
- Severe chronic asthma
- Interstitial lung disease
- Cystic fibrosis
- Pulmonary vascular disease
- Primary pulmonary hypertension

The guidelines do not recommend ambulatory oxygen therapy for patients with chronic lung disease and mild hypoxaemia (not on LTOT) and no exercise desaturation. It is also not recommended for patients with chronic heart failure.

5.2   **In accordance with good clinical practice, ambulatory oxygen should only be ordered after appropriate assessment by a respiratory care specialist.**

6.   CHANGES TO A PATIENT'S REQUIREMENTS

A Patient's Oxygen Needs

6.1   If for any reason, a clinician wishes to alter the patient's regime, he will need to inform the patient and complete a new order for home oxygen and send this to the supplier. The supplier will make the necessary arrangements to adjust or provide new equipment, as appropriate. **The supplier will not be able to make these changes until a revised order for home oxygen has been received.**

Holiday Arrangements and Attendance at School or Workplace

6.2   A clinician may also wish to make arrangements for a secondary order for oxygen therapy - that is, for delivery to a location other than the patient's home. For example, where a patient remains able to attend school or the workplace or where a patient wishes to go on holiday within England and Wales

6.3   In these circumstances, the clinician will need to complete a secondary order, providing details of the address for delivery of the equipment. In the case of holidays, details should be given for the period in which this equipment is needed. The supplier will make the necessary arrangements to install and remove this equipment, subject to prior agreement by those concerned (for example, school, employer, hotel etc).

6.4   The supplier is **not** responsible or required to secure agreement to provide home oxygen equipment in a location other than a patient's home. This will need to be obtained by the patient or patient's family in relation to holiday accommodation or the patient's workplace. Agreement to the provision of oxygen equipment in schools may be arranged through the School Health Service. **The supplier will be unable to provide oxygen equipment in a location other than the patient's home unless prior agreement has been obtained.**

6.5   Current arrangements for the provision of oxygen therapy to patients at home will continue in Scotland - that is, pharmacy contractors providing a cylinder service and the concentrator service delivered under contract with a separate supplier. PCTs for England/LHBs in Wales will be advised as to arrangements for patients wishing to visit Scotland - for example, for holidays or to stay with friends or relatives.

6.6   The arrangements set out in paragraph 6.3 do not apply to patients wishing to take holidays outside the UK. In these circumstances, patients should seek advice on reciprocal arrangements for health care between the United Kingdom and other countries (this is available in a Department of Health leaflet and on the Department of Health website - www.dh.gov.uk). Patients may also wish to discuss any private arrangements for the provision of oxygen supplies that may be available from their local oxygen service supplier.

Patient's Use of Oxygen

6.7   It is for clinical staff to counsel patients on the need for oxygen therapy and the regime to be followed to achieve the benefits. The supplier will provide equipment to deliver the required flow rate and hours of use specified on the HOOF. However, if a patient or carer continues to adjust equipment to change the flow rate, the supplier will inform the clinician so that the patient can be advised further as to flow rate or for review of oxygen therapy needs. **The supplier cannot change the flow rate specified by a clinician**. If a clinician is concerned that a patient may persist with over use of oxygen, he may wish to put in place monitoring arrangements and discuss these with the supplier, as necessary.

Withdrawal of Home Oxygen Service

6.8   The supplier is contracted to provide the service ordered until he is informed otherwise and, thus, will continue to make a charge for the service until notified that it should be withdrawn. Therefore, it is essential that the supplier is informed as soon as possible where oxygen tharapy is no longer required by a patient - for example, due to the death of a patient or, following assessment or review of a patient's needs, that the patient no longer requires oxygen therapy.

Death of a Patient

6.9   Where a patient receiving home oxygen therapy dies, his GP practice or a member of the clinical specialist team treating the patient, as appropriate, should advise the relevant PCT for England, LHB for Wales, so that arrangements can be made for withdrawal of this service by the PCT for England, LHB for Wales.

Where a Patient discontinues oxygen therapy

6.10   Where, following review of need, home oxygen therapy is no longer required by a patient, his GP practice or a member of the clinical specialist team treating the patient, as appropriate, should advise the relevant PCT for England, LHB for Wales, so that arrangements can be made for withdrawal of this service by the PCT for England, LHB for Wales.

Removal of Oxygen Equipment from a Patient's Home

6.11   A supplier may be requested to remove equipment from a patient's home by

6.11.1   the patient's GP practice or a member of the clinical specialist team treating the patient or

6.11.2   a person authorised by the relevant PCT for England, LHB for Wales or

6.11.3   a patient or patient's relative or carer. Where a patient, a patient's relative or carer requests removal of equipment, the supplier is required to inform the clinician who has ordered the service and the relevant PCT for England, LHB for Wales immediately of the details and date of receipt of the request.

6.12   The PCT for England, LHB for Wales should inform the Pricing Authority of withdrawal of the service where

6.12.1   a GP practice or a member of a specialist team has informed the PCT for England, LHB for Wales that a patient has died or has discontinued oxygen therapy and/or where the GP practice or member of the specialist team has informed the PCT for England, LHB for Wales that the supplier has been requested to remove equipment from the patient's home or

6.12.2   the supplier has informed the PCT for England, LHB for Wales that he has received a request from the patient, the patient's relative or carer to remove equipment from the patient's home or

6.12.3   where a person authorised by the PCT for England, LHB for Wales has requested the supplier to remove equipment from the patient's home.

6.13   When informing the Pricing Authority of the withdrawal of the service, the PCT for England, LHB for Wales, should include the date of any request to the supplier to remove equipment from a patient's home.

6.14   The supplier is required to remove the equipment within 14 days of receiving a request for removal.

7.   CLAIMS FOR PAYMENT

7.1   Each oxygen service supplier listed at section 9 will be able to access the Pricing Authority website and submit oxygen payment claims at any time within the first 10 calendar days of the month following that in which the home oxygen service has been provided.

7.2   In Wales, claims should be submitted to the relevant LHB or the LHB's nominated representative body.

8.   TRANSITIONAL ARRANGEMENTS FOR THE PAYMENT OF CONTRACTORS CONTINUING TO PROVIDE AN OXYGEN SERVICE BETWEEN 1 FEBRUARY 2006 AND 31 MARCH 2007

8.1   From 1 February 2006, the suppliers listed at section 9 will provide home oxygen to all patients for whom a clinician orders an oxygen therapy service for the first time on or after this date.

8.2   However, the following transitional arrangements will operate for the payment of claims by contractors continuing to provide a home oxygen service to existing patients who, at 1 February 2006, are awaiting transfer to a new supplier. These arrangements will continue until 31 March 2007.

Claims made by a current concentrator service supplier for the supply of this service to existing patients between 1 February 2006 and the date of a patient's transfer to the new supplier

8.3   Where a current concentrator service supplier continues to provide this service to a patient after 1 February 2006 to a date agreed with the patient and the new supplier for transfer to the new supplier, as now the appropriate claims form should continue to be sent to the Pricing Authority not later than the fifth day of the month following that in which the supply was made.

8.4   Payment for supply of an oxygen concentrator service to existing patients during this transitional period will continue at the same contract rates in place prior to 1 February 2006.

HOME OXYGEN THERAPY SERVICE

8.5   Current concentrator service suppliers are required to inform the Pricing Authority immediately of the date of transfer to the new supplier of any existing patients receiving this service prior to 1 February 2006.

Claims made by a pharmacy contractor providing a cylinder service between 1 February 2006 and the date of a patient's transfer to the new service supplier

8.6   An FP10 (WP10 in Wales) prescription for cylinder oxygen may be issued and dispensed beyond 1 February 2006 within the validity of the prescription in line with arrangements set out in section 8.2.

8.7   Where a pharmacy contractor continues to provide a cylinder service for a patient after 1 February 2006 until a date on which a patient is transferred to the new supplier, the following arrangements will apply.

Supply of Oxygen Equipment

8.8   Where a pharmacy contractor continues to supply oxygen cylinders, masks and other equipment to a patient after 1 February 2006, the basic price of approved oxygen equipment will be as set out in Part X, Section 8 of the Drug Tariff as at 31 January 2006. That is:-

Basic Price of Approved Oxygen Equipment

8.9   Basic Price for the supply of a mask, when prescribed after the initial order on a separate prescription form

Intersurgical 010 Mask, 28%	97p
Ventimask Mk IV, 28%	145p
Intersurgical 005 Mask	78p
Venticaire Mask	71p
Venticaire Venturi Mask 28%	92p

8.10   Basic Price for

Oxygen BP, cylinder	1360 litres	858p
Oxygen BP, composite cylinder with integral headset to specification 02 *	1360 litres	948p

* The supply of these cylinders is limited. They should only be supplied where their use is part of the local home oxygen therapy service or where specifically indicated for an individual patient. The Department of Health is aware of the areas where supply of these cylinders is part of local arrangements.

8.11   Basic Price for;

Oxygen BP, composite cylinder with integral headset *	2122 litres	1340p

* These cylinders are not available from all suppliers.

Claims for Prescriptions Dispensed

8.12   Where a pharmacy contractor has dispensed a prescription for cylinder oxygen, he may submit a claim to the Pricing Authority up until 5 April 2007. Claims submitted after that date will not be considered.

Delivery and Collection of Cylinders and Loan of Headsets to Patients

8.13   Where a pharmacy contractor continues to undertake the delivery and collection of oxygen cylinders and other equipment and provides a headset on loan to a patient, he will be reimbursed for these services, under local arrangements. A pharmacy contractor should continue to make returns in accordance with local arrangements with the relevant PCT for England, LHB for Wales.

Note: different local arrangements with a PCT for England and LHB for Wales may apply.

8.14   The recovery of empty cylinders from patients and their prompt return to the supplier for refilling is essential to maintain adequate supplies for the use of patients, particularly during the period when patients transfer to a new supplier. The efficient use of cylinders supplies will support the management of change and pharmacy contractors are reminded of the importance of ensuring that as few empty cylinders as possible remain in circulation.

Collection of Cylinders and Sets Following Transfer of a Patient to the New Supplier

8.15   Where a patient is transferred to a new supplier - and where the patient or patient's representative fails to return equipment supplied by the pharmacy contractor - the onus of collecting it rests on the pharmacy contractor. A contractor should submit any claim relating to the collection of cylinders and/or sets, in accordance with local arrangements, within one month of being informed by the PCT for England, LHB for Wales that the patient has transferred to a new supplier.

Claims for Compensation for Financial Loss in Respect of Oxygen Equipment

8.16   Where a pharmacy contractor suffers financial loss as a result of the act or default of a person causing the loss or damage to oxygen equipment loaned, the pharmacy contractor should inform the relevant PCT for England, LHB for Wales of such financial loss. In this paragraph, the expression "person" means the person supplied, the patient concerned, members of his household, or the authorities of an institution to which the equipment is delivered, as the case may be.

8.17   Necessary out of pocket expenses incidentally involved in the repair or replacement of the equipment, such as postal or carriage paid, should also be met. Reimbursement of the loss will depend on local PCT for England and LHB for Wales arrangements.

Claims for Fees relating to the Decommissioning of Authorised Headsets held by a Pharmacy Contractor

8.18   A pharmacy contractor who provided an oxygen cylinder service on or after 30 September 2005 may submit a claim to the local PCT for England, (LHB for Wales), for a one-off payment for the withdrawal from service (or decommissioning) of authorised headsets purchased by the pharmacy contractor.

8.19   Pharmacy contractors who continue to provide a home oxygen service to patients after 31 July 2006, as part of the transition to the new service arrangements, may submit a claim for headsets by the required date for receipt of claims (see paragraphs 8.24 and 8.25). Where a pharmacy contractor has made a claim, and is continuing to provide an oxygen service to a patient that includes use of an authorised headset purchased by the contractor, he or she should contact the local PCT for England, LHB for Wales, to discuss arrangements relating to the continued use and maintenance of the headset.

8.20   A pharmacy contractor may submit a claim for an authorised headset purchased by the contractor, subject to the headset being available for use, or in use, by a patient on or after 30 September 2005.

8.21   A pharmacy contractor may submit a claim in respect of each new headset purchased before 1 July 2004 or each new or reconditioned headset purchased on or after 1 July 2004. Authorised new or reconditioned headsets purchased on or after 1 July 2004 may attract a higher decommissioning fee than headsets purchased before this date.

8.22   The PCT for England, LHB for Wales, will consider a claim where the pharmacy contractor has obtained prior PCT or LHB authorisation to purchase the headset. The PCT for England, LHB for Wales, will also consider a claim where authorisation to purchase headsets has been included as part of alternative arrangements agreed between the pharmacy contractor and the PCT for England, LHB for Wales, for the provision of this service.

8.23   The PCT for England, LHB for Wales, will not consider any claim in respect of unauthorised headsets purchased by a pharmacy contractor or in respect of any headset held in the pharmacy that was unfit for use after 30 September 2005. A pharmacy contractor should not submit a claim for an unauthorised headset under these arrangements where s/he has submitted a claim to the PCT for England, LHB for Wales, in accordance with paragraphs 8.16-8.17.

HOME OXYGEN THERAPY SERVICE

8.24 A pharmacy contractor should submit written claims for payment of decommissioning fees on the relevant claim form. This is available on the NHS Business Services Authority Prescription Pricing Division (NHSBSA PPD) website (see www.ppa.nhs.uk) or the Pharmaceutical Services Negotiating Committee (PSNC) website (see www.psnc.org.uk). In Wales, this form is available from the local LHB.

8.25 A pharmacy contractor should submit any claim (by post or e-mail) to the local PCT for England, LHB for Wales, on or before 31 December 2006. A PCT for England, LHB for Wales, will not consider any claim received after this date.

8.26 No payment will be made to a pharmacy contractor until after the closing date for receipt of claims by the PCT for England, LHB for Wales, to allow the PCT or LHB to consider and authorise all claims submitted by that date.

8.27 Further information relating to a claim for the decommissioning of headsets purchased by pharmacy contractors is available from the PSNC or the local PCT for England, LHB for Wales.

8.28 The PCT for England, LHB for Wales, may seek further written information or documentary evidence from a pharmacy contractor to support authorisation of payment of a claim. This may include a requirement on the pharmacy contractor to provide proof of purchase of a headset or PCT or LHB inspection of the equipment at the pharmacy.

8.29 Where unsupported by evidence, the PCT or LHB may reduce the payment claimed by a contractor or may seek to recover any overpayments. Therefore, pharmacy contractors are advised to retain equipment and/or any related documentary evidence as any request or inspection made by a PCT for England, LHB for Wales, may be made or carried out on or before 31 March 2007.

9. HOME OXYGEN SERVICE SUPPLIERS

Oxygen Service Region

1. North West

(includes PCTs in the North West SHA)

Air Products plc
2 Millenium Gate
Westmere Drive
Crewe
Cheshire
CW1 6AP

Tel 0800 373580
Fax 0800 214709
(Free of Charge)

2. North East

(includes PCTs in the North East SHA)

Linde Gas UK Home Care
Unit 2
Port of Tyne
(North Side)
South Shields
NE33 5SP

Tel 0808 2020999
Fax 0191 4974340
(Free of Charge)

HOME OXYGEN THERAPY SERVICE

3. Yorkshire & Humberside
(includes PCTs in Yorkshire and The Humber SHA)

Air Products plc
2 Millenium Gate
Westmere Drive
Crewe
Cheshire
CW1 6AP

Tel 0800 373580
Fax 0800 214709
(Free of Charge)

4. East Midlands
(includes PCTs in the East Midlands SHA)

Air Products plc
2 Millenium Gate
Westmere Drive
Crewe
Cheshire
CW1 6AP

Tel 0800 373580
Fax 0800 214709
(Free of Charge)

5. West Midlands
(includes PCTs in the West Midlands SHA)

Air Products plc
2 Millenium Gate
Westmere Drive
Crewe
Cheshire
CW1 6AP

Tel 0800 373580
Fax 0800 214709
(Free of Charge)

6. Eastern England
(includes PCTs in East of England SHA)

BOC Medical
Vitalair Team
Customer Service Centre
Priestley Road
Worsley
Manchester
M28 2UT

Tel 0800 136603
Fax 0800 1699989
(Free of Charge)

7. SW London, Thames Valley, Hants & Isle of Wight
(includes PCTs in London SHA and South Central SHA)

Allied Respiratory
Charles House
Enterprise Drive
Four Ashes
Wolverhampton
WV10 7DF

Tel 0500 823773
Fax 0800 7814610
(Free of Charge)

X

HOME OXYGEN THERAPY SERVICE

8. SE London, Kent, Surrey & Sussex
(includes PCTs in London SHA and South East Coast SHA)

Allied Respiratory
Charles House
Enterprise Drive
Four Ashes
Wolverhampton
WV10 7DF

Tel 0500 823773
Fax 0800 7814610
(Free of Charge)

9. London North
(includes PCTs in the London SHA)

Air Products plc
2 Millenium Gate
Westmere Drive
Crewe
Cheshire
CW1 6AP

Tel 0800 373580
Fax 0800 214709
(Free of Charge)

10. South West
(includes PCTs in the South West SHA)

BOC Medical
Vitalair Team
Customer Service Centre
Priestley Road
Worsley
Manchester
M28 2UT

Tel 0800 136603
Fax 0800 1699989
(Free of Charge)

11. Wales
(LHBs in Wales)

Air Products plc
2 Millenium Gate
Westmere Drive
Crewe
Cheshire
CW1 6AP

Tel 0800 373580
Fax 0800 214709
(Free of Charge)

RESCINDED - INTENTIONALLY BLANK

This Part has been rescinded and is intentionally blank.

RESCINDED - INTENTIONALLY BLANK

This Page is Intentionally Blank

ESSENTIAL SMALL PHARMACIES SCHEME (ESPS)

For England, ESPS arrangements will continue until 31 March 2006 for those pharmacy contractors in receipt of ESPS payments as at 1 November 2005. A Standard Form LPS has been developed for those meeting similar criteria to current ESPS provisions to provide services after 1 April 2006. Details are set out in Local Pharmaceutical Services (Essential Small Pharmacies) Directions 2005, available on DH website at www.dh.gov.uk/localpharmaceuticalservices Provided conditions are met Primary Care Trusts will enter into ESPLPS agreements with such pharmacies.

For those pharmacies not transferring to the new arrangements (ESPLPS), which were previously designated ESPS as "special consideration" cases and those ESPS pharmacies that dispensed less than 6,000 items per annum, ESPS arrangements shall continue until 31 March 2007.

For Wales, the ESPS arrangements will continue.

ESPS arrangements for those pharmacy contractors qualifying for ESPS payments from April 2005 are as follows:

1.   **Interpretation**

In this Part -

"Authority" means the PCT for England and LHB for Wales in whose locality the premises are located;

"Contractor" means only the pharmacy contractor whose name is included in a pharmaceutical list of the Authority;

"pharmacy" means a pharmacy at premises from which the contractor supplies pharmaceutical services;

"premises" means the premises from which the contractor provides pharmaceutical services;

"year" means the period from 1 April in any one year to 31 March of the following year.

2.   **Entitlement**

2.1 Where, in any year -

    2.1.1 the pharmacy dispenses fewer than 26,400 prescriptions; and

    2.1.2 that pharmacy is more than 1 kilometre by the nearest practicable route available to the public on foot from the next nearest pharmacy or is less than 1 kilometre but previously qualified as a special consideration case and the circumstances of the pharmacy remain unchanged; and

    2.1.3 in the case of pharmacy which has, in the year immediately preceding that year, dispensed fewer than 6,000 prescriptions, the authority certifies in writing at the beginning of that year that the pharmacy is essential to the proper provision of pharmaceutical services, the contractor shall, subject to the following subparagraphs, be entitled to ESPS payments calculated in accordance with paragraph 3 below.
(Note. No new special consideration cases will be entertained).

2.2   A contractor shall be entitled to claim ESPS payments in 2005/06 if, on or before 31 January 2005, he estimates, on the basis of the number of prescriptions dispensed in the preceding twelve months or having regard to any special circumstances, that the number of items to be dispensed in the next year will be less than 26,400.

2.3   The contractor shall apply to the Authority for ESPS payments, in the form specified (Form ESPS1 for contractors on the list not less than 10 months at 31 January 2005 and Form ESPS2 for those on list less than 10 months) on or before 31 January 2005.

2.4   On 1 April 2005, or as soon as practicable thereafter, but before any payment is made, the contractor shall declare to the Authority his estimate of the number of prescriptions dispensed by the pharmacy in the year just ended, if the Authority is satisfied that -

    2.4.1 that number is less than 26,400

    2.4.2 that the number of prescriptions to be dispensed in the year to which the claim relates is unlikely to exceed 26,400 and

2.4.3 the conditions set out in sub-paragraph 2.1.2 and 2.1.3 above are met, payments shall be made by the Authority in accordance with paragraph 3 , subject to the conditions in sub-paragraphs 2.5 and 2.6.

2.5   The Authority, will as soon in the current financial year as they have available the Pricing Authority figure of prescriptions dispensed by the contractor during the preceding financial year, compare this with the contractor's declared estimated figure (sub-paragraph 2.4 above) and if the PA figure of prescriptions dispensed in the previous financial year is 26,400 or more, the ESPS payments made so far in the current financial year shall be recovered from the contractor in the 3 months following that in which the last ESPS payment was made.

2.6   Where, at any time in any year during which ESPS payments are made to the contractor in respect of a pharmacy.

2.6.1 the number of prescriptions dispensed by that pharmacy exceeds 26,400 the contractor shall be deemed not to have been entitled to ESPS payments for that year in respect of that pharmacy, and any such payment made to him in that year shall be recovered from the remuneration due to him in the 3 months immediately following the month in which the number of prescriptions dispensed reached 26,400.

2.6.2 a second contractor begins to provide pharmaceutical services from a pharmacy at premises which are less than 1 kilometre by the nearest practicable route available to the public on foot from the premises of the first contractor, payment to the first contractor shall continue at the full rate for the remainder of the year and will then cease.

2.6.3 in a case to which sub-paragraph 2.1.3 applies, the Authority decides that the pharmacy is no longer essential, it shall notify the contractor and after the date of that notification no further ESPS payments shall be paid in that year in respect of that pharmacy.

2.7   For Wales, where the provision by the contractor of pharmaceutical services from any premises has just begun, the preceding sub-paragraphs shall be modified as follows:

In England, where the provision by the contractor of pharmaceutical services from any premises has begun after 31 January 2005 and before 31 October 2005, or the Authority is satisfied there is a substantial change of circumstances such as to entitle the contractor to claim ESPS, the preceding sub-paragraphs shall be modified as follows, but these provisions are not available to pharmacies beginning services by virtue of Regulation 35(3):-

2.7.1   the contractor may apply to the Authority for ESPS payments, in the form specified (Form ESPS2) at any time during the year;

2.7.2 he shall be entitled to ESPS payments if -

2.7.2.1 in the case of a contractor who is providing services from premises from which, immediately before the day on which he began to provide those services, those services were provided by another contractor, the number of prescriptions dispensed in the twelve months immediately preceding that day was less than 26,400;

2.7.2.2 in any other case, he estimates, and the Authority is satisfied that, less than 26,400 prescriptions will be dispensed in the first twelve months of the provision of pharmaceutical services, and

2.7.2.3 in any case the condition in sub-paragraph 2.1.2 is satisfied;

2.7.3 any entitlement shall begin -

2.7.3.1 if the claim is made within 3 months of the entry on the list in question, from the date of entry;

2.7.3.2 in any case, from the date on which the application is made.

2.8   For England, no payment under these arrangements will be payable after 31 March 2006, except payments that represent adjustments appropriate to the year ended 31 March 2006.

ESSENTIAL SMALL PHARMACIES SCHEME (ESPS)

3.   Payments

3.1   From 1 April 2006, ESPS payments shall be the difference between one-twelfth of the target payment (£59,016) and the remuneration due (i.e. professional fees as in Part IIIA and any payments made under Part VIA but excluding payments made under Part IIIA 2.F), subject to para 3.3 below. See worked example.

3.2   Payments shall be made in arrears.

3.3   From 1 April 2006, the maximum monthly payment shall be £4,279. If in any month the contractor is entitled to more than the maximum payment, the amount due shall be carried forward and paid in the following month, again subject to the maximum monthly payment applicable to that second month.

3.4   Any over, or any under, ESPS payment shall be if necessary, corrected in the remuneration paid in the first month of the following year.

3.5   Where a contractor normally provides pharmaceutical services at a pharmacy for less than 35 hours a week, any ESPS payment shall be calculated by reference to the following formula:

3.5.1   Average hours/35 x payments appropriate to a full-time pharmacy with the same prescription volume, as determined by the Secretary of State for Health as respects England and the National Assembly for Wales as respects Wales.

4.   Worked Example

4.1 Month 1.

April   calculate 1/12 of target payment £59,016

make ESPS payment of the difference between calculated amount and remuneration due.

4.2 Month 2.

May   calculate 2/12 of target payment £59,016

make ESPS payment of the difference between calculated amount and sum of total payment of remuneration due plus ESPS made in month 1 and remuneration due in month 2.

4.3 Month 3.

June   calculate 3/12 of target payment £59,016

make ESPS payment of difference between calculated amount and sum of total payments made in months 1 and 2 and remuneration due in month 3.

ESSENTIAL SMALL PHARMACIES SCHEME (ESPS)

This Page is Intentionally Blank

PAYMENTS IN RESPECT OF PRE-REGISTRATION TRAINEES

1.   From 1 April 2005 a grant of £16,440 is payable to pharmacy contractors who provide the pre-registration training experience needed by pharmacy graduates and certain undergraduates for admission to the Royal Pharmaceutical Society of Great Britain's Register of Pharmaceutical Chemists. The grants are payable at annual rates, determined annually in respect of each pre-registration training place filled by a pharmacy graduate or an undergraduate on a sandwich course recognised by the Royal Pharmaceutical Society of Great Britain as pre-registration training.

2.   Pharmacy contractors who have undertaken to provide pre-registration training should submit a claim to the PCT for England and LHB for Wales at the start of the training period. PCTs for England and LHBs for Wales will arrange for the payment to be made monthly in arrears. Contractors MUST notify the PCT for England and LHB for Wales immediately in writing if the arrangement to provide pre-registration training ceases.

XIII

This Page is Intentionally Blank

REWARD SCHEME - FRAUDULENT PRESCRIPTION FORMS

Payments to chemists who claim a payment under Regulation 59(1) of the National Health Service (Pharmaceutical Services) Regulations 2005 for England and The National Health Service (Pharmaceutical Services)(Amendment)(Wales) Regulations 2005.

The Scheme allows chemists to claim a financial reward where they have identified a fraudulent prescription form and thereby either prevented fraud or contributed with valuable information to the investigation of fraud. A reward is payable where:

• fraudulent activity can be proven

• the conditions for the scheme are met as set out below.

Slightly different versions of the Scheme apply in England and Wales.

PART I: ENGLAND

The NHSBSA, Counter Fraud and Security Management Division (Referred to below as the Authority) is responsible for receiving and considering claims for reward payments in England.

The Scheme applies to all claims which are received by the Authority on or after 7 May 2003.

Retention and Reporting Reward: claims where a chemist -

(a)   has not provided the drugs, medicines or listed appliances ordered on the fraudulent prescription form, or

(b)   has provided the drugs, medicines or listed appliances ordered on the fraudulent prescription form, but had reason to believe at the time or subsequently came to have reason to believe that the form is fraudulent,

and reports this to the relevant authorities as laid out below.

The chemist will be eligible for a payment of £70, where all the conditions for *either* the retention element of the reward *or* the reporting element of the reward are met. Only one reward will be payable for each dispensing occasion.

The conditions for the *retention* element of the reward are:

i   the drugs, medicines or listed appliances specified on the fraudulent prescription form have not been provided, the prescription form has been retained by the chemist, and the Primary Care Trust has been informed as soon as practicable, in accordance with Regulation 18B(1)(i);

ii   a claim is made by contacting the Authority as soon as practicable, normally within 7 days of the form having been presented. A claim form provided by the Authority must be completed and returned to the Authority, along with the original prescription form, normally within 28 days of the form having been presented; and

iii   the form presented as a prescription form was not a genuine order for the person named on the form. An order would not be a genuine order if, for example, it had been stolen or counterfeited and not signed by an authorised prescriber; or had been altered otherwise than by the authorised prescriber by whom it was issued.

The conditions for the *reporting* element of the reward are:

i   the drugs, medicines or listed appliances specified on the fraudulent prescription form have been dispensed, but the chemist has reason to believe at the time or subsequently comes to have reason that the order is not genuine;

ii   the chemist has notified the Primary Care Trust as soon as practicable, in accordance with Regulation 18B(1)(ii);

iii   a claim is made by contacting the Authority as soon as practicable, normally within 7 days of the form having been presented. A claim form provided by the Authority must be completed and returned to the Authority along with the original prescription form, normally within 28 days of the form having been presented;

iv   a detailed explanation of why the chemist felt it necessary to dispense must be included on the claim form. A reward will only be payable where the Authority is satisfied that the chemist had good and sufficient reasons to dispense; and

v   the form presented as a prescription form was not a genuine order for the person named on the form. An order would not be a genuine order if, for example, it had been stolen or counterfeited and not signed by an authorised prescriber; or had been altered otherwise than by the authorised prescriber by whom it was issued.

Where the time-limits for either contacting the Authority and the Primary Care Trust or for returning a claim form to the Authority, as specified above, are exceeded, the Authority will nevertheless consider a claim if there are exceptional circumstances justifying the delay.

Pharmacists who are eligible to claim a reward under the scheme should contact:

England
Patient Fraud Support Unit
NHSBSA, CFSMS
2nd Floor Sandyford House
Archbold Terrace
Jesmond
Newcastle Upon Tyne
NE2 1DB
Freephone: 0800-068-6161
Tel: 0191-2046300

PART II: WALES

Health Solutions Wales (Velindre NHS Trust) (referred to below as HSW) is responsible for receiving and considering claims for reward payments in Wales.

The Scheme applies to all claims which are received by HSW on or after 1 February 2003.

Retention and Reporting Reward: claims where a chemist -

(a)   has not provided the drugs, medicines or listed appliances ordered on the fraudulent prescription form,
        or

(b)   has provided the drugs, medicines or listed appliances ordered on the fraudulent prescription form, but had reason to believe at the time or subsequently came to have reason to believe that the form is fraudulent,

and reports this to the relevant authorities as laid out below.

The chemist will be eligible for a payment of £70, where all the conditions for *either* the retention element of the reward *or* the reporting element of the reward are met. Only one reward will be payable for each dispensing occasion.

The conditions for the retention element of the reward are:

i   the drugs, medicines or listed appliances specified on the fraudulent prescription form have not been provided, the prescription form has been retained by the chemist, and the Local Health Board has been informed immediately, in accordance with regulation 18B(1)(i);

ii   a claim is made by contacting the Local Health Board as soon as practicable, normally within 7 days of the form having been presented. A claim form provided by the Local Health Board must be completed and returned to HSW, along with the original prescription form, normally within 28 days of the form having been presented; and

iii   the form presented as a prescription form was not a genuine order for the person named on the form. An order would not be a genuine order if, for example, it had been stolen or

REWARD SCHEME - FRAUDULENT PRESCRIPTION FORMS

counterfeited and not signed by an authorised prescriber; or had been altered otherwise than by the authorised prescriber by whom it was issued.

The conditions for the reporting element of the reward are:

i the drugs, medicines or listed appliances specified on the fraudulent prescription form have been dispensed, but the chemist believes at the time or subsequently comes to believe that the order is not genuine;

ii the chemist has notified the Local Health Board as soon as practicable, and in any case within 14 days of the order being presented to the chemist, in accordance with regulation 18B(1)(ii);

iii a claim is made by contacting the Local Health Board as soon as practicable. A claim form provided by the Local Health Board must be completed and returned to HSW along with the original prescription form, normally within 28 days of the form having been presented;

iv a detailed explanation of why the chemist felt it necessary to dispense must be included on the claim form. A reward will only be payable where HSW is satisfied that the chemist had good and sufficient reasons to dispense; and

v the form presented as a prescription form was not a genuine order for the person named on the form. An order would not be a genuine order if, for example, it had been stolen or counterfeited and not signed by an authorised prescriber; or had been altered otherwise than by the authorised prescriber by whom it was issued.

Where the time-limits for either contacting HSW and the Local Health Board or for returning a claim form to HSW, as specified above, are exceeded, HSW will nevertheless consider a claim if there are exceptional circumstances justifying the delay.

Pharmacists who are eligible to claim a reward under the scheme should contact:

Wales
Margaret Willis
Health Solutions Wales
Brunel House
Fitzalan Road
Cardiff
CF24 0HA
Tel: 029 2050 0500

XIV

REWARD SCHEME - FRAUDULENT PRESCRIPTION FORMS

This Page is Intentionally Blank

BORDERLINE SUBSTANCES

Borderline Substances

In certain conditions some foods and toilet preparations have characteristics of drugs and the Advisory Committee on Borderline Substances advises as to the circumstances in which such substances may be regarded as drugs. The Advisory Committee's recommendations are listed below. Prescriptions issued in accordance with the Committee's advice and endorsed "ACBS" will normally not be investigated.

Manufacturers wishing to notify changes to their products should contact the ACBS by post: c/o NICE, MidCity Place, 71 High Holborn, Holborn. WC1V 6NA.

LIST A

This is an alphabetical index of products which the ACBS has recommended for the management of the conditions shown under each product.
General Practitioners are reminded that the Advisory Committee on Borderline Substances recommends products on the basis that they may be regarded as drugs for the treatment of specified conditions. Doctors should satisfy themselves that the products can be safely prescribed, that patients are adequately monitored and that, where necessary, expert hospital supervision is available. Prescriptions for products recommended by the Committee should be endorsed "ACBS".
Note: The Committee has recommended a number of products as complete feeds for certain conditions. They may be prescribed both as sole sources of nutrition and as necessary nutritional supplements prescribable on medical grounds.

Definitions

1. The Committee has defined proven lactose or sucrose intolerance as "A condition of intolerance to an intake of the relevant disaccharide confirmed by:

(i)   demonstrated clinical benefit of the effectiveness of the disaccharide free diet;
      and

(ii) the presence of reducing substances and/or excessive acid (1.00pH) in the stools, a low concentration of
      the correspondent disaccharidase enzyme on intestinal biopsy, or by breath tests or lactose tolerance tests."

2. The Committee has defined proven whole protein sensitivity as "Intolerance to whole protein, proven by at least two withdrawal and challenge tests, as suggested by an accurate dietary history."

3. The Committee has defined dysphagia as that associated with "Intrinsic disease of the oesophagus, eg. oesophagitis; neuromuscular disorders, eg. multiple sclerosis and motor neurone disease; major surgery and/or radiotherapy for cancer of the upper digestive tract; protracted severe inflammatory disease of the upper disgestive tract, eg. Stevens-Johnson Syndrome and epidermolysis bullosa."

XV

BORDERLINE SUBSTANCES

LIST A

ALCOHOLIC BEVERAGES
See: Rectified Spirit

ALEMBICOL-D (MCT OIL)
Steatorrhoea associated with cystic fibrosis of the pancreas, intestinal lymphangiectasia, surgery of the intestine, chronic liver disease, liver cirrhosis, other proven malabsorption syndromes, a ketogenic diet in the management of epilepsy and in type 1 hyperlipoproteinaemia.

AMINOGRAN FOOD SUPPLEMENT
Phenylketonuria

AMINOGRAN PKU TABLETS
For use in the dietary management of phenylketonuria. Not to be prescribed for any child under 8 years of age.

ANALOG MSUD
See: MSUD ANALOG

ANALOG RVHB
See: XMET ANALOG

ANALOG XLYS
See: XLYS ANALOG

ANALOG XMET, THRE, VAL, ISOLEU
See: XMTVI ANALOG

ANALOG XP
See: XP ANALOG

ANALOG XP LPC
See: XP ANALOG LCP

ANALOG XPHEN, TYR
See: XPHEN, TYR ANALOG

ANALOG XPHEN, TYR, MET
See: XPTM ANALOG

APROTEN GLUTEN-FREE AND LOW-PROTEIN PRODUCTS
See: Gluten-Free and Low-Protein Products.

ARNOTT'S GLUTEN-FREE PRODUCTS
See: Gluten-Free Products.

A.S. SALIVA ORTHANA
Patients suffering from xerostomia (dry mouth) as a result of having or having undergone radiotherapy or sicca syndrome.

AVEENO BABY COLLOIDAL

AVEENO BATH OIL

AVEENO COLLOIDAL

AVEENO CREAM

AVEENO LOTION
Endogenous and exogenous eczema, xeroderma, ichthyosis and senile pruritus associated with dry skin.

BAKERS DELIGHT
See: Gluten-Free Products

BARKAT GLUTEN-FREE PRODUCTS
See: Gluten-Free Products.

BORDERLINE SUBSTANCES

BI-AGLUT GLUTEN-FREE PRODUCTS
See: Gluten-Free Products.

BIOTENE ORALBALANCE DRY MOUTH SALIVA REPLACEMENT GEL
Patients suffering from xerostomia (dry mouth) as a result of having or having undergone radiotherapy or sicca syndrome.

BIOXTRA GEL MOUTHSPRAY

BIOXTRA MOISTURING GEL
Patients suffering from xerostomia (dry mouth) as a result of having or having undergone radiotherapy or sicca syndrome.

CALOGEN

CALOGEN BANANA

CALOGEN BUTTERSCOTCH

CALOGEN STRAWBERRY
For use in the dietary management of disease-related malnutrition,malabsorption states, or other conditions requiring fortification with a high fat supplement, with or without fluid and electrolyte restrictions.

CALOREEN
Disease related malnutrition, malabsorption states or other conditions requiring fortification with a high or readily available carbohydrate supplement.

CALSHAKE
Disease related malnutrition, malabsorption states or other conditions requiring fortification with a fat/carbohydrate supplement.

CAPRILON
Disorders in which a high intake of MCT is beneficial

CASILAN 90
Biochemically proven hypoproteinaemia.

CLINUTREN DESSERT
As a necessary nutritional supplement prescribed on medical grounds for:
Short bowel syndrome, intractable malabsorption, pre-operative preparation of patients who are undernourished, patients with proven inflammatory bowel disease, following total gastrectomy, dysphagia, bowel fistulae, disease-realated malnutrition, continuous ambulatory peritoneal dialysis (CAPD) and haemodialysis. Not suitable for any child under 3 years; maximum recommended amount of 3 units for 3+ to 6 years.

CLINUTREN FRUIT
As a necessary nutritional supplement prescribed on medical grounds for:
Short bowel syndrome, intractable malabsorption, pre-operative preparation of patients who are undernourished, patients with proven inflammatory bowel disease, following total gastrectomy, dysphagia, bowl fistulae, disease-related malnutrition.   Not suitable for any child under 3 years; maximum recommended amount of 3 units for 3+ to 6 years.

CLINUTREN 1.5

CLINUTREN 1.5 FIBRE
For use as the sole source of nutrition or as a necessary nutritional supplement prescribed on medical grounds for:
Short bowel syndrome, intractable malabsorption, pre-operative preparation of patients who are undernourished, proven inflammatory bowel disease, following total gastrectomy, dysphagia and disease related malnutrition.

CLINUTREN ISO
For use as the sole source of nutrition or as a necessary nutritional supplement prescribed on medical grounds for:
Short bowel syndrome, intractable malabsorption, pre-operative preparation of patients who are undernourished, patients with proven inflammatory bowel disease, following total gastrectomy, dysphagia, bowel fistulae, disease-related malnutrition. Not suitable for any child under 3 years; not suitable as a sole source of nutrition for patients under 6 years; maximum recommended amount of 3 units for 3+ to 6 years.

XV

BORDERLINE SUBSTANCES

CLINUTREN JUNIOR
For use as the sole source of nutrition, or as a necessary nutritional supplement prescribed on medical grounds for:
Short bowel syndrome, intractable malabsorption, pre-operative preparation of patients who are undernourished, patients with proven inflammatory bowel disease, following total gastrectomy, dysphagia, bowel fistulae, disease-related malnutrition, growth failure in children aged 1-10 years. Not to be prescribed for any child under one year.

CLINUTREN THICKENER

CLINUTREN THICKENED DRINKS
Thickening of foods and fluids in dysphagia. Not to be used for children under three years of age.

COLIEF
Is indicated for: the relief of symptoms associated with lactose intolerance, provided that lactose intolerance is confirmed by the presence of reducing substances and/or excessive acid in stools, a low concentration of the corresponding disaccharide enzyme on intestinal biopsy or by breath hydrogen test or lactose intolerance test.

COMMINUTED CHICKEN MEAT (SHS)
Carbohydrate intolerance in association with possible or proven intolerance of milk, glucose and galactose intolerance.

COMPLAN SHAKE
As a necessary nutritional supplement prescribed on medical grounds for:
Short bowel syndrome, intractable malabsorption, pre-operative preparation of patients who are undernourished, patients with proven inflammatory bowel disease, following total gastrectomy, dysphagia, bowel fistulae and disease related malnutrition.

CORN FLOUR AND CORN STARCH
Hypoglycaemia associated with glycogen storage disease.

COVERING CREAMS AND CONCEALMENT OF BIRTH MARKS

Covermark Classic Foundation	Keromask Finishing Powder
Covermark Finishing Powder	Keromask Masking Cream
Dermacolor Camouflage Cream	Veil Cover Cream
Dermacolor Fixing Powder	Veil Finishing Powder

For post operative scars and other deformities and as adjunctive therapy in the relief of emotional disturbance due to disfiguring skin disease, such as vitiligo.

COVERMARK PRODUCTS
See: Covering Creams

COW & GATE PEPTI
For the dietary management in established cows' milk protein intolerance with/without proven secondary lactose intolerance.

COW & GATE PEPTI-JUNIOR (formerly PEPTI-JUNIOR)
Disaccharide and/or whole protein intolerance, or where amino acids and peptides are indicated in conjunction with MCT.

DELPH SUN LOTION SPF30
Protection from UV radiation in abnormal cutaneous photosensitivity resulting from genetic disorders or photodermatoses, including vitiligo and those resulting from radiotherapy, chronic or recurrent herpes simplex labialis.

DERMACOLOR CAMOUFLAGE SYSTEM
See: Covering Creams

DEXTROSE
Glycogen storage disease and sucrose/isomaltose intolerance.

DIALAMINE
Oral feeding where essential amino acid supplements are required, for example chronic renal failure, hypoproteinaemia, wound fistula leakage with excessive protein loss, conditions requiring a controlled nitrogen intake and haemodialysis.

BORDERLINE SUBSTANCES

DIETARY SPECIALS
See: Gluten-Free Products

DISINFECTANTS (ANTISEPTICS)
May be prescribed on FP10 only when ordered in such quantities and with such directions as are appropriate for the treatment of patients, but not if ordered for general hygienic purposes.

DUOBAR (strawberry, toffee, neutral)
Disease related malnutrition, malabsorption states or other conditions requiring fortification with a fat/carbohydrate supplement.

DUOCAL (LIQUID, MCT POWDER AND SUPER SOLUBLE)
Disease related malnutrition, malabsorption states or other conditions requiring fortification with a fat/carbohydrate supplement.

E45 EMOLLIENT BATH OIL

E45 EMOLLIENT WASH CREAM
Endogenous and exogenous eczema, xeroderma, ichthyosis and senile pruritus associated with dry skin.

E45 LOTION
Symptomatic relief of dry skin conditions, such as those associated with atopic eczema and contact dermatitis.

E45 SUN BLOCK SPF 50
Protection from UV radiation in abnormal cutaneous photosensitivity resulting from genetic disorders or photodermatoses, including vitiligo, and those resulting from radiotherapy; chronic or recurrent herpes simplex labialis.

EASIPHEN
For use in the dietary management of proven phenylketonuria in older children (above 8 years) and adults.

ELEMENTAL 028 (FLAVOURED AND UNFLAVOURED)

ELEMENTAL 028 EXTRA

ELEMENTAL 028 EXTRA (LIQUID)
For use as the sole source of nutrition or as a necessary nutritional supplement prescribed on medical grounds for:
Short bowel syndrome, intractable malabsorption, patients with proven inflammatory bowel disease, bowel fistulae. Not to be prescribed for any child under one year; use with caution for young children up to five years of age.

EMSOGEN (FLAVOURED AND UNFLAVOURED)
For use as the sole source of nutrition or as a necessary nutritional supplement prescribed on medical grounds for:
Short bowel syndrome, intractable malabsorption, patients with proven inflammatory bowel disease, bowel fistulae. Not to be prescribed for any child under one year; use with caution for young children up to five years of age.

ENER-G GLUTEN-FREE AND LOW-PROTEIN PRODUCTS
See: Gluten-Free and Low-protein Products

ENER-G LOW-PROTEIN PRODUCTS
See: Low-Protein Products

ENER-G XANTHAN GUM
For use in the dietary management of gluten sensitive enteropathies, inlcuding steatorrhoea due to gluten-sensitivity, coeliac disease, and dermatitis herpetiformis.

ENERGIVIT
For infants requiring additional energy, vitamins, minerals and trace elements following a protein restricted diet.

ENFAMIL AR
Significant reflux disease. For use not in excess of a 6-month period. Not to be used in conjunction with any other thickener or antacid product.

ENFAMIL LACTOFREE
Proven lactose intolerance.

XV

BORDERLINE SUBSTANCES

ENLIVE PLUS
As a necessary nutritional supplement prescribed on medical grounds for:
Disease related malnutrition, short bowel syndrome, intractable malabsorption, inflammatory bowel disease, bowel fistulae, dysphagia, following total gastrectomy and for pre-operative preparation of patients who are malnourished. It is not recommended for children under 1 year of age and should be used with caution in children under 5 years of age.

ENMIX PLUS COMMENCE
As a necessary nutritional supplement prescribed on medical grounds for:
Short bowel syndrome, intractable malabsorption, pre-operative preparation of patients who are undernourished, patients with proven inflammatory bowel disease, following total gastrectomy, dysphagia, bowel fistulae, and disease-related malnutrition. Not to be prescribed for any child under one year; use with caution for young children up to five years of age.

ENRICH
For use as the sole source of nutrition or as a necessary nutritional supplement prescribed on medical grounds for:
Short bowel syndrome, intractable malabsorption, pre-operative preparation of patients who are undernourished, patients with proven inflammatory bowel disease, following total gastrectomy, dysphagia, disease-related malnutrition. Not to be prescribed for any child under one year; use with caution for young children up to five years of age.

ENRICH PLUS
For use as a nutritional supplement for patients with disease-related malnutrition, continuous ambulatory peritoneal dialysis (CAPD) and haemodialysis, short bowel syndrome, intractable malabsorption, dysphagia, proven inflammatory bowel disease, bowel fistulae, gastrectomy and for pre-operative preparation of patients who are undernourished. Not to be prescribed for any child under one year; use with caution for young children up to five years of age.

ENSHAKE (BANANA, CHOCOLATE, STRAWBERRY AND VANILLA FLAVOURS)
Disease related malnutrition, malabsorption states or other conditions requiring fortification with a fat/carbohydrate supplement. Not suitable for children under 1 year.

ENSURE

ENSURE 500ml READY TO HANG (VANILLA FLAVOUR ONLY)
As a necessary nutritional supplement prescribed on medical grounds for:
Disease-related malnutrition, intractable malasorption, total gastrectomy, proven inflammatory bowel disease, and pre-operative preparation of patients who are undernourished. Not to be prescribed for any child under two years; use with caution for young children up to five years of age

ENSURE PLUS COMMENCE

ENSURE PLUS LIQUID FEED

ENSURE PLUS YOGHURT STYLE
As a necessary nutritional supplement prescribed on medical grounds for:
Short bowel syndrome, intractable malabsorption, pre-operative preparation of patients who are undernourished, patients with proven inflammatory bowel disease, following total gastrectomy, dysphagia, bowel fistulae, disease-related malnutrition, continuous ambulatory peritoneal dialysis (CAPD), and haemodialysis. Not to be prescribed for any child under one year; use with caution for young children up to five years of age.

FARLEY'S SOYA FORMULA
Proven lactose and associated sucrose intolerance in pre-school children, galactokinase deficiency, galactosaemia and cow's milk protein intolerance.

FATE LOW PROTEIN PRODUCTS
See: Low-Protein Products

FOODLINK COMPLETE
As a necessary nutritional supplement prescribed on medical grounds for:
Short bowel syndrome, intractable malabsorption, pre-operative preparation of patients who are undernourished, patients with proven inflammatory bowel disease, following total gastrectomy, dysphagia, bowel fistulae, disease-related malnutrition. Not to be prescribed for any child under one year; use with caution for young children up to five years of age.

BORDERLINE SUBSTANCES

FORMANCE
As a necessary nutritional supplement prescribed on medical grounds for:
Short bowel syndrome, intractable malabsorption, pre-operative preparation of patients who are undernourished, patients with proven inflammatory bowel disease, following total gastrectomy, dysphagia, bowel fistulae, disease-related malnutrition, continuous ambulatory peritoneal dialysis (CAPD), and haemodialysis. Not to be prescribed for any child under one year; use with caution for young children up to five years of age.

FORTI RANGE STARTER PACK
See: FORTISIP RANGE STARTER PACK

FORTICARE
As a nutritional supplement for patients with pancreatic cancer

FORTICREME
See: FORTICREME COMPLETE

FORTICREME COMPLETE (formerly FORTICREME)
As a necessary nutritional supplement prescribed on medical grounds for:
Short bowel syndrome, intractable malabsorption, pre-operative preparation of patients who are undernourished, patients with proven inflammatory bowel disease, following total gastrectomy, dysphagia, bowel fistulae, disease-related malnutrition, continuous ambulatory peritoneal dialysis (CAPD) and haemodialysis. Not to be prescribed for any child under one year; use with caution for young children up to five years of age.

FORTIFRESH
For use as the sole source of nutrition or as a necessary nutritional supplement prescribed on medical grounds for:
Short bowel syndrome, intractable malabsorption, pre-operative preparation of patients who are undernourished, patients with proven inflammatory bowel disease, following total gastrectomy, dysphagia, bowel fistulae, disease-related malnutrition. Not to be prescribed for any child under one year; use with caution for young children up to five years of age.

FORTIJUCE

FORTIJUCE STARTER PACK
As a necessary nutritional supplement prescribed on medical grounds for:
Short bowel syndrome, intractable malabsorption, pre-operative preparation of patients who are undernourished, patients with proven inflammatory bowel disease, following total gastrectomy, dysphagia, bowel fistulae, disease-related malnutrition. Not to be prescribed for any child under one year; use with caution for young children up to five years of age.

FORTIMEL
As a necessary nutritional supplement prescribed on medical grounds for:
Short bowel syndrome, intractable malabsorption, pre-operative preparation of patients who are undernourished, patients with proven inflammatory bowel disease, following total gastrectomy, dysphagia, bowel fistulae, disease-related malnutrition. Not to be prescribed for any child under one year; use with caution for young children up to five years of age.

FORTINI

FORTINI MULTI FIBRE
For use as a necessary nutritional supplement prescribed on medical grounds for:
Disease-related malnutrition and growth failure. Not to be prescribed for any child under one year.

FORTISIP BOTTLE

FORTISIP MULTIFIBRE
As a necessary nutritional supplement prescribed on medical grounds for:
Short bowel syndrome, intractable malabsorption, pre-operative preparation of patients who are undernourished, patients with proven inflammatory bowel disease, following total gastrectomy, dysphagia, bowel fistulae, disease-related malnutrition. Not to be prescribed for any child under one year; use with caution for young children up to five years of age.

XV

BORDERLINE SUBSTANCES

FORTISIP PROTEIN

FORTISIP PROTEIN STARTER PACK
> Approved for short bowel syndrome, intractable malabsorption, pre-operative preparation of patients who are undernourished, proven inflammatory bowel disease, following total gastrectomy, bowel fistulae, disease-related malnutrition and dysphagia.

FORTISIP RANGE STARTER PACK (formerly FORTI RANGE STARTER PACK)
> As a necessary nutritional supplement prescribed on medical grounds for:
> Short bowel syndrome, intractable malabsorption, pre-operative preparation of patients who are undernourished, patients with proven inflammatory bowel disease, following total gastrectomy, dysphagia, bowel fistulae, disease-related malnutrition. Not to be prescribed for any child under one year; use with caution for young children up to five years of age.

FREBINI
> For use as the sole source of nutrition or as a necessary nutritional supplement prescribed on medical grounds for children aged 1-10 years or 8-30kg for:
> Short bowel syndrome, intractable malabsorption, pre-operative preparation of patients who are undernourished, patients with proven inflammatory bowel disease, following total gastrectomy, dysphagia, bowel fistulae, disease-related malnutrition and/or growth failure. Not to be prescribed for any child under one year of age.

FREBINI ENERGY

FREBINI ENERGY DRINK (STRAWBERRY AND BANANA FLAVOURS)

FREBINI ENERGY FIBRE DRINK

FREBINI ORIGINAL FIBRE (formerly FREBINI ORIGINAL FIBRE PROTEIN)
> As a sole source of nutrition, or as a nutritional supplement for children aged 1-6 years with disease-related malnutrition and/or growth failure, proven inflammatory bowel disease, following total gastrectomy, short bowel syndrome, intractable malabsorption, dysphagia, bowel fistulae, and for the pre-operative preparation of patients who are malnourished. Not to be prescribed for any child under one year.

FREBINI ORIGINAL FIBRE PROTEIN
> See: FREBINI ORIGINAL FIBRE

FREBINI ENERGY FIBRE
> As a sole source of nutrition, or as a nutritional supplement for children aged 1-10 years with disease-related malnutrition and/or growth failure, proven inflammatory bowel disease, following total gastrectomy, short bowel syndrome, intractable malabsorption, dysphagia, bowel fistulae, and for the pre-operative preparation of patients who are malnourished. Not to be prescribed for any child under one year.

FRESUBIN ENERGY

FRESUBIN ENERGY FIBRE SIP FEED

FRESUBIN ENERGY FIBRE (NEUTRAL) TUBE FEED
> For use as the sole source of nutrition or as a necessary nutritional supplement prescribed on medical grounds for:
> Short bowel syndrome, intractable malabsorption, pre-operative preparation of patients who are undernourished, patients with proven inflammatory bowel disease, following total gastrectomy, dysphagia, bowel fistulae, disease-related malnutrition. Not to be prescribed for any child under one year; use with caution for young children up to five years of age.

FRESUBIN HP ENERGY
> As a necessary nutritional supplement prescribed on medical grounds for:
> Short bowel syndrome, intractable malabsorption, pre-operative preparation of patients who are undernourished, patients with proven inflammatory bowel disease, following total gastrectomy, dysphagia, bowel fistulae, disease-related malnutrition continuous ambulatory peritoneal dialysis (CAPD), and haemodialysis. Not to be prescribed for any child under one year; use with caution for young children up to five years of age.

BORDERLINE SUBSTANCES

FRESUBIN LIQUID AND SIP FEEDS
For use as the sole source of nutrition or as a necessary nutritional supplement prescribed on medical grounds for:
Short bowel syndrome, intractable malabsorption, pre-operative preparation of patients who are undernourished, patients with proven inflamatory bowel disease, following total gastrectomy, dysphagia, bowel fistulae, disease-related malnutrition and Refsum's Disease. Not to be prescribed for any child under one year; use with caution for young children up to five years of age.

FRESUBIN PROTEIN ENERGY DRINK
As a necessary nutritional supplement prescribed on medical grounds for:
Short bowel syndrome, intractable malabsorption, pre-operative preparation of patients who are undernourished, patients with proven inflammatory bowel disease, following total gastrectomy, dysphagia, bowel fistulae, disease-related malnutrition continuous ambulatory peritoneal dialysis (CAPD), and haemodialysis. Not to be prescribed for any child under one year; use with caution for young children up to five years of age.

FRESUBIN 1000 COMPLETE
For use as the sole source of nutrition or as a necessary nutritional supplement prescribed on medical grounds for:
Short bowel syndrome, intractable malabsorption, pre-operative preparation of patients who are undernourished, patients with proven inflammatory bowel disease, following total gastrectomy, dysphagia, bowel fistula, disease-related malnutrition. Not to be prescribed for any child under one year; use with caution for young children up to five years of age.

FRESUBIN 1200 COMPLETE
For use as the sole source of nutrition or as a necessary nutritional supplement prescribed on medical grounds for:
Short bowel syndrome, intractable malabsorption, pre-operative preparation of patients who are undernourished, patients with proven inflammatory bowel disease, following total gastrectomy, bowel fistulae, disease-related malnutrition. Not to be prescribed for any child under five years of age.

FRUCTOSE
Proven glucose/galactose intolerance.

GADSBYS GLUTEN FREE PRODUCTS
See: Gluten-Free Products.

GALACTOMIN 17
Proven lactose intolerance in pre-school children, galactosaemia and galactokinase deficiency.

GALACTOMIN 19 (FRUCTOSE FORMULA)
Glucose plus galactose intolerance.

GENERAID
Patients with chronic liver disease and/or porto-hepatic encephalopathy.

GENERAID PLUS
Children over one year of age with hepatic disorders.

GLANDOSANE
Patients suffering from xerostomia (dry mouth) as a result of having or having undergone radiotherapy or sicca syndrome.

GLUCOSE
Glycogen storage disease and sucrose/isomaltose intolerance.

GLUTAFIN GLUTEN-FREE PRODUCTS
See: Gluten-Free Products.

GLUTAFIN SELECT GLUTEN-FREE PRODUCTS
See: Gluten-Free Products.

GLUTANO GLUTEN-FREE PRODUCTS
See: Gluten-Free Products.

BORDERLINE SUBSTANCES

GLUTEN-FREE PRODUCTS (Not necessarily low-protein, lactose or sucrose free).
* For established gluten enteropathy with coexisting established wheat sensitivity only

Aproten gluten-free flour
Arnott's gluten-free rice cookies
Baker's Delight wheat, gluten and dairy free bread
Barkat brown rice pizza crust
Barkat gluten-free bread mix
Barkat gluten-free brown rice bread
Barkat gluten-free wheat-free multi grain bread
Barkat gluten-free white rice bread
Barkat white rice pizza crust
Bi-Aglut gluten-free biscuits
Bi-Aglut gluten-free cracker toast
Bi-Aglut gluten-free crackers
Bi-Aglut gluten-free pastas (fusilli, lasagne, macaroni, penne, spaghetti)
Dietary Specials gluten-free brown bread mix
Dietary Specials gluten-free corn bread mix
Dietary Specials gluten-free cracker bread
Dietary Specials gluten-free digestive biscuits
Dietary Specials gluten-free fibre mix
Dietary Specials gluten-free high fibre crackers
Dietary Specials gluten-free hoops tea biscuits
Dietary Specials gluten-free multigrain sliced loaf
Dietary Specials gluten-free part baked bloomer
Dietary Specials gluten-free part baked brown loaf
Dietary Specials gluten-free part baked white baguettes
Dietary Specials gluten-free part baked white buns
Dietary Specials gluten-free part baked white loaf
Dietary Specials gluten-free part baked white rolls
Dietary Specials gluten-free pasta (fusilli, penne, spaghetti)
Dietary Specials gluten-free pastry mix
Dietary Specials gluten-free pizza bases
Dietary Specials gluten-free savory biscuits
Dietary Specials gluten-free sweet biscuits
Dietary Specials gluten-free white bread mix
Dietary Specials gluten-free white cake mix
Dietary Specials gluten-free white mix
Dietary Specials gluten-free white multigrain sliced loaf
Ener-G gluten-free brown rice bread
Ener-G gluten-free brown rice pasta (lasagne, macaroni, spaghetti)
Ener-G gluten-free cookies (vanilla flavour)
Ener-G gluten-free dinner rolls
*   Ener-G gluten-free pizza bases
Ener-G gluten-free rice loaf
Ener-G gluten-free rice pasta (cannelloni, lasagne, macaroni, shells, small shells, spaghetti, tagliatelle, vermicelli)
Ener-G gluten-free Seattle brown loaf
*   Ener-G gluten-free Seattle brown rolls (hamburger)
*   Ener-G gluten-free Seattle brown rolls (hot dog)
*   Ener-G gluten-free six flour loaf
Ener-G gluten-free tapioca bread
Ener-G gluten-free white rice bread
Ener-G gluten-free xanthan gum
Gadsbys gluten-free white bread
Gadsbys gluten-free white bread flour
Gadsbys gluten-free white rolls
Gadsbys gluten-free white sliced bread
*   Glutafin Crisp Bread
Glutafin gluten-free biscuits
Glutafin gluten-free crackers

BORDERLINE SUBSTANCES

GLUTEN-FREE PRODUCTS (Not necessarily low-protein, lactose or sucrose free).
* For established gluten enteropathy with coexisting established wheat sensitivity only

      Glutafin gluten-free digestive biscuits
      Glutafin gluten-free high fibre crackers
      Glutafin gluten-free pasta (lasagne, long-cut spaghetti, macaroni penne, shells, spirals, tagliatelle nests)
      Glutafin gluten-free pizza base
      Glutafin gluten-free savoury biscuits
      Glutafin gluten-free savoury shorts
      Glutafin gluten-free shortbread biscuit
      Glutafin gluten-free sweet biscuits (without chocolate or sultanas)
      Glutafin gluten-free tea biscuits
  * Glutafin gluten-free wheat-free bread mix
  * Glutafin gluten-free wheat-free cake mix
  * Glutafin gluten-free wheat-free fibre bread mix
      Glutafin gluten-free wheat-free fibre loaf (sliced and unsliced)
      Glutafin gluten-free wheat-free fibre mix
      Glutafin gluten-free wheat-free fibre rolls
  * Glutafin gluten-free wheat-free pastry mix
      Glutafin gluten-free wheat-free white loaf (sliced and unsliced)
      Glutafin gluten-free wheat-free white mix
      Glutafin gluten-free wheat-free white rolls
      Glutafin Select gluten-free bread mix
      Glutafin Select gluten-free cake mix
      Glutafin Select gluten-free fibre bread mix
      Glutafin Select gluten-free fibre loaf (sliced and unsliced)
      Glutafin Select gluten-free fibre mix
      Glutafin Select gluten-free fibre rolls
      Glutafin Select gluten-free fresh bread
      Glutafin Select gluten-free part-baked fibre loaf
      Glutafin Select gluten-free part-baked fibre rolls
      Glutafin Select gluten-free part-baked long fibre rolls
      Glutafin Select gluten-free part-baked long white rolls
      Glutafin Select gluten-free part-baked white loaf
      Glutafin Select gluten-free part-baked white rolls
      Glutafin Select gluten-free pastry mix
      Glutafin Select gluten-free seeded loaf
      Glutafin Select gluten-free white loaf (sliced and unsliced)
      Glutafin Select gluten-free white mix
      Glutafin Select gluten-free white rolls
      Glutano gluten-free biscuits
      Glutano gluten-free crackers, crackers snack pack
      Glutano gluten-free crispbread
      Glutano gluten-free flour mix
      Glutano gluten-free par-baked (baguette, rolls, white sliced bread)
      Glutano gluten-free pasta (animal shapes, macaroni, spaghetti, spirals, tagliatelle)
      Glutano gluten-free shortcake rings
      Glutano gluten-free wheat-free digestive biscuit
      Glutano gluten-free wholemeal bread (sliced), wholemeal bread (sliced) snack pack
      Glutano gluten-free wholemeal par-baked bread
      Gratis gluten-free pasta (alphabets, macaroni, shells, short cut spaghetti, spirals)
      Heron Foods Organic gluten-free bread mix
      Heron Foods Organic gluten-free hi-fibre bread mix
  * Heron Foods Organic gluten-free wheat-free bread/cake mix
  * Heron Foods Organic gluten-free wheat-free hi-fibre bread mix
      Innovative Solutions brown rice flour
      Innovative Solutions potato flour
      Innovative Solutions tapioca flour
      Innovative Solutions white rice flour
      Juvela gluten-free bread rolls

XV

BORDERLINE SUBSTANCES

GLUTEN-FREE PRODUCTS (Not necessarily low-protein, lactose or sucrose free).
* For established gluten enteropathy with coexisting established wheat sensitivity only

Juvela gluten-free crispbread
Juvela gluten-free digestive biscuits
Juvela gluten-free fibre bread rolls
Juvela gluten-free fibre loaf (sliced and unsliced)
Juvela gluten-free fibre mix
Juvela gluten-free fresh sliced white loaf
Juvela gluten-free harvest mix
Juvela gluten-free lasagne
Juvela gluten-free loaf (sliced and unsliced)
Juvela gluten-free mix
Juvela gluten-free part-baked bread rolls
Juvela gluten-free part-baked fibre bread rolls
Juvela gluten-free part-baked fibre loaf
Juvela gluten-free part-baked loaf
Juvela gluten-free pasta (fusilli, lasagne, macaroni, spaghetti)
Juvela gluten-free pizza base
Juvela gluten-free savoury biscuits
Juvela gluten-free sweet biscuits
Juvela gluten-free tagliatelle
Juvela gluten-free tea biscuits
Lifestyle gluten-free bread rolls
Lifestyle gluten-free brown bread
Lifestyle gluten-free high fibre bread
Lifestyle gluten-free high fibre bread rolls
Lifestyle gluten-free white bread
Livwell sliced brown bread
Livwell sliced white bread
Livwell white baguette
Livwell white rolls
Orgran bread mix
Orgran gluten-free buckwheat spirals pasta
Orgran gluten-free corn lasagne, corn spaghetti, corn spirals pasta
Orgran gluten-free crispbread corn, crispbread rice
Orgran gluten-free organic brown rice spirals
Orgran gluten-free pizza & pastry mix
Orgran gluten-free rice spaghetti, rice spirals
Orgran gluten-free rice and millet spirals
Orgran gluten-free ris o'mais (rice and maize) lasagne, ris o'mais spaghetti, ris o'mais spirals
Orgran gluten-free split pea & soya pasta shells
Orgran ris 'o' mais macaroni
Orgran self-raising flour
Pleniday gluten-free bread (sliced country loaf, petit pain (par-baked), rustic loaf sliced)
Pleniday gluten-free pasta (conchigli, penne, rigate, tagliatelli)
Pleniday sesame rolls
Polial gluten-free biscuits
* Proceli brown rice bread
* Proceli pizza bases
* Proceli sliced white bread
Pure gluten-free blended flour
Pure xantham gum
Rite-Diet gluten-free fibre mix
Rite-Diet gluten-free fibre rolls
Rite-Diet gluten-free fibre bread (sliced and unsliced)
Rite-Diet gluten-free white bread (sliced and unsliced)
Rite-Diet gluten-free white mix
Riet-Diet gluten-free white rolls
Rite-Diet gluten-free part-baked fibre loaf
Rite-Diet gluten-free 2 part-baked long fibre rolls
Rite-Diet gluten-free 2 part-baked long white rolls

BORDERLINE SUBSTANCES

GLUTEN-FREE PRODUCTS (Not necessarily low-protein, lactose or sucrose free).
* For established gluten enteropathy with coexisting established wheat sensitivity only
>   Rite-Diet gluten-free part-baked white loaf
>   Schar gluten-free biscuits
>   Schar gluten-free bread
>   Schar gluten-free bread mix
>   Schar gluten-free bread rolls
>   Schar gluten-free brown bread ertha
>   Schar gluten-free cake mix
>   Schar gluten-free crackers
>   Schar gluten-free cracker toast
>   Schar gluten-free crispbread
>   Schar gluten-free flour mix for cooking
>   Schar gluten-free french bread (baguette)
>   Schar gluten-free frollini tea biscuits
>   Schar gluten-free grissini breadsticks
>   Schar gluten-free pasta (alphabet pasta, bavette, fusilli, lasagne, macaroni, penne, spaghetti)
>   Schar gluten-free pizza base
>   Schar gluten-free savoy biscuits
>   Schar gluten-free wheat-free biscottini
>   Schar gluten-free wheat-free bread buns (white)
>   Schar gluten-free wheat-free lunch rolls
>   Schar gluten-free white bread
>   Schar gluten-free wholemeal bread
>   Schar gluten-free wholemeal flour mix
>   Sunnyvale gluten-free mixed grain sourdough bread
>   Tritamyl gluten-free brown bread mix
>   Tritamyl gluten-free flour mix
>   Tritamyl gluten-free white bread mix
>   Ultra gluten-free baguette
>   Ultra gluten-free bread
>   Ultra gluten-free bread rolls
>   Ultra gluten-free crackerbread
>   Ultra gluten-free high fibre bread
>   Ultra gluten-free pasta (tagliatelle, spaghetti, penne, fusili)
>   Ultra gluten-free pizza base
>   Ultra gluten-free sweet biscuits
>   Valpiform gluten-free and wheat free pastry mix
>   Valpiform gluten-free bread mix
>   Valpiform gluten-free country loaf
>   Valpiform gluten-free crac'form toast
>   Valpiform gluten-free crisp rolls
>   Valpiform gluten-free maxi baguettes
>   Valpiform gluten-free pastry mix
>   Valpiform gluten-free petites baguettes
>   Wellfoods gluten-free burger buns
>   Wellfoods gluten-free flour alternative
>   Wellfoods gluten-free loaf
>   Wellfoods gluten-free pizza bases
>   Wellfoods gluten-free rolls
>   Wellfoods gluten-free sliced loaf

>   For established gluten enteropathy

GRATIS GLUTEN-FREE PRODUCTS
>   See: Gluten-Free Products

HARIFEN PRODUCTS
>   See: Low Protein Products

BORDERLINE SUBSTANCES

HCU EXPRESS (formerly VITAFLO - HCU EXPRESS)
A nutritional supplement designed for patients with Homocystinuria (HCU); this is a Methionine-free powder protein substitute approved for patients over 8 years old.

HCU GEL (formerly VITAFLO HCU GEL)
A methionine free protein substitute for use in the dietary management of homocystinuria in children between the ages 12 months and 10 years of age.

HCU-LV (UNFLAVOURED AND TROPICAL FLAVOUR)
For the dietary management of hypermethioninaemia or vitamin B6 non-responsive homocystinuria in children over 8 years and adults.

HERON FOODS
See: Gluten-Free Products

INFATRINI
Disease-related malnutrition, malabsorption, and growth failure in infancy.

INFASOY
Proven lactose and associated sucrose intolerance in pre-school children, galactokinase deficiency, glactosaemia and proven whole cows milk sensitivity.

INNOVATIVE SOLUTIONS PRODUCTS
See: Gluten-Free Products

INSTANT CAROBEL
Thickening feeds in the treatment of vomiting.

ISOMIL
Proven lactose intolerance in pre-school children, galactokinase deficiency, galactasaemia and proven whole cows milk sensitivity.

ISOSOURCE ENERGY
For use as the sole source of nutrition or as a necessary nutritional supplement prescribed on medical grounds for:
Short bowel syndrome, intractable malabsorption, pre-operative preparation of patients who are undernourished, patients with proven inflammatory bowel disease, following total gastrectomy, dysphagia, bowel fistulae, disease-related malnutrition. Not to be prescribed for any child under one year; use with caution for young children up to fives years of age.

ISOSOURCE ENERGY FIBRE
A high energy nutritionally complete enteral tube feed liquid with fibre presribed on medical grounds for:-
Dietary management of patients with short bowel syndrome, intractable malabsorption, pre-operative preparation of patients who are undernourished, inflammatory bowel disease, following total gastrectomy, dysphagia and disease related malnutrition. It can also be recommended for patients requiring high energy intake or a fluid restricted diet.

ISOSOURCE FIBRE
For use as the sole source of nutrition or as a necessary nutritional supplement prescribed on medical grounds for:
Short bowel syndrome, intractable malabsorption, pre-operative preparation of patients who are undernourished, patients with proven inflammatory bowel disease, following total gastrectomy, dysphagia, bowel fistulae, disease-related malnutrition. Not to be prescribed for any child under one year; use with caution for young children up to fives years of age.

ISOSOURCE JUNIOR
A nutritionally complete feed approved for disease related malnutrition, short bowel syndrome, intractable malabsorption, pre-operative preparation of patients who are malnourished, proven inflammatory bowel disease, following total gastrectomy, dysphagia and growth failure from 1 to 6 years of age and 8 to 20kg.

ISOSOURCE STANDARD
For use as the sole source of nutrition or as a necessary nutritional supplement prescribed on medical grounds for:
Short bowel syndrome, intractable malabsorption, pre-operative preparation of patients who are undernourished, patients with proven inflammatory bowel disease, following total gastrectomy, dysphagia, bowel fistulae, disease-related malnutrition. Not to be prescribed for any child under one year; use with caution for young children up to fives years of age.

BORDERLINE SUBSTANCES

JEVITY
> For use as the sole source of nutrition or as a necessary nutritional supplement prescribed on medical grounds for:
> Short bowel syndrome, intractable malabsorption, pre-operative preparation of patients who are undernourished, patients with proven inflammatory bowel disease, following total gastrectomy, dysphagia, disease-related malnutrition. Not to be prescribed for any child under one year; use with caution for young children up to five years of age.

JEVITY PLUS
> For use as the sole source of nutrition or as a necessary nutritional supplement prescribed on medical grounds for:
> Short bowel syndrome, intractable malabsorption, pre-operative preparation of patients who are undernourished, patients with proven inflammatory bowel disease, following total gastrectomy, dysphagia, bowel fistulae, disease-related malnutrition. Not recommended for any child under ten years of age.

JEVITY PROMOTE
> For use as the sole source of nutrition or as a necessary nutritional supplement prescribed on medical grounds for:
> Short bowel syndrome, intractable malabsorption, pre-operative preparation of patients who are undernourished, patients with proven inflammatory bowel disease, following total gastrectomy, dysphagia, bowel fistulae, disease-related malnutrition. Not to be prescribed for children less than two years of age. Use with caution in children under ten years of age.

JEVITY 1.5 KCAL
> For use as the sole source of nutrition or as a necessary nutritional supplement prescribed on medical grounds for:
> Short bowel syndrome, intractable malabsorption, pre-operative preparation of patients who are undernourished, patients with proven inflammatory bowel disease, following total gastrectomy, dysphagia, disease-related malnutrition, bowel fistulae.

JUVELA GLUTEN-FREE PRODUCTS
> See: Gluten-Free Products.

JUVELA LOW-PROTEIN PRODUCTS
> See: Low-Protein Products

KEROMASK
> See: Covering creams.

KINDERGEN
> Complete nutritional support or supplementary feeding for infants and children with chronic renal failure who are receiving peritoneal rapid overnight dialysis.

L-ARGININE SUPPLEMENT FOR UREA CYCLE DISORDERS (S.H.S.)
> Urea cycle disorders other than arginase deficiency, such as hyperammonaemia types I and II, citrullaemia, arginossuccinic aciduria, and deficiency of N-acetyl glutamate synthetase.

LIFESTYLE GLUTEN-FREE PRODUCTS
> See: Gluten-Free Products.

LIQUIGEN
> Steatorrhoea associated with cystic fibrosis of the pancreas, intestinal lymphangiectasia, surgery of the intestine, chronic liver disease, liver cirrhosis, other proven malabsorption syndromes, a ketogenic diet in the management of epilepsy and in type 1 hyperlipoproteinaemia.

LIVWELL PRODUCTS
> See: Gluten Free Products

LOCASOL
> Calcium intolerance

LOPHLEX (UNFLAVOURED, ORANGE FLAVOUR AND BERRY FLAVOUR)

LOPHLEX LQ (ORANGE, BERRY AND CITRUS FLAVOURS)
> For use in the dietary management of proven phenylketonuria in older children (over 8 years) and adults (includes use in pregnant women).

LOPROFIN LOW-PROTEIN PRODUCTS
> See: Low-Protein Products

XV

BORDERLINE SUBSTANCES

LOPROFIN PKU DRINK
  Phenylketonuria

LOW-PROTEIN PRODUCTS
        Aproten low-protein biscuits
        Aproten low-protein bread mix
        Aproten low-protein crispbread
        Aproten low-protein pastas (anellini, ditalini, rigatini, spaghetti, tagliatelle)
        Ener-G low-protein egg replacer
        Ener-G low-protein pasta (lasagne, macaroni, large shells, small shells, spaghetti)
        Ener-G low-protein rice bread
        Fate low-protein all-purpose mix
        Fate low-protein cake mix
        Fate low-protein chocolate flavour cake mix
        Fate low-protein potato mix
        Harifen Low Protein Cracker Toast
        Harifen White Chip Cookies
        Juvela low-protein bread rolls
        Juvela low-protein chocolate chip, cinnamon and orange flavour cookies
        Juvela low-protein loaf (sliced and unsliced)
        Juvela low-protein mix
        Juvela low-protein pizza base
        Loprofin low-protein breakfast cereal
        Loprofin low-protein chocolate flavour cream biscuits
        Loprofin low-protein chocolate, orange and vanilla flavour cream wafers
        Loprofin low-protein cinnamon and chocolate chip cookies
        Loprofin low-protein crackers
        Loprofin low-protein crunch bar
        Loprofin low-protein egg replacer
        Loprofin low-protein egg white replacer
        Loprofin low-protein fibre bread (sliced and unsliced)
        Loprofin low-protein herb crackers
        Loprofin low-protein loaf (sliced and unsliced)
        Loprofin low-protein mix
        Loprofin low-protein part baked rolls
        Loprofin low-protein pasta (long-cut spaghetti, macaroni penne, spirals, vermicelli, lasagne)
        Loprofin low-protein rice
        Loprofin low-protein snack pot
        Loprofin low-protein sweet biscuits
        Loprofin low-protein white bread rolls
        Milupa low-protein drink
        PK Foods Aminex low-protein biscuits
        PK Foods Aminex low-protein cookies
        PK Foods Aminex low-protein rusks
        PK Foods low-protein crispbread
        PK Foods low-protein pasta spirals
        PK Foods low-protein white sliced bread
        PKU-Gel
        Promin low-protein burger mix
        Promin low-protein cous cous
        Promin low-protein hot breakfast (apple & cinnamon, banana, chocolate and original flavours)
        Promin low-protein imitation rice
        Promin low-protein imitation rice pudding (apple, banana, strawberry and original flavours)
        Promin low-protein lasagne sheets
        Promin low-protein pasta (alphabets, macaroni, shells, short cut spaghetti, spirals)
        Promin low-protein pasta in sauce (cheese and broccoli, tomato pepper and herb flavours)
        Promin low-protein pastameal
        Promin low-protein tricolour pasta (alphabets, shells, spirals)
        Rite-Diet low-protein baking mix.
        Rite-Diet low-protein flour mix
        Ultra low-protein canned brown bread
        Ultra low-protein canned white bread

BORDERLINE SUBSTANCES

LOW-PROTEIN PRODUCTS

>Ultra PKU biscuits
>Ultra PKU bread
>Ultra PKU cookies
>Ultra PKU flour mix
>Ultra PKU pizza base
>Ultra PKU savoy biscuits
>Valpiform low-protein cookies with chocolate nuggets and hazelnut flavour
>Valpiform low-protein savory bites (herbs flavour)
>Valpiform low-protein savory bites (tomato flavour)
>Valpiform low-protein shortbread biscuits
>Vita-Bite
>Inherited metabolic disorders, renal or liver failure requiring a low-protein diet

L-TYROSINE SUPPLEMENT FOR PHENYLKETONURIA
Maternal Phenylketonurics who have low plasma tyrosine levels

LUBORANT SALIVA REPLACEMENT
Patients suffering from xerostomia (dry mouth) as a result of having or having undergone radiotherapy or sicca syndrome.

MAPLEFLEX (UNFLAVOURED)
A leucine, isoleucine and valine free mix for use in the dietary management of MSUD approved for patients aged between 1 and 10 years.

MAXIJUL LIQUID

MAXIJUL SUPER SOLUBLE
Disease related malnutrion, malabsorption states or other conditions requiring fortification with a high or readily available carbohydrate supplement.

MAXISORB
Biochemically proven or clinical evidence of protein deficiency, and if recommended by a renal unit.

MCT FEED STEP 1
For the dietary management of fat malabsorption in disorders of fatty acid oxidation.

MCT PEPDITE

MCT PEPDITE 1+
Disorders in which a high intake of MCT is beneficial

MEDIUM-CHAIN TRIGLYCERIDE (MCT) OIL
Steatorrhoea associated with cystic fibrosis of the pancreas, intestinal lymphangiectasia, surgery of the intestine, chronic liver disease, liver cirrhosis, other proven malabsorption syndromes, in a ketogenic diet in the management of epilepsy and in type 1 hyperlipoproteinaemia.

METABOLIC MINERAL MIXTURE
Mineral supplement in synthetic diets.

MILUPA LOW-PROTEIN DRINK
Inherited disorders of amino acid metabolism in childhood.

MINAPHLEX FLAVOURED & UNFLAVOURED
For use in the dietary management of children with phenylketonuria.

MODULEN IBD
For the sole source of nutrition during the active phase of Crohn's disease, and for nutritional support during the remission phase in patients who are malnourished. Not to be prescribed for any child under one year; use with caution for young children up to five years of age. This product may be flavoured with NESTLE NUTRITION FLAVOUR MIX.

MONOGEN
Long chain acyl-coa dehydrogenase deficiency (LCAD), carnitine palmitayl transferase deficiency (CPTD), and primary and secondary lipoprotein lipase deficiency

XV

BORDERLINE SUBSTANCES

MSUD AID III
Maple syrup urine disease (MSUD) and related conditions when it is necessary to limit the intake of branched chain amino acids

MSUD ANALOG (formerly ANALOG MSUD)
Maple Syrup Urine Disease

MSUD EXPRESS (formerly VITAFLO - MSUD EXPRESS)
This is a protein substitute for maple syrup urine disease in children over the age of 8.

MSUD GEL
For use in the dietary management of Maple syrup urine disease in children aged between 1 and 10 years.

MSUD MAXAMAID

MSUD MAXAMUM
Maple syrup urine disease

NEOCATE

NEOCATE ACTIVE (UNFLAVOURED AND BLACKCURRANT FLAVOUR)

NEOCATE ADVANCE (UNFLAVOURED, BANANA VANILLA FLAVOUR AND STRAWBERRY VANILLA FLAVOUR)
Proven whole protein intolerance, short bowel syndrome, intractable malabsorption, and other gastrointestinal disorders where an elemental diet is specifically indicated.

NEPRO (CAN, READY TO HANG AND TETRAPAK)
Patients with chronic renal failure who are on haemodialysis or complete ambulatory peritoneal dialysis (CAPD), or patients with cirrhosis or other conditions requiring a high energy, low fluid, low electrolyte diet.

NESTARGEL
Thickening of foods in the treatment of vomiting.

NESTLE NUTRITION FLAVOUR MIX
For use with VANILLA-FLAVOURED PEPTAMEN and MODULEN IBD.

NOVASOURCE FORTE
For use as the sole source of nutrition, or as a necessary nutritional supplement prescribed on medical grounds for:
Short bowel syndrome, intractable malabsorption, pre-operative preparation of patients who are undernourished, patients with proven inflammatory bowel disease, following total gastrectomy, dysphagia, bowel fistulae, disease-realted malnutrition, neoplasia-related cachexia. Not to be prescribed for any child under one year; use with caution for young children up to five years of age.

NOVASOURCE GI CONTROL
For use as the sole source of nutrition, or as a necessary nutritional supplement prescribed on medical grounds for:
Short bowel syndrome,intractable malabsorption, pre-operative preparation of patients who are undernourished, patients with proven inflammatary bowel disease, following total gastrectomy, dysphagia, bowel fistulae, disease-related malnutrition. Not to be prescribed for any child under one year, use with caution for young children up to five years of age.

NUTILIS
Thickening of foods in dysphagia. Not to be prescribed for children under one year old except in cases of failure to thrive.

NUTRAMIGEN 1
Disaccharide and/or whole protein intolerance where additional MCT is not indicated

NUTRAMIGEN 2
Established whole protein sensitivity and/or disaccharide intolerance in patients over 6 months in age.

NUTRINI
For use as the sole source of nutrition or as a necessary nutritional supplement prescribed on medical grounds for:
Short bowel syndrome, intractable malabsorption, pre-operative preparation of patients who are undernourished, dysphagia, bowel fistulae, disease-related malnutrition and/or growth failure. Not to be prescribed for any child under one year.

BORDERLINE SUBSTANCES

NUTRINI ENERGY
For use as the sole source of nutrition or as a necessary nutritional supplement prescribed on medical grounds for:
Short bowel syndrome, intractable malabsorption, pre-operative preparation of patients who are undernourished, patients with proven inflammatory bowel disease, following total gastrectomy, dysphagia, bowel fistulae, disease-related malnutrition and/or growth failure. Not to be prescribed for any child under one year.

NUTRINI ENERGY MULTIFIBRE
It is indicated for:
Short bowel syndrome, intractable malabsorption, pre operative preparation of undernourished patients, total gastrectomy, dysphagia, disease related malnutrition and growth failure.

NUTRINI LOW ENERGY MULTIFIBRE
It is indicated for:
Short bowel syndrome, intractable malabsorption, pre operative preparation of undernourished patients, total gastrectomy, dysphagia, disease related malnutrition and growth failure.

NUTRINI MULTIFIBRE
For use as the sole source of nutrition or as a necessary nutritional supplement prescribed on medical grounds for:
Short bowel syndrome, intractable malabsorption, pre-operative preparation of patients who are undernourished, patients with proven inflammatory bowel disease , following total gastrectomy, dysphagia, bowel fistulae, disease-related malnutrition and/or growth failure. Not to be prescribed for any child under one year.

NUTRIPREM 2

NUTRIPREM 2 LIQUID
Suitable for catch-up growth in pre-term infants (ie less than 35 weeks at birth) and small for gestational age infants, until 6 months corrected age.

NUTRISON 1000 COMPLETE MULTI FIBRE
For dietary management of disease related malnutrition in patients with low energy and/or low fluid requirements

NUTRISON 1200 COMPLETE MULTI FIBRE
Approved for short bowel syndrome, intractable malabsorption, pre-operative preparation of patients who are undernourished, proven inflammatory bowel disease, following total gastrectomy, disease-related malnutrition and dysphagia.

NUTRISON ENERGY
As a necessary nutritional supplement prescribed on medical grounds for:
Short bowel syndrome, intractable malabsorption, pre-operative preparation of patients who are undernourished, patients with proven inflammatory bowel disease, following total gastrectomy, dysphagia, bowel fistulae, disease-related malnutrition. Not to be prescribed for any child under one year; use with caution for young children up to five years of age.

NUTRISON ENERGY MULTIFIBRE
For use as the sole source of nutrition or as a necessary nutritional supplement prescribed on medical grounds for:
Short bowel syndrome, intractable malabsorption, pre-operative preparation of patients who are undernourished, patients with proven inflammatory bowel disease, following total gastrectomy, dysphagia, bowel fistulae, disease-related malnutrition. Not to be prescribed for any child under one year; use with caution for young children up to five years of age.

NUTRISON MCT
As a necessary nutritional supplement prescribed on medical grounds for:
Short bowel syndrome, intractable malabsorption, pre-operative preparation of patients who are undernourished, patients with proven inflammatory bowel disease, following total gastrectomy, dysphagia, bowel fistulae, disease-related malnutrition. Not to be prescribed for any child under one year; use with caution for young children up to five years of age.

BORDERLINE SUBSTANCES

NUTRISON MULTIFIBRE
For use as the sole source of nutrition or as a necessary nutritional supplement prescribed on medical grounds for:
Short bowel syndrome, intractable malabsorption, pre-operative preparation of patients who are undernourished, patients with proven inflammatory bowel disease, following total gastrectomy, dysphagia, bowel fistulae, disease-related malnutrition. Not to be prescribed for any child under one year; use with caution for young children up to five years of age.

NUTRISON PROTEIN PLUS

NUTRISON PROTEIN PLUS MULTIFIBRE
For use as dietary management of disease related malnutrition.

NUTRISON SOYA
For use as the sole source of nutrition or as a necessary nutritional supplement prescribed on medical grounds for:
Short bowel syndrome, intractable malabsorption, pre-operative preparation of patients who are undernourished, patients with proven inflammatory bowel disease, following total gastrectomy, dysphagia, bowel fistulae, disease-related malnutrition, cows milk protein and lactose intolerance. Not to be prescribed for any child under one year; use with caution for young children up to five years of age.

NUTRISON STANDARD
For use as the sole source of nutrition or as a necessary nutritional supplement prescribed on medical grounds for:
Short bowel syndrome, intractable malabsorption, pre-operative preparation of patients who are undernourished, patients with proven inflammatory bowel disease, following total gastrectomy, dysphagia, bowel fistulae, disease-related malnutrition. Not to be prescribed for any child under one year; use with caution for young children up to five years of age.

ORALBALANCE DRY MOUTH SALIVA REPLACEMENT GEL
See: Biotene Oralbalance

ORGRAN GLUTEN-FREE PRODUCTS
See: Gluten-Free Products

OSMOLITE
For use as the sole source of nutrition or as a necessary nutritional supplement prescribed on medical grounds for:
Short bowel syndrome, intractable malabsorption, pre-operative preparation of patients who are undernourished, patients with proven inflammatory bowel disease, following total gastrectomy, dysphagia, bowel fistulae, disease-related malnutrition. Not to be prescribed for any child under one year; use with caution for young children up to five years of age.

OSMOLITE PLUS
For use as the sole source of nutrition or as a necessary nutritional supplement prescribed on medical grounds for:
Short bowel syndrome, intractable malabsorption, pre-operative preparation of patients who are undernourished, patients with proven inflammatory bowel disease, following total gastrectomy, dysphagia, bowel fistulae, disease-related malnutrition. Not recommended for any child under ten years of age.

PAEDIASURE
For use as the sole source of nutrition or as a necessary nutritional supplement prescribed on medical grounds for children aged 1-10 years or 8-30kg for:
Short bowel syndrome, intractable malabsorption, pre-operative preparation of patients who are undernourished, dysphagia, bowel fistulae, disease-related malnutrition and/or growth failure. Not to be prescribed for any child under one year.

PAEDIASURE PLUS
For use as the sole source of nutrition, or as a necessary nutritional supplement prescribed on medical grounds for children aged 1-10 years or 8-30kg for:
Short bowel syndrome, intractable malasorption, pre-operative preparation of patients who are undernourished, dysphagia, bowel fistulae, disease-related malnutrition, and/or growth failure. Not to be prescribed for any child under one year.

BORDERLINE SUBSTANCES

PAEDIASURE PLUS WITH FIBRE (TETRAPAK AND TUBE FEED)
As a sole source of nutrition, or as a nutritional supplement for children aged 1-10 years or 8-30kg with disease-related malnutrition and/or growth failure, short bowel syndrome, intractable malabsorption, dysphagia, bowel fistulae, and for the pre-operative preparation of patients who are malnourished. Not to be prescribed for any child under one year.

PAEDIASURE WITH FIBRE
For use as the sole source of nutrition, or as a necessary nutritional supplement prescribed on medical grounds for children aged 1-10 years or 8-30kg for:
Short bowel syndrome, intractable malasorption, pre-operative preparation of patients who are undernourished, dysphagia, bowel fistulae, disease-realted malnutrition, and/or growth failure. Not to be prescribed for any child under one year.

PAEDIATRIC SERAVIT
Vitamin and mineral supplement in restrictive therapeutic diets in infants and children.

PEPDITE

PEPDITE 1+
Disaccharide and/or whole protein intolerance, or where amino acids or peptides are indicated in conjunction with MCT.

PEPDITE 1+ (BANANA FLAVOUR)
Whole protein intolerance, or where amino acids or peptides are indicated in conjunction with MCT.

PEPTAMEN (FLAVOURED AND UNFLAVOURED)
For use as the sole source of nutrition or as a necessary nutritional supplement prescribed on medical grounds for:
Short bowel syndrome, intractable malabsorption, patients with proven inflammatory bowel disease, bowel fistulae. Not to be prescribed for any child under one year; use with caution for young children up to five years of age. This product may be flavoured with NESTLE NUTRITION FLAVOUR MIX.

PEPTAMEN JUNIOR
For use as the sole source of nutrition or as a necessary nutritional supplement for children aged 1-10 years prescribed on medical grounds for:
Short bowel syndrome, intractable malabsorption, patients with proven inflammatory bowel disease, bowel fistulae.

PEPTI-JUNIOR
See: COW & GATE PEPTI-JUNIOR

PEPTISORB
For use as the sole source of nutrition or as a necessary nutritional supplement prescribed on medical grounds for:-
Short bowel syndrome, intractable malabsorption, patients with proven inflammatory bowel disease, bowel fistulae. Not to be prescribed for any child under one year; use with caution for young children up to five years of age.

PERATIVE
As a necessary nutritional supplement prescribed on medical grounds for:
Short bowel syndrome, intractable malabsorption, pre-operative preparation of patients who are undernourished, patients with proven inflammatory bowel disease, following total gastrectomy, bowel fistulae, disease-related malnutrition. Not to be prescribed for any child under five years of age.

PHLEXY-10 EXCHANGE SYSTEM (BAR, CAPSULES AND DRINK MIX)
Phenylketonuria

PHLEXY-10 TABLETS
For Phenylketonuria only

PHLEXY-VITS

PHLEXY-VITS TABLETS
For use as a vitamin and mineral component of restricted therapeutic diets for older children, from the age of around eleven years, and adults with phenylketonuria and similar amino acid abnormalities.

PK AID 4
Phenylketonuria

XV

BORDERLINE SUBSTANCES

PK FOODS LOW-PROTEIN PRODUCTS
See: Low-Protein Products

PK FOODS LOW-PROTEIN RANGE (FLOUR MIX, EGG REPLACER, CHOCOLATE CHIP COOKIES, CINNAMON COOKIES, ORANGE COOKIES, JELLY MIX DESSERT ORANGE FLAVOUR, JELLY MIX DESSERT CHERRY FLAVOUR)
Phenylketonuria

PKU 2 (MILUPA)
Phenylketonuria

PKU 3 (MILUPA)
Phenylketonuria (not normally to be prescribed for a child below about 8 months old.)

PKU COOLER 15 (formerly PKU EXPRESS COOLER)
For use in the dietary management of phenylketonuria.

PKU COOLER 20
For use in the dietary management of phenylketonuria.

PKU EXPRESS
Phenylketonuria

PKU EXPRESS COOLER
See: PKU COOLER 15

PKU-GEL
As part of the low-protein dietary management of phenylketonuria in children aged one to ten years. Not recommended for children under one year of age.

PKU START
For use in the dietary management of phenylketonuria.

PLENIDAY GLUTEN-FREE PRODUCTS
See: Gluten-Free Products.

POLIAL GLUTEN-FREE PRODUCTS
See: Gluten-Free Products.

POLYCAL LIQUID
Disease related malnutrition, malabsorption states or other conditions requiring fortification with a high or readily available carbohydrate supplement.

POLYCOSE POWDER
Disease related malnutrition, malabsorption states or other conditions requiring fortification with a high or readily available carbohydrate supplement.

PREGESTIMIL
Disaccharide and/or whole protein intolerance, or where amino acids or peptides are indicated in conjunction with MCT.

PREJOMIN (MILUPA)
Disaccharide and/or whole protein intolerance where additional MCT is not indicated

PREMCARE
Suitable for catch-up growth in pre-term infants (ie less than 35 weeks at birth) and small for gestational age infants, until 6 months post-natal age.

PRO-CAL
Disease-related malnutrition, malabsorption states or other conditions requiring fortification with a fat/carbohydrate supplement. Not to be prescribed for any child under one year; use with caution for young children up to five years of age.

PROCELI PRODUCTS
See: Gluten-Free Products

PROMIN LOW-PROTEIN PRODUCTS
See: Low-Protein Products

BORDERLINE SUBSTANCES

PRO-MOD
  Biochemically proven hypoproteinaemia.

PROSOBEE LIQUID AND POWDER
  Proven lactose and associated sucrose intolerance in pre-school children, glactokinase deficiency, galactosaemia and proven whole cows milk sensitivity.

PROSURE
  As a nutritional supplement for patients with pancreatic cancer.

PROSURE 500ml READY TO HANG
  As a nutritional supplement for patients with pancreatic cancer.

PROTIFAR
  Biochemically proven hypoproteinaemia.

PROVIDE XTRA
  As a necessary nutritional supplement prescribed on medical grounds for:
  Short bowel syndrome, intractable malabsorption, pre-operative preparation of patients who are undernourished, patients with proven inflammatory bowel disease, following total gastrectomy, dysphagia, bowel fistulae, disease-related malnutrition. Not to be prescribed for any child under one year; use with caution for young children up to five years of age.

PURE GLUTEN-FREE PRODUCTS
  See: Gluten-Free products

PURE XANTHAN GUM
  For use in the dietary management of gluten-sensitive enteropathies, including steatorrhoea due to gluten-sensitivity, coeliac disease, and dermatitis herpetiformis.

QUICKCAL
  Disease-related malnutrition, malabsorption states or other conditions requiring fortification with a fat/carbohydrate supplement. Not to be prescribed for any child under one year; use with caution for young children up to five years of age.

RECTIFIED SPIRIT
  Where the therapeutic qualities of alcohol are required rectified spirit (suitably flavoured and diluted) should be prescribed.

RENAMIL
  Chronic renal failure. Not suitable for infants and young children under one year of age.

RENAPRO
  Dialysis and hypoproteinaemia. Not suitable for infants and children under one year of age.

RENILON 7.5
  For use as a necessary nutritional supplement prescribed on medical grounds for:
  Short bowel syndrome, intractable malabsorption, pre-operative preparation of patients who are undernourished, patients with proven inflammatory bowel disease, following total gastrectomy, bowel fistulae, disease-related malnutrition. Not to be prescribed for any child under three years of age.

RESOURCE 2.0 FIBRE
  For use as the sole source of nutrition, or as a necessary nutritional supplement prescribed on medical grounds for:
  Short bowel syndrome, intractable malabsorption, pre-operative preparation of patients who are undernourished, patients with proven inflammatory bowel disease, following total gastrectomy, dysphagia, bowel fistulae, disease-related malnutrition. Not to be prescribed for any child under 6 years of age; use with caution for children up to ten years of age.

RESOURCE BENEFIBER
  As a necessary nutritional supplement prescribed on medical grounds for:
  Short bowel syndrome, intractable malabsorption, pre-operative preparation of patients who are undernourished, patients with proven inflammatory bowel disease, following total gastrectomy, bowel fistulae, disease-related malnutrition. Not to be prescribed for any child under five years of age.

XV

BORDERLINE SUBSTANCES

RESOURCE DESSERT FRUIT (APPLE, APPLE-PEACH, APPLE-STRAWBERRY)
As a necessary nutritional supplement prescribed on medical grounds for:
Short bowel syndrome, intractable malasorption, pre-operative preparation of patients who are undernourished, patients with proven inflammatory bowel disease, following total gastrectomy, dysphagia, bowel fistulae, disease-related malnutrition, continuous ambulatory peritoneal dialysis (CAPD) and haemodialysis. Not to be prescribed for any child under one year; use with caution for young children up to five years of age.

RESOURCE DESSERT ENERGY (formerly RESOURCE ENERGY DESSERT)
As a necessary nutritional supplement prescribed on medical grounds for:
Short bowel syndrome, intractable malasorption, pre-operative preparation of patients who are undernourished, patients with proven inflammatory bowel disease, following total gastrectomy, dysphagia, bowel fistulae, disease-related malnutrition, continuous ambulatory peritoneal dialysis (CAPD) and haemodialysis. Not to be prescribed for any child under one year; use with caution for young children up to five years of age.

RESOURCE ENERGY DESSERT
See: RESOURCE DESSERT ENERGY

RESOURCE FRUIT FLAVOUR DRINK
Nutritionally balanced medical food, formulated to prevent or correct malnutrition in patients requiring a non-milk tasting, lactose free and fat free nutritional supplement.

RESOURCE PROTEIN (FORMERLY RESOURCE PROTEIN EXTRA)
As a necessary nutritional supplement prescribed on medical grounds for:
Short bowel syndrome, intractable malasorption, pre-operative preparation of patients who are undernourished, patients with proven inflammatory bowel disease, following total gastrectomy, dysphagia, bowel fistulae and disease-related malnutrition suitable as a supplement for patients over 3 years, 1 to 3 units per day under appropriate medical/dietetic supervision.

RESOURCE PROTEIN EXTRA
See: RESOURCE PROTEIN

RESOURCE SHAKE NUTRITIONAL SUPPLEMENT
As a necessary nutritional supplement prescribed on medical grounds for:
Disease-related malnutrition, short bowel syndrome, intractable malabsorption, proven inflammatory bowel disease, bowel fistalae, dysphagia. May also be used for pre-operative preparation of undernourished patients and after total gastrectomy

RESOURCE SUPPORT
As a nutritional supplement for patients with pancreatic cancer.

RESOURCE THICKENED SQUASH AND RESOURCE READY THICKENED DRINKS
Dyphagia. Not suitable for infants and children under one year of age.

RESOURCE THICKENUP WITHOUT VITAMINS AND MINERALS
Thickening of foods in dysphagia. Not to be prescribed for children under three years of age.

RITE-DIET GLUTEN-FREE AND LOW-PROTEIN PRODUCTS
See: Gluten-Free and Low-Protein Products.

SALIVEZE

SALIVIX PASTILLES
Patients suffering from xerostomia (dry mouth) as a result of having or having undergone radiotherapy or sicca syndrome.

SCANDISHAKE MIX FLAVOURED AND UNFLAVOURED
Disease related malnutrition, malabsorption states or other conditions requiring fortification with a fat/carbohydrate supplement.

SCHAR GLUTEN-FREE PRODUCTS
See: Gluten-Free Products

SHS FLAVOUR MODJUL
For use with any unflavoured product based on peptides or amino acids.

SHS FLAVOUR SACHETS
For use with SHS unflavoured amino acid and peptide based products.

BORDERLINE SUBSTANCES

SLO DRINKS (ORANGE, BLACKCURRANT, LEMON AND PEACH FLAVOURS)
For the dietary management of dysphagia.

SMA HIGH ENERGY
Disease-related malnutrition, malabsorption and growth failure in infancy.

SMA LF
Proven lactose intolerance

SMA STAYDOWN
For use in significant reflux disease, for use not in excess of a 6 month period and not to be used in conjunction with any other thickener or antacid product.

SNO-PRO DRINK
Phenylketonuria, chronic renal failure, and other inborn errors of metabolism

SONDALIS 1.5 LIQUID FEED

SONDALIS FIBRELIQUID FEED

SONDALIS ISO LIQUID FEED
For use as the sole source of nutrition or as necessary nutritional supplements prescribed on medical grounds for:
Short bowel syndrome, intractable malabsorption, pre-operative preparation of patients who are undernourished, patients with proven inflammatory bowel disease, following total gastrectomy, dysphagia, bowel fistulae, disease-related malnutrition.
Not to be prescribed for any child under one year; use with caution for young children up to five years of age.

SPECTRABAN ULTRA
Protection from UV radiation in abnormal cutaneous photosensitivity resulting from genetic disorders or photodermatoses, including vitiligo and those resulting from radiotherapy; chronic or recurrent herpes simplex labialis.

SUNNYVALE PRODUCTS
See: Gluten-Free Products

SUNSENSE ULTRA (EGO)
Protection from UV radiation in abnormal cutaneous photosensitivity resulting from genetic disorders or photodermatoses, including vitiligo, and those resulting from radiotherapy; chronic or recurrent herpes simplex labialis.

SUPLENA LIQUID NUTRITION
Patients with chronic or acute renal failure who are not undergoing dialysis; patients with chronic or acute liver disease with fluid restriction; other conditions requiring a high energy, low protein, low electrolyte, low volume enteral feed.

SURVIMED OPD
As a necessary nutritional supplement prescribed on medical grounds for:
Short bowel syndrome, intractable malabsorption, pre-operative preparation of patients who are undernourished, patients with proven inflammatory bowel disease, following total gastrectomy, dysphagia, bowel fistulae, disease-related malnutrition and/or growth failure. Not to be prescribed for any child under one year; use with caution for young children up to five years of age.

TENTRINI

TENTRINI ENERGY
As indicated for:-
Short bowel syndrome, intractable malabsorption, pre operative preparation of undernourished patients, inflammatory bowel disease, total gastrectomy, bowel fistulae, dysphagia, disease related malnutrition and growth failure.

TENTRINI ENERGY MULTI FIBRE

TENTRINI MULTI FIBRE
As indicated for:-
Short bowel syndrome, intractable malabsorption, pre operative preparation of undernourished patients, inflammatory bowel disease, total gastrectomy, dysphagia, disease related malnutrition and growth failure.

XV

BORDERLINE SUBSTANCES

THICK AND EASY

THICK AND EASY DAIRY

THIXO-D
   Thickening of foods in dysphagia. Not to be prescribed for children under one year old except in cases of failure to thrive.

THIXO-D LOW-CAL
   Thickening feeds in the treatment of vomiting and dysphagia.

TRITAMYL PRODUCTS
   See: Gluten-Free Products

TWOCAL HN
   For use as the sole source of nutrition or as a necessary nutritional supplement prescribed on medical grounds for:
   Short bowel syndrome, intractable malabsorption, pre-operative preparation of patients who are undernourished, patients with proven inflammatory bowel disease, following total gastrectomy, dysphagia, bowel fistulae, disease-related malnutrition. Not to be prescribed for any child under six years of age; use with caution in children up to 10 years of age with appropriate dietetic or medical supervision.

TYR EXPRESS
   For the dietary management of Tyrosinaemia in patients aged 8 years and over.

TYR GEL (formerly VITAFLO - TYR GEL)
   A Tyrosine and Phenylalanine free protein substitute for use in the dietary management of Tyrosinaemia, approved for patients between the ages 12 months and 10 years.

ULTRA GLUTEN-FREE AND LOW-PROTEIN PRODUCTS
   See: Gluten-Free and Low-Protein Products

ULTRA PKU LOW-PROTEIN PRODUCTS
   See: Low-Protein Products

UVISTAT LIPSCREEN SPF 50

UVISTAT SUNCREAM SPF 30
   Protection from UV radiation in abnormal cutaneous photosensitivity resulting from genetic disorders or photodermatoses, including vitiligo and those resulting from radiotherapy; chronic or recurrent herpes simplex labialis.

VALPIFORM GLUTEN-FREE AND LOW-PROTEIN PRODUCTS
   See: Gluten-Free and Low-Protein Products

VASELINE DERMACARE CREAM

VASELINE DERMACARE LOTION
   Endogenous and exogenous eczema, xeroderma, icthyosis and senile pruritis associated with dry skin.

VEGENAT MED (APPLE, CHICKEN, CHICKPEAS, CHOCOLATE, CURRY CHICKEN, FISH, FISH AND VEGETABLES, HAM, HONEY, LEMON, LENTILS, ORANGE, RICE AND LEMON, SAVOURY, VEAL, VEGETABLES, WINTER VEGETABLES AND RICE WITH APPLE FLAVOURS)
   As a necessary nutritional supplement prescribed on medical grounds for:
   Short bowel syndrome, intractable malabsorption, pre-operative preparation of patients who are undernourished, patients with proven inflammatory bowel disease, following total gastrectomy, dysphagia and disease-related malnutrition.

VEIL COVER CREAM

VEIL FINISHING POWDER
   See: Covering Creams

VITA-BITE
   Inherited metabolic disorders, renal or liver failure requiring a low protein diet. Not recommended for any child under one year of age.

VITAFLO FLAVOUR PAC
   Specifically designed to use in conjunction with Vitaflo's Inborn Error range of protein substitutes.

BORDERLINE SUBSTANCES

VITAFLO - HCU EXPRESS
See: HCU EXPRESS

VITAFLO HCU GEL
See: HCU GEL

VITAFLO - ISOLEUCINE AMINO ACID SUPPLEMENT
Supplements for maple syrup urine disease.

VITAFLO - MSUD EXPRESS
See: MSUD EXPRESS

VITAFLO - TYR GEL
See: TYR GEL

VITAFLO - VALINE AMINO ACID SUPPLEMENT
Supplements for maple syrup urine disease.

VITAJOULE
Disease related malnutrition, malabsorption states or other conditions requiring fortification with a high or readily available carbohydrate supplement.

VITAMIN & MINERAL PREPARATIONS
Only in the management of actual or potential vitamin or mineral deficiency; not to be prescribed as dietary supplements or "pick-me-ups".

VITAPRO
Biochemically proven hypoproteinaemia.

VITAQUICK
Thickening of foods in dysphagia. Not to be prescribed for children under one year old except in cases of failure to thrive.

VITASAVOURY
Disease-related malnutrition, malabsorption states or other conditions requiring fortification with a fat/ carbohydrate supplement. Not to be prescribed for any child under one year; use with caution for young children up to five years of age.

WELLFOODS GLUTEN-FREE PRODUCTS
See: Gluten-Free Products

WYSOY
Proven lactose and associated sucrose intolerance in pre-school children, galactokinase deficiency, galactosaemia and proven whole cows milk sensitivity.

XLEU ANALOG

XLEU FALADON

XLEU MAXAMAID
Isovaleric acidaemia

XLYS ANALOG (formerly ANALOG XLYS)
Hyperlysinaemia

XLYS LOW TRY ANALOG (formerly XLYS TRY LOW ANALOG)
Type 1 glutaric aciduria

XLYS LOW TRY MAXAMAID
Glutaric aciduria

XLYS MAXAMAID
Hyperlysinaemia

XLYS, TRY LOW ANALOG
See: XLYS LOW TRY ANALOG

XV

BORDERLINE SUBSTANCES

XMET ANALOG (formerly ANALOG RVHB)
Hypermethioninaemia, homocystinuria

XMET HOMIDON
Homocystinuria or hypermethioninaemia

XMET MAXAMAID

XMET MAXAMUM
Hypermethioninaemia, homocystinuria

XMET, THRE, VAL, ISOLEU MAXAMAID
See: XMTVI MAXAMAID

XMET, THRE, VAL, ISOLEU MAXAMUM
See: XMTVI MAXAMUM

XMTVI ANALOG (formerly ANALOG XMET, THRE, VAL, ISOLEU)
Methylmalonic acidaemia, propionic acidaemia

XMTVI ASADON
Methylmalonic acidaemia or propionic acidaemia

XMTVI MAXAMAID (formerly XMET, THRE, VAL, ISOLEU MAXAMAID)
Methylmalonic acidaemia and propionic acidaemia

XMTVI MAXAMUM (formerly XMET, THRE, VAL, ISOLEU MAXAMUM)
Methylmalonic acidaemia and propionic acidaemia

XP ANALOG (formerly ANALOG XP)
Phenylketonuria

XP ANALOG LCP (formerly ANALOG XP LPC)
Phenylketonuria in infants and children under two years of age.

XP MAXAMAID (ORANGE AND UNFLAVOURED)

XP MAXAMAID CONCENTRATE
Phenylketonuria

XP MAXAMUM (ORANGE AND UNFLAVOURED)
Phenylketonuria. Not to be prescribed for children under 8 years old.
Tyrosinaemia

XPHEN, TYR ANALOG (formerly ANALOG XPHEN, TYR)
Tyrosinaemia

XPHEN TYR MAXAMAID

XPT TYROSIDON
Tyrosinaemia where plasma methionine levels are normal

XPTM ANALOG (formerly ANALOG XPHEN, TYR, MET)
Tyrosinaemia

XPTM TYROSIDON
Tyrosinaemia type 1 where plasma levels are above normal

BORDERLINE SUBSTANCES

LIST B

This is a cross index listing clinical conditions and the products which the ACBS has approved for the management of those conditions. It is essential to consult LIST A for more precise guidance.

LIST B

AMINO ACID METABOLIC DISORDERS AND SIMILAR PROTEIN DISORDERS

Histidinaemia
Homocystinuria
Low-Protein Products
Maple Syrup Urine Disease
Phenylketonuria
Synthetic Diets
Tyrosinaemia

BIRTHMARKS
See: Disfiguring Skin Lesions

BOWEL FISTULAE

Clinutren 1.5
Clinutren Dessert (as a supplement)
Clinutren Fruit (as a supplement)
Clinutren ISO
Clinutren Junior
Complan Shake (as a supplement)
Elemental 028
Elemental 028 Extra
Elemental 028 Extra (Liquid)
Emsogen
Enlive Plus (as a supplement)
Enmix Plus Commence (as a supplement)
Enrich
Enrich Plus
Ensure
Ensure 500ml Ready to Hang (Vanilla Flavour only)
Ensure Plus Liquid Feed (as a supplement)
Ensure Plus Commence (as a supplement)
Ensure Plus Yoghurt Style (as a supplement)
Foodlink Complete
Formance (as a supplement)
Forticreme Complete (as a supplement)
Fortifresh
Fortijuce (as a supplement)
Fortijuce Starter Pack (as a supplement)
Fortimel (as a supplement)
Fortisip Bottle (as a supplement)
Fortisip Multifibre (as a supplement)
Fortisip Protein
Fortisip Protein Starter Pack
Fortisip Range Starter Pack (as a supplement)
Frebini
Frebini Energy
Frebini Energy Drink (Strawberry and Banana Flavours)
Frebini Enegy Fibre
Frebini Energy Fibre Drink
Frebini Original Fibre
Fresubin Energy

XV

BORDERLINE SUBSTANCES

BOWEL FISTULAE

Fresubin Energy Fibre Sip Feed
Fresubin Energy Fibre (Neutral) Tube Feed
Fresubin HP Energy (as a supplement)
Fresubin Liquid and Sip Feeds
Fresubin Protein Energy Drink (as a supplement)
Fresubin 1000 Complete
Fresubin 1200 Complete
Isosource Energy
Isosource Fibre
Isosource Standard
Jevity
Jevity 1.5kcal
Jevity Plus
Jevity Promote
Modulen IBD
Novasource Forte
Novasource GI Control
Nutrini
Nutrini Energy
Nutrini Multifibre
Nutrison Energy (as a supplement)
Nutrison Energy Multifibre
Nutrison MCT (as a supplement)
Nutrison Multifibre
Nutrison Standard
Osmolite
Osmolite Plus
Paediasure
Paediasure Plus
Paediasure with Fibre
Paediasure Plus with Fibre
Peptamen
Peptamen Junior
Peptisorb
Perative (as a supplement)
Provide Xtra (as a supplement)
Renilon 7.5
Resource 2.0 Fibre
Resource Benefiber (as a supplement)
Resource Dessert Fruit (as a supplement)
Resource Dessert Energy (as a supplement)
Resource Protein (as a supplement)
Resource Shake Nutritional Supplement
Sondalis 1.5 Liquid Feed
Sondalis Fibre Liquid Feed
Sondalis Iso Liquid Feed
Survimed OPD (as a supplement)
Tentrini
Tentrini Energy
TwoCal HN

CALCIUM INTOLERANCE

Locasol

BORDERLINE SUBSTANCES

CARBOHYDRATE MALABSORPTION

for definition of lactose or sucrose intolerance, see page 435

        Pro-Cal
        QuickCal
        Vitasavoury

See: Synthetic Diets
        Malabsorption States

a)   <u>Disaccharide intolerance</u> (without isomaltose intolerance)
        Caloreen
        Cow & Gate Pepti-Junior
        Duocal (Liquid and Super Soluble)
        Maxijul Liquid
        Maxijul Super Soluble
        Nutramigen 1
        Nutramigen 2
        Nutrison Soya
        Pepdite
        Pepdite 1+
        Polycal (Liquid & Powder)
        Polycose Powder
        Pregestimil
        Prejomin
        Pro-Cal
        QuickCal
        Vitajoule
        Vitasavoury

See: Lactose intolerance
        Lactose with associated sucrose intolerance

b)   <u>Isomaltose intolerance</u>
        Glucose

c)   <u>Glucose + galactose intolerance</u>
        Comminuted Chicken Meat (SHS)
        Fructose
        Galactomin 19 (Fructose Formula)

d)   <u>Lactose intolerance</u>
        Colief
        Comminuted Chicken Meat (SHS)
        Cow & Gate Pepti
        Enfamil Lacto free
        Farley's Soya Formula
        Galactomin 17
        Infasoy
        Isomil Powder
        Nutramigen 1
        Nutrison Soya
        Pepdite
        Pepdite 1+
        Pepdite 1+ (Banana Flavour)
        Pregestimil
        Prejomin
        Prosobee liquid and powder
        SMA LF
        Wysoy

XV

BORDERLINE SUBSTANCES

CARBOHYDRATE MALABSORPTION
e) <u>Lactose with associated sucrose intolerance</u>
Comminuted Chicken Meat (SHS)
Cow & Gate Pepti-Junior
Farley's Soya Formula
Galactomin 17
Infasoy
Nutramigen 1
Nutrison Soya
Pregestimil
Prejomin
Prosobee liquid and powder
Wysoy

f) <u>Sucrose intolerance</u>
Glucose (dextrose)
See: Synthetic Diets
Malabsorption
Lactose with associated sucrose intolerance

CARNITINE PALMITOYL TRANSFERASE DEFICIENCY (CPTD)
Monogen

COELIAC DISEASE
See: Gluten-Sensitive Enteropathies

CONTINUOUS AMBULATORY PERITONEAL DIALYSIS (CAPD)
See: Dialysis

CYSTIC FIBROSIS
See: Malabsorption

DERMATITIS
Aveeno Baby Colloidal
Aveeno Bath Oil
Aveeno Colloidal
Aveeno Cream
Aveeno Lotion
E45 Emollient Bath Oil
E45 Emollient Wash Cream
E45 Lotion
Vaseline Dermacare Cream
Vaseline Dermacare Lotion

DERMATITIS HERPETIFORMIS
See: Gluten-Sensitive Enteropathies.

DIALYSIS
Nutritional Supplements for Haemodialysis or Continuous Ambulatory Peritoneal Dialysis
(CAPD) patients.
Clinutren Dessert
Enrich Plus
Ensure Plus Commence
Ensure Plus Liquid Feed
Ensure Plus Yoghurt Style
Formance
Forticreme Complete
Fresubin HP Energy
Fresubin Protein Energy Drink

BORDERLINE SUBSTANCES

DIALYSIS

> Kindergen
> Nepro
> Renapro
> Resource Dessert Fruit
> Resource Dessert Energy
> Suplena

DISACCHARIDE INTOLERANCE
   See: Carbohydrate malabsorption

DISFIGURING SKIN LESIONS (BIRTHMARKS, MUTILATING LESIONS, AND SCARS)

> Covermark Classic Foundation
> Covermark Finishing Powder
> Dermacolor Camouflage Cream
> Dermacolor Fixing Powder
> Keromask Finishing Powder
> Keromask Masking Cream
> Veil Cover Cream
> Veil Finishing Powder

DYSPHAGIA

for definition, see page 435

> Clinutren 1.5
> Clinutren 1.5 Fibre
> Clinutren Dessert (as a supplement)
> Clinutren Fruit (as a supplement)
> Clinutren ISO
> Clinutren Junior
> Clinutren Thickened Drinks
> Clinutren Thickener
> Complan Shake (as a supplement)
> Enfamil AR
> Enlive Plus (as a supplement)
> Enmix Plus Commence (as a supplement)
> Enrich
> Enrich Plus
> Ensure
> Ensure 500ml Ready to Hang (Vanilla Flavour only)
> Ensure Plus Commence (as a supplement)
> Ensure Plus Liquid Feed (as a supplement)
> Ensure Plus Yoghurt Style (as a supplement)
> Foodlink Complete
> Formance (as a supplement)
> Forticreme Complete (as a supplement)
> Fortifresh
> Fortijuce (as a supplement)
> Fortijuce Starter Pack (as a supplement)
> Fortimel (as a supplement)
> Fortisip Bottle (as a supplement)
> Fortisip Multifibre (as a supplement)
> Fortisip Protein
> Fortisip Protein Starter Pack
> Fortisip Range Starter Pack (as a supplement)
> Frebini
> Frebini Energy
> Frebini Energy Drink (Strawberry and Banana Flavours)
> Frebini Energy Fibre
> Frebini Energy Fibre Drink
> Frebini Original Fibre

XV

BORDERLINE SUBSTANCES

DYSPHAGIA

Fresubin Energy
Fresubin Energy Fibre Sip Feed
Fresubin Energy Fibre (Neutral) Tube Feed
Fresubin HP Energy (as a supplement)
Fresubin Liquid and Sip Feeds
Fresubin Protein Energy Drink (as a supplement)
Fresubin 1000 Complete
Isosource Energy
Isosource Energy Fibre
Isosource Fibre
Isosource Junior
Isosource Standard
Jevity
Jevity Plus
Jevity Promote
Jevity 1.5kcal
Modulen IBD
Novasource Forte
Novasource GI Control
Nutilis (as a thickener)
Nutrini
Nutrini Energy
Nutrini Energy Multifibre
Nutrini Low Energy Multifibre
Nutrini Multifibre
Nutrison Energy (as a supplement)
Nutrison Energy Multifibre
Nutrison MCT (as a supplement)
Nutrison Multifibre
Nutrison Soya
Nutrison Standard
Nutrison 1200 Complete Multi Fibre
Osmolite
Osmolite Plus
Paediasure
Paediasure Plus
Paediasure Plus with Fibre
Paediasure with Fibre
Provide Xtra (as a supplement)
Resource 2.0 Fibre
Resource Benefiber
Resource Dessert Fruit (as a supplement)
Resource Dessert Energy (as a supplement)
Resource Junior (as a supplement)
Resource Protein (as a supplement)
Resource Shake Nutritional Supplement
Resource ThickenUp without Vitamins and Minerals
Resource Thickened Squash and Resource Ready Thickened Drinks
Slo Drinks (Orange, Blackcurrant, Lemon and Peach Flavours)
SMA Staydown
Sondalis 1.5 Liquid Feed
Sondalis Fibre Liquid Feed
Sondalis ISO Liquid Feed
Survimed OPD (as a supplement)
Tentrini
Tentrini Energy
Tentrini Energy Multi Fibre

BORDERLINE SUBSTANCES

DYSPHAGIA

> Tentrini Multi Fibre
> Thick and Easy (as a thickener)
> Thick and Easy Dairy
> Thixo-D (as a thickener)
> Thixo-D Low-Cal (as a thickener)
> TwoCal HN
> Vegenat Med (as a supplement)
> Vitaquick (as a thickener)

ECZEMA
> See: Dermatitis

EPILEPSY (KETOGENIC DIET IN)

> Alembicol D
> Liquigen
> Medium-chain triglyceride oil (MCT)

FLAVOURING FOR USE WITH ANY UNFLAVOURED PRODUCT BASED ON PEPTIDES OR AMINO ACIDS

> SHS Flavour Modjul
> SHS Flavour Sachet

GALACTOKINASE DEFICIENCY AND GALACTOSAEMIA

> Farley's Soya Formula
> Galactomin 17
> Infasoy
> Isomil Powder
> Prosobee Liquid and Powder
> Wysoy

GASTRECTOMY (TOTAL)

> Clinutren 1.5
> Clinutren 1.5 Fibre
> Clinutren Dessert (as a supplement)
> Clinutren Fruit (as a supplement)
> Clinutren ISO
> Clinutren Junior
> Complan Shake (as a supplement)
> Enlive Plus (as a supplement)
> Enmix Plus Commence (as a supplement)
> Enrich
> Enrich Plus
> Ensure
> Ensure 500ml Ready to Hang (Vanilla Flavour only)
> Ensure Plus Commence (as a supplement)
> Ensure Plus Liquid Feed (as a supplement)
> Ensure Plus Yoghurt Style (as a supplement)
> Foodlink Complete
> Formance (as a supplement)
> Forticreme Complete (as a supplement)
> Fortifresh
> Fortijuce (as a supplement)
> Fortijuce Starter Pack (as a supplement)
> Fortimel (as a supplement)
> Fortisip Bottle (as a supplement)
> Fortisip Multifibre (as a supplement)
> Fortisip Protein
> Fortisip Protein Starter Pack

XV

BORDERLINE SUBSTANCES

GASTRECTOMY (TOTAL)
Fortisip Range Starter Pack (as a supplement)
Frebini
Frebini Energy
Frebini Energy Drink (Strawberry and Banana Flavours)
Frebini Energy Fibre
Frebini Energy Fibre Drink
Frebini Original Fibre
Fresubin Energy
Fresubin Energy Fibre Sip Feed
Fresubin Energy Fibre (Neutral) Tube Feed
Fresubin HP Energy (as a supplement)
Fresubin Liquid and Sip Feeds
Fresubin Protein Energy Drink (as a supplement)
Fresubin 1000 Complete
Fresubin 1200 Complete
Isosource Energy
Isosource Energy Fibre
Isosource Fibre
Isosource Junior
Isosource Standard
Jevity
Jevity Plus
Jevity Promote
Jevity 1.5kcal
Modulen IBD
Novasource Forte
Novasource GI Control
Nutrini Energy
Nutrini Energy Multifibre
Nutrini Low Energy Multifibre
Nutrini Multifibre
Nutrison Energy (as a supplement)
Nutrison Energy Multifibre
Nutrison MCT (as a supplement)
Nutrison Multifibre
Nutrison Soya
Nutrison Standard
Nutrison 1200 Complete Multi Fibre
Osmolite
Osmolite Plus
Perative (as a supplement)
Provide Xtra (as a supplement)
Renilon 7.5
Resource 2.0 Fibre
Resource Benefiber
Resource Dessert Fruit (as a supplement)
Resource Dessert Energy (as a supplement)
Resource Junior (as a supplement)
Resource Protein (as a supplement)
Resource Shake Nutritional Supplement
Sondalis 1.5 Liquid Feed
Sondalis Fibre Liquid Feed
Sondalis ISO Liquid Feed
Survimed OPD (as a supplement)
Tentrini
Tentrini Energy
Tentrini Energy Multi Fibre

BORDERLINE SUBSTANCES

GASTRECTOMY (TOTAL)

    Tentrini Multi Fibre
    TwoCal HN
    Vegenat Med (as a supplement)

GLUCOSE/GALACTOSE INTOLERANCE

    Comminuted Chicken Meat (SHS)
    Galactomin 19 (Fructose Formula)
See: Carbohydrate Malabsorption

GLUTARIC ACIDURIA

    XLYS, Low TRY Analog
    XLYS LOW TRY Maxamaid

GLUTEN-SENSITIVE ENTEROPATHIES

    Aproten gluten-free flour
    Arnott's gluten-free rice cookies
    Baker's Delight wheat, gluten and dairy free bread
    Barkat brown rice pizza crust
    Barkat gluten-free bread mix
    Barkat gluten-free brown rice bread
    Barkat gluten-free wheat-free multi grain bread
    Barkat gluten-free white rice bread
    Barkat white rice pizza crust
    Bi-Aglut gluten-free biscuits
    Bi-Aglut gluten-free cracker toast
    Bi-Aglut gluten-free crackers
    Bi-Aglut gluten-free pastas (fusilli, lasagne, macaroni, penne, spaghetti)
    Dietary Specials gluten-free brown bread mix
    Dietary Specials gluten-free corn bread mix
    Dietary Specials gluten-free cracker bread
    Dietary Specials gluten-free digestive biscuits
    Dietary Specials gluten-free fibre mix
    Dietary Specials gluten-free high fibre crackers
    Dietary Specials gluten-free hoops tea biscuits
    Dietary Specials gluten-free multigrain sliced loaf
    Dietary Specials gluten-free part baked bloomer
    Dietary Specials gluten-free part baked brown loaf
    Dietary Specials gluten-free part baked white baguettes
    Dietary Specials gluten-free part baked white buns
    Dietary Specials gluten-free part baked white loaf
    Dietary Specials gluten-free part baked white rolls
    Dietary Specials gluten-free pasta (fusilli, penne, spaghetti)
    Dietary Specials gluten-free pastry mix
    Dietary Specials gluten-free pizza bases
    Dietary Specials gluten-free savory biscuits
    Dietary Specials gluten-free sweet biscuits
    Dietary Specials gluten-free white bread mix
    Dietary Specials gluten-free white cake mix
    Dietary Specials gluten-free white mix
    Dietary Specials gluten-free white multigrain sliced loaf
    Ener-G gluten-free brown rice bread
    Ener-G gluten-free brown rice pasta (lasagna, macaroni, spaghetti)
    Ener-G gluten-free cookies (vanilla flavour)
    Ener-G gluten-free dinner rolls
    Ener-G gluten-free rice loaf
    Ener-G gluten-free rice pasta (cannelloni, lasagna, macaroni, shells, small shells, spaghetti, tagliatelle, vermicelli)
    Ener-G gluten-free Seattle brown loaf

BORDERLINE SUBSTANCES

GLUTEN-SENSITIVE ENTEROPATHIES
    Ener-G gluten-free tapioca bread
    Ener-G gluten-free white rice bread
    Ener-G gluten-free xanthan gum
    Gadsbys gluten-free white bread
    Gadsbys gluten-free white bread flour
    Gadsbys gluten-free white rolls
    Gadsbys gluten-free white sliced bread
    Glutafin gluten-free biscuits
    Glutafin gluten-free crackers
    Glutafin gluten-free digestive biscuits
    Glutafin gluten-free high fibre crackers
    Glutafin gluten-free pasta (lasagne, long-cut spaghetti, macaroni penne, shells, spirals, tagliatelle nests)
    Glutafin gluten-free pizza base
    Glutafin gluten-free savoury biscuits
    Glutafin gluten-free savoury shorts
    Glutafin gluten-free shortbread biscuit
    Glutafin gluten-free sweet biscuits (without chocolate or sultanas)
    Glutafin gluten-free tea biscuits
    Glutafin gluten-free wheat-free fibre loaf (sliced and unsliced)
    Glutafin gluten-free wheat-free fibre mix
    Glutafin gluten-free wheat-free fibre rolls
    Glutafin gluten-free wheat-free white loaf (sliced and unsliced)
    Glutafin gluten-free wheat-free white mix
    Glutafin gluten-free wheat-free white rolls
    Glutafin Select gluten-free bread mix
    Glutafin Select gluten-free cake mix
    Glutafin Select gluten-free fibre bread mix
    Glutafin Select gluten-free fibre loaf (sliced and unsliced)
    Glutafin Select gluten-free fibre mix
    Glutafin Select gluten-free fibre rolls
    Glutafin Select gluten free fresh bread
    Glutafin Select gluten-free part-baked fibre loaf
    Glutafin Select gluten-free part-baked fibre rolls
    Glutafin Select gluten-free part-baked long fibre rolls
    Glutafin Select gluten-free part-baked long white rolls
    Glutafin Select gluten-free part-baked white loaf
    Glutafin Select gluten-free part-baked white rolls
    Glutafin Select gluten-free seeded loaf
    Glutafin Select gluten-free pastry mix
    Glutafin Select gluten-free white loaf (sliced and unsliced)
    Glutafin Select gluten-free white mix
    Glutafin Select gluten-free white rolls
    Glutano gluten-free biscuits
    Glutano gluten-free crackers, crackers snack pack
    Glutano gluten-free crispbread
    Glutano gluten-free flour mix
    Glutano gluten-free par-baked (baguette, rolls, white sliced bread)
    Glutano gluten-free pasta (animal shapes, macaroni, spaghetti, spirals, tagliatelle)
    Glutano gluten-free shortcake rings
    Glutano gluten-free wheat-free digestive biscuit
    Glutano gluten-free wholemeal bread (sliced), wholemeal bread (sliced) snack pack
    Glutano gluten-free wholemeal par-baked bread
    Gratis gluten-free pasta (alphabets, macaroni, shells, short cut spaghetti, spirals)
    Heron Foods Organic gluten-free bread mix
    Heron Foods Organic gluten-free hi-fibre bread mix
    Innovative Solutions brown rice flour

BORDERLINE SUBSTANCES

GLUTEN-SENSITIVE ENTEROPATHIES

Innovative Solutions potato flour
Innovative Solutions tapioca flour
Innovative Solutions white rice flour
Juvela gluten-free bread rolls
Juvela gluten-free crispbread
Juvela gluten-free digestive biscuits
Juvela gluten-free fibre bread rolls
Juvela gluten-free fibre loaf (sliced and unsliced)
Juvela gluten-free fibre mix
Juvela gluten-free fresh sliced white loaf
Juvela gluten-free harvest mix
Juvela gluten-free lasagne
Juvela gluten-free loaf (sliced and unsliced)
Juvela gluten-free mix
Juvela gluten-free part-baked bread rolls
Juvela gluten-free part-baked fibre bread rolls
Juvela gluten-free part-baked fibre loaf
Juvela gluten-free part-baked loaf
Juvela gluten-free pasta (fusilli, lasagne, macaroni, spaghetti)
Juvela gluten-free pizza base
Juvela gluten-free savoury biscuits
Juvela gluten-free sweet biscuits
Juvela gluten-free tagliatelle
Juvela gluten-free tea biscuits
Lifestyle gluten-free bread rolls
Lifestyle gluten-free brown bread
Lifestyle gluten-free high fibre bread
Lifestyle gluten-free high fibre bread rolls
Lifestyle gluten-free white bread
Livwell sliced brown bread
Livwell sliced white bread
Livwell white baguette
Livwell white rolls
Orgran bread mix
Orgran gluten-free buckwheat spirals pasta
Orgran gluten-free corn lasagne, corn spaghetti, corn spirals pasta
Orgran gluten-free crispbread corn, crispbread rice
Orgran gluten-free organic brown rice spirals
Orgran gluten-free pizza & pastry mix
Orgran gluten-free rice spaghetti, rice spirals
Orgran gluten-free rice and millet spirals
Orgran gluten-free ris o'mais (rice and maize) lasagne, ris o'mais spaghetti, ris o'mais spirals
Orgran gluten-free split pea & soya pasta shells
Orgran ris 'o' mais macaroni
Orgran self-raising flour
Pleniday gluten-free bread (sliced country loaf, petit pain (par baked), rustic loaf sliced)
Pleniday gluten-free pasta (conchigli, penne, rigate, tagliatelli)
Pleniday sesame rolls
Polial gluten-free biscuits
Pure gluten-free blended flour
Pure xanthan gum
Rite-Diet gluten-free fibre mix
Rite-Diet gluten-free fibre rolls
Rite-Diet gluten-free fibre bread (sliced and unsliced)
Rite-Diet gluten-free white bread (sliced and unsliced)
Rite-Diet gluten-free white mix
Riet-Diet gluten-free white rolls

BORDERLINE SUBSTANCES

GLUTEN-SENSITIVE ENTEROPATHIES

Rite-Diet gluten-free part-baked fibre loaf
Rite-Diet gluten-free 2 part-baked long fibre rolls
Rite-Diet gluten-free 2 part-baked long white rolls
Rite-Diet gluten-free part-baked white loaf
Schar gluten-free biscuits
Schar gluten-free bread
Schar gluten-free bread mix
Schar gluten-free bread rolls
Schar gluten-free brown bread ertha
Schar gluten-free cake mix
Schar gluten-free crackers
Schar gluten-free cracker toast
Schar gluten-free crispbread
Schar gluten-free flour mix for cooking
Schar gluten-free french bread (baguette)
Schar gluten-free frollini tea biscuits
Schar gluten-free grissini breadsticks
Schar gluten-free pasta (alphabet pasta,bavette, fusilli, lasagne, macaroni, penne, spaghetti)
Schar gluten-free pizza base
Schar gluten-free savoy biscuits
Schar gluten-free wheat-free biscottini
Schar gluten-free wheat-free bread buns (white)
Schar gluten-free wheat-free lunch rolls
Schar gluten-free white bread
Schar gluten-free wholemeal bread
Schar gluten-free wholemeal flour mix
Sunnyvale gluten-free mixed grain sourdough bread
Tritamyl gluten-free brown bread mix
Tritamyl gluten-free flour mix
Tritamyl gluten-free white bread mix
Ultra gluten-free baguette
Ultra gluten-free bread
Ultra gluten-free bread rolls
Ultra gluten-free crackerbread
Ultra gluten-free high fibre bread
Ultra gluten-free pasta (tagliatelle, spaghetti, penne, fusili)
Ultra gluten-free pizza base
Ultra gluten-free sweet biscuits
Valpiform gluten-free and wheat free pastry mix
Valpiform gluten-free bread mix
Valpiform gluten-free country loaf
Valpiform gluten-free crac'form toast
Valpiform gluten-free crisp rolls
Valpiform gluten-free maxi baguettes
Valpiform gluten-free pastry mix
Valpiform gluten-free petites baguettes
Wellfoods gluten-free burger buns
Wellfoods gluten-free flour alternative
Wellfoods gluten-free loaf
Wellfoods gluten-free pizza bases
Wellfoods gluten-free rolls
Wellfoods gluten-free sliced loaf

GLUTEN-SENSITIVE ENTEROPATHIES WITH COEXISTING ESTABLISHED WHEAT SENSITIVITY

Ener-G gluten-free pizza bases
Ener-G gluten-free Seattle brown rolls (hamburgers)
Ener-G gluten-free Seattle brown rolls (hot dogs)

BORDERLINE SUBSTANCES

GLUTEN-SENSITIVE ENTEROPATHIES WITH COEXISTING ESTABLISHED WHEAT SENSITIVITY
Ener-G gluten-free six flour loaf
Glutafin Crisp Bread
Glutafin gluten-free wheat-free bread mix
Glutafin gluten-free wheat-free cake mix
Glutafin gluten-free wheat-free fibre bread mix
Glutafin gluten-free wheat-free pastry mix
Heron Foods Organic gluten-free wheat-free bread/cake mix
Heron Foods Organic gluten-free wheat-free hi-fibre bread mix
Proceli brown rice bread
Proceli pizza bases
Proceli sliced white bread

GLYCOGEN STORAGE DISEASE
Caloreen
Corn Flour or Corn Starch
Dextrose
Glucose
Maxijul Liquid (Orange flavour only)
Maxijul Super Soluble
Polycal (Liquid & Powder)
Polycose Powder
Pro-Cal
QuickCal
Vitajoule
Vitasavoury

GROWTH FAILURE (DISEASE RELATED)
Clinutren Junior
Fortini
Fortini Multi Fibre
Frebini
Frebini Energy
Frebini Energy Drink (Strawberry and Banana Flavours)
Frebini Energy Fibre
Frebini Energy Fibre Drink
Frebini Original Fibre
Nutrini
Nutrini Energy
Nutrini Energy Multifibre
Nutrini Low Energy Multifibre
Nutrini Multifibre
Paediasure
Paediasure Plus
Paediasure Plus with Fibre
Paediasure with Fibre
SMA High Energy
Survimed OPD
Tentrini
Tentrini Energy
Tentrini Energy Multi Fibre
Tentrini Multi Fibre

HAEMODIALYSIS
See: Dialysis

HISTIDINAEMIA
See: Low-Protein Products
          Synthetic Diets

XV

BORDERLINE SUBSTANCES

HOMOCYSTINURIA

HCU Express
HCU Gel
HCU-LV (Unflavoured and Tropical Flavour)
Vitaflo Flavour Pac
XMET Analog
XMET Homidon
XMET Maxamaid
XMET Maxamum

See: Low-Protein Products
Synthetic Diets

HYPERLIPOPROTEINAEMIA TYPE 1

Alembicol-D (MCT Oil)
Liquigen
Medium chain triglyceride oil

HYPERLYSINAEMIA

XLYS Analog
XLYS Maxamaid

HYPERMETHIONINAEMIA

HCU-LV (Unflavoured and Tropical Flavour)
XMET Analog
XMET Homidon
XMET Maxamaid
XMET Maxamum

HYPOGLYCAEMIA

Corn Flour or Corn Starch
See: Glycogen Storage Disease

HYPOPROTEINAEMIA

Casilan 90
Dialamine
Maxisorb
Pro-Mod
Protifar
Renapro
Vitapro

INFLAMMATORY BOWEL DISEASE

Clinutren 1.5
Clinutren 1.5 Fibre
Clinutren Dessert (as a supplement)
Clinutren Fruit (as a supplement)
Clinutren ISO
Clinutren Junior
Complan Shake (as a supplement)
Elemental 028
Elemental 028 Extra
Elemental 028 Extra (Liquid)
Emsogen
Enlive Plus (as a supplement)
Enmix Plus Commence (as a supplement)
Enrich
Enrich Plus
Ensure

BORDERLINE SUBSTANCES

INFLAMMATORY BOWEL DISEASE

Ensure 500ml Ready to Hang (Vanilla Flavour only)
Ensure Plus Commence (as a supplement)
Ensure Plus Liquid Feed (as a supplement)
Ensure Plus Yoghurt Style (as a supplement)
Foodlink Complete
Formance (as a supplement)
Forticreme Complete (as a supplement)
Fortifresh
Fortijuce (as a supplement)
Fortijuce Starter Pack (as a supplement)
Fortimel (as a supplement)
Fortisip Bottle (as a supplement)
Fortisip Multifibre (as a supplement)
Fortisip Protein
Fortisip Protein Starter Pack
Fortisip Range Starter Pack (as a supplement)
Frebini
Frebini Energy
Frebini Energy Drink (Strawberry and Banana Flavours)
Frebini Energy Fibre
Frebini Energy Fibre Drink
Frebini Original Fibre
Fresubin Energy
Fresubin Energy Fibre Sip Feed
Fresubin Energy Fibre (Neutral) Tube Feed
Fresubin HP Energy (as a supplement)
Fresubin Liquid & Sip Feeds
Fresubin Protein Energy Drink (as a supplement)
Fresubin 1000 Complete
Fresubin 1200 Complete
Isosource Energy
Isosource Energy Fibre
Isosource Fibre
Isosource Junior
Isosource Standard
Jevity
Jevity Plus
Jevity Promote
Jevity 1.5kcal
Modulen IBD
Novasource Forte
Novasource GI Control
Nutrini Energy
Nutrini Multifibre
Nutrison Energy (as a supplement)
Nutrison Energy Multifibre
Nutrison MCT (as a supplement)
Nutrison Multifibre
Nutrison Soya
Nutrison Standard
Nutrison 1200 Complete Multi Fibre
Osmolite
Osmolite Plus
Peptamen
Peptamen Junior
Peptisorb
Perative (as a supplement)

BORDERLINE SUBSTANCES

INFLAMMATORY BOWEL DISEASE

> Provide Xtra (as a supplement)
> Renilon 7.5
> Resource 2.0 Fibre
> Resource Benefiber
> Resource Dessert Fruit (as a supplement)
> Resource Dessert Energy (as a supplement)
> Resource Junior (as a supplement)
> Resource Protein (as a supplement)
> Resource Shake Nutritional Supplement
> Sondalis 1.5 Liquid Feed
> Sondalis Fibre Liquid Feed
> Sondalis ISO Liquid Feed
> Survimed OPD (as a supplement)
> Tentrini
> Tentrini Energy
> Tentrini Energy Multi Fibre
> Tentrini Multi Fibre
> TwoCal HN
> Vegenat Med (as a supplement)

INTESTINAL LYMPHANGIECTASIA

INTESTINAL SURGERY
> See: Malabsorption

ISOMALTOSE INTOLERANCE
> See: Carbohydrate Malabsorption

ISOVALERIC ACIDAEMIA

> XLEU Analog
> XLEU Faladon
> XLEU Maxamaid

LACTOSE INTOLERANCE
> See: Carbohydrate Malabsorption

LIPOPROTEIN LIPASE DEFICIENCY (PRIMARY AND SECONDARY)

> Monogen

LIVER FAILURE

> Alembicol D
> Aminex low-protein biscuits
> Aminex low-protein cookies
> Aminex low-protein rusks
> Aproten low-protein biscuits
> Aproten low-protein bread mix
> Aproten low-protein cake mix
> Aproten low-protein crispbread
> Aproten low-protein pasta (anellini, ditalini, rigatini, spaghetti, tagliatelle)
> Ener-G low-protein egg replacer
> Ener-G low-protein pasta (lasagne, macaroni, large shells, small shells, spaghetti)
> Ener-G low-protein rice bread
> Fate low-protein all-purpose mix
> Fate low-protein cake mix
> Fate low-protein chocolate flavour cake mix
> Generaid
> Generaid Plus
> Harifen white chip cookies
> Juvela low-protein bread rolls

BORDERLINE SUBSTANCES

LIVER FAILURE
Juvela low-protein chocolate chip, orange and cinnamon flavour cookies
Juvela low-protein loaf
Juvela low-protein mix
Juvela low-protein pizza base
Liquigen
Loprofin low-protein breakfast cereal
Loprofin low-protein chocolate flavour cream biscuits
Loprofin low-protein chocolate, orange and vanilla flavour cream wafers
Loprofin low-protein cinnamon and chocolate chip cookies
Loprofin low-protein crackers
Loprofin low-protein egg replacer
Loprofin low-protein egg white replacer
Loprofin low-protein fibre bread (sliced and unsliced)
Loprofin low-protein loaf (sliced and unsliced)
Loprofin low-protein mix
Loprofin low-protein part baked rolls
Loprofin low-protein pasta (long-cut spaghetti, macaroni penne, spirals, vermicelli, lasagne)
Loprofin low-protein rice
Loprofin low-protein sweet biscuits
Loprofin low-protein white rolls
Medium chain triglyceride (MCT) oil
Nepro
Promin low-protein burger mix
Promin low-protein pasta (alphabets, macaroni, shells, short cut spaghetti, spirals)
Promin low-protein pastameal
Promin low-protein tricolour pasta (alphabets, shells and spirals)
Rite-Diet low-protein baking mix
Rite-Diet low-protein flour mix
Suplena
Ultra low-protein canned brown bread
Ultra low-protein canned white bread
Ultra PKU biscuits
Ultra PKU bread
Ultra PKU cookies
Ultra PKU flour mix
Ultra PKU pizza base
Ultra PKU savoy biscuits
Valpiform low-protein cookies with chocolate nuggets and hazelnut flavour
Valpiform low-protein shortbread biscuits
Vita-Bite

LONG CHAIN ACYL-COA DEHYDROGENASE DEFICIENCY (LCAD)
Monogen

LOW-PROTEIN PRODUCTS
Aproten low-protein biscuits
Aproten low-protein bread mix
Aproten low-protein crispbread
Aproten low-protein pasta (anellini, ditalini, rigatini, spaghetti, tagliatelle)
Ener-G low-protein egg replacer
Ener-G low-protein pasta (lasagne, macaroni, large shells, small shells, spaghetti)
Ener-G low-protein rice bread
Fate low-protein all-purpose mix
Fate low-protein cake mix
Fate low-protein chocolate flavour cake mix
Fate low-protein potato mix
Harifen low protein cracker toast

XV

LOW-PROTEIN PRODUCTS

Harifen white chip cookies
Juvela low-protein bread rolls
Juvela low-protein chocolate chip, orange and cinnamon flavour cookies
Juvela low-protein loaf
Juvela low-protein mix
Juvela low-protein pizza base
Loprofin low-protein breakfast cereal
Loprofin low-protein chocolate flavour cream biscuits
Loprofin low-protein chocolate, orange and vanilla flavour cream wafers
Loprofin low-protein cinnamon and chocolate chip cookies
Loprofin low-protein crackers
Loprofin low-protein crunch bar
Loprofin low-protein egg replacer
Loprofin low-protein egg white replacer
Loprofin low-protein fibre bread (sliced and unsliced)
Loprofin low-protein herb crackers
Loprofin low-protein loaf (sliced and unsliced)
Loprofin low-protein mix
Loprofin low-protein part baked rolls
Loprofin low-protein pasta (long-cut spaghetti, macaroni penne, spirals, vermicelli, lasagne)
Loprofin low-protein rice
Loprofin low-protein snack pot
Loprofin low-protein sweet biscuits
Loprofin low-protein white bread rolls
Milupa low-protein drink
PK Foods Aminex low-protein biscuits
PK Foods Aminex low-protein cookies
PK Foods Aminex low-protein rusks
PK Foods low-protein crispbread
PK Foods low-protein pasta spirals
PK Foods low-protein white sliced bread
PKU-Gel
Promin low-protein burger mix
Promin low-protein cous cous
Promin low-protein hot breakfast (apple & cinnamon, banana, chocolate and original flavours)
Promin low-protein imitation rice
Promin low-protein imitation rice pudding (apple, banana, strawberry and original flavours)
Promin low-protein lasagne sheets
Promin low-protein pasta (alphabets, macaroni, shells, short cut spaghetti, spirals)
Promin low-protein pasta in sauce (cheese and broccoli, tomato pepper and herb flavours)
Promin low-protein pastameal
Promin low-protein tricolour pasta (alphabets, shells, spirals)
Rite-Diet low-protein baking mix
Rite-Diet low-protein flour mix
Ultra low-protein canned brown bread
Ultra low-protein canned white bread
Ultra PKU biscuits
Ultra PKU bread
Ultra PKU cookies
Ultra PKU flour mix
Ultra PKU pizza base
Ultra PKU savoy biscuits
Valpiform low-protein cookies with chocolate nuggets and hazelnut flavour
Valpiform low-protein savory bites (herbs flavour)
Valpiform low-protein savory bites (tomato flavour)
Valpiform low-protein shortbread biscuits
Vita-Bite
Inherited metabolic disorders, renal or liver failure requiring a low-protein diet.

BORDERLINE SUBSTANCES

MALABSORPTION STATES
(See also: gluten-sensitive enteropathies, liver failure, carbohydrate malabsorption, intestinal lymphangiectasia, milk intolerance and synthetic diets)

a)   Protein sources
- Caprilon
- Comminuted Chicken Meat (SHS)
- Duocal (Liquid & Super Soluble)
- Maxisorb
- MCT Pepdite
- MCT Pepdite 1+
- Neocate
- Neocate Active (unflavoured and blackcurrant flavour)
- Neocate Advance (Unflavoured, banana vanilla flavour and strawberry vanilla flavour)
- Pepdite
- Pepdite 1+
- Pepdite 1 + (Banana Flavour)

b)   Fat sources
- Alembicol D
- Calogen
- Calogen Banana
- Calogen Butterscotch
- Calogen Strawberry
- Caprilon
- Liquigen
- MCT Feed Step 1
- MCT Pepdite
- MCT Pepdite 1+
- Medium chain triglyceride oil
- Pro-Cal
- QuickCal
- Vitasavoury

c)   Carbohydrate sources
- Caloreen
- Maxijul Liquid
- Maxijul Super Soluble
- Novasource GI Control
- Novasource GI Forte
- Nutrini Energy
- Nutrini Multifibre
- Polycal (Liquid & Powder)
- Polycose Powder
- Pro-Cal
- QuickCal
- Renilon 7.5
- Resource Benefiber
- Vitajoule
- Vitasavoury

d)   Fat/Carbohydrate sources
- Calshake
- Duobar (strawberry, toffee, neutral)
- Duocal (Liquid, MCT Powder & Super Soluble)
- Enshake (Banana, Chocolate, Strawberry and Vanilla Flavours)
- Scandishake Mix Flavoured and Unflavoured

XV

BORDERLINE SUBSTANCES

MALABSORPTION STATES

e)   Complete Feeds
     For use as the sole source of nutrition or as necessary nutritional supplements prescribed on
     medical grounds
     Caprilon
     Clinutren 1.5
     Clinutren 1.5 Fibre
     Clinutren ISO
     Clinutren Junior
     Cow & Gate Pepti-Junior
     Elemental 028
     Elemental 028 Extra
     Elemental 028 Extra (Liquid)
     Emsogen
     Enrich
     Ensure
     Ensure 500ml Ready to Hang (Vanilla Flavour only)
     Foodlink Complete
     Fortifresh
     Frebini
     Frebini Energy
     Frebini Energy Drink (Strawberry and Banana Flavours)
     Frebini Energy Fibre
     Frebini Energy Fibre Drink
     Frebini Original Fibre
     Fresubin Energy
     Fresubin Energy Fibre Sip Feed
     Fresubin Energy Fibre (Neutral) Tube Feed
     Fresubin Liquid and Sip Feeds
     Fresubin 1000 Complete
     Fresubin 1200 Complete
     Infatrini
     Isosource Energy
     Isosource Energy Fibre
     Isosource Fibre
     Isosource Standard
     Jevity
     Jevity Plus
     Jevity Promote
     Jevity 1.5kcal
     MCT Pepdite
     MCT Pepdite 1+
     Modulen IBD
     Novasource Forte
     Novasource GI Control
     Nutrini
     Nutrini Energy
     Nutrini Energy Multi Fibre
     Nutrini Low Energy Multi Fibre
     Nutrini Multifibre
     Nutrison Energy Multifibre
     Nutrison Multifibre
     Nutrison Soya
     Nutrison Standard
     Nutrison 1200 Complete Multi Fibre
     Osmolite
     Paediasure
     Paediasure with Fibre
     Paediasure Plus
     Paediasure Plus with Fibre

BORDERLINE SUBSTANCES

MALABSORPTION STATES

Pepdite
Pepdite 1+
Pepdite 1+ (Banana Flavour)
Peptamen
Peptamen Junior
Peptisorb
Pregestimil
Reabilan
Resource 2.0 Fibre
SMA High Energy
Sondalis 1.5 Liquid Feed
Sondalis Fibre Liquid Feed
Sondalis ISO Liquid Feed
Tentrini
Tentrini Energy
Tentrini Energy Multi Fibre
Tentrini Multi Fibre
TwoCal HN

f)   Nutritional supplements
Necessary nutritional supplements prescribed on medical grounds (products should be labelled to state that they are to be taken under dietetic supervision and that a maximum of x mls containing 80g protein (approximately y cans/packs) may be taken per day)
Clinutren Dessert
Clinutren Fruit
Complan Shake
Enlive Plus
Enmix Plus Commence (as a supplement)
Enrich Plus
Ensure Plus Commence
Ensure Plus Liquid Feed
Ensure Plus Yoghurt Style
Formance
Forticreme Complete
Fortijuce
Fortijuce Starter Pack
Fortimel
Fortisip Bottle
Fortisip Multifibre
Fortisip Protein
Fortisip Protein Starter Pack
Fortisip Range Starter Pack (as a supplement)
Fresubin HP Energy
Fresubin Protein Energy Drink
Nutrison Energy
Nutrison MCT
Perative
Provide Xtra
Renilon 7.5
Resource Benefiber
Resource Dessert Fruit (Apple, Apple-Peach and Apple-Strawberry Flavours)
Resource Protein
Resource Shake Nutritional Supplement
Survimed OPD
Vegenat Med (as a supplement)

g)   Minerals
Metabolic Mineral Mixture

BORDERLINE SUBSTANCES

MALABSORPTION STATES

h) Vitamins - as appropriate
   See: Synthetic Diets

i) Vitamins and Minerals
          Energivit
          Paediatric Seravit

MALNUTRITION (DISEASE RELATED)

Calogen
Calogen Banana
Calogen Butterscotch
Calogen Strawberry
Caloreen
Calshake
Clinutren 1.5
Clinutren 1.5 Fibre
Clinutren Dessert (as a supplement)
Clinutren Fruit (as a supplement)
Clinutren ISO
Clinutren Junior
Complan Shake (as a supplement)
Duobar (strawberry, toffee, neutral)
Duocal (Liquid, MCT Powder & Super Soluble)
Enlive Plus (as a supplement)
Enmix Plus Commence (as a supplement)
Enrich
Enrich Plus
Enshake (Banana, Chocolate, Strawberry and Vanilla Flavours)
Ensure
Ensure 500ml Ready to Hang (Vanilla Flavour only)
Ensure Plus Commence (as a supplement)
Ensure Plus Liquid Feed (as a supplement)
Ensure Plus Yoghurt Style (as a supplement)
Foodlink Complete
Formance (as a supplement)
Forticreme Complete (as a supplement)
Fortifresh
Fortijuce (as a supplement)
Fortijuce Starter Pack (as a supplement)
Fortimel (as a supplement)
Fortini (as a supplement)
Fortini Multi Fibre (as a supplement)
Fortisip Bottle (as a supplement)
Fortisip Multifibre (as a supplement)
Fortisip Protein
Fortisip Protein Starter Pack
Fortisip Range Starter Pack (as a supplement)
Frebini
Frebini Energy
Frebini Energy Drink (Strawberry and Banana Flavours)
Frebini Energy Fibre
Frebini Energy Fibre Drink
Frebini Original Fibre
Fresubin Energy
Fresubin Energy Fibre Sip Feed
Fresubin Energy Fibre (Neutral) Tube Feed
Fresubin HP Energy (as a supplement)

BORDERLINE SUBSTANCES

MALNUTRITION (DISEASE RELATED)

Fresubin Liquid & Sip Feeds
Fresubin Protein Energy Drink (as a supplement)
Fresubin 1000 Complete
Fresubin 1200 Complete
Infatrini
Isosource Energy
Isosource Energy Fibre
Isosource Fibre
Isosource Junior
Isosource Standard
Jevity
Jevity Plus
Jevity Promote
Jevity 1.5kcal
Maxijul Liquid
Maxijul Super Soluble
Modulen IBD
Novasource Forte
Novasource GI Control
Nutrini
Nutrini Energy
Nutrini Energy Multifibre
Nutrini Low Energy Multifibre
Nutrini Multifibre
Nutrison Energy (as a supplement)
Nutrison Energy Multifibre
Nutrison MCT (as a supplement)
Nutrison Multifibre
Nutrison Protein Plus
Nutrison Protein Plus Multifibre
Nutrison Soya
Nutrison Standard
Nutrison 1000 Complete Multi Fibre
Nutrison 1200 Complete Multi Fibre
Osmolite
Osmolite Plus
Paediasure
Paediasure Plus
Paediasure Plus with Fibre
Paediasure with Fibre
Perative (as a supplement)
Polycal (Liquid & Powder)
Polycose Powder
Pro-Cal
Provide Xtra (as a supplement)
QuickCal
Renilon 7.5
Resource 2.0 Fibre
Resource Benefiber
Resource Dessert Fruit (as a supplement)
Resource Dessert Energy (as a supplement)
Resource Fruit Flavour Drink
Resource Junior (as a supplement)
Resource Protein (as a supplement)
Resource Shake Nutritional Supplement
Scandishake Mix Flavoured and Unflavoured
SMA High Energy
Sondalis 1.5 Liquid Feed
Sondalis Fibre Liquid Feed
Sondalis ISO Liquid Feed

BORDERLINE SUBSTANCES

MALNUTRITION (DISEASE RELATED)
Survimed OPD (as a supplement)
Tentrini
Tentrini Energy
Tentrini Energy Multi Fibre
Tentrini Multi Fibre
TwoCal HN
Vegenat Med (as a supplement)
Vitajoule
Vitasavoury

MAPLE SYRUP URINE DISEASE
Mapleflex (Unflavoured)
MSUD Aid III
MSUD Analog
MSUD Express
MSUD Gel
MSUD Maxamaid
MSUD Maxamum
Vitaflo - Valine Amino Acid (as a supplement)
Vitaflo - Isoleucine Amino Acid (as a supplement)
See: Low-Protein Products
        Synthetic Diets

METHYLMALONIC ACIDAEMIA
XMTVI Analog
XMTVI Asadon
XMTVI Maxamaid
XMTVI Maxamum

MILK PROTEIN SENSITIVITY
Comminuted Chicken meat (SHS)
Cow & Gate Pepti
Farley's Soya Formula
Infasoy
Isomil Powder
Nutramigen 1
Prosobee Liquid and Powder
Wysoy
See: Synthetic Diets.

NUTRITIONAL SUPPORT FOR ADULTS
(for precise conditions for which these products have been approved see the product listing in List A)
A   Nutritionally complete feeds
    For use as the sole source of nutrition or as necessary nutritional supplements prescribed on
    medical grounds
    a)   Gluten Free
                    Clinutren Junior
                    Foodlink Complete
                    Fortifresh
                    Fresubin Energy
                    Fresubin Energy Fibre Sip Feed
                    Fresubin Energy Fibre (Neutral) Tube Feed
                    Fresubin Liquid and Sip Feeds
                    Fresubin 1000 Complete
                    Fresubin 1200 Complete
                    Nutrison Energy Multifibre
                    Nutrison Multifibre
                    Nutrison Standard
                    Paediasure Plus
                    Sondalis ISO Liquid Feed

BORDERLINE SUBSTANCES

NUTRITIONAL SUPPORT FOR ADULTS

b)   <u>Lactose and Gluten Free</u>
                  Enrich
                  Ensure
                  Ensure 500ml Ready to Hang (Vanilla Flavour only)
                  Nutrison Soya
                  Osmolite
                  Osmolite Plus
                  Sondalis 1.5 Liquid Feed

c)   <u>Containing Fibre</u>
                  Clinutren 1.5 Fibre
                  Enrich
                  Fresubin Energy Fibre Sip Feed
                  Fresubin Energy Fibre (Neutral) Tube Feed
                  Fresubin Isofibre
                  Isosource Energy Fibre
                  Isosource Fibre
                  Jevity
                  Jevity Plus
                  Jevity Promote
                  Jevity 1.5kcal
                  Novasource Forte
                  Novasource GI Control
                  Nutrini Energy
                  Nutrini Energy Multifibre
                  Nutrini Low Energy Multifibre
                  Nutrini Multifibre
                  Nutrison Energy Multifibre
                  Nutrison Multifibre
                  Paediasure with Fibre
                  Resource 2.0 Fibre
                  Sondalis Fibre Liquid Feed

d)   <u>Elemental Feeds</u>
                  Elemental 028
                  Elemental 028 Extra
                  Elemental 028 Extra (Liquid)
                  Emsogen
                  Peptamen
                  Peptamen Junior
                  Peptisorb

B   <u>Nutritional Source Supplements</u>
See: <u>Synthetic Diets</u>
        Malabsorption States

a)   <u>General Supplements</u>
Necessary nutritional supplements prescribed on medical grounds for the diseases in List A (products should be labelled to state that they are to be taken under dietetic supervision and that a maximum of xmls containing 80g protein (approximately y cans/packs) may be taken per day)
                  Clinutren Dessert
                  Clinutren Fruit
                  Complan Shake
                  Enlive Plus
                  Enmix Plus Commence (as a supplement)
                  Enrich Plus
                  Ensure Plus Commence
                  Ensure Plus Liquid Feed
                  Ensure Plus Yoghurt Style
                  Foodlink Complete
                  Formance
                  Forticare
                  Forticreme Complete

XV

BORDERLINE SUBSTANCES

NUTRITIONAL SUPPORT FOR ADULTS

Fortijuce
Fortijuce Starter Pack
Fortimel
Fortini
Fortini Multi Fibre
Fortisip Bottle
Fortisip Multifibre
Fortisip Range Starter Pack
Fresubin HP Energy
Fresubin Protein Energy Drink
Fresubin 1000 Complete
Fresubin 1200 Complete
Nutrison Energy
Nutrison MCT
Perative
Prosure
Prosure 500ml Ready to Hang
Provide Xtra
Renilon 7.5
Resource Dessert Fruit
Resource Dessert Energy
Resource Junior
Resource Protein
Resource Support
Survimed OPD
Vegenat Med

b)   Carbohydrates

Caloreen	(Low electrolyte content)
Maxijul Liquid	
Maxijul Super Soluble	
Polycal (Liquid & Powder)	(Low electrolyte content)
Polycose Powder	
Pro-Cal	
QuickCal	
Resource Benefiber	
Vitajoule	
Vitasavoury	

c)   Fat

Alembicol D
Calogen
Calogen Banana
Calogen Butterscotch
Calogen Strawberry
Liquigen
MCT Oil

d)   Fat/Carbohydrate sources

Calshake	
Duobar (strawberry, toffee, neutral)	
Duocal (Liquid, MCT Powder & Super Soluble)	(Low electrolyte content)
Scandishake Mix Flavoured and Unflavoured	

e)   Nitrogen Sources

Casilan 90	(Whole protein based, low sodium)
Maxisorb	
Pro-Mod	(Whey protein based, low sodium)

f)   Minerals

Metabolic mineral mixture

BORDERLINE SUBSTANCES

PHENYLKETONURIA

Aminex low-protein biscuits
Aminex low-protein cookies
Aminex low-protein rusks
Aminogran food supplement
Aminogran PKU tablets
Aproten low-protein biscuits
Aproten low-protein bread mix
Aproten low-protein cake mix
Aproten low-protein crispbread
Aproten low-protein pasta (anellini, ditalini, rigatini, spaghetti, tagliatelle)
Easiphen
Ener-G low-protein egg replacer
Ener-G low-protein pasta (lasagne, macaroni, large shells, small shells, spaghetti)
Fate low-protein potato mix
Harifen low protein cracker toast
Harifen white chip cookies
Juvela low-protein bread rolls
Juvela low-protein chocolate chip; orange and cinnamon flavour cookies
Juvela low-protein loaf (sliced and unsliced)
Juvela low-protein mix
Lophlex (unflavoured, orange flavour and berry flavour)
Lophlex LQ (Orange, Berry and Citrus Flavours)
Loprofin low-protein breakfast cereal
Loprofin low-protein chocolate flavour cream biscuits
Loprofin low-protein chocolate, orange and vanilla flavour cream wafers
Loprofin low-protein cinnamon and chocolate chip cookies
Loprofin low-protein crackers
Loprofin low-protein egg replacer
Loprofin low-protein fibre bread (sliced and unsliced)
Loprofin low-protein loaf (sliced and unsliced)
Loprofin low-protein mix
Loprofin low-protein part baked rolls
Loprofin low-protein pasta (long-cut spaghetti, macaroni penne, spirals, vermicelli)
Loprofin low-protein sweet biscuits
Loprofin low-protein white rolls
Loprofin PKU Drink
L-Tyrosine Supplement
Metabolic Mineral Mixture
Minaphlex Flavoured & Unflavoured
Phlexy-10 Exchange System (Bar, Capsules & Drink Mix)
Phlexy-10 Tablets
Phlexy-Vits
Phlexy-Vits Tablets
PK Foods low-protein chocolate chip cookies
PK Foods low-protein cinnamon cookies
PK Foods low-protein crispbread
PK Foods low-protein egg replacer
PK Foods low-protein flour mix
PK Foods low-protein jelly mix dessert cherry flavour
PK Foods low-protein jelly mix dessert orange flavour
PK Foods low-protein orange cookies
PK Foods low-protein pasta spirals
PK Foods low-protein white sliced bread
PK Aid 4
PKU 2 (Milupa)
PKU 3 (Milupa)

BORDERLINE SUBSTANCES

PHENYLKETONURIA

PKU Cooler 15
PKU Cooler 20
PKU Express
PKU-Gel
PKU Start
Promin low-protein burger mix
Promin low-protein cous cous
Promin low-protein hot breakfast (apple & cinnamon, banana, chocolate and original flavours)
Promin low-protein lasagne sheets
Promin low-protein imitation rice pudding (apple, banana, strawberry and original flavours)
Promin low-protein pasta (alphabets, macaroni, shells, short-cut spaghetti, spirals)
Promin low-protein pasta in sauce (cheese and broccoli, tomato pepper and herb flavours)
Promin low-protein pastameal
Promin low-protein tricolour pasta (alphabets, shells, spirals)
Rite-Diet low-protein baking mix
Rite-Diet low-protein flour mix
Sno-Pro Drink
Ultra low-protein canned white bread
Ultra PKU biscuits
Ultra PKU bread
Ultra PKU cookies
Ultra PKU flour mix
Ultra PKU pizza base
Ultra PKU savoy biscuits
Valpiform low-protein cookies which chocolate nuggets and hazelnut flavour
Valpiform low-protein shortbread biscuits
XP Analog
XP Analog LCP
XP Maxamaid
XP Maxamaid Concentrate
XP Maxamum

See: Low-Protein Products
         Synthetic Diets

PHOTODERMATOSES (SKIN PROTECTION IN)

Delph Sun Lotion SPF 30
E45 Sun Block SPF 50
Spectraban Ultra
Sunsense Ultra (Ego)
Uvistat Lipscreen SPF 50
Uvistat Suncream SPF 30

PROPIONIC ACIDAEMIA

XMTVI Analog
XMTVI Asadon
XMTVI Maxamaid
XMTVI Maxamum

PROTEIN INTOLERANCE

See: Amino Acid Metabolic Disorders
         Low-Protein Products
         Milk Protein Sensitivity
         Synthetic Diets
         Whole Protein Sensitivity

PRURITUS
See: Dermatitis

PSORIASIS
See: Scaling of the Scalp

BORDERLINE SUBSTANCES

REFSUM'S DISEASE
  See: Fresubin Liquid and Sip Feeds

RENAL DIALYSIS
  See: Dialysis

RENAL FAILURE

Aminex low-protein biscuits
Aminex low-protein cookies
Aminex low-protein rusks
Aproten low-protein biscuits
Aproten low-protein bread mix
Aproten low-protein cake mix
Aproten low-protein crispbread
Aproten low-protein pasta (anellini, ditalini, rigatini, spaghetti, tagliatelle)
Dialamine
Ener-G low-protein egg replacer
Ener-G low protein pasta (lasagne, macaroni, large shells, small shells, spaghetti)
Ener-G low-protein rice bread
Fate low-protein all-purpose mix
Fate low-protein cake mix
Fate low-protein chocolate flavour cake mix
Juvela low-protein bread rolls
Juvela low-protein chocolate chip, orange and cinnamon flavour cookies
Juvela low-protein loaf
Juvela low-protein mix
Juvela low-protein pizza base
Kindergen
Loprofin low-protein breakfast cereal
Loprofin low-protein cinnamon and chocolate chip cookies
Loprofin low-protein chocolate flavour cream biscuits
Loprofin low-protein chocolate, orange and vanilla flavour cream wafers
Loprofin low-protein crackers
Loprofin low-protein egg replacer
Loprofin low-protein egg white replacer
Loprofin low-protein fibre bread (sliced and unsliced)
Loprofin low-protein loaf (sliced and unsliced)
Loprofin low-protein mix
Loprofin low-protein part-baked rolls
Loprofin low-protein pasta (long-cut spaghetti, macaroni penne, spirals, vermicelli)
Loprofin low-protein rice
Loprofin low-protein sweet biscuits
Loprofin low-protein white rolls
Nepro
Promin low-protein burger mix
Promin low-protein pasta (alphabets, macaroni, shells, short-cut spaghetti, spirals)
Promin low-protein pastameal
Promin low-protein tricolour pastas (alphabets, shells, spirals)
Renamil
Rite-Diet low-protein baking mix
Rite-Diet low-protein flour mix
Sno-Pro drink
Suplena
Ulltra low-protein canned brown bread
Ultra low-protein canned white bread
Ultra PKU biscuits
Ultra PKU bread
Ultra PKU cookies
Ultra PKU flour mix
Ultra PKU pizza base

XV

BORDERLINE SUBSTANCES

RENAL FAILURE
Ultra PKU savoy biscuits
Valpiform low-protein cookies with chocolate nuggets and hazelnut flavour
Valpiform low-protein shortbread biscuits
Vita-Bite

SHORT BOWEL SYNDROME
See: Malabsorption

SICCA SYNDROME
A.S. Saliva Orthana
Biotene Oralbalance Dry Mouth Saliva Replacement Gel
BioXtra Gel Mouthspray
BioXtra Moisturising Gel
Glandosane
Luborant Saliva Replacement
Saliveze
Salivix Pastilles

SYNTHETIC DIETS
(for precise conditions for which these products have been approved see the product listing in List A)

a)   Fat
Alembicol D
Calogen
Calogen Banana
Calogen Butterscotch
Calogen Strawberry
Liquigen
Medium chain triglyceride oil
Pro-Cal
QuickCal
Vitasavoury

b)   Carbohydrate
Caloreen
Maxijul Liquid
Maxijul Super Soluble
Polycal (Liquid & Powder)
Polycose Powder
Pro-Cal
QuickCal
Vitasavoury
Vitajoule

c)   Fat/Carbohydrate
Calshake
Duobar (strawberry, toffee, neutral)
Duocal (Liquid, MCT Powder & Super Soluble)
Enshake (Banana, Chocolate, Strawberry and Vanilla Flavours)
Scandishake Mix Flavoured and Unflavoured

d)   Minerals
Metabolic Mineral Mixture

e)   Protein Sources
See: Malabsorption states

f)   Vitamins - as appropriate
See: Malabsorption States
Nutritional Support for Adults

g)   Vitamins and Minerals
Paediatric Seravit
Phlexy-Vits
Phlexy-Vits Tablets

BORDERLINE SUBSTANCES

TYROSINAEMIA

Tyr Express
Tyr Gel
XPHEN, TYR Analog
XPHEN TYR Maxamaid
XPT Tyrosidon
XPTM Analog
XPTM Tyrosidon

UREA CYCLE DISORDERS

L-Arginine Supplement for urea cycle disorders. (S.H.S.)

VITILIGO

Covermark Classic Foundation
Covermark Finishing Powder
Dermacolor Camouflage Cream
Dermacolor Fixing Powder
Keromask Finishing Powder
Keromask Masking Cream
Veil Cover Cream
Veil Finishing Powder

VOMITING IN INFANCY

Instant Carobel
Nestargel

WHOLE PROTEIN SENSITIVITY

for definition, see page 435
Caprilon
Cow & Gate Pepti-Junior
MCT Pepdite 1+
Neocate
Neocate Active (unflavoured and blackcurrant flavour)
Neocate Advance (unflavoured, banana vanilla flavour and strawberry vanilla flavour)
Nutramigen 1
Nutramigen 2
Pepdite
Pepdite 1+
Pepdite 1+ (Banana Flavour)
Pregestimil
Prejomin

XEROSTOMIA

A.S. Saliva Orthana
Biotene Oralbalance Dry Mouth Saliva Replacement Gel
BioXtra Gel Mouthspray
BioXtra Moisturising Gel
Glandosane
Luborant Saliva Replacement
Saliveze
Salivix Pastilles

XV

BORDERLINE SUBSTANCES

LIST C

LIST C

The products which have been considered by the ACBS and may not be prescribed on Form FP10, are now included in Part XVIIIA.

NOTES ON CHARGES

NOTES ON CHARGES FOR DRUGS AND APPLIANCES PAYABLE UNDER REGULATIONS MADE UNDER SECTION 77(1) OF THE NATIONAL HEALTH SERVICE ACT 1977

(i)   Information about the number of charges payable is in paragraph 11 - with examples of the application of the charging arrangements in paragraph 12.

(ii) Where the arrangements or charge rates differ between England and Wales, provisions for England (ie set out in regulations made in England) apply to prescriptions dispensed by community pharmacists, appliance contractors and dispensing doctors in agreement with Primary Care Trusts (PCT) in England. Provisions for Wales (ie set out in regulations made in Wales) apply to prescriptions dispensed by community pharmacists, appliance contractors and dispensing doctors in agreement with Local Health Boards (LHB) in Wales. The cost of prescription prepayment certificates (PPCs) will apply in accordance with the normal address of the patient. Details are in paragraph 6.

(iii) Any PPC or exemption certificate issued in England, Northern Ireland, Scotland or Wales is valid across the UK.

(iv) In the following paragraphs, where no separate provision for Wales is noted, the same provisions apply in England and Wales.

1.   CHARGES PAYABLE

£6.65 (England) for each prescription item, preparation or type of appliance including each anklet, legging, knee-cap, below-knee, above knee or thigh stocking (In Wales £3.00). No charge is payable for <u>Oxygen concentrators</u> from 1 April 1992.

2.   PHARMACY AND APPLIANCE CONTRACTORS

Unless a completed declaration of entitlement to exemption or remission (paragraphs 4 and 5) is made on the prescription form, a charge is payable for each drug or appliance supplied, including each piece of elastic hosiery.

In order to secure exemption of or remission from prescription charges when presenting a prescription form to a pharmacy, or appliance contractor, the patient, or a person on his behalf, must complete the declaration on the back of the prescription form. The regulations have now been changed to require them to do so.

Patients, or their representatives, are also required to sign the prescription form to declare that a charge has been paid. Charges are retained by the dispensing practitioner whose payment for provision of pharmaceutical services is adjusted accordingly.

3.   DISPENSING DOCTORS

Unless a completed declaration of entitlement to exemption or remission (paragraphs 4 and 5) is made on the prescription form, the charges set out at (1) above are payable in respect of each item supplied by a dispensing doctor. In order to secure exemption or remission from prescription charges when presenting a prescription form to a dispensing doctor, the patient, or a person on his behalf, must complete the declaration on the back of the prescription form. The regulations have now been changed to require them to do so.

Patients, or their representatives, are also required to sign the prescription form to declare that a charge has been paid. Charges are retained by the dispensing practitioner whose payment for provision of pharmaceutical services is adjusted accordingly.

When an item dispensed by a dispensing doctor is delivered to a patient outside the surgery, every reasonable effort should be made to obtain a signed declaration from the patient that they have either paid the charge or are exempt.

However, there will be occasions when repeat prescriptions are delivered to points outside the surgery, or for example for collection from village shops to rural areas. Where a patient is exempt from charges and it is not practical for the patient to sign the form, a dispensing doctor or responsible member of the practice team should mark the reverse of the form as "remote delivery" and sign the form.

XVI

NOTES ON CHARGES

4. PEOPLE ENTITLED TO EXEMPTION

Provided that the appropriate declaration is received, a charge is not payable to the pharmacist, appliance contractor or dispensing doctor for drugs or appliances, including elastic hosiery, supplied for:

4.1 Children aged under 16;

4.2 Young people aged 16, 17 or 18 in qualifying full-time education;

4.3 In Wales, people aged under 25;

4.4 People aged 60 and over.

4.5 People holding a valid exemption certificate, which is issued to:

    4.5.1 expectant mothers;

    4.5.2 women who have borne a child or women who have given birth to a child in the last 12 months;

    4.5.3 people suffering from the following specified conditions who have a valid exemption certificate:

- permanent fistula (for example, caecostomy, colostomy, laryngostomy or ileostomy) requiring continuous surgical dressing;

- a form of hypoadrenalism (for example, Addison's Disease) for which specific substitution therapy is essential;

- diabetes insipidus and other forms of hypopituitarism;

- diabetes mellitus, except where treatment is by diet alone;

- hypoparathyroidism;

- myasthenia gravis;

- myxoedema (that is, hypothyroidism requiring thyroid hormone replacement);

- epilepsy requiring continuous anti-convulsive therapy;

- a continuing physical disability which means they cannot go out without the help of another person.

4.6 War pensioners holding a War Pension exemption certificate for prescriptions needed for treating their accepted disablement;

4.7 People who have purchased a Prescription Prepayment Certificate (PPC), which is valid at the point of dispensing.

5. NO PRESCRIPTION CHARGE EXEMPTION DECLARATION NEEDED FROM CERTAIN PATIENTS

1. In England from 1 April 2005, and in Wales from 1 August 2005 certain patients exempt on age grounds (aged under 16 in England or under 25 in Wales, or aged 60 or over) are no longer required to make a declaration of entitlement to claim exemption from prescription charges. (This means that certain patients do not have to complete any part of the exemption declaration i.e. will not have to fill in Part 1, 2, 3 or sign the declaration. In such cases pharmacists will not have to complete any part of the patient declaration.)

2. This easement applies only to patients (and representatives acting on behalf of patients) whose date of birth is automatically printed out on a hard copy paper prescription or inserted into an electronic prescription by an appropriate computer system that stores the patient's NHS care record. This easement also applies to repeat prescriptions (both electronic and paper) in the same way.

3. Those patients who are given an electronic prescription and who claim exemption from prescription charges on age grounds but whose date of birth is not held on the NHS care record will have to continue to make an exemption declaration. The same will also apply to those patients who are given hand written prescription forms where the date of birth is inserted manually.

NOTES ON CHARGES

6. PEOPLE ENTITLED TO REMISSION

6.1   People, and their partners, receiving Income Support or Income-based Jobseeker's Allowance;

6.2   People aged under 60 who are the partner of somebody getting Pension Credit guarantee credit;

6.3   People and their partner whose family income for tax credits is £15,050 or less (the limit is valid until 31 March 2007) and:

    6.3.1   they get Working Tax Credit (WTC) and Child Tax Credit (CTC); or

    6.3.2   they get WTC with a disability or severe disability element; or

    6.3.3   they are not eligible for WTC but get CTC.

6.4   HM Revenue & Customs send information to the NHSBSA, Help with Health Costs about people getting tax credits who are entitled to remission. Help with Health Costs send exemption certificates to these people. The certificate can be used as evidence of their entitlement to remission.

6.5   People and their partners who are named on an NHS Charges certificate HC2 because they are entitled to full help through the NHS Low Income Scheme.

6.6   Leaflet HC11and the equivalent HC11W in Wales provides information for patients about help with health costs within the respective countries. HC11 is on the Department of Health's website at www.dh.gov.uk\helpwithhealthcosts. HC11W is also available at www.wales.gov.uk/healthforms.

6.7   Leaflet HC12 and the equivalent HC12W in Wales provides information for patients about NHS charges and optical voucher values within the respective countries. HC12 is on the Department of Health's website at www.dh.gov.uk\helpwithhealthcosts. HC12W is also available at www.wales.gov.uk/healthforms.

6.8   Copies of both HC11 (HC11W in Wales) and HC12 (HC12W in Wales) should be made available to patients. They may be ordered free of charge from your PCT in England and requested from your LHB in Wales, or direct from:

In England

- Department of Health, PO Box 777, London, SE1 6XH, by letter;

- 01623 724 524 by fax;

- 08701 555 455 by telephone;

- doh@prolog.uk.com by email

In Wales

- Welsh Assembly Government, PO Box 2000, St. Helens, WA11 9XY by letter;

- 01942 271 717 by fax;

- 01623 724 233 by telephone;

- welshassembly@prolog.uk.com by email

XVI

7. PRESCRIPTION CHARGE REFUND PROCEDURE

1. This guidance applies to refunds of prescription charges in England and Wales only. Patients enquiring about getting a refund paid in Scotland should call the following number

Scotland - 0131 275 6076

Or they can write to: Practitioner Services (Pharmacy Repayments), 1 South Gyle Crescent, Edinburgh, EH12 9EB, Scotland

NOTES ON CHARGES

Security of forms

2. Prescription refund and receipt forms are secure items and should not be left in locations where they may be accessed by the public. They should be locked away when not required. Only authorised staff may process prescription refunds. If a pad or a form disappears, or cannot be accounted for, report this urgently to the Primary Care Trust (in England) or Business Services Centre (in Wales). Pharmacists should be alert to the possibility of misuse of the forms.

When to issue Prescription refund and receipt forms

3. Only issue a prescription refund form and receipt when the patient (or representative) requests this (but see paragraph 8 below) or is in genuine doubt about whether they might be exempt from prescription charges, or they have applied (or are thinking about applying) for a prescription charge exemption certificate or prepayment certificate.

4. When a patient (or representative) states they do not have to pay prescription charges because they are in an exempted group or hold a pre-payment certificate, they are not required to pay a charge simply because they do not have any evidence of entitlement. If they are prepared to sign to say they are exempt, they should complete and sign the declaration on the reverse of the prescription form. The "evidence not seen" box should be crossed, as per normal Point of Dispensing check procedures.

5. Only issue a prescription refund form and receipt at the time the prescription charge is paid. Later requests may be an attempt to get a second form to obtain a double refund fraudulently. If the patient or their representative is persistent in their request and they have grounds why they do not have a prescription refund and receipt, they should be advised to write to NHSBSA, Help with Health Costs, Sandyford House, Newcastle Upon Tyne, NE2 1DB or ring 0845 8501166, to explain why they were unable to obtain an FP57. Their Review Section will examine the claim and will either send a payment directly to the patient or advise the patient why they do not qualify.

6. If a receipt is required by a carer or representative, for example to show that the charge was paid, a till receipt may be sufficient proof. Only if a refund may be required should the patient be issued with a prescription refund and receipt.

Issuing prescription refund and receipt forms

7. Part A must be fully completed by the dispenser or an authorised member of staff. There must be no alterations to the amounts or the quantities in Part A. If a mistake is made, then start again with a new form and cross through the discarded form in such a way that it cannot be used and write, "CANCELLED" diagonally across it. The dispenser can initial any other alterations elsewhere on the form. Any forms which have been discarded due to alterations or mistakes in Part A should be kept for audit purposes.

8. The dispenser's stamp and date of payment must be on the form with the patient's name and address, the rate of prescription charge paid per item, the number of charges paid and the total paid.

Pharmacies processing forms for refunds

9. Patients should preferably return the prescription refund and receipt form to the community pharmacy that issued it. However, if this is not possible they may take the form to the most convenient pharmacy (normally in the country where the charge was paid.)

10. Community pharmacists should accept the claim even if the form was issued by a hospital or other NHS organisation. If a dispensing doctor or appliance contractor has taken a payment and the patient requires a refund the dispensing doctor or appliance contractor must provide the patient with a prescription refund and receipt. The patient should go to a community pharmacy to obtain the refund.

11. Pharmacists in England may make refunds for prescription refund and receipt forms issued in England, Scotland or Wales. The paid form will be sent to the NHSBSA, Prescription Pricing Division (In England). Pharmacists in Wales may make prescription refunds on Welsh receipt and refund forms (WP57) only. The paid form should be sent to Powys LHB via the Business Services Centre local offices (In Wales) in the normal way.

12. When a patient presents a prescription refund and receipt form for payment, the pharmacist (or any member of staff who would normally collect a prescription charge) should check the following:

- serial number on the form to ensure it is in the same format as the forms held by that pharmacy;

- that there are no alterations to the amounts or quantities in Part A and the form appears genuine, e.g. there is no white border indicating that it is a "home produced" copy.

NOTES ON CHARGES

13. If the form is not in order the pharmacist should phone the NHSBSA, Counter Fraud and Security Management Division fraud line number 08702 400100 (In England) and CFS Wales on 01495 745844 (In Wales).

14. If the form is in order, take the following steps:

- Check that the claim is being made within three months of the date the charge was paid, or the patient has an authorised form (LIS04(P)) from NHSBSA, Help with Health Costs

- Request evidence of entitlement to exemption or sight of form LIS04(P) authorising payment

- Check that the evidence relates to the patient

- Check that the evidence covers the date the charge was paid

- Note on the form what was produced, e.g. tax credit exemption certificate

- Note on the form the reference number on the exemption document (where applicable) e.g. 1234365

- Note on the form the LIS04(P) form reference number and date

- The person claiming the refund must print their name and address (i.e. the representative's details where appropriate)

- Pay the amount shown in Part A of the form

- Obtain signature of patient, or representative, and date for the cash

- Ensure that you, or the member of staff authorised to make refunds sign and print their name on the FP57/WP57 form.

Time Limit for making claims

15. A refund must be claimed within 3 months of the date on which the prescription charge was paid (e.g. if charge is paid 1 January, the refund must be claimed by 31 March). If more than 3 months have elapsed between the time the charge was paid and the prescription refund and receipt form is presented for payment, the refund may not be paid unless the patient has a form LIS04(P).

16. In the event of a late claim, patients will need to send the prescription refund and receipt form to NHSBSA, Help with Health Costs, Sandyford House, Newcastle Upon Tyne NE2 1DB and explain why they did not claim the refund within the 3 month time limit. Their Review Section will examine the claim and either authorise a refund by sending form LIS04(P) or advise the patient why they do not qualify.

Old style forms

17. You may be presented with the FP57/WP57 (0403) version of the form. If a patient does produce a 0403 form, the refund may be paid as long as either the form is presented within three months of the charge being paid, or the patient has an authorised form LIS04(P).

8.   PREPAYMENT CERTIFICATES (PPCs)

In England, patient can buy a PPC:

8.1   Over the internet, using their debit or credit card, at www.ppa.org.uk/ppc;

8.2   Over the telephone, using their debit or credit card, by calling 0845 850 0030;

8.3   By post, making payment by cheque, postal order, or their debit or credit card by completing the PPC application form (FP95);

8.4   At a pharmacy registered to sell PPCs on behalf of the NHSBSA. A list of pharmacies registered to sell PPCs can be found at www.ppa.org.uk/ppc.

PPCs may start up to one month earlier or one month later than the NHSBSA, Help with Health Costs receive the application.

Doctors and pharmacists could greatly assist any patient who makes frequent payments for prescriptions by drawing attention to the availability of PPCs. These certificates cost £95.30 (England) for one year or £34.65 (England) for four months. (In Wales, £43.09 for one year or £15.69 for four months.)

XVI

NOTES ON CHARGES

They are worthwhile for anyone requiring more than 14 prescription items in 12 months or 5 items in four months. For the convenience of patients, pharmacists are asked to hold PPC application forms FP95 (which are also available from PCTs) or WP95(Wales).

In Wales, patients may refer to their local Business Service Centre to obtain PPCs, the telephone numbers of which are as follows:

> Cardiff 029 2040 2402
> Carmarthen 01267 225 225
> Flintshire 01352 700 227
> Gwent 01495 765 065
> Swansea 01792 458 066.

9. BULK PRESCRIPTION

Charges are not payable in respect of "bulk" prescriptions for schools or institutions supplied in accordance with the Regulations See Note 9, Part VIII (page 70).

10. CONTRACEPTIVE SERVICES

No charge is payable for contraceptive substances and listed contraceptive appliances for women prescribed on FP10 or any of its variants.

The great majority of family planning prescriptions will be for contraceptive devices (See Part IXA) spermicidal gels, creams, films, pessaries and aerosols; or those systemic drugs promoted as contraceptives which are listed below: prescriptions for those products will not be specially marked and a prescription charge should not be levied.

Prescriptions for other drugs - If the prescription is for contraceptive purposes the prescriber should mark the item with the symbol ♀ (or endorse the item in another way which makes it clear that the prescription is for contraceptive purposes) and a prescription charge should not be levied for any items so marked. In the absence of such an endorsement by the prescriber, the normal prescription charge will apply to that item.

Where a dispensing doctor paid on the Drug Tariff basis supplies for contraceptive purposes a drug which is not on the list he should mark the item with the symbol ♀ (or endorse the item in another way which makes it clear that the prescription is for contraceptive purposes) on the prescription form before it is submitted for pricing.

List of Contraceptive Drugs to be Dispensed Free of Charge:

Bi Novum	Mercilon
Brevinor	Microgynon 30
Cerazette	Microgynon 30 ED
Cilest	Micronor
Depo-Provera 150mg/ml	Mirena System
Desogestrel Tablets 75microgram	Minulet
Evra	Norgeston
Femodene	Noriday
Femodene ED	Norimin
Femodette	Norinyl-1
Femulen	Noristerat Injection
Implanon	Ovranette
Levonelle 1500	Ovysmen
Levonelle One-Step	Synphase
Levonorgestrel Tablets 1.5mg	Triadene
Loestrin 20	Tri-Minulet
Loestrin 30	Trinordiol
Logynon	Trinovum
Logynon ED	Yasmin
Marvelon	
Medroxyprogesterone Acetate Injection (Aqueous Suspension) 150mg/5ml	

NOTES ON CHARGES

11. NOTES ON THE NUMBER OF CHARGES PAYABLE

11.1 SINGLE PRESCRIPTION CHARGE PAYABLE

Unless the patient claims exemption a single prescription charge is payable where:

11.1.1   The same drug or preparation is supplied in more than one container.

11.1.2   Different strengths of the same drug are ordered as separate prescriptions on the same prescription form (see also paragraph 12.4.2).

11.1.3   More than one appliance of the same type (other than hosiery*) is supplied.

11.1.4   A set of parts making up a complete appliance is supplied.

11.1.5   Drugs are supplied in powder form with the solvent separate for subsequent admixing.

11.1.6   A drug is supplied with a dropper, throat brush, or vaginal applicator.

11.1.7   Several flavours of the same preparation are supplied.

More than one prescription charge is payable where:

11.2 MULTIPLE PRESCRIPTION CHARGES PAYABLE

11.2.1   Different drugs, types of dressing or appliances are supplied.

11.2.2   Different formulations or presentations of the same drug or preparation are prescribed (but see 12.4.2) and supplied.

11.2.3   Additional parts are supplied together with a complete set of apparatus or additional dressing(s) together with a dressing pack.

11.2.4   More than one piece of elastic hosiery* is supplied.

*   (Anklet, legging, knee-cap, below-knee, above knee or thigh stocking).

12. EXAMPLES OF APPLICATION OF PRESCRIPTION CHARGE ARRANGEMENTS

"NO CHARGE" ITEM

The number of "no charge" items (ie items which are counted as prescriptions for pricing purposes but which do not carry a prescription charge) should be included on the invoice submitted with the prescription forms to the Pricing Authority.

12.1 LIQUIDS

Required by the prescriber to be supplied in more than one container. Certain preparations, if extemporaneously dispensed, may be subject to additional fees, (see Part IIIA paragraph 2).

		Professional Fees	Number of Prescription Charges	No Charge Prescriptions
Ammonium Chloride	300ml x 3	1	1	-
Boric Acid Eye Lotion	100ml x 2	1	1	-
Chloramphenicol Ear Drops	10ml x 2	1	1	-
Ferric Chloride Gargle	200ml x 2	1	1	-
Hydrogen Peroxide Ear Drops	10ml x 3	1	1	-
Lead Lotion	200ml x 3	1	1	-
Sulphacetamide Sodium Eye Drops	10ml x 2	1	1	-

XVI

NOTES ON CHARGES

		Professional Fees	Number of Prescription Charges	No Charge Prescriptions
12.2	**INJECTIONS**			
12.2.1	**Dispensed in powder form with solvent**			
	Amoxil Inj. Powder 500mg x 1	2	1	1
	Water for Injection 5ml x 1			
	Digoxin Amps 0.5mg x 10	2	1	1
	Normal Saline Amps 5ml x 10			
12.2.2	Influenza Vaccine (2 different strains in separate ampoules)	2	1	1

		Professional Fees	Number of Prescription Charges	No Charge Prescriptions
12.3	**TABLETS, CAPSULES, OINTMENTS, etc. - Different strengths of the same drug ordered as separate prescriptions at the same time**			
	Dithranol ½% in Lassar's Paste			
	Dithranol 1% in Lassar's Paste	3	1	2
	Dithranol 1½% in Lassar's Paste			
	Phenindione Tabs 50mg/one three times daily, 90	2	1	1
	Phenindione Tabs 10mg/one three times daily, 90			
	Phenindione Tabs 50mg/one in the morning, 30	2	1	1
	Phenindione Tabs 10mg/three at night, 90			
	Sulphacetamide Eye Drops 10%	2	1	1
	Sulphacetamide Eye Drops 30%			

		Professional Fees	Number of Prescription Charges	No Charge Prescriptions
12.4	**TABLETS, CAPSULES, etc.**			
12.4.1	**Different formulations or presentations of the same drug ordered as separate prescriptions**			
	Indocid Caps	2	2	-
	Indocid R Caps			
	Camcolit 250 Tabs	2	2	-
	Camcolit 400 Tabs sustained release			
	Bezalip Tabs 200mg	2	2	-
	Bezalip Mono Tabs			
	Prednisolone Tabs 1mg	2	2	-
	Prednisolone Tabs 2.5mg enteric coated			
	Trasicor Tabs	2	2	-
	Slow Trasicor Tabs			

NOTES ON CHARGES

			Professional Fees	Number of Prescription Charges	No Charge Prescriptions
12.4.2	**Strength required not listed** - should be ordered as the required strength and dispensed and priced by a combination of two different strengths and/or presentations. Tolanase Tabs - 350mg x 60				
	Contractor endorses	100mg x 60 } 250mg x 60 }	2	1	1
	Prothiaden - 100mg x 100 Contractor endorses				
		Caps 25mg x 100 } Tabs 75mg x 100 }	2	1	1

		Professional Fees	Number of Prescription Charges	No Charge Prescriptions
12.5	**COMBINATION PACKS**			
	Biotene Oralbalance Dry Mouth System	3	3	-
	Canesten Combi	2	2	-
	Canesten Cream Combi	2	1	1
	Canesten Oral and Cream Duo	2	2	-
	Climagest Tablets	2	2	-
	Cyclo-Progynova Tabs 1mg or 2mg	2	2	-
	Cyclo-Progynova Tabs 1mg (prescribed } Cyclo-Progynova Tabs 2mg together) }	4	3	1
	Didronel PMO 90 day Treatment Pack	2	2	-
	Diocalm Complete (Capsules and Powder Sachets)	2	2	-
	Ecostatin Twin Pack	2	2	-
	Elleste Duet Tablets 1mg or 2mg	2	2	-
	Estracombi TTS	2	2	-
	Evorel Pak	2	2	-
	Evorel Sequi	2	2	-
	Femapak 40 or 80	2	2	-
	Femoston Tablets 1/10, 2/10 or 2/20	2	2	-
	Femoston Tablets 2/10 (prescribed } Femoston Tablets 2/20 together) }	3	2	1
	FemSeven Sequi	2	2	-
	FemTab Sequi Tablets	2	2	-
	Germoloids Complete	2	2	-
	Gyno-Daktarin Combipack	2	2	-
	Gyno-Pevaryl 150 Combipack	2	2	-
	Gyno-Pevaryl 1 CP Pack	2	2	-
	Heliclear Triple Pack	3	3	-
	Helicobacter Test Hp-Plus	2	2	-
	Hytrin Starter Pack	2	1	1
	Hytrin-BPH Starter Pack	3	1	2
	Migraleve Complete Tablets (formerly Duo Pack)	2	2	-
	Napratec Combination Pack Tablets	2	2	-
	Neurontin Titration Pack	2	2	-
	Niaspan MR Titration Pack	3	1	2
	Norprolac Starter Pack	2	1	1
	Novofem Tablets	2	2	-
	Nuvelle Tablets	2	2	-
	Premique Cycle	2	2	-
	Prempak-C 0.625	2	2	-
	Prempak-C 1.25	2	2	-

XVI

NOTES ON CHARGES

	Professional Fees	Number of Prescription Charges	No Charge Prescriptions
Rehidrat Multipack	3	1	2
Tridestra	3	2	1
Trisequens	3	2	1
Tritace Titration Pack	3	1	2

		Professional Fees	Number of Prescription Charges	No Charge Prescriptions
12.6	**MULTIPLES OF SAME APPLIANCE OF SAME OR DIFFERING SIZE**			
Crepe Bandages	2 x 5cm	1	1	-
Open-Wove Bandages	1 x 2.5cm			
	1 x 5cm	1	1	-
	1 x 7.5cm			

	Professional Fees	Number of Prescription Charges	No Charge Prescriptions
12.7 SET OF APPLIANCES OR DRESSINGS			
Atomizer	1	1	-
Douche	1	1	-
Hypodermic Syringe	1	1	-
Multiple Pack Dressing No.1	1	1	-
Portable Urinal	1	1	-
Suprapubic Belt	1	1	-
Higginson's Enema Syringe	1	1	-

	Professional Fees	Number of Prescription Charges	No Charge Prescriptions
12.8 SETS OF APPLIANCES ORDERED WITH EXTRA PARTS			
Hypodermic Syringes } Hypodermic Needles	2	2	-
Multiple Pack Dressing No.2 } Absorbent Cotton 25g	2	2	-
Portable Urinal } Spare Sheaths 2	2	2	-

	Professional Fees	Number of Prescription Charges	No Charge Prescriptions
12.9 DIFFERENT APPLIANCES			
Lint 25g Absorbent Cotton 25g } Gauze 90cm x 1m	3	3	-

NOTES ON CHARGES

	Professional Fees	Number of Prescription Charges	No Charge Prescriptions
12.10 DRUGS ORDERED WITH DRUG TARIFF APPLIANCES			
Ametop Gel 4% Dispensing Pack (12 tubes 1.5g Gel and 15 Opsite Flexigrid Dressings)	2	2	-
Intal Spincaps } Spinhaler }	2	2	-

	Professional Fees	Number of Prescription Charges	No Charge Prescriptions
12.11 DRUGS PACKED WITH NON DRUG TARIFF APPLIANCES* (including metered aerosols with refills)			
Betadine Vaginal Preparation:-			
Pessaries (with applicator)	1	1	-
V.C. Kit	1	1	-
Syntaris Nasal Spray	1	1	-
Verrugon Ointment (Composite Pack)	1	1	-

* (These appliances are being allowed because they are packed with drug/preparation).

	Professional Fees	Number of Prescription Charges	No Charge Prescriptions
12.12 ELASTIC HOSIERY			
1 pr Knee-caps - One Way Stretch	1	2	-
1 pr Thigh Stockings - Class II	1	2	-
1 pr Spare Suspenders	1	1	-
1 Suspender Belt	1	1	-

	Professional Fees	Number of Prescription Charges	No Charge Prescriptions
12.13 LYMPHOEDEMA GARMENTS			
2 x Jobst Elvarex Custom Fit Class 1 Thigh High Stockings	1	1	-
1 x Jobst Elvarex Custom Fit Class 1 Thigh High Stocking } 1 x Jobst Elvarex Custom Fit Class 2 Thigh High Stocking }	2	2	-
2 x Jobst Elvarex Custom Fit Class 1 Thigh High Stockings with Class 1 Body Bandage	2	2	-
1 x Jobst Elvarex Custom Fit Class 1 Thigh High Stockings with silicone band	1	1	-
1 x Jobst Elvarex Custom Fit Class 1 Gauntlet to Wrist with four Class 1 fingers	1	1	-

XVI

NOTES ON CHARGES

	Professional Fees	Number of Prescription Charges	No Charge Prescriptions
12.14 MISCELLANEOUS			
12.14.1 Preparation supplied as separate parts for admixing as required for use			
Chlorhexidine 0.2% Aqueous Solution - 400ml) }			
Sodium Fluoride 2% Aqueous Solution - 400ml) }	2	1	1
12.14.2 Preparation having various flavours			
Dioralyte Natural			
Dioralyte Blackcurrant }	2	1	1
12.14.3 Different but related preparations			
Aminogran Food Supplement	1	1	-
Rite-Diet Gluten Free Flour			
Rite-Diet Gluten Free Bread }	2	2	
Migraleve Tabs, yellow	1	1	-
Migraleve Tabs, pink	1	1	-
Migraleve Tabs, yellow and pink	2	2	-
Triptafen-M Tabs			
Triptafen Tabs }	2	2	-
12.14.4 Eye, Ear and Nasal Drops (supplied with dropper bottles, or with a separate dropper where appropriate) (See Part IV.Containers)	1	1	-
12.14.5 A drug in powder form together with a solvent in the same packs (Treatment Pack) (2 vials of powder and 2 vials of solvent)			
Actinac	2	1	1
12.14.6 Oxygen			
Oxygen Therapy Set with cylinder(s)	1	1	-
Oxygen Cylinders	1	1	-
(See Part X, Home Oxygen Therapy Service)			
12.14.7 Trusses			
Spring Truss Inguinal - Single	1	1	-
Elastic Band Truss Scrotal-Double	1	1	-
12.14.8 Vaginal Creams and Applicators*			
Ortho Creme			
Vaginal Applicator - Type 1 }	2	-	2
Sultrin (Triple Sulfa) Cream			
Vaginal Applicator - Type 1 }	2	1	1
Applicator Vaginal			
Type 1 (Ortho)	1	-	1
Type 2 (Durex)	1	-	1

*   (No attempt should be made to determine whether or not the applicator is required for use with a contraceptive)

DENTAL PRESCRIBING

List of Preparations approved by the Secretary of State for Health as respects England and the National Assembly for Wales as respects Wales which may be prescribed on form FP10(D) by Dentists for National Health Service patients

Aciclovir Cream BP
Aciclovir Oral Suspension BP 200mg/5ml
Aciclovir Tablets BP 200mg
Amoxicillin Capsules BP
Amoxicillin Oral Powder DPF
Amoxicillin Oral Suspension BP (includes sugar-free formulation)
Amphotericin Lozenges BP
Ampicillin Capsules BP
Ampicillin Oral Suspension BP
Artificial Saliva DPF
Artificial Saliva Substitutes as listed below (to be prescribed only for indications approved by ACBS)
   # AS Saliva Orthana
   # Biotene Oralbalance
   # Bioxtra
   # Glandosane
   # Saliveze
   # Salivix
Ascorbic Acid Tablets BP
Aspirin Tablets Dispersible BP
Azithromycin Oral Suspension 200mg/5ml DPF

Benzydamine Mouthwash BP 0.15%
Benzydamine Oromucosal Spray BP 0.15%

Carbamazepine Tablets BP
Carmellose Gelatin Paste DPF (a medical device listed in Part IXA)
Cefalexin Capsules BP
Cefalexin Oral Suspension BP
Cefalexin Tablets BP
Cefradine Capsules BP
Cefradine Oral Solution DPF
Chlorhexidine Gluconate 1% Gel DPF
Chlorhexidine Mouthwash BP 0.2% w/v
Chlorhexidine Oral Spray DPF
Chlorphenamine Tablets BP
Choline Salicylate Dental Gel BP
Clindamycin Capsules BP

Diazepam Oral Solution BP 2mg/5ml
Diazepam Tablets BP
Diflunisal Tablets BP
Dihydrocodeine Tablets BP 30mg
Doxycycline Capsules BP 100mg
Doxycycline Tablets 20mg DPF

Ephedrine Nasal Drops BP
Erythromycin Ethyl Succinate Oral Suspension BP (includes sugar-free formulation)
Erythromycin Ethyl Succinate Tablets BP
Erythromycin Stearate Tablets BP
Erythromycin Tablets BP

Fluconazole Capsules 50mg DPF
Fluconazole Oral Suspension 50mg/5ml DPF

Hydrocortisone Cream BP 1%
Hydrocortisone Oromucosal Tablets BP
Hydrocortisone and Miconazole Cream DPF
Hydrocortisone and Miconazole Ointment DPF
Hydrogen Peroxide Mouthwash BP

Ibuprofen Oral Suspension BP sugar free
Ibuprofen Tablets BP

Lidocaine 5% Ointment DPF

Menthol and Eucalyptus Inhalation BP 1980
Metronidazole Oral Suspension DPF
Metronidazole Tablets BP
Miconazole Oromucosal Gel BP 24mg/ml
Mouth-wash Solution - tablets DPF

Nitrazepam Tablets BP
Nystatin Ointment BP
Nystatin Oral Suspension BP (includes sugar-free formulation)
Nystatin Pastilles BP 100,000 units

Oxytetracycline Tablets BP

*Paracetamol Oral Suspension BP (includes sugar-free formulation)
Paracetamol Tablets BP
Paracetamol Tablets Soluble BP
Penciclovir Cream DPF
Pethidine Tablets BP
Phenoxymethylpenicillin Oral Solution BP
Phenoxymethylpenicillin Tablets BP
Promethazine Hydrochloride Tablets BP
Promethazine Oral Solution BP

Sodium Chloride Mouthwash Compound BP
Sodium Fluoride Mouthwash BP
Sodium Fluoride Oral Drops BP
Sodium Fluoride Tablets BP
Sodium Fluoride Toothpaste 0.619% DPF, 1.1% DPF
Sodium Fusidate Ointment BP

Temazepam Oral Solution BP
Temazepam Tablets BP
Tetracycline Tablets BP
Triamcinolone Dental Paste BP

Vitamin B Tablets Compound Strong BPC

\#   These products have Advisory Committee on Borderline Substances approval for patients suffering dry mouth as a result of having (or having undergone) radiotherapy or sicca syndrome.

*   The title covers strengths of 120mg/5ml and 250mg/5ml, it is therefore necessary to specify the strength required.

This Page is Intentionally Blank

NURSE PRESCRIBERS' FORMULARY FOR COMMUNITY PRACTITIONERS (IN WALES DISTRICT NURSES AND HEALTH VISITORS)

Part XVIIB(i)
List of preparations as determined by the Secretary of State for Health as respects England and the National Assembly for Wales as respects Wales which may be prescribed by Community Practitioner Nurse Prescribers on Form FP(10)P (Forms WP10 (CN) and WP10 (PN) in Wales) for NHS patients under Section 41(1)(d) of the National Health Service Act 1977.

Community Practitioner Nurse Prescribers (in Wales district nurses and health visitors) who have completed the necessary training may only prescribe items appearing in the Nurse Prescribers' Formulary for Community Practitioners list set below.

NURSE PRESCRIBERS' FORMULARY FOR COMMUNITY PRACTITIONERS

See Also: Drug Tariff Part 1, 2, 3; Note 7 to Part IXA, B, C and Note 1 to Part IXR
Nurses are recommended to prescribe generically, except where this would not be clinically appropriate or where there is no approved generic name.

1   Only in quantities up to 100

2   Except pack sizes that are not to be prescribed under the NHS (See Part XVIIIA)

3   Except for indications and doses that are POM

4   Notes for Nurse Prescribers in Family Planning Clinics - Where it is not appropriate for nurse prescribers in family planning clinics to prescribe contraceptive devices using Form FP10(P) (forms WP10(CN) and WP10(PN) in Wales), they may prescribe using the same system as doctors in the clinic.

Medicinal Preparations
Almond Oil Ear Drops BP
Arachis Oil Enema NPF
[1] Aspirin Tablets Dispersible 300mg BP
Bisacodyl Suppositories BP (includes 5mg and 10mg strengths)
Bisacodyl Tablets BP
Cadexomer-Iodine Ointment NPF
Cadexomer-Iodine Paste NPF
Cadexomer-Iodine Powder NPF
Catheter Maintenance Solution Chlorhexidine NPF
Catheter Maintenance Solution Sodium Chloride NPF
Catheter Maintenance Solution 'Solution G' NPF
Catheter Maintenance Solution 'Solution R' NPF
Chlorhexidine Gluconate Alcoholic Solutions containing at least 0.05%
Chlorhexidine Gluconate Aqueous Solutions containing at least 0.05%
Choline Salicylate Dental Gel BP
Clotrimazole Cream 1% BP
Co-danthramer Capsules NPF
Co-danthramer Capsules Strong NPF
Co-danthramer Oral Suspension NPF
Co-danthramer Oral Suspension Strong NPF
Co-danthrusate Capsules BP
Co-danthrusate Oral Suspension NPF
Crotamiton Cream BP
Crotamiton Lotion BP
Dimeticone barrier creams containing at least 10%
Dimeticone Lotion 4%

Docusate Capsules BP
Docusate Enema NPF
Docusate Enema Compound BP
Docusate Oral Solution BP
Docusate Oral Solution Paediatric BP
Econazole Cream 1% BP
Emollients as listed below:
   Aqueous Cream BP
   Arachis Oil BP
   Cetraben Emollient Cream
   Decubal Clinic
   Dermamist
   Diprobase Cream
   Diprobase Ointment
   Doublebase
   E45 Cream
   Emulsifying Ointment BP
   Gammaderm Cream
   Hydromol Cream
   Hydromol Ointment
   Hydrous Ointment BP
   Keri Therapeutic Lotion
   Lipobase
   Liquid and White Soft Paraffin Ointment NPF
   Neutrogena Dermatological Cream
   Oilatum Cream
   Paraffin White Soft BP
   Paraffin Yellow Soft BP
   Ultrabase
   Unguentum M
   Zerobase Cream

XVIIB

NURSE PRESCRIBERS' FORMULARY FOR COMMUNITY PRACTITIONERS (IN WALES DISTRICT NURSES AND HEALTH VISITORS)

Emollient Bath Additives as listed below:
Alpha Keri Bath Oil
Ashbourne Emollient Medicinal Bath Oil
[2]Balneum
Cetraben Emollient Bath Additive
Dermalo Bath Emollient
Diprobath
Hydromol Emollient
Imuderm Bath Oil
Oilatum Emollient
Oilatum Junior Emollient Bath Additive
Oilatum Gel
Folic Acid 400 microgram/5ml Oral Solution NPF
Folic Acid Tablets 400 micrograms BP
Glycerol Suppositories BP
[3]Ibuprofen Oral Suspension BP
[3]Ibuprofen Tablets BP
Ispaghula Husk Granules BP
Ispaghula Husk Granules Effervescent BP
Ispaghula Husk Oral Powder BP
Lactulose Solution BP
Lidocaine Gel BP
Lidocaine Ointment BP
Lidocaine and Chlorhexidine Gel BP
Macrogol Oral Powder Compound NPF
Macrogol Oral Powder Compound
Half-Strength NPF (Movicol-Half)
Macrogol Oral Powder NPF
Magnesium Hydroxide Mixture BP
Magnesium Sulphate Paste BP
Malathion Alcoholic Lotions (containing at
least 0.5%)
Malathion Aqueous Lotions (containing at
least 0.5%)
Mebendazole Oral Suspension NPF
Mebendazole Tablets NPF
Methylcellulose Tablets BP
Miconazole Cream 2% BP
Miconazole Oromucosal Gel BP
Mouthwash Solution-tablets NPF
Nicotine Inhalation Cartridge for Oromucosal
Use NPF
Nicotine Lozenge NPF
Nicotine Medicated Chewing Gum NPF
Nicotine Nasal Spray NPF
Nicotine Sublingual Tablets NPF
Nicotine Transdermal Patches NPF

Prescriber should specify brand and strength to be
dispensed
Releasing nicotine over 16 hours:
Nicorette Patches
Releasing nicotine over 24 hours:
Boots NRT Patches
NiQuitin CQ Patches
Nicotinell TTS Patches
Nystatin Oral Suspension BP
Nystatin Pastilles BP
Olive Oil Ear Drops BP
Paracetamol Oral Suspension BP
(includes120mg/5ml and 250mg/5ml strengths
both of which are available as sugar-free
formulations)
[1] Paracetamol Tablets BP
Paracetamol Tablets Soluble BP
(includes 120mg and 500mg tablets)
Permethrin Cream NPF
Phenothrin Alcoholic Lotion NPF
Phenothrin Aqueous Lotion NPF
Phosphate Suppositories NPF
Phosphates Enema BP
Piperazine and Senna Powder NPF
Povidone-Iodine Solution BP
Senna Granules Standardised BP
Senna Oral Solution NPF
Senna Tablets BP
Senna and Ispaghula Granules NPF
Sodium Chloride Solution Sterile BP
Sodium Citrate Compound Enema NPF
Sodium Picosulfate Capsules NPF
Sodium Picosulfate Elixir NPF
Spermicidal Contraceptives as listed below:
Ortho-Creme Cream
Orthoforms Pessaries
Sterculia Granules NPF
Sterculia and Frangula Granules NPF
Titanium Ointment BP
Water for Injection
Zinc Cream BP
Zinc Ointment BP
Zinc and Castor Oil Ointment BP
Zinc Oxide and Dimeticone Spray NPF
Zinc Oxide Impregnated Medicated Stocking NPF
Zinc Paste bandage, BP 1993
Zinc Paste and Calamine Bandage
Zinc Paste, Calamine and Clioquinol Bandage BP
1993
Zinc Paste and Ichthammol Bandage BP 1993

Appliances and Reagents (Including Wound Management Products)

All Appliances and Reagents included in this list must comply with the description, specifications, sizes, packs and quantities as specified in the relevant entry in Part IX of the Drug Tariff

Appliances as listed in Part IXA (including Contraceptive Devices[4])

Incontinence Appliances as listed in Part IXB

Stoma Appliances and Associated Products as listed in Part IXC

Chemical Reagents, as listed in Part IXR

NURSE & PHARMACIST INDEPENDENT PRESCRIBING

From April 2006, the Nurse Prescribers' Extended Formulary is discontinued. From May 2006, Nurse Independent Prescribers (formerly known as Extended Formulary Nurse Prescribers) are able to prescribe any licensed medicine for any medical condition, including some Controlled Drugs - see below.

Pharmacist Independent Prescribers can also prescribe similarly, but currently cannot prescribe any Controlled Drug independently.

Nurse Independent Prescribers and Pharmacist Independent Prescribers:

- must work within their own level of professional competence and expertise

- are recommended to prescribe generically, except where this would not be clinically appropriate or where there is no approved generic name;

Nurse Independent Prescribers are also able to prescribe independently the following list of **Controlled Drugs**, solely for the medical conditions indicated:

Drug	Indication	Route of Administration
Buprenorphine	Transdermal use in palliative care	Transdermal
Chlordiazepoxide hydrochloride	Treatment of initial or acute withdrawal symptoms caused by the withdrawal of alcohol from persons habituated to it	Oral
Codeine phosphate	N/A	Oral
Co-phenotrope	N/A	Oral
Diamorphine hydrochloride	Use in palliative care, pain relief in respect of suspected myocardial infarction or for relief of acute or severe pain after trauma, including in either case post-operative pain relief	Oral or parenteral
Diazepam	Use in palliative care, treatment of initial or acute withdrawal symptoms caused by the withdrawal of alcohol from persons habituated to it, tonic-clonic seizures	Oral, parenteral or rectal
Dihydrocodeine tartrate	N/A	Oral
Fentanyl	Transdermal use in palliative care	Transdermal
Lorazepam	Use in palliative care, tonic-clonic seizures	Oral or parenteral
Midazolam	Use in palliative care, tonic-clonic seizures	Parenteral or buccal
Morphine hydrochloride	Use in palliative care, pain relief in respect of suspected myocardial infarction or for relief of acute or severe pain after trauma, including in either case post-operative pain relief	Rectal
Morphine sulphate	Use in palliative care, pain relief in respect of suspected myocardial infarction or for relief of acute or severe pain after trauma, including in either case post-operative pain relief	Oral, parenteral or rectal
Oxycodone hydrochloride	Use in palliative care	Oral or parenteral administration in palliative care

XVIIB

For the purposes of nurse independent prescribing, palliative care means the care of patients with advanced, progressive illness.

NURSE & PHARMACIST INDEPENDENT PRESCRIBING

Nurse Independent Prescribers & Pharmacist Independent Prescribers:

- can prescribe licensed medicines independently for uses outside their licensed indications (so-called 'off-licence' or 'off-label'). They must accept clinical/legal responsibility for that prescribing, and should only prescribe off-licence/off-label where it is accepted clinical practice;

- may prescribe any appliances/dressings that are listed in Part IX of the Drug Tariff;

- must not prescribe drugs and other substances listed in Part XVIIIA of the Drug Tariff at NHS expense;

- may prescribe drugs listed in Part XVIIIB of the Drug Tariff at NHS expense, but only in the specified circumstances, and/or for the specified patient groups listed in the Drug Tariff;

- must not prescribe unlicensed medicines;

- may prescribe borderline substances, which have been approved by the Advisory Committee on Borderline Substances (ACBS). A list of ACBS approved products and the circumstances under which they can be prescribed, can be found in part XV of the Drug Tariff. Although this is a non-mandatory list, Nurse Independent Prescribers should normally restrict their prescribing of borderline substances to items on the ACBS approved list.

Up-to-date information and guidance on nurse independent prescribing is available on the Department of Health website at www.dh.gov.uk/nonmedicalprescribing and at www.dh.gov.uk/PolicyAndGuidance/MedicinesPharmacyAndIndustry/Prescriptions

For Wales it is available at
http://www.wales.nhs.uk/sites3/page.cfm?orgid=371&pid=14547

NATIONAL OUT-OF-HOURS FORMULARY

THE FORMULARY CORE DRUG LIST

The following National Out-of-Hours Core Formulary contains the *minimum* list of drugs that patients should be able to access. Exact mechanisms for the provision of these drugs should be decided locally, taking into account existing treatment protocols. **(England only. At the time of going to press the National Assembly for Wales had not adopted the formulary)**

Guidance and information on template PGDs can be found on the website:http://www.pgd.nhs.uk/

Drug	Comment	Oral			
		Child	Adult	Inject able	Other
ANALGESIA					
Codeine or equivalent	Oral formulations to be supplied as a full course to appropriately treat the presenting condition. Codeine preferred as it has a dual role for pain relief and diarrhoea.		Y		
Diamorphine	Diamorphine is preferred for its use in both cardiac pain and palliative care.			Y	
Non Steroidal Anti-Inflammatory Drug (NSAID)	Oral formulations to be supplied as a full course to appropriately treat the presenting condition. The exact preparation(s) should be decided after local negotiation. Intramuscular injection of a NSAID may avoid the need for controlled drug use.	Y	Y	Y	
Paracetamol	Supply as a full course to appropriately treat the presenting condition.	Y	Y		
ASTHMA					
Inhaled Ipratropium	Supply as a full course to appropriately treat the presenting condition.				Y
Inhaled Salbutamol or equivalent	Supply as a full course to appropriately treat the presenting condition.				Y
Prednisolone	Oral formulations to be supplied as a full course to appropriately treat the presenting condition. Soluble tablets may be preferable for dual use in children and adults.	Y	Y		
Spacer Device	Or nebuliser device.				Y
CARDIAC EMERGENCIES					
Adrenaline/Epinephrine	Strength/formulation suitable for treatment of cardiac arrest.			Y	
Aspirin	For use in all patients with suspected Myocardial Infarction unless contraindicated or already taken.		Y		
Atropine	For use in cardiac emergencies.			Y	
Diamorphine				Y	

Drug	Comment	Oral			
		Child	Adult	Inject able	Other
Furosemide	Supply as a full course to appropriately treat the presenting condition. Full course of oral tablets is expected to be 7 days maximum.		Y	Y	
Glyceryl Trinitrate Sub-lingual	Supply as a full course to appropriately treat the presenting condition.		Y		
ALLERGY/ANAPHYLAXIS					
Adrenaline/Epinephrine	Strength/formulation suitable for treatment of anaphylaxis.			Y	
Hydrocortisone	Hydrocortisone sodium succinate can be used for anaphylaxis, asthma and hypoadrenalism.			Y	
Chlorphenamine	Supply as a full course to appropriately treat the presenting condition.	Y	Y	Y	
Non-Sedating Antihistamine	Supply as a full course to appropriately treat the presenting condition. Choice of preparation to be decided locally.		Y		
DIABETIC EMERGENCIES					
Glucagon Injection	Current recommendation is for both Glucose IV and Glucagon to be carried. Children may not respond to Glucagon so are more likely to need glucose. Patients not responding should be admitted.			Y	
Glucose				Y	
OPIOID OVERDOSE					
Naloxone	Any patient with an opioid overdose should be admitted to hospital, as repeated doses may be required.			Y	
GASTROINTESTINAL					
Antacid	Supply as a full course to appropriately treat the presenting condition taking into account manufacturers' pack sizes.		Y		
Domperidone	Supply as a full course to appropriately treat the presenting condition (see also metoclopramide).		Y		
Glycerol Suppositories	Included for immediate symptom relief (may be suitable for use by other healthcare professionals).				Y
Anti-Spasmodic Agent	Supply as a full course to appropriately treat the presenting condition.		Y		
Loperamide	Supply as a full course to appropriately treat the presenting condition.		Y		
Metoclopramide	Included as there is no parenteral formulation of domperidone			Y	
Oral Rehydration Sachets	Supply as a full course to appropriately treat the presenting condition.	Y			

NATIONAL OUT-OF-HOURS FORMULARY

Drug	Comment	Oral			
		Child	Adult	Inject able	Other
Phosphate Enema	Included for immediate symptom relief (may be suitable for use by other healthcare professionals).				Y
Prochlorperazine	Oral formulations to be supplied as a full course to appropriately treat the presenting condition.		Y	Y	Y
PSYCHIATRIC EMERGENCIES/CNS					
Diazepam	Supply as a full course to appropriately treat the presenting condition. Course length to be decided locally taking into account local policies and guidelines. Small quantities may be more appropriate. An appropriate rectal formulation to be included.	Y	Y	Y	Y
Haloperidol	Supply as a full course to appropriately treat the presenting condition. May also be used for treatment of severe nausea and vomiting.		Y	Y	
Procyclidine	Supply as a full course to appropriately treat the presenting condition.		Y	Y	
OBSTETRIC AND GYNAECOLOGY					
Levonorgestrel 1500	Full course to be supplied - included as current evidence suggests early treatment is appropriate.		Y		
Syntometrine Injection	Rarely used but essential to have available for intra or post partum obstetric emergencies. Special storage arrangements may be necessary.			Y	
PALLIATIVE CARE DRUGS					
Diamorphine				Y	
Cyclizine				Y	
Dexamethasone	It is expected that these drugs would be part of a special tamper proof palliative care pack that would be locally available. Local discussions will be necessary to determine appropriate access. The quantities supplied should be enough to allow appropriate symptom relief until formal review by palliative care team or General Practitioner.		Y		
Hyoscine Butylbromide				Y	
Ketorolac/Diclofenac				Y	
Methotrimeprazine/ Levomepromazine				Y	
Midazolam				Y	

XVIIC

NATIONAL OUT-OF-HOURS FORMULARY

Drug	Comment	Oral			
		Child	Adult	Inject able	Other
LOCAL ANTIBIOTIC CHOICE					
Following local discussion, antibiotics should be made available to appropriately treat the conditions listed below. Choice of preparation(s) should take into account local resistance patterns.					
Cellulitis and other skin infections	Supply as a full course to appropriately treat the presenting condition. Choice of preparation(s) should be made after local discussion taking into account local resistance patterns.	Y	Y		
Respiratory infections		Y	Y		
Upper respiratory tract infections		Y	Y		
Urinary tract infections		Y	Y		
INFECTION					
Bacterial conjunctivitis	Supply as a full course to appropriately treat the presenting condition. Choice of preparation(s) should be made after local discussion taking into account local resistance patterns.				Y
Candidiasis (Topical)	Included for immediate symptom relief.				Y
Herpes Zoster	Supply as a full course to appropriately treat the presenting condition. Choice of preparation to be decided locally. Included as current evidence suggest early treatment is appropriate.		Y		
Benzylpenicillin	For immediate treatment of meningococcal meningitis or septicaemia. Patients with suspected meningitis should be transferred to hospital urgently.			Y	
MISCELLANEOUS					
Sodium chloride for injection/ infusion	Also to include IV giving set and canula			Y	
Water for injection	For dissolving injectable drugs.			Y	
Blood glucose testing sticks	Use where **diagnosis** cannot safely wait e.g. to identify patients who have urgent treatment needs or who should be admitted to hospital.				Y
Urine testing sticks	Use where **diagnosis** cannot safely wait e.g. to identify patients who have urgent treatment needs or who should be admitted to hospital.				Y
DRUGS WHERE SPECIAL ARRANGEMENTS MAY BE APPROPRIATE					
Oxygen	It may be appropriate for some organisations to keep a supply of oxygen. Alternatively, local discussion and specific arrangements will need to be made for the delivery of oxygen.				

DRUGS AND OTHER SUBSTANCES NOT TO BE PRESCRIBED UNDER THE NHS PHARMACEUTICAL SERVICES

Part XVIIIA reproduces Schedule 1 to the National Health Service (General Medical Services Contracts) (Prescription of Drugs etc.) Regulations 2004.

10.10 Cleaning and Disinfecting Solution
10.10 Rinsing and Neutralising Solution
10 Day Slimmer Tablets
10 Hour Capsules
4711 Cologne
Abidec Capsules
Acarosan Foam
Acarosan Moist Powder
Acclaim Flea Control Aerosol Plus
Acnaveen Bar
Acne Aid Bar
Actal Suspension
Actal Tablets
Actifed Compound Linctus
Actifed Cough Relief
Actifed Expectorant
Actifed Linctus with Codeine
Actifed Syrup
Actifed Tablets
Actomite
Actonorm Gel
Actonorm Powder
Actonorm Tablets
Actron Tablets
Adpack Europe Gamolenic Acid (GLA) Capsules
Adreno-Lyph Plus Tablets
Adult Cough Balsam (Cupal)
Adult Meltus Cough & Catarrh Linctus
Adult Tonic Mixture (Thornton & Ross)
Advanced Nutrition Bee Pollen Granules
Advanced Nutrition Bee Propolis Tablets
Advanced Nutrition Chromium Compound Liquid
Advanced Nutrition Ener-B NSL Gel
Advanced Nutrition Herbal Aloe Juice
Advanced Nutrition L-Arginine Capsules
Advanced Nutrition Linseed Oil
Advanced Nutrition Silica-Organic Capsules
Advanced Nutrition Sulphur Capsules
Advanced Nutrition Vitamin E Capsules
Aerocide 2 Spray 400ml
Afrazine Nasal Drops
Afrazine Nasal Spray
Afrazine Paediatric Nasal Drops
Agarol Emulsion
Agiolax Granules
Airbal Breathe Easy Vapour Inhaler
AL Tablets
Alagbin Tablets
Alcin Tablets
Alcon Salette Aerosol Saline Solution
Aletres Cordial (Potters)
Alexitol Sodium Suspension 360 mg/5 ml
Alexitol Sodium Tablets
Algipan Rub
Algipan Tablets
Alka-Donna P Mixture
Alka-Donna P Tablets
Alka-Donna Suspension
Alka-Donna Tablets
Alka Mints

Alka-Seltzer Tablets
Alket Powders
All Clear Shampoo
All Fours Cough Mixture (Harwood)
All Fours Mixture (Glynwed Wholesale Chemists)
All Fours Mixture (Roberts Laboratories)
Allbee with C Capsules
Allbee with C Elixir
Aller-eze Plus Tablets
Aller-eze Tablets
Allinson's Wholemeal Flour
Almasilate Tablets 500 mg
Almay Aftersun Soother
Almay Face Powder
Almay Sun Protection Cream SPF 12
Almay Ultra Protection Lotion SPF 12
Almazine Tablets 1mg
Almazine Tablets 2.5 mg
Aloin Tablets 40 mg
Alophen Pills
Alpine Tea
Alprazolam Tablets 0.25mg
Alprazolam Tablets 0.5mg
Alprazolam Tablets 1 mg
Altacaps
Altacite Plus Tablets
Altacite Suspension
Altacite Tablets
Altelave Liquid
Aludrox Gel
Aludrox Liquid
Aludrox M H Suspension
Aludrox S A Suspension
Aludrox Tablets
Aluhyde Tablets
Aluminium Hydroxide & Silicone Suspension
Aluminium Phosphate Gel
Aluminium Phosphate Tablets 400 mg
Alupent Expectorant Mixture
Alupent Expectorant Tablets
Aluphos Gel
Aluphos Tablets
Alupram Tablets 2 mg
Alupram Tablets 5 mg
Alupram Tablets 10 mg
Aluzyme Tablets
Alzed Tablets
Ambre Solaire Cream Factor 8
Ambre Solaire Cream Factor 10
Ambre Solaire High Protection Cream SPF10
Ambre Solaire High Protection Milk SPF 12
American Nutrition Strezz B-Vite Tablets
Ami - 10 Rinsing and Storage Solution
Amiclear Contact Lens Cleanser Tablets
Amidose Saline Solution 30 ml
Amin-Aid
Amisyn Tablets
Ammonium Chloride and Morphine Mixture BP
Amplex Mint Capsules
Amplex Mouthwash

XVIIIA

DRUGS AND OTHER SUBSTANCES NOT TO BE PRESCRIBED UNDER THE NHS PHARMACEUTICAL SERVICES

Amplex Original Capsules
Anadin Analgesic Capsules Maximum Strength
Anadin Analgesic Tablets
Anadin Extra Analgesic Tablets
Anadin Extra Soluble
Anadin Ibuprofen Tablets
Anadin Paracetamol Tablets
Anadin Tablets Soluble
Anaflex Cream
Andrews Answer
Andrews Antacid Tablets
Andrews Liver Salts Effervescent Powder
Andrews Liver Salts (Diabetic Formula)
     Effervescent Powder
Andursil Liquid
Andursil Tablets
Anestan Bronchial Tablets
Anethaine Cream
Aneurone Mixture
Angiers Junior Aspirin Tablets
Angiers Junior Paracetamol Tablets
Anorvit Tablets
Antasil Liquid
Antasil Tablets
Anthisan Cream
Antistin-Privine Nasal Drops
Antistin-Privine Nasal Spray
Antitussive Linctus (Cox)
Antoin Tablets
Antussin Liquid (Sterling Winthrop)
Anxon Capsules 15 mg
Anxon Capsules 30 mg
Anxon Capsules 45 mg
Aperient Tablets (Brome & Schimmer)
Aperient Tablets (Kerbina)
Apodorm Tablets 2.5 mg
Apodorm Tablets 5 mg
APP Stomach Powder
APP Stomach Tablets
Applefords Gluten-Free Rice Cakes
Arnica Lotion
Arocin Capsules
Arret Capsules
Ascorbef Tablets
Ascorbic Acid & Hesperidin Capsules (Regent
     Laboratories)
Asilone Antacid Liquid
Asilone Antacid Tablets
Asilone Orange Tablets
Askit Capsules
Askit Powders
Askit Tablets
Aspergum Chewing Gum Tablets 227 mg
Aspirin Chewing-Gum Tablets 227 mg
Aspirin Tablets, Effervescent Soluble 300 mg
Aspirin Tablets, Effervescent Soluble 500 mg
Aspirin Tablets, Slow (Micro-Encapsulated) 648 mg
Aspro Clear Extra Tablets
Aspro Clear Tablets
Aspro Extra Strength Tablets 500 mg
Aspro Junior Tablets
Aspro Microfined Tablets
Aspro Paraclear Junior Tablets
Aspro Paraclear Tablets

Asthma Tablets (Cathay)
Astral Moisturising Cream
Astroplast Analgesic Capsules
Atensine Tablets 2 mg
Atensine Tablets 5 mg
Atensine Tablets 10 mg
Ativan Tablets 1 mg
Ativan Tablets 2.5 mg
Atrixo
Audax Ear Drops
Autan Insect Repellent
Aveeno Baby
Aveeno Bar
Aveeno Bar Oilated
Aveeno Emulave Bar
Aveenobar
Ayrtons Analgesic Balm
Ayrtons Macleans Formula Tablets

B Complex Capsules (Rodale)
B Complex Super Capsules (Rodale)
B Extra Tablets (British Chemotherapeutic
     Products)
Babezone Syrup
Baby Chest Rub Ointment (Cupal)
Babylix Syrup
Babysafe Tablets
Badedas Bath Gelee
Balm of Gilead (Robinsons)
Balm of Gilead Cough Mixture (Wicker Herbal
     Stores)
Balm of Gilead Liquid (Culpeper)
Balm of Gilead Mixture (Potters)
Balneum Bath Treatment 150ml pack
Balneum Plus Bath Treatment 150ml pack
Banfi Hungarian Hair Tonic
Banimax Tablets
Barker's Liquid of Life Solution
Barker's Liquid of Life Tablets
Barkoff Cough Syrup
Barnes - Hind Cleaning and Soaking Solution
Barnes - Hind Intensive Cleaner
Barnes - Hind No 4 Cleaner
Barnes - Hind Wetting and Soaking Solution
Bausch and Lomb Cleaning Tablets
Bausch and Lomb Concentrated Cleaner (for Hard
     Lenses)
Bausch and Lomb Daily Lens Cleaner
Bausch and Lomb Saline Solution
Bausch and Lomb Soaking and Wetting Solution
Bayer Aspirin Tablets 300 mg
BC500 Tablets
BC500 with Iron Tablets
BC500 Vitamin Sachets effervescent
Becosym Forte Tablets
Becosym Syrup
Becosym Tablets
Becotab Tablets
Bee Health Propolis Capsules
Beecham Analgesic Cream
Beechams Catarrh Capsules
Beechams Day Nurse Capsules
Beechams Day Nurse Syrup
Beechams Night Nurse Capsules

DRUGS AND OTHER SUBSTANCES NOT TO BE PRESCRIBED UNDER THE NHS PHARMACEUTICAL SERVICES

Beechams Night Nurse Cold Remedy
Beechams Pills
Beechams Powders
Beechams Powders Capsule Form
Beechams Powders Mentholated
Beechams Powders Tablet Form
Beehive Balsam
Bekovit Tablets
Belladonna and Ephedrine Mixture, Paediatric, BPC
Bellocarb Tablets
Bemax Natural Wheatgerm
Benadon Tablets 20 mg
Benadon Tablets 50 mg
Benafed Linctus
Benerva Compound Tablets
Benerva Injection 25 mg/ml
Benerva Injection 100 mg/ml
Benerva Tablets 3 mg
Benerva Tablets 10 mg
Benerva Tablets 25 mg
Benerva Tablets 50 mg
Benerva Tablets 100 mg
Benerva Tablets 300 mg
Bengers Food
Bengue's Balsam
Benylin Chesty Coughs Original
Benylin Children's Coughs
Benylin Children's Cough Linctus
Benylin Cough & Congestion
Benylin Day & Night Tablets
Benylin Day & Night Cold Treatment
Benylin Dry Coughs Original
Benylin Expectorant
Benylin Fortified Linctus
Benylin Mentholated Cough & Decongestant Linctus
Benylin Non-Drowsy Cough Linctus
Benylin Paediatric
Benylin with Codeine
Benzedrex Inhaler
Benzoin Inhalation BP
Bepro Cough Syrup
Beres Drops Plus
Bergasol After Sun Soother
Bergasol Ultra Protection Tanning Lotion
Best Royal Jelly Capsules
Beta Carotene Capsules (Nutri Imports & Exports)
Biactol Anti-Bacterial Face Wash
Bile Beans Formula 1 Pill
Bio-Antioxidant Tablets
Biocare Acidophilus Powder
Biocare AD206 (Adreno-Zyme) Capsules
Biocare Allicin Compound Capsules
Biocare Amino-Plex Capsules
Biocare Artemisia Compound Capsules
Biocare ATP Factor Capsules
Biocare Beetroot Concentrate (Bioflavour Complex) Capsules
Biocare Beta-Carotene Capsules
Biocare Betaine HCL/Pepsin Capsules 200/100mg
Biocare BGF Bifidophilus Growth Factor Powder
Biocare Bio Acidophilus Milk Free Capsules
Biocare Bio-A Emulsifying Liquid

Biocare Biogard Capsules
Biocare Bio-Cysteine Capsules
Biocare Bio-Magnesium Capsules 100mg
Biocare Bio-Manganese Capsules
Biocare Bio-Plex Powder
Biocare Butyric Acid Compound Capsules
Biocare Calcidophilus Capsules
Biocare Calcium EAP2 Capsules
Biocare Candistatin Capsules
Biocare Catalase Compound Liquid
Biocare Cervagyn Vaginal Cream
Biocare Cellguard Forte Capsules
Biocare CG233 Capsules
Biocare Children's Multi Vitamin/Mineral Capsules
Biocare Cholesteraze Capsules
Biocare Chromium Polynicotinate Liquid
Biocare Colleginase Capsules
Biocare Colon Care Capsules
Biocare Cystoplex Powder
Biocare Dermasorb Skin Cream
Biocare Digestaid Capsules
Biocare DMSA Capsules
Biocare Efaplex Linseed/GLA Blend Capsules
Biocare Enteroplex Powder
Biocare Eradicin Forte Capsules
Biocare Femforte Capsules
Biocare Garlicin Capsules
Biocare GLA Complex Tablets
Biocare GLA/Co Q10 Catalase Capsules
Biocare Glutenzyme Capsules
Biocare Hep 194 (Hepaguard) Capsules
Biocare HCL Pepsin Capsules
Biocare Histazyme Capsules
Biocare IMU Power Pack
Biocare Int B2 Bifidophilus Bacterium Powder
Biocare Iron EAP2 Capsules
Biocare Kalmar Capsules
Biocare Lactase Enzyme Liquid
Biocare Ligazyme Capsules
Biocare Linseed Oil Emulsifying Capsules
Biocare Lipazyme Capsules
Biocare Lipo-Plex Capsules
Biocare Lipo-Plex Co-Q10 EPA/DHA Capsules
Biocare Magnesium Calcium 2:1 Capsules
Biocare Magnesium EAP2 Capsules
Biocare Mega GLA Complex Capsules 163mg
Biocare Molybdenum Liquid
Biocare Multi-Mineral Complex Capsules
Biocare Multivitamin Mineral Capsules
Biocare Mycopryl 250 Junior Strength Capsules
Biocare Mycopryl 400 Capsules
Biocare Mycopryl 680 Capsules
Biocare N-Acetyl Glucosamine Capsules
Biocare NT 188 (Neurotone) Capsules
Biocare Organic Selenium Capsules 100mcg
Biocare Oxy-B15 Complex Capsules
Biocare Oxyplex Tablets
Biocare Oxy Pro Liquid
Biocare Pancrogest Capsules
Biocare Paracidin (Citricidal) Oral Drops
Biocare Permatrol Capsules
Biocare Pit-Enzyme Capsules
Biocare Polyzyme Capsules
Biocare Polyzyme Forte & Acidophilus Capsules

XVIIIA

DRUGS AND OTHER SUBSTANCES NOT TO BE PRESCRIBED UNDER THE NHS PHARMACEUTICAL SERVICES

Biocare Polyzyme Forte Capsules
Biocare Potassium Ascorbate Capsules
Biocare Prolactazyme Capsules
Biocare Prolactazyme Tablets
Biocare Reduced Glutathione Capsules
Biocare Replete Sachets
Biocare Sea Plasma Capsules 500mg
Biocare Selenium Complex Tablets 50mcg
Biocare Selenium Liquid
Biocare Shiitake Mushroom Extract Capsules
Biocare Spectrumzyme Capsules
Biocare TH207 (Thyro-Zyme) Capsules
Biocare Thioproline Capsules
Biocare Uritol Capsules
Biocare Vegi-Dophilus Capsules
Biocare Vitamin B6 Capsules
Biocare Vitamin B Compound Capsules
Biocare Vitamin B12 Timed Release Capsules
Biocare Vitamin C Capsules
Biocare Vitamin C Magnesium Ascorbate Powder
Biocare Vitamin E Emulsifying Capsules
Biocare Vyta Mins Capsules
Biocare Zinc Tablets
Bio-Carotene Softgel Capsules
Bioflav Complex Tablets
Bioflav Complex + C Tablets
Bioflavonoid C Capsules
Bio-Glandin 25 Capsules
Bio Harmony Sachets
Bio-Health Buffered C500 Capsules
Bio-Health Extra Calcium Capsules
Bio-Health Zinc Gluconate Capsules
Bio-Light Slimming Food Supplement
Bio-Quinone Q10 Softgel Capsules
Bio-Quinone Q10 Super Softgel Capsules
Bioscal Hair Formula
Bio Science Basic Health AM Capsules
Bio Science Basic Health PM Capsules
Bio Science Bio-C Powder
Bio Science Cal-Mag Alkaline Capsules
Bio Science Chelated Cal-Mag Compound
    Capsules
Bio Science Chelated Zinc Capsules
Bio Science Full Spectrum Aminos Powder
Bio Science Lipid Enzyme Capsules
Bio Science Lo-pH Complete Spectrum Digestive
    Enzyme Capsules
Bio Science Lo-pH Digestive Enzyme Capsules
Bio Science MSM Organic Sulphur Capsules
Bio Science Non-Acidic Sustained Release Vitamin
    C Tablets
Bio Science Organic Iron Capsules
Bio Science Pro Enzyme Capsules
Bio Science Pyroxidal 5 Phosphates Capsules
Bio Science Selenium Plus Capsules
Bio Science Timed Release Vitamin C Tablets
Bio Science Vitamin B1 Capsules
Bio Science Vitamin B3 Nicotinamide Capsules
Bio Science Vitamin B5 Calcium Pantothenate
    Capsules
Bio Science Vitamin B6 Capsules
Bio Science Vitamin E Capsules
Bio-Selenium + Zinc Tablets
Bio-Strath Drops

Bio-Strath Elixir
Biovital Tablets
Biovital Vitamin Tonic
Birley's Antacid Powder
Bis-Mag Lozenge
Bis-Peps Tablets
Bisma-Calna Cream
Bisma-Rex Powder
Bisma-Rex Tablets
Bismag Antacid Powder
Bismag Tablets
Bismuth Compound Lozenges BPC
Bismuth Dyspepsia Lozenges
Bismuth Pepsin and Pancreatin Tablets
Bismuth, Soda and Pepsin Mixture
Bisodol Antacid Powder
Bisodol Extra Tablets
Bisodol Tablets
Bisolvomycin Capsules
Bisolvon Elixir
Bisolvon Tablets
Blackcurrant Cough Elixir (Thornton & Ross)
Blackcurrant Seed Oil Capsules
Blackcurrant Syrup Compound (Beben)
Blackmore's Acidophilus & Pectin Tablets
Blackmore's Bio C Tablets
Blackmore's Celloid CS36 Calcium Sulphate
    Tablets
Blackmore's Celloid IP82 Iron pH Tablets
Blackmore's Celloid SS69 Sodium Sulphate
    Tablets
Blackmore's Citrus C & AcerolaTablets
Blackmore's Duocelloid PP/MP Tablets
Blackmore's Duocelloid PS/MP Tablets
Blackmore's Duocelloid S/CF Tablets
Blackmore's Duocelloid SP/S Tablets
Blackmore's Echinacea ACE + Zinc Tablets
Blackmore's Hypericum Tablets
Blackmore's Sodical Plus Tablets
Blandax Suspension
Blavig Tablets
Blood Tonic Mixture (Thompsons)
Boldolaxine Tablets
Bonemeal Calfos, Vit A Ester, Vit D Tablets
Bonomint Chewing Gum
Bonomint Tablets
Booth's Cough & Catarrh Elixir
Boots Aromatherapy Massage Oil
Boots Baby Oil
Boots Cold Relief Powder for Solution
Boots Compound Laxative Syrup of Figs
Boots Cough Relief for Adults
Boots Glucosamine Sulphate Capsules
Boots Glycerin & Blackcurrant Soothing Cough
    Relief
Boots Hard Lens Soaking Solution
Boots Hard Lens Wetting Solution
Boots Health Salts
Boots Indigestion Plus Mixture
Boots Indigestion Powder
Boots Lip Salve
Boots Menthol & Wintergreen Embrocation
Boots Nasal Spray
Boots No 7 Vitamin E Skin Cream

DRUGS AND OTHER SUBSTANCES NOT TO BE PRESCRIBED UNDER THE NHS PHARMACEUTICAL SERVICES

Boots Orange Drink
Boots Soft Lens Cleaning Solution
Boots Soft Lens Comfort Solution
Boots Soft Lens Soaking Solution
Boots Soya Milk
Boots Vapour Rub Ointment
Boston Lens Cleaning Solution
Boston Lens Wetting and Soaking Solution
Box's Balm of Gilead Cough Mixture
Bravit Capsules
Bravit Tablets
Breoprin Tablets 648 mg
Brewers Yeast Super B Tablets (Rodale)
Brewers Yeast Tablets (3M Health Care)
Brewers Yeast Tablets (Phillips Yeast Products)
Bricanyl Compound Tablets
Bricanyl Expectorant
Brogans Cough Mixture
Brogans Cough Syrup
Bromazepam Tablets 1.5 mg
Bromazepam Tablets 3 mg
Bromazepam Tablets 6 mg
Bromhexine Hydrochloride Elixir 4 mg/5 ml
Bromhexine Hydrochloride Tablets 8 mg
Bronalin Decongestant
Bronalin Dry Cough Linctus
Bronalin Expectorant
Bronalin Paediatric Cough Syrup
Bronchial & Cough Mixture (Worthington Walter)
Bronchial Balsam (Cox)
Bronchial Catarrh Syrup (Rusco)
Bronchial Cough Mixture (Evans Medical)
Bronchial Emulsion (Three Flasks) (Thornton & Ross)
Bronchial Emulsion AS Extra Strong (Ayrton Saunders)
Bronchial Mixture (Rusco)
Bronchial Mixture Extra Strong (Cox)
Bronchial Mixture Sure Shield Brand
Bronchial Tablets (Leoren)
Bronchialis Mist Liquid (Industrial Pharmaceutical Services)
Bronchialis Mist Nig Double Strength (Phillip Harris Medical)
Bronchisan Childrens Cough Syrup
Bronchisan Cough Syrup
Broncholia Mixture
Bronchotone Solution
Bronkure Cough & Bronchitis Mixture (Jacksons)
Brontus Syrup
Brontus Syrup for Children
Brontussin Cough Suppressant Mixture
Brooklax Tablets
Brotizolam Tablets 0.125 mg
Brotizolam Tablets 0.25 mg
Bufferin Tablets
Build-Up (Nestle Health Care)
Buttercup Baby Cough Linctus
Buttercup Syrup
Buttercup Syrup Honey and Lemon

Cabdrivers Adult Linctus
Cabdrivers Diabetic Linctus

Cabdrivers Junior Linctus
Cabdrivers Nasal Decongestant Tablets
Cadbury's Coffee Compliment
Cafadol Tablets
Caffeine & Dextrose Tablets
Cal-A-Cool Aftersun Moisturising Cream
Caladryl Cream
Caladryl Lotion
Calamage
Calcia Calcium Supplement Tablets
Calcimax Syrup
Calcinate Tablets
Calcium Syrup (Berk Pharmaceuticals)
Calendolon Ointment
California Syrup of Figs
Calpol Extra Tablets
Calpol Infant Suspension
Calpol Six Plus Suspension
Calpol Tablets
Calsalettes Sugar Coated Tablets
Calsalettes Uncoated Tablets
Camfortix Linctus P1
Camphor Spirit
Candacurb Capsules
Candacurb-E Capsules
Canderel Intense Sweetener Spoonful
Candermyl Liposome Cream
Cantaflour
Cantamac Tablets
Cantamega 1000 Tablets
Cantamega 2000 Divided Dose Tablets ¼ Size
Cantamega 2000 Naturtab Tablets
Cantassium Amino M.S. Tablets
Cantassium Discs
Cantassium Fructose
Cantassium Multivitamin Tablets
Capramin Tablets
Caprystatin Capsules
Carbellon Tablets
Carbo-Cort Cream
Carisoma Compound Tablets
Carnation Coffeemate
Carnation Slender Meal Replacement (All Flavours)
Carrzone Powder
Carters Little Pills
Carylderm Shampoo
Cascara Evacuant Liquid Mixture
Cascara Tablets BP
Castellan No 10 Cough Mixture
Catarrh & Bronchial Syrup (Thornton & Ross)
Catarrh Cough Syrup (Boots)
Catarrh Mixture (Herbal Laboratories)
Catarrh Syrup for Children (Boots)
Catarrh Tablets (Cathay)
Catarrh-Ex Tablets
Ce-Cobalin Syrup
Ceeyees Tablets
Celaton Rejuvenation Tablets
Celaton CH3 Strong & Calm Tablets
Celaton CH3 Triplus Tablets
Celaton CH3 + Ease & Vitality Tablets
Celaton Whole Wheat Germ Capsules
Celavit 1 Powder

XVIIIA

DRUGS AND OTHER SUBSTANCES NOT TO BE PRESCRIBED UNDER THE NHS
PHARMACEUTICAL SERVICES

Celavit 2 Powder
Celavit 3 Powder
Celevac Granules
Centrax Tablets 10 mg
Cephos Powders
Cephos Tablets
Cetaphil Lotion
Charabs Tablets
Charvita Tablets
Cheroline Cough Linctus
Cherry Bark Cough Syrup Childrens (Loveridge)
Cherry Bark Linctus Adults (Loveridge)
Cherry Cough Balsam (Herbal Laboratories)
Cherry Cough Linctus (Savoury & Moore)
Cherry Cough Mixture (Rusco)
Cherry Flavoured Extract of Malt (Distillers)
Chest & Cough Tablets (Brome & Schimmer)
Chest & Cough Tablets (Kerbina)
Chest & Throat Tablets No 8,000 (English Grains)
Chest Pills (Brome & Schimmer)
Chest Tablets (Kerbina)
Chesty Cough Syrup (Scott & Browne)
Chickweed Ointment
Chilblain Tablets (Boots)
Child's Cherry Flavoured Linctus (Cupal)
Children's Blackcurrant Cough Syrup (Rusco)
Children's Cherry Cough Syrup (Thornton & Ross)
Children's Cough Linctus (Ransoms)
Children's Cough Mixture (Beecham)
Children's Cough Mixture (Loveridge)
Children's Cough Syrup (Ayrton Saunders)
Children's Cough Syrup (Cox)
Children's Cough Syrup (Evans Medical)
Children's Cough Syrup (Thornbers)
Children's Medicine Liquid (Hall's)
Children's Phensic Tablets
Children's Wild Cherry Cough Linctus (Evans Medical)
Chilvax Tablets
Chlorasol Sachets
Chocolate Laxative Tablets (Isola)
Chocovite Tablets
Christy's Rich Lanolin
Christy's Skin Emulsion
Cidal
Cidex Longlife
Cidex Sterilising Solution
Cinnamon Essence Medicinal Mixture (Langdale)
Cinnamon Tablets Medicinal (Langdale)
Cinota Drops
Citrosan Powder
Claradin Effervescent Tablets
Clara's Kitchen Gluten-Free Porridge
Clarityn Allergy
Clarkes Blood Mixture
Clean and Soak
Cleansing Herb Dried (Potters)
Cleansing Herbs (Brome & Schimmer)
Cleansing Herbs Powder (Dorwest)
Clen-Zym Tablets
Clerz Lubricating and Rewetting Eye Drops
Clerz Lubricating Cleaning and
Clinique Clarifying Lotion
Clinique Continuous Coverage

Clinique Crystal Clear Cleaning Oil
Clinique Dramatically Different Moisturising Lotion
Clinique Facial Mild Soap
Clinisan Skin Cleansing Foam
Clinisan Skin Cleansing Foam Aerosol 500ml
Clorazepate Dipotassium Capsules 7.5 mg
Clorazepate Dipotassium Capsules 15 mg
Clorazepate Dipotassium Tablets 15 mg
Co-op Aspirin Tablets BP 300 mg
Co-op Bronchial Mixture
Co-op Halibut Liver Oil Capsules BP
Co-op Paracetamol Tablets BP 500 mg
Co-op Soluble Aspirin Tablets BP 300 mg
Cobalin H Injection 250 mcg/ml
Cobalin H Injection 1000 mcg/ml
Cobalin Injection 100 mcg/ml
Cobalin Injection 250 mcg/ml
Cobalin Injection 500 mcg/ml
Cobalin Injection 1000 mcg/ml
Coda - Med Tablets
Cod Liver Oil & Creosote Capsules (5 Oval) (R P Scherer)
Cod Liver Oil & Creosote Capsules (10 Oval) (R P Scherer)
Cod Liver Oil Caps 10 Minims (Woodward)
Cod Liver Oil High Potency Capsules (R P Scherer)
Cod Liver Oil with Malt Extract & Hypophosphite Syrup (Distillers)
Cod Liver Oil 0.3 ml Capsules (R P Scherer)
Cod Liver Oil 0.6 ml Capsules (R P Scherer)
Codalax
Codalax Forte
Codanin Analgesic Tablets
Codis Soluble Tablets
Codural Tablets
Cojene Tablets
Cold & Influenza Capsules (Regent Laboratories)
Cold & Influenza Mixture (Boots)
Cold & Influenza Mixture (Davidson)
Cold & Influenza Mixture (Rusco)
Cold & Influenza Mixture (Thornton & Ross)
Cold Relief (Blackcurrant Flavour) Granular Powder (Boots)
Cold Relief Capsules (Scott & Bowne)
Cold Relief Tablets (Boots)
Cold Tablets (Roberts)
Coldrex Powder
Coldrex Tablets
Colgard Emergency Essence (Lane Health Products)
Colgate Dental Cream with MFP Fluoride
Colgate Disclosing Tablets
Collins Elixir
Colocynth & Jalap Tablets Compound BPC 1963
Colocynth Compound Pills BPC 1963
Cologel Liquid
Comfort Sachets
Communion Wafers
Complan
Comploment Continus Tablets
Compound Fig Elixir BP
Compound Rhubarb Oral Powder BP
Compound Rhubarb Tincture BP
Compound Syrup of Glycerophosphates BPC 1963

DRUGS AND OTHER SUBSTANCES NOT TO BE PRESCRIBED UNDER THE NHS PHARMACEUTICAL SERVICES

Compound Syrup of Hypophosphites BPC 1963
Comtrex Capsules
Comtrex Liquid
Comtrex Tablets
Concavit Capsules
Concavit Drops
Concavit Injection
Concavit Syrup
Confiance Dietary Supplement Tablets
Congreves Balsamic Elixir
Constipation Herb Dried (Potters)
Constipation Herbs (Hall's)
Constipation Herbs (Mixed Herbs) (Brome & Schimmer)
Constipation Mixture No 105 (Potters)
Contac 400 Capsules
Contac Coughcaps
Contactaclean Cleaning Solution
Contactasoak Disinfecting and Soaking Solution
Contactasol O2 Care Solution
Contactasol Complete Care All-In-One Solution
Contactasol Solar Saline Spray
Contactasol Wetting Solution
Copholco Cough Syrup
Copholcoids
Coppertone Apres Plage Aftersun Milk
Coppertone Children's Cream SPF25
Coppertone Children's Lotion SPF15
Coppertone Dark Tanning Lotion SPF4
Coppertone Sun Tanning Lotion SPF6
Coppertone Water Resistant Tanning Cream SPF8
Co-QIO Tablets
Core Level Adrenal Tablets
Core Level Auto Sym Tablets
Core Level C Timed Release Tablets
Core Level Health Reserve Tablets
Core Level Ilioduodenal Tablets
Core Level Magnesium Tablets
Core Level Zinc Tablets
Corrective Tablets (Ayrton Saunders)
Correctol Tablets
Cosalgesic Tablets
Cosylan Syrup
Coterpin Syrup
Cough & Bronchitis Mixture (Davidson)
Cough & Cold Mixture (Beecham)
Cough Balsam (Abernethy's)
Cough Balsam (Thornbers)
Cough Expectorant Elixir (Regent Laboratories)
Cough Linctus (Sanderson's)
Cough Linctus Alcoholic (Thomas Guest)
Cough Linctus for Children (Boots)
Cough Medicine for Infants & Children Solution (Boots)
Cough Mixture (Tingles)
Cough Mixture Adults (Thornton & Ross)
Cough Mixture Adults (Wicker Herbal Stores)
Cough Syrup Best (Diopharm)
Cough Tablets (Kerbina)
Country Basket Rice Cakes
Covermark Removing Cream
Covonia Bronchial Balsam Linctus
Cow & Gate Babymeals Stage One
Cow & Gate Baby Milk Plus

Cow & Gate Follow-On Babymilk Step Up
Cow & Gate Junior Meal
Cow & Gate Olvarit Stage Two Main Course
Cow & Gate Premium Baby Food
Cox Pain Tablets
Crampex Tablets
Cranberry Juice
Cream of Magnesia Tablets 300 mg
Cremaffin Emulsion
Cremalgin Balm
Creosote Bronchial Mixture (Loveridge)
Crookes One-a-Day Multivitamins with Iron
Crookes One-a-Day Multivitamins without Iron
Crookes Wheat Germ Oil Capsules
Croupline Cough Syrup (Roberts)
Crusha Milk Shake Syrup
Cullen's Headache Powders
Culpepper Healing Ointment
Culpepper Rheumatic Cream
Cupal Health Salts
Cupal Nail Bite Lotion
Cuprofen Soluble Tablets
Cuprofen Tablets
Cuticura Medicated Foam Bath
Cuticura Talcum Powder
Cyanocobalamin Solution (any strength)
Cytacon Liquid
Cytacon Tablets
Cytamen 250 Injection
Cytamen 1000 Injection
Cytoplan Acidophilus Capsules (Milk Free)
Cytoplan Acidophilus/Bifidophilus 50%/50% Capsules
Cytoplan Aloe Vera Concentrate
Cytoplan Betaine & Pepsin Capsules 345mg/10mg
Cytoplan Bifidophilus Extra Tablets
Cytoplan Biotin Capsules 100mcg
Cytoplan Children's Chewable Mineral/Vitamin Tablets
Cytoplan Choline/Inositol Capsules 250mg/250mg
Cytoplan Co-Factor Compound Plus Capsules
Cytoplan Cytocleanse Formula Capsules
Cytoplan Cytomin Mineral/Vitamin Tablets
Cytoplan Cytoplex Tablets
Cytoplan Cytophilus Milk Free Capsules
Cytoplan De-Toxifying Compound Capsules
Cytoplan Dolomite Magnesium Carbon Calcium Carbon Tablets
Cytoplan EPA Capsules
Cytoplan Iron Extra Tablets
Cytoplan Lecithin Capsules
Cytoplan Magnesium Ascorbic Capsules
Cytoplan Magnesium/Calcium Capsules 250mg/250mg
Cytoplan Magnesium Citric Capsules
Cytoplan Magnesium Complex Capsules
Cytoplan Manganese Complex Capsules
Cytoplan Multex Multivitamin and Mineral Formulation
Cytoplan Pantothenic Acid Tablets
Cytoplan Potassium Pantothenate Capsules
Cytoplan Pryoxidal-5-pH Complex Capsules
Cytoplan Selenium Capsules
Cytoplan Supermag-Plus Capsules

DRUGS AND OTHER SUBSTANCES NOT TO BE PRESCRIBED UNDER THE NHS PHARMACEUTICAL SERVICES

Cytoplan Vitamin A Capsules
Cytoplan Vitamin C 1000mg + Bioflavour 50mg
   Capsules
Cytoplan Vitamin C Powder
Cytoplan Vitamin E Capsules
Cytoplan Zinc Lozenge Wafers

Dakin's Golden Vitamin Malt Syrup
Daktarin Cream 15g
Daktarin Powder
Daktarin Twin Pack
Dalivit Capsules
Dalivit Syrup
Dalmane Capsules 15 mg
Dalmane Capsules 30 mg
Dansac Skin Lotion
Davenol Linctus
Daxaids Tablets
Day-Vits Multivitamin & Mineral Tablets
Dayovite
De Witt's Analagesic Pills
De Witt's Antacid Powder
De Witt's Antacid Tablets
De Witt's Baby Cough Syrup
De Witt's Cough Syrup
De Witt's PL Pills
Dead Sea Natural Mineral Soap
Deakin & Hughes Cough & Cold Healer Mixture
Deakin's Fever & Inflammation Remedy Mixture
Delax Emulsion
Delial Lotion SPF2
Delial Lotion SPF6 Water Resistant
Delimon
Deltasoralen Bath Lotion
Dencyl Spansules
Dentakit Toothache First Aid Kit
Dentu-Hold Liquid
Derbac C Shampoo
Derbac Soap
Derl Dermatological Soap
Dermablend Chromatone Fade Creme Plus
Dermablend Cleanser/Remover
Dermablend Maximum Moisturiser
Dermablend Quick Fix Concealment Stick
Dermacolor Body Cover
Dermacolor Cleansing Cream
Dermacolor Cleansing Lotion
Dermacolor Cleansing Milk
Dermacolor 6 Colour Palette
Dermacolor Creme Effective No.2
Dermacolor Fixier Spray
Dermacolor Skin Plastic
Dermacort Cream
Dermalex Skin Lotion
Dermidex Dermatological Cream
Dermo-Care Soapless Soap
Desiccated Liver Tablets
Desiccated Liver USNF Tablets
Detox Tablets (Hursdrex)
Dettox Antibacterial Cleanser
Dextro Energy Glucose Tablets
Dextrogesic Tablets
Dextromethorphan Hydrobromide Solution
   3.75 mg/5 ml

Dextromethorphan Hydrobromide Solution
   7.5 mg/5 ml
Dextromethorphan Hydrobromide Syrup
   6.6 mg/5 ml
Dextromethorphan Hydrobromide Syrup
   13.5 mg/5 ml
Dextropropoxyphene & Paracetamol Dispersible
   Tablets
Dextropropoxyphene & Paracetamol Soluble
   Tablets
DF 118 Elixir
DF 118 Tablets
DGL 1 Suspension
DGL 2 Suspension
DGT 1 Tablets
DGT 2 Tablets
DHL Rheumatic Massage Cream
Diabetic Bronal Syrup
Dialar Forte Syrup 5 mg/5 ml
Dialar Syrup 2 mg/5 ml
Dialume Capsules 500 mg
Diazepam Capsules, Slow 10 mg
Diazepam Elixir 5 mg/5 ml
Diazepam Oral Solution 5mg/5ml
Diazepam Oral Suspension 5mg/5ml
Dietade Diabetic Jam
Dietade Diabetic Marmalade
Dietade Diabetic Squash
Dietade Dietary Foods Fruit Sugar
Dietade Fruit Sugar
Dietade Jelly Crystals
Digesprin Antacid Tablets
Digestells Lozenges
Dihydroxyaluminium Sodium Carbonate Tablets
Dijex Liquid
Dijex Tablets
Dimotane Expectorant
Dimotane Expectorant DC
Dimotane with Codeine Elixir
Dimotane with Codeine Paediatric Elixir
Dimotapp Elixir
Dimotapp Elixir Paediatric
Dimotapp LA Tablets
Dimotapp P Tablets
Dimyril Linctus
Dinnefords Gripe Mixture
Diocalm Ultra Capsules
Dioctyl Ear Drops
Disprin Direct Tablets
Disprin Extra Tablets
Disprin Solmin Tablets
Disprin Tablets
Disprinex Tablets
Disprol Infant Suspension
Disprol Junior Tablets Soluble
Distalgesic Soluble Tablets
Distalgesic Tablets
Ditemic Spansules
Do-Do Linctus
Do-Do Tablets
Dolasan Tablets
Doloxene Capsules
Doloxene Compound Pulvules
Dolvan Tablets

DRUGS AND OTHER SUBSTANCES NOT TO BE PRESCRIBED UNDER THE NHS
PHARMACEUTICAL SERVICES

Dorbanex Capsules
Dorbanex Liquid
Dorbanex Liquid Forte
Dormonoct Tablets 1 mg
Dove Cleansing Bar
Dr Brandreth's Pills
Dr D E Jongh's Cod Liver Oil with Malt Extract &
    Vitamins Fortified Syrup
Dr William's Pink Pills
Dragon Balm
Drastin Tablets
Dristan Decongestant Tablets with Antihistamine
Dristan Nasal Spray
Droxalin Tablets
Dry Cough Linctus (Scott & Bowne)
Dual-Lax Extra Strong Tablets
Dual-Lax Tablets
Dubam Cream
Dubam Spray Relief
Dulca Tablets
Dulcodos Tablets
Dulco-Lax Suppositories
Dulco-Lax Tablets
Duo-Gastritis Mixture (Baldwin's)
Duphalac Syrup
Duralin Capsules Extra Strength
Duralin Tablets
Dusk Insect Repellent Cream
Duttons Cough Mixture
Dynese Aqueous Suspension
Dynese Tablets
D001 Capsules
D002 Capsules
D004 Capsules
D006 Capsules
D007 Capsules
D009 Capsules
D010 Capsules
D011 Capsules
D012 Capsules
D013 Capsules
D014 Capsules
D017 Capsules
D018 Capsules
D019 Capsules
D020 Capsules
D021 Capsules
D024 Capsules
D029 Capsules
D030 Capsules
D031 Capsules
D032 Capsules
D033 Capsules
D034 Capsules
D036 Capsules

Earex Ear Drops
Earthdust Aged Garlic Tablets
Earthdust Capricin Forte Capsules
Earthdust Formula 1 Capsules
Earthdust Pro-Biotic New Complex Powder
Earthdust Super-Pro-Bifidus Powder
Earthdust Super-Pro-Dophilus Powder

Earthlore Vitamin B Compound Tablets
Ecologic 315 Granules
Ecdilyn Syrup
Educol Tablets
Efamol
Efamol Capsules
Efamol Marine Capsules
Efamol Oil
Efamol Plus Capsules
Efamol Plus Evening Primrose Oil & Coenzyme
    Q10 Capsules
Efamol PMP
Efamolia Enriched Moisture Cream
Efamolia Moisture Cream
Efamolia Night Cream
Efavite Tablets
Efavite Vitamin & Zinc Supplement Tablets
Effer-C Tablets
Effico Syrup
Elagen
Eldermint Cough Mixture (Herbal Laboratories)
Elgydium Toothpaste
Elizabeth Arden Flawless Finish
Elizabeth Arden Sunblock Cream Factor 15
Elizabeth Arden Sunscience Superblock
    Cream spf 34
Elkamol Tablets
Ellimans Universal Embrocation
Elsan Blue Liquid
Emuwash
Endet Powders
Ener-G Gluten-free and Soya-free Macaroon
    Cookies
Ener-G Gluten-free Rice and Peanut-Butter
    Cookies
Ener-G Gluten-free Rice Walnut Cookies
Energen Starch Reduced Crispbread
Enfamil Human Milk Fortifier
English Grains Mixed Gland Compound Tablets
English Grains Red Kooga Multivitamins & Minerals
Engran HP Tablets
Engran Tablets
Eno Fruit Salts
Enzyme Process Achol Tablets
Enzyme Process Enzastatin Tablets
Enzyme Process Liver Tablets
Enzyme Process Pancreas 523 Tablets
Enzyme Process Pro-T-Compound Tablets
Enzyme Process Vitamin B12 + Liver Tablets
EP Tablets
EPOC Capsules
Equagesic Tablets
Equisorb High Fibre Guar Bread Rolls
Eskamel Cream
Eskornade Spansule Capsules
Eskornade Syrup
Eso-Col Cold Treatment Tablets
Esoterica Fortified Cream
Essentia Special E Cream
Ester-C Powder
Ester-C Tablets
Euhypnos Capsules 10 mg
Euhypnos Elixir 10 mg/5 ml
Euhypnos Forte Capsules 20 mg

XVIIIA

DRUGS AND OTHER SUBSTANCES NOT TO BE PRESCRIBED UNDER THE NHS PHARMACEUTICAL SERVICES

Evacalm Tablets 2 mg
Evacalm Tablets 5 mg
Evans Cough Balsam
Evening Primrose Oil
Evening Primrose Oil Capsules
Evian Mineral Water
Evident Disclosing Cream
Ex-Lax Chocolate Laxative Tablets
Ex-Lax Pills
Expectorant Cough Mixtures (Beecham)
Expulin Cough Linctus
Expulin Decongestant Linctus for Babies &
    Children
Expulin Paediatric Cough Linctus
Extil Compound Linctus
Extravite Tablets
Extren Tablets
Exyphen Elixir
E001 Capsules
E015 Capsules
E018 Capsules
E021 Capsules
E031 Capsules
E032 Capsules

Fade Out Skin Lightening Cream
Fairy Household Liquid
Falcodyl Linctus
Falkamin
Fam Lax Tablets
Famel Expectorant
Famel Linctus
Famel Original Linctus
Family Cherry Flavoured Linctus (Cupal)
Family Health Multivitamin Tablets
Family Herbal Pills
Fanalgic Syrup
Fanalgic Tablets
Farex Fingers
Farley's Farex Weaning Food
Farley's First Milk
Farley's Follow-On Milk
Farley's Premcare Ready-to-Feed
Farleys Rusks
Farley's Tea Timer
Father Pierre's Monastery Herbs
Fe-Cap C Capsules
Feac Tablets
Feen-a-Mint Tablets
Fefol Spansule Capsules
Fefol-Vit Spansules
Fefol Z Spansule Capsules
Femafen Capsules
Femerital Tablets
Femeron Cream
Feminax Tablets
Fendamin Tablets
Fennings Adult Cooling Powders
Fennings Children's Cooling Powders
Fennings Little Healers Pills
Fennings Mixture
Fennings Soluble Junior Aspirin Tablets
Fenox Nasal Drops

Fenox Nasal Spray
Feospan Spansule Capsules
Ferfolic SV Tablets
Ferfolic Tablets
Fergluvite Tablets
Fergon Tablets
Ferraplex B Tablets
Ferrlecit Tablets/Dragees
Ferrocap Capsules
Ferrocap F-350 Capsules
Ferroglobin B12 Vitamin/Mineral Compound
Ferrograd C Tablets
Ferrol
Ferrol Compound Mixture
Ferromyn B Elixir
Ferromyn B Tablets
Ferrous Gluconate Compound Tablets
Ferrous Sulphate Compound Tablets BP
Fesovit Spansules
Fesovit Z Spansules
Fibre Biscuits
Fibrosine Analgesic Balm
Fiery Jack Cream
Fiery Jack Ointment
Filetti Sensitive Skin Soap
Finasteride 1mg Tablets
Fine Fare Aspirin Tablets 300 mg
Fine Fare Hot Lemon Powders
Fink Linusit Gold Pure Golden Linseeds
Flar Capsules
Flavelix Syrup
Flexcare Soft Lens Solution
Flexsol Solution
Flora Margarine
Floradix Formula Liquid
Floradix Tablets
Floral Arbour Tablets (Cathay)
Flucaps
Flunitrazepam Tablets 1 mg
Fluralar Capsules 15 mg
Fluralar Capsules 30 mg
Flurazepam Capsules 15 mg
Flurazepam Capsules 30 mg
Flurazepam Hydrochloride Capsules 15 mg
Flurazepam Hydrochloride Capsules 30 mg
Flu-Rex Tablets
Flurex Bedtime Cold Remedy
Flurex Capsules
Flurex Decongestant Inhalant Capsules
Flurex Hot Lemon Concentrate
Flurex Tablets
Folex-350 Tablets
Folicin Tablets
Folped
Foresight Tablets Mineral Formula
Foresight Tablets Vitamin (Multivitamins)
Formula M.E. (Multiple Elevator) No 1 Capsules
Formula M.E. (Multiple Elevator) No 2 Capsules
Formula M.E. (Multiple Elevator) No 3 Capsules
Formule B Spot Treatment Roll On
Formulix
Forprin Tablets
Fortagesic Tablets
Fortespan Spansules

DRUGS AND OTHER SUBSTANCES NOT TO BE PRESCRIBED UNDER THE NHS PHARMACEUTICAL SERVICES

Fort-E-Vite Capsules
Fort-E-Vite 1000 Capsules
Fort-E-Vite Cream
Fort-E-Vite Plus Capsules
Fort-E-Vite Super Plus Capsules
Fortison Low Sodium
Fortral Capsules 50 mg
Fortral Injection
Fortral Suppositories
Fortral Tablets 25 mg
Fortral Tablets 50 mg
Fortris Solution
Fosfor Syrup
Franol Expectorant
Franolyn Sed Liquid
Frisium Capsules 5 mg
Frisium Capsules 10 mg
Frisium Capsules 20 mg
FSC Betaine HCL Capsules
FSC Beta Plus Capsules
FSC Evening Primrose Oil + Vitamin E Cream
FSC Lactobacillus Acidophilus Capsules
FSC Multivitamin Addlife For Over 50s Capsules
FSC Natural Vitamin E Capsules
FSC Organic Linseed Oil Capsules
FSC Super B-Supreme High-Potency Tablets
FSC Super Calcium 200mg + Vitamin
  A & D Tablets
FSC Vitamin B6 Tablets
FSC Vitamin D 400u
Fybranta Tablets
Fynnon Calcium Aspirin Tablets
Fynnon Salt

G Brand Linctus
Galake Tablets
Gale's Honey
Galfer-Vit Capsules
Galloway's Baby Cough Linctus
Galloway's Bronchial Cough Care
Galloway's Bronchial Expectorant
Galloway's Cough Syrup
Gammolin Capsules
Gamophase Gamolenic Acid Capsules
Gamophen
Gastalar Tablets
Gastric Ulcer Tablets No 1001
Gastrils Pastilles
Gastritabs
Gastrovite Tablets
Gatinar Syrup
Gaviscon Granules
Gaviscon 250 Tablets
Gelusil Lac Powder
Gelusil Tablets
Genasprin Tablets
Genatosan
Gentian Acid Mixture with Nux Vomica
Gentian Alkaline Mixture with Nux Vomica
Gentian & Rhubarb Mixture BPC
Georges Vapour Rub Ointment
Gericaps Capsules
Gericare Multivitamin & Mineral Capsules

Gerimax Original Korean Panax Ginseng with
  Vitamins, Minerals and Amino Acid.
Geriplex Capsules
Germolene Ointment
Gevral Capsules
Gevral Tablets
Ginkgo Biloba Extract Capsules 40mg
Ginkgo Biloba Liquid
Givitol Capsules
Gladlax Tablets
Glemony Balsam (Baldwin's)
Glenco Elixir
Gluca-Seltzer Effervescent Powder
Glucodin
Glutafin Gluten-Free Chocolate Chip Cookies
Glutafin Gluten-Free Custard Cream Biscuits
Glutafin Gluten-Free Gingernut Cookies
Glutafin Gluten-Free Milk Chocolate Biscuits
Glutafin Gluten-Free Milk Chocolate Digestive
  Biscuits
Glutafin Gluten-Free Shortcake Biscuits
Glutano Gluten-Free Chocolate Hazelnut Wafer
  Bar
Glutano Gluten-Free Muesli
Glutano Gluten-Free Pretzel
Glutano Gluten-Free Wafer
Glutano Gluten-Free Wafer, Cream Filled
Glycerin Honey & Lemon Cough Mixture (Isola)
Glycerin Honey & Lemon Linctus (Boots)
Glycerin Honey & Lemon Linctus with Ipecacuanha
  (Boots)
Glycerin Lemon & Honey and Ipecacuanha
  (Thomas Guest)
Glycerin Lemon & Honey Linctus (Rusco)
Glycerin Lemon & Honey Syrup (Cupal)
Glycerin Lemon & Honey Syrup (Thomas Guest)
Glycerin Lemon & Honey Syrup (Waterhouse)
Glycerin Lemon & Ipecacuanha Cough Mixture
  (Isola)
Glykola Infants Elixir
Glykola Tonic
Glymiel Hand Care
Goat's Milk Spray Dried Powder
Goddard's White Oils Embrocation
Golden Age Vitamin & Mineral Capsules
Golden Health Feverfew Tablets
Golden Health Super Sea Kelp Tablets
Golden Health Tablets (Kerbina)
Golden Health Tablets (Brome & Schimmer)
Gon Tablets
Gonfalcon Tablets
Grangewood Insomnia Tablets
Granogen
Granose Liquid Soya Milk
Granose Soya Yogert
Granoton Emulsion
Gratis Gluten-Free Tricolour Pasta
Gregovite C Tablets
GS Tablets
Guaiphenesin Syrup (any strength)
Guanor Expectorant
Gynovite Plus Nutritional Supplement Tablets

DRUGS AND OTHER SUBSTANCES NOT TO BE PRESCRIBED UNDER THE NHS PHARMACEUTICAL SERVICES

H-Pantoten Tablets
Hactos Chest & Cough Mixture (Thomas Hubert)
Halaurant Syrup
Halcion Tablets 0.125 mg
Halcion Tablets 0.25 mg
Haliborange Syrup
Haliborange Tablets
Halibut Liver Oil A & D Capsules (Rodale)
Halibut Oil A & D Capsules (GR Lane Health
     Products)
Halin Tablets
Halocaps Inhalant Capsules
Halycitrol Emulsion
Harvestime Malt Extract with Cod Liver Oil and
     Butterscotch
Hayphryn Nasal Spray
HC45 Cream
Head and Shoulders Shampoo
Health Aid Children's Multivitamin + Mineral Tablets
Health Aid DL-Phenylalanine Tablets 500mg
Health Aid Dolomite Tablets
Health Aid Eczema Oil
Health Aid EPO Forte Capsules 1000mg
Health Aid Halibut Liver Oil Capsules
Health Aid Magnesium & Calcium Tablets
Health Aid Multivitamins & Minerals Tablets
Health Aid Super Cod Liver Oil Capsules
Health Aid Super Lecithin Capsules
Health Aid Vitamin A Capsules
Health Aid Vitamin A + D Capsules
Health Aid Vitamin B6 Tablets Prolonged Release
Health Aid Vitamin B Complex Supreme Tablets
Health Aid Vitamin C Tablets
Health Aid Vitamin E Capsules
Health Aid Vitamin E Cream
Health Aid Vitamin E Hand and Body Lotion
Health Aid Vitamin E Natural Capsules
Health Aid Vitamin E Oil
Health Aid Zinc Sulphate Tablets 200mg
Health Aid Zinc Tablets 10mg
Healthaid Glucosamine Sulphate Tablets
Healthcrafts Aminochel Calcium Tablets
Healthcrafts Aminochel Chelated Magnesium
     Tablets
Healthcrafts Aminochel Zinc Tablets 1.3mg
Healthcrafts Aminochel Zinc Tablets 5mg
Healthcrafts Arteroil Tablets
Healthcrafts Betacarotene Capsules
Healthcrafts Brewers Yeast Tablets
Healthcrafts Calcium + Vitamin D Chewable Tablets
Healthcrafts Calcium Chewable Tablets
Healthcrafts Calcium Pantothenate Super Tablets
Healthcrafts Cod Liver Oil Capsules
Healthcrafts Cod Liver Oil Compleat Tablets
Healthcrafts Dolomite Tablets 500mg
Healthcrafts EPA Forte Capsules
Healthcrafts High Strength Starflower Oil
Healthcrafts Kelp Tablets
Healthcrafts Lecithin Capsules
Healthcrafts Multivitamin Chewable Tablets
Healthcrafts Multivitamin + Iron & Calcium Tablets
Healthcrafts Natural Vitamin C 1g Tablets (High
     Potency)

Healthcrafts Prolonged Release Nutrition Mega-B6
     Tablets
Healthcrafts Prolonged Release Nutrition Mega B-
     Complex Tablets
Healthcrafts Prolonged Release Nutrition Mega C
     1500 Tablets
Healthcrafts Prolonged Release Nutrition Mega
     Multis Tablets
Healthcrafts Vitamin E Capsules
Healthcrafts Vitamin E Capsules High-Potency
Healthcrafts Vitamin E Capsules Mega
Healthcrafts Vitamin E Capsules Super
Healthcrafts Vitamin E Natural Oil
Healthcrafts Vitamin E One-A-Day Capsules
Healthcrafts Zinc One-A-Day Capsules
Healtheries Rice Crispbread
Healthilife Dolomite Tablets 60mg
Healthilife Halibut Oil Capsules
Healthilife Rutin Tablets 60mg
Healthilife Sunflower Seed Oil Capsules 500 mg
Healthilife Vitamin A Capsules
Healthilife Vitamin E Soya Free Capsules
Healthilife Wild Sea Kelp Tablets 300mg
Healthlink High Zinc + Manganese Formula 1
     Capsules
Healthlink Loosemore Herbal Capsules
Healthlink Magnesium Acetate Capsules
Healthlink Psyllium Husks
Health Perception Glucosamine Tablets
Health + Plus Absorb Plus Capsules
Health + Plus Absorb Plus Tablets
Health + Plus Chromium GTF & B3 Tablets
Health + Plus Complex B Tablets
Health + Plus Co-Q Plus Tablets
Health + Plus Dolomite + D Tablets
Health + Plus E500 Tablets
Health + Plus Immunade Tablets
Health + Plus Multiminerals Tablets
Health + Plus Multivite Tablets
Health + Plus Nutrient Pack, Metabolic Pack
Health + Plus Pregnancy Pack
Health + Plus Selenium Tablets 50mcg
Health + Plus Super B6 + Zinc Tablets
Health + Plus Super C1000 Tablets + Bioflavour
Health + Plus Supercholine Tablets
Health + Plus Vitamin E Capsules High-Potency
Health + Plus VV Pack
Health + Plus Ziman Plus (Manganese & Zinc)
     Tablets
Health Salts (Wicker Herbal Stores)
Health Tonic Mixture (Hall's)
Healthwise Halibut Oil Capsules
Healthwise Vitamin E Capsules
Heart Shape Indigestion Tablets
Heath & Heather Feverfew Tablets
Heath & Heather Garlic Perles (Odourless)
Hedamol Capsules
Hedex Extra Caplets
Hedex Plus Capsules
Hedex Seltzer Granules
Hedex Soluble Granules
Hedex Tablets
Heinz Weight Watcher Baked Beans
Hemingways Catarrh Syrup

DRUGS AND OTHER SUBSTANCES NOT TO BE PRESCRIBED UNDER THE NHS
PHARMACEUTICAL SERVICES

Hemoplex Injection
Hepacon B12 Injection
Hepacon B-Forte Injection
Hepacon Liver Extract Injection
Hepacon-Plex
Hepanorm Tablets
Herbal Aperient Tablets (Cathay)
Herbal Aperient Tablets (Kerbina)
Herbal Bronchial Cough Tablets (English Grains)
Herbal Laboratories Feverfew Tablets
Herbal Laxative Naturtabs
Herbal Pile Tablets
Herbal Quiet Nite Sleep Naturtabs
Herbal Syrup (Baldwin's)
Herbalene Herbs
Hermesetas (blue)
Hermesetas Gold
Hermesetas Light
Hermesetas Liquid Sweetener
Hermesetas Sprinkle Sweet
Hexidin Solution
Hi-g-ah Tea
Higher Nature Paraclear Capsules
Hi-pro Liver Tablets
Hill's Adult Balsam
Hill's Balsam Children's Mixture for Chesty Coughs
Hip C Rose Hip Syrup
Hismanal Tablets 10-tablet pack
Histalix Expectorant
Hofels Cardiomax Garlic Pearles
Hofels Garlic Pearles
Hofels One-A-Day Garlic Pearles
Hofels One-A-Day Neo Garlic Pearles
Honey & Molasses Cough Mixture (Lane Health
   Products)
Hot Blackcurrant Cold Remedy (Beechams)
Hot Lemon Cold Remedy (Beechams)
Hot Lemon Cold Treatment (Scott & Bowne)
Hot Measure Solution (Reckitt & Colman)
Hydrex Hand Rub
Hydrocare Boiling/Rinsing Solution
Hydrocare Cleaning and Soaking Solution
Hydrocare Preserved Saline Solution
Hydrocare Protein Remover Tablets
Hydroclean Solution
Hydron Europe Cleaning Solution
Hydron Europe Comfort Soaking Solution
Hydron Europe Solusal
Hydron Europe Solution Comfort
Hydrosoak Disinfecting and Soaking Solution
Hydrosol Comfort Solution
Hymosa Vitamin E Cream
Hypomultiple Capsules
Hypon Tablets

Iberet 500 Tablets
Iberol Tablets
Ibrufhalal Tablets
ICC Analgesic Tablets
Idoloba Tablets
Iliadin Mini Nasal Drops
Iliadin Mini Paediatric Nasal Drops
Imarale Agba Suspension

Imarale Omode Suspension
Imedeen Skin Regenerating Tablets
Imedeen Tablets
Imodium Capsules Pharmacy Packs 8 and 12
   Capsules
Importal
Imuderm Body Wash
Imuderm Hand & Face Wash
Imuderm Shower Gel
Inabrin Tablets 200 mg
Indian Brandy Solution
Indigestion Mixture (Boots)
Indigestion Mixture (Thornton & Ross)
Indigestion Mixture (William Ransom)
Indigo Indigestion Lozenges
Infa-Care Baby Bath
Infaderm Baby Bath
Infaderm Baby Cream
Infaderm Baby Hair Wash
Infaderm Baby Lotion
Influenza and Cold Mixture 2315 (Wright Layman &
   Umney)
Inhalit Liquid Inhalation
Innoxa Concealing Cream
Innoxa Creme Satin Foundation
Innoxa Finishing Touch Loose Powder
Innoxa Foundation
Innoxa Moisturised Liquid Make-up
Innoxa Sensitive/Dry Range: Enriched Moisture
   Cream
Innoxa Sensitive/Normal Range: Creamy
   Moisturiser
Innoxa Young Solution Spot Gel
Inoven Caplets
Iodinated Glycerol Elixir 60 mg/ 5 ml
Iodised Vitamin Capsules
Iodo-Ephedrine Mixture
Ionax Scrub
Ipecacuanha Pills 20 mg
Ipecacuanha & Morphine Mixture BP
Ipecacuanha & Squill Linctus Paediatric BPC
Ipsel Hygienic Babysalve
Irofol C
Iron & Brewers Yeast Tablets (3M Health Care)
Iron & Vitamin Tablets (Davidson)
Iron Formula Tablets (Rodale)
Iron Jelloids Tablets
Iron Tonic Tablets (Boots)
Ironorm Capsules
Ironorm Tonic
Ironplan Capsules
Isoaminile Linctus
Isocal
Ivy Tablets (Ayrton Saunders)

Jaap's Health Salts
Jacksons All Fours Cough Mixture
Jacksons Febrifuge
Jambomins Tablets
Jenners Suspension
Jenners Tablets
Jochem Hormone Hair Preparation
Johnson & Johnson Baby Bath

DRUGS AND OTHER SUBSTANCES NOT TO BE PRESCRIBED UNDER THE NHS PHARMACEUTICAL SERVICES

Johnson & Johnson Baby Cream
Johnson & Johnson Baby Lotion
Johnson & Johnson Baby Oil
Johnson & Johnson Baby Powder
Johnson & Johnson Baby Shampoo
Johnson & Johnson Baby Sunblock Stick
Johnson & Johnson Prickly Heat Powder
Jolen Creme Bleach
Jordans Crunchy Bar
Junamac
Jung Junipah Tablets
Jungle Formula Insect Repellent Gel
Jungle Formula Insect Repellent Pump Spray
Junior Cabdrivers Linctus
Junior Disprin Tablets
Junior Disprol Tablets
Junior Ex-Lax Chocolate Tablets
Junior Lemsip Powder
Junior Meltus Cough & Catarrh Linctus
Junior Mucron Liquid
Junior Paraclear Tablets
Junior Tablets (Rodale)
Juno-Junipah Mineral Salts
Juvel Elixir
Juvel Tablets
Juvela Gluten-Free Mince Pies
Juvela Gluten-Free Sage & Onion Stuffing Mix
Juvela Low-Protein Savoury Snack

Kamillosan Baby Cleansing Bar
K'An Herbal Preparations
Kaodene Suspension
Kaopectate
Karvol Capsules
Kelsoak 2 Solution
Kelvinol 2 Wetting Solution
Kenco Instant Decaffeinated Coffee
Kendales Adult Cough Syrup
Kendales Cherry Linctus
Kentogam Gamolenic Acid Capsules
Kest Tablets
Ketazolam Capsules 15 mg
Ketazolam Capsules 30 mg
Ketazolam Capsules 45 mg
Keybells Linctus of Glycerine, Lemon & Ipecacuanha
Kingo Cough Syrup
Koladex Tablets
Kolanticon Tablets
Kolanticon Wafers
Kolantyl Gel
Kolorex Capsules
Kolynos Denture Fixative
Krauses Cough Linctus
Kruschen Salts
Kuralax Herbs
Kwai Garlic Tablets
Kylie Skin Guard

Labiton Kola Tonic
Laboprin Tablets
Lac Bismuth Mixture

Lactaid Lactase enzyme for milk drops
Lactaid Lactase enzyme tablets
Lactaid Lactose reduced, skimmed and whole milk UHT
Lacto Calamine
Ladycare No 2 (Menopausal) Tablets
Laevoral
Lamberts Acidophilus Extra Capsules
Lamberts Bee Propolis Tablets
Lamberts Beta Carotene Capsules
Lamberts Betaine HCL/Pepsin Tablets
Lamberts Betasec Tablets
Lamberts Betasec Timed Release Antioxidant Tablets
Lamberts Calcium Extra Tablets
Lamberts Calcium/Magnesium Balance Capsules
Lamberts Calcium & Magnesium Chelates Tablets
Lamberts Calcium 500/Magnesium 250 Amino Acid Chelated Tablets
Lamberts Calcium/Magnesium/Zinc Orotates Capsules
Lamberts Caprylic Acid Tablets
Lamberts Chelating Mega Mineral Complex Tablets
Lamberts Co-Enzyme Q10 Capsules
Lamberts DLPA Complex + Vitamin B & C Capsules
Lamberts Dolomite Tablets
Lamberts Enzygest Capsules
Lamberts EPA Marine Lipid Concentrate Capsules
Lamberts Evening Primrose Oil 250 mg Capsules
Lamberts Evening Primrose Oil 500 mg Capsules
Lamberts Evening Primrose Oil 1000 mg Capsules
Lamberts Gentle Vitamin C Tablets
Lamberts Ginkgo Biloba Extract Tablets
Lamberts Glucosamine Sulphate Tablets
Lamberts GTF Chromium Capsules
Lamberts Health Insurance Plus Tablets
Lamberts High Potency EPA Capsules
Lamberts L-Carnitine Capsules
Lamberts L-Carnitine Tablets
Lamberts L-Glutamic Acid Powder
Lamberts L-Glutamine Capsules
Lamberts L-Glutathione Complex Capsules
Lamberts L-Histidine HCL Capsules
Lamberts L-Isoleucine Capsules
Lamberts L-Leucine Capsules
Lamberts L-Threonine 500mg Capsules
Lamberts Magnesium Amino Acid Chelated Tablets
Lamberts Magnesium Orotate Capsules
Lamberts Magnesium Sustained Release Tablets
Lamberts Magnesium Sustained Release Timed Release Tablets
Lamberts Mega Mineral Compound Tablets
Lamberts Mega 3 Vitamins/Minerals Tablets
Lamberts Multi-Max Tablets
Lamberts Natural Vitamin E Capsules
Lamberts One Daily Vitamin/Mineral Tablets
Lamberts Playfair Tablets
Lamberts PMT Supplement Optivite Tablets
Lamberts Protein Deficiency Formula Capsules
Lamberts Protein Deficiency Formula Powder
Lamberts Pycnogenol Capsules
Lamberts Pyridoxal-5-Phosphate Capsules
Lamberts Pyridoxal-5-Phosphate Plus Capsules
Lamberts Selenium Capsules

DRUGS AND OTHER SUBSTANCES NOT TO BE PRESCRIBED UNDER THE NHS PHARMACEUTICAL SERVICES

Lamberts Selenium Tablets
Lamberts Senior Capsules
Lamberts Super Acidophilus Plus Capsules
Lamberts Taurine Capsules
Lamberts Ultra Detoxifying Capsules
Lamberts Vitamin B-50 Complex Capsules
Lamberts Vitamin B-50 Complex Tablets
Lamberts Vitamin B-100 Complex Tablets
Lamberts Vitamin C Ascorbic Acid & Calcium
    Ascorbate Crystals
Lamberts Vitamin C Ascorbic Acid Powder
Lamberts Vitamin C & Bioflav Tablets
Lamberts Vitamin C Calcium Ascorbate Crystals
Lamberts Vitamin C-Time Bioflav Timed-Release
    Tablets
Lamberts Vitamin E 200 D-Alpha Tablets
Lamberts Vitamin E 200 D-Alpha/Selenium Tablets
Lamberts Vitamin E 400 D-Alpha/Selenium Tablets
Lamberts Vitamin/Mineral Compound Tablets
Lamberts Zinc Citrus Capsules
Lamberts Zinc Gluconate Tablets
Lamberts Zinc Tablets
Lanacane Cream
Lanacort Cream
Lanacort Ointment
Lance B & C Tablets
Lancome Nutrix Cream
Lane's Cut-a-Cough
Lane's Laxative Herb Tablets
Lane's Sage and Garlic Catarrh Remedy
Lanes Glanolin Capsules 250/500
Lanes LecigranGranules
Lantigen B
Larkhall Acidophilus 500 Tablets
Larkhall B13 Zinc Tablets
Larkhall Beta Carotene Capsules
Larkhall Calcimega 500 Tablets
Larkhall DLPA 375 Tablets
Larkhall Dolomite Tablets
Larkhall Folic Acid Tablets 100mcg
Larkhall Folic Acid Tablets 500mcg
Larkhall L-Carnitine Capsules
Larkhall Magnesium Orotate B13 Tablets
Larkhall Selenium Supplement Tablets
Larkhall Vitamin C Naturtabs 1000mg Buffered
Lavender Bath
Laxaliver Pills
Laxatabs Leoren
Laxipurg Tablets
Laxoberal Elixir
LC 65 Cleaning Solution
Lecithin Capsules
Ledercort Cream
Lederplex Capsules
Lederplex Liquid
Lejfibre Biscuit
Lemeze Cough Syrup
Lemon Eno Powder
Lemon Flu-Cold Concentrated Syrup
Lemon Glycerine & Honey Cough Syrup
    Compound (Carter Bond)
Lemon Glycerine & Honey Lung Mixture (Whitehall
    Laboratories)

Lemon Glycerine & Ipecac Cough Syrup
    Compound (Carter Bond)
Lemon Juice, Glycerine & Honey A S Syrup (Ayrton
    Saunders)
Lemon Linctus 1-472
Lem-Plus Capsules
Lem-Plus Hot Lemon Drink
Lemsip Expectorant
Lemsip Flu Strength
Lemsip Lemcaps Cold Relief Capsules
Lemsip Linctus
Lemsip Flu Strength Night Time Formula
Lemsip Powder
Lendormin Tablets 0.125 mg
Lendormin Tablets 0.25 mg
Lensept Solution
Lensine 5 All in One Solution
Lensplus Sterile Saline Spray
Lensrins Solution
Leoren Tonic Tablets
Lexotan Tablets 1.5 mg
Lexotan Tablets 3 mg
Lexotan Tablets 6 mg
Libraxin Tablets
Librium Capsules 5 mg
Librium Capsules 10 mg
Librium Tablets 5 mg
Librium Tablets 10 mg
Librium Tablets 25 mg
Librofem Tablets
Lifeplan Acidophilus Capsules
Lifeplan Boron 3 Tablets
Lifeplan Cod Liver Oil One-A-Day Capsules
Lifeplan DL-Phenylalanine (DLPA) Tablets 500
Lifeplan Dolomite Tablets 500mg
Lifeplan Dolomite Tablets 800mg
Lifeplan Dolomite (Natural) Tablets
Lifeplan Super Galanol Starflower Capsules
Lifeplan Vitamin B6 Tablets
Lightning Cough Remedy Solution (Potters)
Limbitrol Capsules "5"
Limbitrol Capsules "10"
Linctifed Expectorant
Linctifed Expectorant Paediatric
Linctoid C
Linituss
Linoleic Acid
Linus Vitamin C Powder
Lipoflavonoid Capsules
Lipotriad Capsules
Lipotriad Liquid
Liqufruta Blackcurrant Cough Medicine
Liqufruta Honey & Lemon Cough Medicine
Liqufruta Medica
Liqufruta Medica Garlic Flavoured Cough Medicine
Liquid Formula (Food Concentrate) (Rodale)
Liquid Paraffin & Phenolphthalein Emulsion BP
Liquid Paraffin Emulsion with Cascara BPC
Liquifilm Wetting Solution
Listerine Antiseptic Mouthwash
Listermint Mouthwash
Liver Herbs (Hall's)
Livibron Mixture
Lloyds Cream (Odour Free)

XVIIIA

DRUGS AND OTHER SUBSTANCES NOT TO BE PRESCRIBED UNDER THE NHS
PHARMACEUTICAL SERVICES

Lloyds Heat Spray
Loasid Tablets
Lobak Tablets
Lofthouse's Original Fisherman's Friend Honey
  Cough Syrup
Logado
London Herb and Spice Herbal Tea Bags
Loramet Capsules 1 mg
Loramet Tablets 0.5 mg
Loramet Tablets 1 mg
Lotil Facial Cream
Lotussin Cough Syrup
L-Threonine Capsules
L-Threonine Tablets
Lucozade
Luma Bath Salts
Lung Balsam (Rusco)
Lyons Ground Coffee Beans
Lypsyl Lemon
Lypsyl Mint
Lypsyl Original
Lysaldin

M & B Children's Cough Linctus
MA4 Herbal Fruit Concentrate Paste
MA572 Tablets
Maalox Concentrate Suspension
Maalox Plus Tablets
Mackenzies Smelling Salts
Maclean Indigestion Powder
Maclean Indigestion Tablets
Macleans Toothpaste
Magaldrate Tablets
Magnesium Citrus Tru-Fil Capsules
Magnesium Glycerophos Tablets
Magnesium OK Tablets
Mainstay Pure Cod Liver Oil
Male Gland Double Strength Supplement Tablets
Male Sex Hormone Tablets (Diopharm)
Malinal Plus Tablets
Malinal Suspension 500 mg/5 ml
Malinal Tablets 500 mg
Malt Extract with Cod Liver Oil & Chemical Food
  (Distillers)
Malt Extract with Cod Liver Oil BPC &
  Hypophosphites (Distillers)
Malt Extract with Cod Liver Oil BPC Soft Extract
  (Jeffreys Miller)
Malt Extract with Haemoglobin & Vitamins Syrup
  (Distillers)
Malt Extract with Halibut Liver-Oil Syrup (Distillers)
Malvern Water
Mandarin Tablets
Manna Herbal Rheumapainaway Tablets
Marly Skin
Marvel
Matthew Cough Mixture
Maturaplus Tablets
Maws Sterilising Tablets
Max Factor Face Powder
Max Factor Pan-Stik
Maxivits Tablets
Medathlon Aspirin Tablets 300 mg

Medazepam Capsules 5 mg
Medazepam Capsules 10 mg
Medex Elixir
Mediclean Soft Lens Solutions
Medilax Tablets
Medinol Over 6 Paracetamol Oral Suspension
Medinol Under 6 Paracetamol Junior Suspension
Medipain Tablets
Medised Suspension
Medised Tablets
Medisoak Soft Lens Solution
Meditus Syrup
Medocodene Tablets
Meggeson Dyspepsia Tablets
Melissin Syrup
Melo Brand Glycerin Lemon & Honey with Ipecac
Meloids Lozenges
Meltus Adult Dry Cough Elixir
Meltus Adult Expectorant
Meltus Baby Cough Linctus
Meltus Honey and Lemon Cough Linctus
Meltus Junior Expectorant
Memo Boost Capsules
Menopace Capsules
Menthacol Liquid
Menthells Pellet/Pill
Menthol & Benzoin Inhalation BP
Menthol & Eucalyptus (M in P) Pastilles (Thomas
  Guest)
Menthol Inhalation
Mentholated Balsam (Loveridge)
Mentholated Balsam (Savory & Moore)
Mentholated Balsam (Wright Laymen & Umney)
Mentholated Balsam Mixture (Pilsworth
  Manufacturing)
Mentholatum Balm
Mentholatum Deep Freeze Spray
Mentholatum Deep Heat Massage Liniment
Mentholatum Deep Heat Maximum Strength Rub
Mentholatum Deep Heat Rub
Mentholatum Nasal Inhaler
Mercurochrome Solution
Metatone
Micaveen
Midro-Tea Powder
Migrafen Tablets
Mijex Cream
Milgard Baby Cleansing Milk
Milk of Magnesia Tablets
Mil-Par Suspension
Milton Sterilising Tablets
Milumil Baby Milk
Milupa 7 Cereal Breakfast
Milupa Aptamil Baby Milk
Milupa Braised Steak & Vegetable Infant Food
Milupa Camomile Infant Drink
Milupa Cauliflower Cheese Special Infant Food
Milupa Country Chicken & Vegetable Casserole
Milupa Fennel Variety Infant Drink
Milupa Forward Follow-On Milk
Milupa Harvest Muesli Breakfast
Milupa Infant Dessert, Banana & Apple Yoghurt
Milupa Infant Dessert, Caribbean Fruit
Milupa Infant Dessert, Semolina & Honey

DRUGS AND OTHER SUBSTANCES NOT TO BE PRESCRIBED UNDER THE NHS PHARMACEUTICAL SERVICES

Milupa Infant Tea-Time, Cheese & Tomato
Milupa Modified Yoghurt
Milupa Special Formula HN25
Milupa Sunshine Orange Breakfast
Milupa Vegetable Hotpot Infant Food
Minadex Chewable Vitamin Tablets
Minadex Syrup
Minamino Syrup
Minivits Tablets
Minoxidil Cream
Minoxidil Lotion
Minoxidil Ointment
Minoxidil Solution (for external use)
Mira Flow Cleaning Solution
Mira Flow Soft Lens Solution
Mira Soak Lens Soaking Solution
Mira Sol Soft Lens Solution
Mitchell's Wool Fat Soap
Modifast Nutritionally Complete Supplemented
    Fasting Formula
Mogadon Capsules 5 mg
Mogadon Tablets 5 mg
Moorland Indigestion Tablets
Morning Glory Tablets
Morny Lavender Talc
Mosquito Milk Mosquito Repellent Tropical Formula
Mrs Cullen's Lemsoothe Powder
Mrs Cullen's Powders
Mucofalk Sachets
Mucolex Syrup
Mucolex Tablets
Mu-Cron Junior Syrup
Mu-Cron Tablets
Mucron Liquid
Muflin Linctus
Multi-Vitamin Tablets (English Grains)
Multivitamin Capsules (Regent Laboratories)
Multivitamin Tablets (Approved Prescription
    Services)
Multivitamin Tablets (Chemipharm)
Multivitamin Tablets (Evans Medical)
Multivitamin Tablets (UAC International)
Multivitamin with Mineral Capsules (Potters)
Multivitamin with Minerals Tablets (Chemipharm)
Multivite Pellets
Multone Tablets
My Baby Cough Syrup
Mycocidin Perles
Mycolactine Tablets
Mylanta Liquid
Mylanta Tablets
Myolgin Tablets

N Tonic Syrup (Cupal)
N-300 Capsules
Nair Depilatory Cream
Nanny Goat's Milk Infant Formula
Napca Skin Lotion
Napisan Nappy Treatment
Napoloids Tablets
Napsalgesic Tablets
Nasal Drops for Children (Boots)
Natex 12A Tablets

Natural Bran
Natural Flow Acidophilus Capsules
Natural Flow Amino Acid Complex Capsules
Natural Flow Animal Fun Children's Chewable
    Tablets
Natural Flow Boron + Calcium & Silica Tablets
Natural Flow Calcium Ascorbate Tablets
Natural Flow Calcium & Magnesium Chelated
    Tablets
Natural Flow Candiforte Capsules
Natural Flow Digestive Enzyme Compound Tablets
Natural Flow Dolomite + A & D Tablets
Natural Flow Mega B Complex Tablets
Natural Flow Mega Multi Tablets
Natural Flow Multimineral Tablets
Natural Flow Organic Germanium Capsules
Natural Flow Primedophilus Powder
Natural Flow Probion Bifidus Powder
Natural Flow Probion Tablets
Natural Flow Psyllium Husks
Natural Flow Psyllium Husk Capsules
Natural Flow Selenium Chelated Tablets
Natural Flow Selenium Tablets
Natural Flow Super Vitamin C Complex Tablets
Natural Flow Super Vitamin C Tablets
Natural Flow Tangerine C Chewable Tablets
Natural Flow Thiamin Tablets (Vitamin B1)
Natural Flow Vega Mins Tablets
Natural Flow Vitamin A Tablets
Natural Flow Vitamin C Powder
Natural Flow Zinc Chelated Tablets
Natural Herb Laxative Tablets (Brome & Schimmer)
Natural Herb Laxative Tablets (Kerbina)
Natural Herb Tablets (Dorwest)
Natural Herb Tablets (Kerbina)
Natural Herb Tablets (Lane)
Naturavite Tablets
Nature's Aid Co-Enzyme Q-10 Capsules
Nature's Own Acidophilus Plus Capsules
    (Supreme)
Nature's Own Betacarotene Capsules
Nature's Own Beta Carotene tablets
Nature's Own Calcium Orotate Tablets
Nature's Own Dolomite Tablets
Nature's Own Dolomite-Calcium Carbonate
    Magnesium Carbonate Tablets
Nature's Own Food State Beta Carotene Tablets
Nature's Own Food State Calcium Tablets
Nature's Own Food State "Euro Formula" Vitamin B
    Complex + Vitamin C & MagnesiumTablets
Nature's Own Food State Magnesium Tablets
Nature's Own Food State Selenium Tablets
Nature's Own Food State Vitamin B6 (Pyridox)
    Tablets
Nature's Own Food State Vitamin C Tablets
Nature's Own Food State Vitamin E 300 Tablets
Nature's Own Food State Zinc/Copper Tablets
Nature's Own Multi-Vitamin Tablets
Nature's Own Vitamin B Complex Plus Tablets High
    Potency
Nature's Own Vitamin B6 (Pyridox) Tablets
Nature's Own Vitamin C Ascorbic Acid Powder
Nature's Own Vitamin C as Calcium Ascorbate
    Tablets

DRUGS AND OTHER SUBSTANCES NOT TO BE PRESCRIBED UNDER THE NHS
PHARMACEUTICAL SERVICES

Nature's Own Vitamin C (as Sodium Ascorbate)
    Tablets
Nature's Own Vitamin C with Bioflavonoids
Nature's Own Vitamin E 100 Capsules
Nature's Own Vitamin E 100 Emulsifying Capsules
Nature's Own Vitamin E 200 Capsules
Nature's Own Zinc Orotates
Nature's Plus Calcium/Magnesium Tablets
Nature's Plus Green Magma Powder
Nature's Plus Liquid B Complex & Iron
Nature's Plus Mega C Tablets
Nature's Plus Rutin Tablets 500mg
Nature's Plus Super B50 Capsules
Naturtabs Choline
Naturtabs Nicotinamide
Naturtabs Nicotinic Acid
Naturtabs Paba
Natusan Baby Ointment
Naudicelle
Nella Red Oil Liniment
Neo-Cytamen Injection 250 mcg/ml
Neo-Cytamen Injection 1000 mcg/ml
Neoklenz Powder
Neophryn Nasal Drops
Neophryn Nasal Spray
Nescafe Instant Coffee
Nestle Nativa HA
Nethaprin Expectorant
Neuro Phosphates
Neurodyne Capsules
Neutradol Concentrated Air Deodoriser
Neutradonna Powder
Neutradonna Sed Powder
Neutradonna Sed Tablets
Neutradonna Tablets
Neutrogena Body Oil (Scented and Unscented)
Neutrogena Conditioner
Neutrogena Hand Cream
Neutrogena Lip Care
Neutrogena Liquid
Neutrogena Moisture
Neutrogena Norwegian Formula Body Emulsion
Neutrogena Rainbath Shower and Bath Gel
Neutrogena Shampoo
Neutrogena Soap
Neutrogena Sun Care Lotion SPF 14
Neutrolactis Tablets
New Formula Beechams Powders Capsules
New Life Herbs
New Life Tablets
Newton's Children's Cough Treatment
Newton's Cough Mixture for Adults
Nezcaam Syrup
Nezeril Nose Drops (single dose pipette)
Nicobrevin
Niferex 150 Capsules
Nilbite
Nirolex Expectorant Linctus
Nitrados Tablets 5 mg
Nitrazepam Capsules 5 mg
Nivea
No 177 Tablets (Leoren)
Nobacter Medicated Shaving Foam
Nobrium Capsules 5 mg

Nobrium Capsules 10 mg
Nocold Tablets
Noctamid Tablets 0.5 mg
Noctamid Tablets 1 mg
Noctesed Tablets 5 mg
Noradran Bronchial Syrup
Norgesic Tablets
Normax Capsules
Normison Capsules 10 mg
Normison Capsules 20 mg
Norvits Syrup
Noscapine Linctus BP
Nourkrin Tablets
Novaprin Tablets
Novasil Antacid Tablets
Novasil Antacid Viscous Suspension
Noxzema Medicated Skin Cream
Nucross Coconut Oil
Nulacin Tablets
Numark Multivitamin Tablets
Nurodol Tablets
Nurofen Soluble Tablets
Nurofen Tablets 200 mg
Nurse Sykes Bronchial Balsam
Nurse Sykes Powders
Nu-Soft Baby Oil
Nutricare Beta Carotene Capsules
Nutricare Capricin Capsules
Nutricare Selenium Tablets
Nutricare Vitamin C Tablets
Nutricare Zinc Orotate Tablets
NutriTec Vitamin Mineral Complex Food
    Supplement
Nutrition Associates Beta Carotene Capsules
Nutrition Associates Reduced Glutathione
    Capsules
Nux Vomica Acid Mixture
Nux Vomica Alkaline Mixture
Nux Vomica Elixir BPC
Nylax Tablets
Nytol Tablets

Octovit Tablets
Ocuvite Multivitamin & Mineral Tablets
Oilatum Bar
Oilatum Soap
Olbas Oil
Omeiri Iron Tonic Tablets
Omilcaf Suspension
Onadox 118 Tablets
One Gram C Capsule
Opas Powder
Opas Tablets
Opobly Bailly Pills
Optivite Tablets
Oral B Plaque Check Disclosing Tablets
Orange & Halibut Vitamins (Kirby Warrick
    Pharmaceuticals)
Organidin Elixir
Organidin Solution
Organidin Tablets
Original Indigestion Tablets (Boots)
Orovite 7
Orovite Elixir

DRUGS AND OTHER SUBSTANCES NOT TO BE PRESCRIBED UNDER THE NHS PHARMACEUTICAL SERVICES

Orovite Tablets
Orthoxicol Syrup
Osteocare Calcium & Magnesium Tablets
Ostermilk Complete Formula
Ostermilk Two Milk Powder
Osterprem
Otrivine Nasal Drops 0.05%
Otrivine Nasal Drops 0.1%
Otrivine Nasal Spray 0.1%
Otrivine-Antistin Nasal Drops
Otrivine-Antistin Nasal Spray
Overnight Bedtime Cold Medicine
Owbridge's Cough Mixture
Oxanid Tablets 10 mg
Oxanid Tablets 15 mg
Oxanid Tablets 30 mg
Oxy 5 Acne Lotion
Oxy 10 Acne Lotion
Oxy Clean Facial Wash Gel
Oxy Clean Medicated Cleanser
Oxymetazoline Hydrochloride Nasal Drops 0.025%
Oxymetazoline Hydrochloride Nasal Drops 0.05%
Oxymetazoline Hydrochloride Nasal Spray 0.05%
Oxysept 1 Disinfecting Solution
Oxysept 2 Rinsing, Neutralising and Storing
    Solution
Ozium 500 Air Sanitizer
Ozium 1500 Air Sanitizer
Ozium Air Sanitizer
Ozium 3000

Pacidal Tablets
Pacifene Tablets
Paedo-Sed Syrup
Pain Relief Tablets (Cox)
Pain Relief Tablets (Davidson)
Paldesic Elixir
Pameton Tablets
Panacron Nasal Spray
Panacron Tablets
Panadeine Co Tablets
Panadeine Forte Tablets
Panadeine Soluble Effervescent Tablets
Panadeine Tablets
Panadol Baby & Infant Suspension
Panadol Caplets
Panadol Extra Soluble Tablets
Panadol Extra Tablets
Panadol Junior Sachets
Panadol Soluble Tablets
Panadol Tablets
Panaleve Junior
Panaleve Six Plus Suspension
Panasorb Tablets
Panax 600 Ginseng Tablets
Panerel Tablets
Panets Tablets
Pango Pain Paracetamol Codeine Tablets (Cupal)
Pantene Hair Tonic
Papain Compound Tablets
Paprika Tablets (Kerbina)
Para-Seltzer Effervescent Tablets
Paracetamol & Caffeine Capsules
Paracetamol & Caffeine Tablets

Paracetamol DC Tablets
Paracetamol Tablets Soluble (Boots)
Paracetamol Tablets, Sorbitol Basis 500 mg
Paracets Tablets 500 mg
Paraclear Tablets
Paracodol Capsules
Paracodol Tablets
Paradeine R Tablets
Paragesic Effervescent Tablets
Parahypon Tablets
Parake Tablets
Paralgin Tablets
Paramin Capsules
Paramol Tablets
Paranorm Cough Syrup
Pardale Tablets
Parenamps Intramuscular Injection
Pastilaids Pastilles
Pavacol Cough Syrup
Paxadon Tablets
Paxalgesic Tablets
Paxidal Tablets
Paynocil Tablets
PEM Linctus
Penetrol Inhalant
Pentazocine-Aspirin Compound Tablets
Peplax Peppermint Flavoured Laxative Tablets
Peppermint Indigestion Tablets (Boots)
Pepto-Bismol Suspension
Perform 1 Disinfecting Solution
Perform 2 Rinsing and Neutralising Solution
Pernivit Tablets
Perrier Mineral Water
Persomnia Tablets
Pestroy Flea and Insect Powder
Petrolagar Emulsion Plain
Petrolagar Emulsion with Phenolphthalein
PF Plus Tablets
Pharmacin Capsules
Pharmacin Effervescent Plus C Tablets
Pharmacin Effervescent Tablets 325 mg
Pharmaton Capsules
Pharmidone Tablets
Phenergan Compound Expectorant Linctus
Phenolphthalein Compound Pills BPC
Phenolphthalein Compound Tablets BPC 1963
Phenolphthalein Tablets BP
Phensedyl Cough Linctus
Phensic Tablets
Phensic 2 Tablets
Phenylephrine Hydrochloride Nasal Drops 0.25%
Phenylephrine Hydrochloride Nasal Spray 0.5%
Phillips Brewers Yeast Tablets
Phillips Iron Tonic Tablets
Phillips Tonic Yeast Tablets
Phillips' Toothpaste
Phisoderm
Phisohex System Medicated Face Wash
pHiso-Med Solution
Pholcolix Syrup
Pholcomed D Linctus
Pholcomed Diabetic Forte Linctus
Pholcomed Expectorant
Pholcomed Forte Linctus

DRUGS AND OTHER SUBSTANCES NOT TO BE PRESCRIBED UNDER THE NHS
PHARMACEUTICAL SERVICES

Pholcomed Linctus
Pholcomed Pastilles
Pholtex Syrup
Pholtussa Mixture
Phor Pain
Phor Pain Double Strength
Phosferine Liquid
Phosferine Multi-Vitamin Liquid
Phosferine Tablets
Phygeine Liquid
Phyllosan Tablets
Physeptone Linctus
Pickles Nail Bite Lotion
PIL Food Capsules
Pile Mixture (Ayrton Saunders)
Pile Tablets (Ayrton Saunders)
Pine Bath Milk
Pine Catarrh Drops Lozenges
Piriton Allergy
Piz Buin After Sun Lotion
Piz Buin After Sun Shower Gel
Piz Buin Children's Balm SPF 8
Piz Buin Cream Factor 12
Piz Buin Creme factor 6
Piz Buin Creme factor 8
Piz Buin Factor 4 Cold Air Protection Cream
Piz Buin Glacier Cream SPF 15
Piz Buin Lip Protection Stick SPF 8
Piz Buin Sun Allergy Lotion SPF 12
Piz Buin Sun Protection Lotion SPF 12
Piz Buin SPF 6 Lotion
Piz Buin SPF 8 Lotion
Plax Anti-Plaque Pre-Brushing Rinse
Plenamin Super
Plenivite with Iron Tablets
Pliagel Soft Lens Solution
Plurivite M Tablets
Plurivite Tablets
Poli-grip Denture Fixative Cream
Pollen-Eze Tablets
Polyalk Gel
Polyalk Tablets
Polyvite Capsules
Porosis D Calcium Supplement Tablets
Potaba + 6 Capsules
Potaba + 6 Tablets
Potassium Bromide & Nux Vomica Mixture
   BPC 1963
Potters Household Liniment
Potters Nine Rubbing Oils
Powdered Bran Tablets 2 g
Power Cranberry Juice Capsules
Power Cranberry Juice Concentrated Powder
Power Dolomite Tablets
Power Dophilus Capsules
Power Feverfew Capsules
Power GLA 65 (Borage Oil) Capsules
Power Halibut Liver Oil Capsules
Power Kelp Tablets 500mg
Power Nature Vitamin E Cream
Power Nutrimental 24 Tablets
Power Plus Super Multivitamin and Mineral
   Capsules
Powerin Tablets

PP Tablets
PR Freeze Spray
PR Heat Spray
PR Tablets
Prazepam Tablets 10 mg
PRD 200 Tablets 600 mg
Preflex Solution
Pregaine Shampoo
Pregnacare Capsules
Pregnadon Tablets
Pregnavite Forte Tablets
Pregnavite Forte F Tablets
Prematil with Milupan
Premence-28 Capsules
Premit Tablets 20 mg
Prenatal Dri-Kaps Capsules
Prenatol Anti Stretch Mark Cream
Pre-Nutrison
Primes Premiums Tablets
Prioderm Cream Shampoo
Priory Cleansing Herbs Powder
Probase 3 Cream
Pro-Bifidus Powder (Dairy Free)
Procol Capsules
Proctofibre Tablets
Prodexin Tablets
Pro-Dophilus Powder (Dairy Free)
Proflex Capsules
Proflex Tablets 200 mg
Progress Powder
Propain Tablets
Propecia
Pro-Plus He-Vite Elixir
Proteolised Liver Tablets
Protexin B Powder
Protexin Natural Care Powder
Protexin Natural Care Tablets
Pro-Vitamin A Capsules (Rodale)
Pru Sen Tablet Bar
Prymecare Tablets for Soft and and Gas Permeable
   Lenses
Prymeclean Cleaning Solution for Soft Lenses
Prymesoak Soaking Solution for Soft Lenses
Pulmo Bailly Liquid
Purgoids Tablets
Pyridoxine Tablets, Slow 100 mg

Quest Balanced Ratio Cal-Mag Tablets
Quest Beta Carotene Tablets
Quest Folic Acid with Vitamin B Capsules
Quest Gamma EPA Capsules 1000mg
Quest Herbal Range Feverfew Formula Capsules
Quest Improved Once-A-Day Tablets
Quest Kyolic 350 Tablets
Quest Mega B50 Tablets
Quest Mega B-100 Timed Release Tablets
Quest Mega B Complex Plus 1000mg C Tablets
Quest Multi B Complex Plus 500mg C Tablets
Quest Multi C Complex Tablets
Quest Non-Dairy Acidophilus Plus Capsules
Quest Once-A-Day Tablets
Quest Super Mega B-50 Timed Release Tablets

DRUGS AND OTHER SUBSTANCES NOT TO BE PRESCRIBED UNDER THE NHS PHARMACEUTICAL SERVICES

Quest Super Mega B + C TabletsQuest Super
   Once-A-Day Tablets
Quest Super Once-A-Day Divided Dose Tablets
Quest Synergistic Boron Tablets
Quest Synergistic Iron Capsules
Quest Synergistic Magnesium Tablets
Quest Synergistic Selenium Capsules
Quest Synergistic Zinc Capsules
Quest Vitamin C Tablets
Quest Vitamin C Tablets Sustained Release
Quest Vitamin E Capsules
Quick Action Cough Cure (Brian C Spencer)
Quiet Life Tablets

Rabenhorst Tomato Juice
Radian-B Mineral Bath Liquid
Radian-B Mineral Bath Salts
Radian-B Muscle Lotion
Radian-B Muscle Rub
Ralgex Cream
Ralgex Stick
Rappell Head Louse Repellent Pump Spray
Raspberry Tablets No B039
Rayglo Chest Rub Ointment
Rayglo Laxative Tablets
Reach Mouthwash
Reactivan Tablets
Red Catarrh Pastilles (Baldwin)
Redelan Effervescent Tablets
Redoxon Adult Multivitamin Tablets
Redoxon C Effervescent Tablets 1 g
Redoxon C Tablets 25 mg
Redoxon C Tablets 50 mg
Redoxon C Tablets 200 mg
Redoxon C Tablets 250 mg
Redoxon C Tablets 500 mg
Redoxon Childrens Multivitamins Tablets
Redoxon Effervescent Tablets 1 g
Regaine
Regina Royal Jelly Capsules
Reg-U-Lett Tablets
Relanium Tablets 2 mg
Relanium Tablets 5 mg
Relanium Tablets 10 mg
Relcofen Tablets
Relcol Tablets
Remegel Tablets
Remnos Tablets 5 mg
Remnos Tablets 10 mg
Rennie Tablets
Rennie Gold Tablets
Rennie Plus Tablets
Rennie Rap-Eze Tablets
Replens Vaginal Moisturiser
Please note: For reimbursement purposes the
   product Replens should not be confused with
   the medical device Replens MD listed in Part
   IXA - Appliances
Resolve Granules
Respaton
Retinova
Revlon Nurtrasome Shampoo
Revlon ZP11 Medicated Shampoo

Rheumavit Tablets
Rhuaka Herbal Syrup
Rhuaka Tablets
Rhubarb & Soda Mixture Ammoniated BP
Rhubarb Compound Mixture BPC
Rhubarb Mixture Compound Paediatric BPC
Ribena
Riddovydrin Liquid
Rinurel Linctus
Rinurel Tablets
Rite-Diet Egg White Replacer
Rite-Diet Gluten-Free Baking Powder
Rite-Diet Gluten-Free Banana Cake
Rite-Diet Gluten-Free Bourbon Biscuits
Rite-Diet Gluten-Free Christmas Pudding
Rite-Diet Gluten-Free Half Covered Chocolate
   Digestive Biscuits
Rite-Diet Gluten-Free Coconut Cookies
Rite-Diet Gluten-Free Date and Walnut Cake
Rite-Diet Gluten-Free Gingernut Cookies
Rite-Diet Gluten-Free Muesli Cookies
Rite-Diet Gluten-Free Lemon Madeira Cake
Rite-Diet Gluten-Free Rich Fruit Cake
Rite-Diet Gluten-Free Wheat-Free Mince Pies
Rite-Diet Hot Breakfast Cereal
Robaxisal Forte Tablets
Roberts Aspirin & Caffeine Tablets
Robinsons Baby Rice
Robinsons Instant Baby Foods Baby Breakfast
Robinsons Instant Baby Foods Baby Dessert
Robitussin AC Liquid
Robitussin Cough Soother
Robitussin Cough Soother Junior Formula
Robitussin Expectorant
Robitussin Expectorant Plus
Robitussin Liquid
Robitussin Plus Liquid
Robitussin Syrup
RoC Amino Moisturising Cream
RoC Compact Cleanser
RoC Eye Make-up Remover Lotion
RoC Face Powder Loose
RoC Foundation Cream
RoC High Protection Sun Cream SPF 7/9
RoC Hydra and Body Cream
RoC Hydra Plus
RoC Intensive Hand Cream
RoC Lipo Moisturising Treatment
RoC Lipo Vitamin Treatment
RoC Pre-Tanning Lotion
RoC Soap for Delicate Skin
RoC Soothing After Sun Lotion
RoC Soothing Eye Gel
RoC Treatment Lipstick
RoC Vitamin Cream
Roche Starflower Oil Capsules 500mg
Roche Starflower Oil (GLA) Capsules 250mg
Rock Salmon Cough Mixture
Rohypnol Tablets 1 mg
Roscorbic Effervescent Tablets
Roscorbic Tablets 25 mg
Roscorbic Tablets 50 mg
Roscorbic Tablets 200 mg
Roscorbic Tablets 500 mg

DRUGS AND OTHER SUBSTANCES NOT TO BE PRESCRIBED UNDER THE NHS PHARMACEUTICAL SERVICES

Rose Hip C-100 Capsules
Rose Hip C-200 Capsules
Rose Hip Tablets (English Grains)
Rose Hip Tablets (Potters)
Rose Hip Tablets (Roberts)
Rosemary Bath
Roskens Ultracare 3
Rosmax Syrup
Roter Tablets
Rovigon
RRC1 Cream
Rubelix Syrup
Rubraton B Elixir
Ruby Tonic Tablets (Jacksons)
Rum Cough Elixir
Ruthmol
Rutin Plus Tablets (Gerard)

Safapryn Tablets
Safapryn-Co Tablets
Safflower Seed Oil
Sainsbury's Aspirin Tablets 300mg
Sainsbury's Cold Powders with Blackcurrant
Sainsbury's Hot Lemon Powders
Sainsbury's Indigestion Tablets
Sainsbury's Junior Soluble Aspirin Tablets
Sainsbury's Paracetmaol Tablets 500 mg
Sainsbury's Soluble Aspirin Tablets
St. Clements Fruit Juice Concentrate
Salonair Spray
Salzone Syrup
Salzone Tablets 500 mg
Sanatogen Childrens Vitamins Plus Minerals
Sanatogen Cod Liver Oil Capsules
Sanatogen Garlic Oil Perle One-A-Day
Sanatogen Junior Vitamins Tablets
Sanatogen Multivitamin Plus Iron (Formula One) Tablets
Sanatogen Multivitamins Tablets
Sanatogen Multivitamins & Calcium Tablets
Sanatogen Nerve Tonic Powder
Sanatogen Selected Multivitamins Plus Iron (Formula Two) Tablets
Sanatogen Tonic
Sanatogen Vitamin B6 Capsules
Sanatogen Vitamin E Capsules
Sancos Compound Linctus
Sancos Syrup
Savant Tablets
Savlon Dry Skin Cream
Saxin
SBL Junior Cough Linctus
SBL Soothing Bonchial Linctus
Schar Gluten Free Sponge Cake
Scholl Foot Refresher Spray
Scott's Cod Liver Oil Capsules
Scott's Emulsion
Scott's Husky Biscuits
Seatone Capsules
Seatone Super Strength Capsules
Seaweed Vitamin A Ester BP & Vitamin D BP Capsules (Regent Laboratories)

Seba-Med Cleansing Bar
Seba-Med Cream
Seba-Med Facial Wash
Seba-Med Lotion
Seba-Med Shampoo
Sebbix Shampoo
Secaderm Salve
Seclodin Capsules
Sedazin Tablets 1 mg
Sedazin Tablets 2.5 mg
Seldane Tablets
Selenium ACE Tablets
Selora Sodium-free Salt Substitute
Selsun Soft Conditioner
Senlax Tablets
Senna Laxative Tablets (Boots)
Senna Tablets (Potters)
Senokot Tablets
Senotabs Tablets
Senselle Natural Feminine Moisture
Sensodyne Toothpaste
Serenid D Tablets 10 mg
Serenid D Tablets 15 mg
Serenid Forte Capsules 30 mg
Sergeant's Dust Mite Patrol Powder
Sertin Tablets
Setamol Soluble Tablets
Setlers Extra Strength Tablets
Setlers Liquid
Setlers Tablets
Seven Seas Antioxidant Beta Carotene Capsules
Seven Seas Antioxidant Vitamin E Capsules
Seven Seas Beta Carotene Capsules
Seven Seas Calcium Chewables (Chewable Caps)
Seven Seas Cod Liver Oil
Seven Seas Evening Primrose Oil Capsules
Seven Seas Folic Acid & Vitamin B12 One-A-Day Tablets
Seven Seas Formula 70 Multivitamin- Multimineral Capsules
Seven Seas Garlic Oil Perles
Seven Seas Iron Chewables (Chewable Caps)
Seven Seas Korean Ginseng Capsules
Seven Seas Lecithin Capsules
Seven Seas Magnesium Berries
Seven Seas Malt and Cod Liver Oil
Seven Seas Multivitamin & Mineral Capsules
Seven Seas Natural Vitamin E in Wheatgerm Capsules
Seven Seas Orange Syrup & Cod Liver Oil
Seven Seas Pulse Capsules
Seven Seas Pure Cod Liver Oil Capsules
Seven Seas Pure Starflower Oil
Seven Seas Selenium E & Cod Liver Oil Capsules
Seven Seas Start Right Cod Liver Oil for Babies
Seven Seas Vitamin and Mineral Tonic
Seven Seas Wheatgerm Oil Capsules
Seven Seas Zinc Chewables (Chewable Caps)
Sidros Tablets
Silk-Lax Tablets
Siloxyl Suspension
Siloxyl Tablets
Simeco Suspension
Simeco Tablets

DRUGS AND OTHER SUBSTANCES NOT TO BE PRESCRIBED UNDER THE NHS
PHARMACEUTICAL SERVICES

Simple Hair Conditioner
Simple Moisturising Lotion
Simple Night Cream
Simple Protective Moisture Cream
Simple Refreshing Shower Gel
Simple Shampoo
Simple Soap
Simple Sun Block
Simple Talcum Powder
Sine-Off Tablets
Sinitol Capsules
Sinutab Tablets
Sionon Sweetner
Skin Glow Capsules
Slim-Fast Meal Replacement
SMA Gold Cap Powder and Ready-to- Feed
SMA Powder and Concentrated Liquid
Snufflebabe Vapour Rub
Soaclens Solution
Soframycin Ointment
Softab Soft Lens Care Tablets
Solgar Cartilade Capsules
Solgar Ester-C Tablets
Solgar Evening Primrose Oil
Solgar Glucosamine Sulfate Tablets
Solgar Maxi Coenzyme Q10 Capsules
Solgar Maxi L-Carnitine Tablets
Solgar Provatene Softgel Capsules
Solis Capsules 2 mg
Solis Capsules 5 mg
Solis Capsules 10 mg
Solmin Tablets
Solpadeine Capsules
Solpadeine Forte Tablets
Solpadeine Tablets
Solpadeine Tablets Effervescent
Solprin Tablets
Soluble Aspirin Tablets for Children (Boots)
Soluble Phensic Tablets
Solusol Solution
Sominex Tablets
Somnite Suspension 2.5 mg/5 ml
Somnite Tablets 5 mg
Soquette Soaking Solution
Sovol Liquid
Sovol Tablets
Soya Powder & Nicotinamide Tablets
SP Cold Relief Capsules
Special E Moisture Cream
Special Stomach Powder (Halls)
Spectraban 4 Lotion
SPHP Tablets
SPS Low-Protein Drink
Squill Linctus Opiate BP (Gee's Linctus)
Squill Linctus Opiate, Paediatric, BP
Squire's Soonax Tablets
SR2310 Expectorant
SR Toothpaste (Gibbs)
Staffords Mild Aperient Tablets
Staffords Strong Aperient Tablets
Steradent Mouthwash
Steri-Clens Solution
Steri-Solve Soft Lens Solution
Sterling Health Salts Effervescent

Sterling Indigestion Tablets
Sterling Paracetamol Tablets
Sterogyl Alcoholic Solution
Stomach Aids Tablets
Stomach Mixture (Herbal Laboratories)
Stomach Mixture H138 (Southon Laboratories)
Stomach Powder (Diopharm)
Stomach Tablets (Ulter)
Stop 'N' Grow Nail Biting Deterrent
Street's Cough Mixture
Strengthening Mixture (Hall's)
Stress B Supplement Tablets
Strychnine & Iron Mixture BPC 1963
Strychnine Mixture BPC 1963
Stute Diabetic Blackcurrant Jam
Stute Diabetic Marmalade
Sudafed Co Tablets
Sudafed Expectorant
Sudafed Linctus
Sudafed Nasal Spray
Sudocrem Baby Lotion
Suleo C Shampoo
Sun E45 Lotion SPF8
Sunerven Tablets
Sunnyvale Gluten-Free Rich Plum Pudding
Sun Yums Gluten Free & Dairy Free Almond &
    Coconut Cake
Sun Yums Gluten Free & Dairy Free Banana &
    Sesame Seed Cake
Sun Yums Gluten Free & Dairy Free Carob & Mint
    Cake
Sun Yums Gluten Free & Dairy Free Ginger &
    Pecan Nut Cake
Sun Yums Gluten Free & Dairy Free Jaffa Spice
    Cake
Super Plenamins Tablets
Super Yeast + C Tablets
Superdophilus Powder
Superdrug Health Salts
Superdrug Heat Spray
Supradyn Capsules
Supradyn Effervescent Tablets
Supradyn Tablets for Children
Surbex-T Tablets
Surem Capsules 5 mg
Surem Capsules 10 mg
Surelax Laxative Tablets
Sweetex
Sylopal Suspension
Sylphen Tablets
Syn-Ergel
Syndol Tablets
Syrtussar Cough Syrup

T-Zone Decongestant Tablets
Tabasan Tablets
Tablets No B006
Tablets No B011
Tablets No B015
Tablets No B024
Tablets No B025
Tablets No B029
Tablets No B034

DRUGS AND OTHER SUBSTANCES NOT TO BE PRESCRIBED UNDER THE NHS PHARMACEUTICAL SERVICES

Tablets No B035	Tablets to Formula A274
Tablets No B036	Tablets to Formula A275
Tablets No B037	Tablets to Formula A276
Tablets No B038	Tablets to Formula A277
Tablets No B040	Tablets to Formula A298
Tablets No B041	Tablets to Formula A301
Tablets No B045	Tablets to Formula A316
Tablets No B048	Tablets to Formula BA6
Tablets No B070	Tablets to Formula B10
Tablets No 268A (Potters)	Tablets to Formula B15
Tablets to Formula A10	Tablets to Formula B18
Tablets to Formula A11	Tablets to Formula B19
Tablets to Formula A18	Tablets to Formula B20
Tablets to Formula A19	Tablets to Formula B21
Tablets to Formula A20	Tablets to Formula B22
Tablets to Formula A22	Tablets to Formula B25
Tablets to Formula A23	Tablets to Formula B26
Tablets to Formula A31	Tablets to Formula B29
Tablets to Formula A32	Tablets to Formula B41
Tablets to Formula A33	Tablets to Formula B48
Tablets to Formula A45	Tablets to Formula B51
Tablets to Formula A51	Tablets to Formula B56
Tablets to Formula A63	Tablets to Formula B58
Tablets to Formula A67	Tablets to Formula B64
Tablets to Formula A68	Tablets to Formula B65
Tablets to Formula A69	Tablets to Formula B66
Tablets to Formula A70	Tablets to Formula B67
Tablets to Formula A71	Tablets to Formula B68
Tablets to Formula A105	Tablets to Formula B70
Tablets to Formula A111	Tablets to Formula B71
Tablets to Formula A114	Tablets to Formula B72
Tablets to Formula A120	Tablets to Formula B73
Tablets to Formula A147	Tablets to Formula B74
Tablets to Formula A157	Tablets to Formula B75
Tablets to Formula A158	Tablets to Formula B76
Tablets to Formula A161	Tablets to Formula B77
Tablets to Formula A162	Tablets to Formula B78
Tablets to Formula A164	Tablets to Formula B79
Tablets to Formula A165	Tablets to Formula B80
Tablets to Formula A166	Tablets to Formula B81
Tablets to Formula A167	Tablets to Formula B82
Tablets to Formula A169	Tablets to Formula B83
Tablets to Formula A175	Tablets to Formula B85
Tablets to Formula A183	Tablets to Formula B86
Tablets to Formula A184	Tablets to Formula B87
Tablets to Formula A190	Tablets to Formula B90
Tablets to Formula A195	Tablets to Formula B91
Tablets to Formula A202	Tablets to Formula B93
Tablets to Formula A203	Tablets to Formula B94
Tablets to Formula A213	Tablets to Formula B96
Tablets to Formula A221	Tablets to Formula B98
Tablets to Formula A244	Tablets to Formula B100
Tablets to Formula A245	Tablets to Formula B102
Tablets to Formula A246	Tablets to Formula B104
Tablets to Formula A247	Tablets to Formula B117
Tablets to Formula A248	Tablets to Formula B118
Tablets to Formula A249	Tablets to Formula B120
Tablets to Formula A250	Tablets to Formula B122
Tablets to Formula A264	Tablets to Formula B124
Tablets to Formula A266	Tablets to Formula B128
Tablets to Formula A270	Tablets to Formula B141
Tablets to Formula A271	Tablets to Formula B143
Tablets to Formula A272	Tablets to Formula B145
Tablets to Formula A273	Tablets to Formula B148

DRUGS AND OTHER SUBSTANCES NOT TO BE PRESCRIBED UNDER THE NHS PHARMACEUTICAL SERVICES

Tablets to Formula B156
Tablets to Formula B157
Tablets to Formula B158
Tablets to Formula B160
Tablets to Formula B163
Tablets to Formula B169
Tablets to Formula B178
Tablets to Formula B180
Tablets to Formula B181
Tablets to Formula B182
Tablets to Formula B190
Tablets to Formula B193
Tablets to Formula B207
Tablets to Formula B209
Tablets to Formula B210
Tablets to Formula B211
Tablets to Formula B212
Tablets to Formula B213
Tablets to Formula B214
Tablets to Formula B215
Tablets to Formula B216
Tablets to Formula B217
Tablets to Formula B218
Tablets to Formula B222
Tablets to Formula B223
Tablets to Formula B224
Tablets to Formula B225
Tablets to Formula B227
Tablets to Formula B228
Tablets to Formula B231
Tablets to Formula B234
Tablets to Formula B235
Tablets to Formula B236
Tablets to Formula B243
Tablets to Formula B248
Tablets to Formula B250
Tablets to Formula B251
Tablets to Formula B252
Tabmint Anti-Smoking Chewing Gum Tablets
Tanacet Feverfew 125
Tancolin Childrens Cough Linctus
Tedral Expectorant
Temazepam Gelthix Capsules
Temazepam Planpak
Temazepam Soft Gelatin Gel-Filled Capsules
Tenaset Wash Cream
Tenaset Wash Cream (Unperfumed)
Tensium Tablets 2 mg
Tensium Tablets 5 mg
Tensium Tablets 10 mg
Tercoda Elixir
Tercolix Elixir
Terpalin Elixir
Terperoin Elixir
Terpoin Antitussive
Terrabron
T-Gel Conditioner
Thermogene Medicated Rub
Thixo-D Thickened Drink Mixes
Three Noughts Cough Syrup
Tidmans Bath Sea Salt
Tidman's Sea Salt Coarse
Tiger Balm Liquid
Tiger Balm Red

Tiger Balm White
Timotei Herbal Shampoo
Tinaderm Cream
Titan Hard Cleanser
Tixylix Cough and Cold Linctus
Tixylix Cough Linctus
Tixylix Day-Time Cough Linctus
Tixylix Decongestant Inhalant Capsules
Tolu Compound Linctus Paediatric BP
Tolu Solution BP
Tolu Syrup BP
Tonatexa Mixture
Tonic Tablets (Thomas Guest)
Tonic Wines
Tonivitan A & D Syrup
Tonivitan B Syrup
Tonivitan Capsules
Top C Tablets
Topfit Amino Acid Powder
Topfit L Threonine + Vitamin B6 Capsules 500/12.5mg
Toptabs
Total All Purpose Solution
Total Nutrient Liquid
Totavit D R Capsules
Totolin Paediatric Cough Syrup
Tramil Capsules
Trancoprin Tablets
Transclean Cleaning Solution
Transdrop
Transoak Solution
Transol Solution
Tranxene Capsules 7.5 mg
Tranxene Capsules 15 mg
Tranxene Tablets 15 mg
Triludan Forte Tablets 7-tablet pack
Triludan Tablets 10-tablet pack
Triocos Linctus
Triogesic Elixir
Triogesic Tablets
Triominic Syrup
Triominic Tablets
Triopaed Linctus
Triotussic Suspension
Triovit Tablets
Triple Action Cold Relief Tablets
Tropium Capsules 5 mg
Tropium Capsules 10 mg
Tropium Tablets 5 mg
Tropium Tablets 10 mg
Tropium Tablets 25 mg
Trufree Crispbran
Trufree Tandem IQ Tablets
Trufree Vitamin & Minerals Tablets
Tudor Rose Bay Rhum
Tums Tablets
Tusana Linctus
Tussifans Syrup
Tussimed Liquid
Two-A-Day Iron Jelloids Tablets
Tymasil
Tysons Catarrh Syrup

DRUGS AND OTHER SUBSTANCES NOT TO BE PRESCRIBED UNDER THE NHS
PHARMACEUTICAL SERVICES

Ucerax Tablets
Udenum Gastric Vitamin Powder
Ultracach Analgesic Capsules
Ultradal Antacid Stomach Tablets
Ultralief Tablets
Uncoated Tablets to Formula A323
Uncoated Tablets to Formula A325
Undecyn Capsules
Unguentum Merck Cream 60g
Unicap M Tablets
Unicap T Tablets
Unichem Baby Oil
Unichem Chesty Cough Linctus
Unichem Children's Dry Cough Linctus
Unichem Cod Liver Oil Capsules
Unichem Cold Relief Capsules
Unichem Cold Relief Day-Time Liquid
Unichem Cold Relief Night-Time Liquid
Unichem Cold Relief Powders
Unichem Dry Cough Linctus
Unichem Extract of Malt with Cod Liver Oil
Unichem Multivitamins + Iron Tablets
Unichem Multivitamins & Minerals One-A-Day
    Capsules
Uniflu Tablets
Unigesic Capsules
Unigest Tablets
Unisomnia Tablets 5 mg
United Skin Care Programme (Uni-Derm; Uni-
    Salve; Uni-Wash)
Uvistat Aftersun Lotion
Uvistat Baby Sun Cream SPF 12
Uvistat Cream SPF 4
Uvistat Facial Cream SPF 8
Uvistat Facial Cream SPF 22
Uvistat Lipscreen SPF 5 Lipstick
Uvistat SPF 8 Suncream
Uvistat SPF 10 Suncream
Uvistat Sun Lotion SPF 6
Uvistat Sun Lotion SPF 8

Vadarex Wintergreen Heat Rub
Vagisil Feminine Powder
Valium Capsules 2 mg
Valium Capsules 5 mg
Valium Syrup 2 mg/5 ml
Valium Tablets 2 mg
Valium Tablets 5 mg
Valium Tablets 10 mg
Valonorm Tonic Solution
Valrelease Capsules
Vanamil Tablets
Vantage Baby Shampoo
Vantage Garlic One-A-Day Capsules
Vantage Halibut Fish Oil One-A-Day Capsules
Vantage Sterilising Fluid
Vapex Inhalent
Vaseline Intensive Care Lotion
Vaseline Intensive Care Lotion Herbal and Aloe
Vega Glucosamine Sulphate Capsules
Veganin Tablets
Veno's Adult Formula Cough Mixture
Veno's Cough Mixture
Veno's Honey & Lemon Cough Mixture

Veracolate Tablets
Verdiviton Elixir
Vervain Compound Tablets
Vichy Total Sunscreen
Vicks Coldcare Capsules
Vicks Cremacoat Syrup
Vicks Cremacoat Syrup with Doxylamine Succinate
Vicks Cremacoat Syrup with Guaiphenesin
Vicks Cremacoat Syrup with Paracetamol &
    Dextromethorphan
Vicks Daymed
Vicks Formula 44 Cough Mixture
Vicks Inhaler
Vicks Medinite
Vicks Pectorex Solution
Vicks Sinex Nasal Spray
Vicks Vapo-Lem Powder Sachets
Vicks Vaposyrup Children's Dry Cough
Vicks Vaposyrup for Chesty Coughs
Vicks Vaposyrup for Chesty Coughs and Nasal
    Congestion
Vicks Vaposyrup for Dry Coughs
Vicks Vaposyrup for Dry Coughs and Nasal
    Congestion
Vicks Vapour Rub
Vi-Daylin Syrup
Videnal Tablets
Vigour Aids Tablets
Vigranon B Complex Tablets
Vigranon B Syrup
Vikelp Coated Tablets
Vikonon Tablets
Villescon Liquid
Villescon Tablets
Viobin Octacosanol Tablets 50,000mcg
Viobin Pancreatin Tablets 325mg
Vipro Vegetable Protein
Virvina Elixir
Vitabrit Beta Carotene Capsules
Vita Diem Multi Vitamin Drops
Vita-E 200 (D-Alpha Tocopherol) Capsules
Vita-E Cream
Vita-E Ointment
Vital Dophilus Powder
Vitalia Calcium Formula A + D Tablets
Vitalia Lecithin Capsules High Potency
Vitalia Multivitamins & Minerals Children's
    Chewable Sugar-Free Tablets
Vitalia Multivitamin & Minerals with Iron Tablets
Vitalia Multivitamin & Minerals Tablets without Iron
Vitalia Natural E Capsules
Vitalia Vitamin A Tablets
Vitalia Vitamin B Complex Super Tablets
Vitalia Vitamin B6 Tablets
Vitalia Vitamin C Chewable Tablets
Vitalia Vitamin E Tablets
Vitalia Zinc Amino Acid Chelated Tablets 15mg
Vitalia Zinc Chelated Tablets
Vitalife Vital E Capsules
Vitalife Vitamin B6 Capsules
Vitalife Vitamin B Complex Tablets
Vitalin Tablets
Vitalzymes Capsules
Vitamin & Iron Tonic (Epitone) Solution

DRUGS AND OTHER SUBSTANCES NOT TO BE PRESCRIBED UNDER THE NHS PHARMACEUTICAL SERVICES

Vitamin A & D Capsules BPC 1968 (Regent
    Laboratories)
Vitamin A Ester & Vitamin D2 Capsules (Regent
    Laboratories)
Vitamin A Ester Capsules (Regent Laboratories)
Vitamin A Ester Conc, Alpha Tocopherol Acetate
    Nat Capsules (Regent Laboratories)
Vitamin A 4500 Units & Vitamin D2 Capsules
    (Regent Laboratories)
Vitamin A 6000 Units & Vitamin D2 Capsules
    (Regent Laboratories)
Vitamin A, C & D Tablets (Approved Prescription
    Services)
Vitamin A, D & C Tablets (Regent Laboratories)
Vitamin B Complex Tablets (English Grains)
Vitamin B Complex with Brewer's Yeast Tablets
    (English Grains)
Vitamin B1 Dried Yeast Powder (Distillers)
Vitamin B1 Yeast Tablets (Distillers)
Vitamin B12 Tablets 0.01 mg
Vitamin B12 Tablets 0.025 mg
Vitamin B12 Tablets 0.05 mg
Vitamin B12 Tablets 0.10 mg
Vitamin B12 Tablets 0.25 mg
Vitamin B12 Tablets 0.5 mg
Vitamin B12 Tablets 1 mg
Vitamin C Tablets (G & G Food Supplies)
Vitamin C Tablets Effervescent 1g
Vitamin Capsules (Regent Laboratories)
Vitamin Malt Extract with Orange Juice (Distillers)
Vitamin Mineral Capsules (Regent Laboratories)
Vitamin Tablets No B077
Vitamin Tablets No B081
Vitamin Tablets No B084
Vitaminised Iron & Yeast Tablets (Kirby Warrick
    Pharmaceuticals)
Vita Natura Evening Primrose Oil + Vitamin E
    Tablets
Vitanorm Malt Extract
Vitanorm Malt Extract Syrup
Vitapointe Conditioner
Vitasafe's CF Kaps Tablets
Vitasafe's WCF Kaps Tablets
Vita-Six Capsules
Vitathone Chilblain Tablets
Vitatrop Tablets
Vitavel Powder for Syrup
Vitavel Solution
Vitepron Tablets
Vitorange Tablets
Vitrite Multi-Vitamin Syrup
Vykamin Fortified Capsules

W L Tablets
Wallachol Syrup
Wallachol Tablets
Wate-on Emulsion
Wate-on Emulsion Super
Wate-on Tablets
Wate-on Tablets Super
Wate-on Tonic
Waterhouses All Fours
Wines

Woodwards Nursery Cream
Wrights Glucose with Vitamin D Powder
Wrights Vaporizing Fluid

Xanax Tablets 0.25 mg
Xanax Tablets 0.5 mg
Xanax Tablets 1.0 mg

Yeast & B12 Tablets (English Grains)
Yeast Plus Tablets (Thomas Guest)
Yeast-Vite Tablets
Yellow Phenolphthalein Tablets (any strength)
Yestamin Vitamin B5 Tablets

Zactirin Tablets
Zam Buk Ointment
Zefringe Sachets
Zemaphyte Chinese Herbal Eczema Remedy
Zendium Toothpaste
Zenoxone Cream
Zirtek 7
Zubes Expectorant Cough Syrup
Zubes Original Cough Mixture
Zyriton Expectorant Linctus

XVIIIA

DRUGS AND OTHER SUBSTANCES NOT TO BE PRESCRIBED UNDER THE NHS PHARMACEUTICAL SERVICES

This Page is Intentionally Blank

DRUGS TO BE PRESCRIBED IN CERTAIN CIRCUMSTANCES UNDER THE NHS PHARMACEUTICAL SERVICES

Part XVIIIB reproduces Schedule 2 to the National Health Service (General Medical Services Contracts) (Prescription of Drugs etc.) Regulations 2004.

Drugs in Column 1 of this part may be prescribed for persons mentioned in Column 2, only for the treatment of the purpose specified in Column 3. The Prescriber must endorse the prescription with the reference "SLS".

* "at-risk" means an adult or child patient or a patient over the age of 13 who-
(a) has chronic respiratory disease (including asthma and chronic obstructive pulmonary disease);
(b) has significant cardiovascular disease, excluding an adult or child patient who has hypertension only
(c) has chronic renal disease;
(d) are immunocompromised;
(e) has diabetes mellitus; or
(f) is aged 65 years or over;

Drug	Patient	Purpose
Clobazam	Any patient	Epilepsy
Cyanocobalamin Tablets	A patient who is a vegan or who has a proven vitamin B12 deficiency of dietary origin.	Treatment or prevention of vitamin B12 deficiency.
Locabiotal Aerosol	Any patient	Treatment of infections and inflammation of the oropharynx.
Niferex Elixir 30ml Paediatric Dropper Bottle	Infants born prematurely	Prophylaxis in treatment of iron deficiency
Nizoral Cream	Any patient	Treatment of seborrhoeic dermatitis and pityriasis versicolor

XVIIIB

DRUGS TO BE PRESCRIBED IN CERTAIN CIRCUMSTANCES UNDER THE NHS PHARMACEUTICAL SERVICES

Drug	Patient	Purpose
Oseltamivir (Tamiflu)	(1) *At-risk adult and child patients where-	Treatment of influenza
	(a) It has been determined in accordance with a community based virological surveillance scheme that influenza A or influenza B is circulating in the locality in which the patient resides or is present or was present at the time that the virus was circulating;	
	(b) the patient has an influenza-like illness; and	
	(c) the patient can start therapy within 48 hours of the onset of symptoms.	
	(2) *At-risk patients aged 13 years and older where-	Prophylaxis of influenza
	(a) It has been determined in accordance with a community based virological surveillance scheme that influenza A and influenza B is circulating in the locality in which the patient resides;	
	(b) the patient has been exposed to an influenza-like illness through being in close contact with someone with whom he lives who is or has been suffering from an influenza-like illness;	
	(c) the patient is not effectively protected by vaccination against influenza because- (i) he has not been vaccinated because vaccination is contraindicated; (ii) he has not been vaccinated since the previous influenza season; (iii) he has been vaccinated but it has yet to take effect; or (iv) he has been vaccinated but the vaccine is not well matched to the strain of influenza circulating in the locality in which the patient resides or is or has been present;	

DRUGS TO BE PRESCRIBED IN CERTAIN CIRCUMSTANCES UNDER THE NHS PHARMACEUTICAL SERVICES

Drug	Patient	Purpose
	(d) the patient lives in a residential care establishment and another resident or member of staff of the establishment has an influenza-like illness; and	
	(e) the patient can start prophylaxis within 48 hours of exposure to an influenza-like illness.	
Zanamivir (Relenza)	*At-risk adult patients where-	Treatment of influenza
	(a) It has been determined in accordance with a community based virological surveillance scheme that influenza A or influenza B is circulating in the locality in which the patient resides or is present or was present at the time that the virus was circulating;	
	(b) the patient has an influenza-like illness; and	
	(c) the patient can start therapy within 48 hours of the onset of symptoms	

XVIIIB

DRUGS TO BE PRESCRIBED IN CERTAIN CIRCUMSTANCES UNDER THE NHS PHARMACEUTICAL SERVICES

Drug		Patient	Purpose
The following drugs for the treatment of erectile dysfunction -	a)	a man with erectile dysfunction who on 14 September 1998 was receiving a course of treatment under the Act, the National Health Service (Scotland) Act 1978(a) or the Health and Personal Social Services (Northern Ireland) Order 1972(b) for this condition with any of the following drugs -	Treatment of erectile dysfunction.
Alprostadil (Caverject), (MUSE), (Viridal) Apomorphine Hydrochloride (Uprima) Moxisylyte Hydrochloride (Erecnos) Sildenafil (Viagra) Tadalafil (Cialis) Thymoxamine Hydrochloride (Erecnos) Vardenafil (Levitra)		Alprostadil (Caverject), (MUSE), (Viridal) Apomorphine Hydrochloride (Uprima) Moxisylyte Hydrochloride (Erecnos) Sildenafil (Viagra) Tadalafil (Cialis) Thymoxamine Hydrochloride (Erecnos); or	
	b)	a man who is a national of an EEA State who is entitled to treatment by virtue of Article 7(2) of Council Regulation 1612/68(c) as extended by the EEA Agreement or by virtue of any other enforceable Community right who has erectile dysfunction and was on 14th September 1998 receiving a course of treatment under a national health insurance system of an EEA State for this condition with any of the drugs listed in sub-paragraph (a); or	
	c)	a man who is not a national of an EEA State but who is the member of the family of such a national who has an enforceable Community right to be treated no less favourably than the national in the provision of medical treatment and has erectile dysfunction and was being treated for that condition on 14th September 1998 with any of the drugs listed in sub-paragraph (a); or	
	d)	a man who is suffering from any of the following - diabetes multiple sclerosis Parkinson's disease poliomyelitis prostate cancer severe pelvic injury single gene neurological disease spina bifida spinal cord injury; or	
	e)	a man who is receiving treatment for renal failure by dialysis; or	
	f)	a man who has had the following surgery - prostatectomy radical pelvic surgery renal failure treated by transplant.	

(a) 1978 c.29

(b) SI 1972/1265 (NI 14)

(c) OJ No.L257, 19.10.68, p.22 (OJ/SE 1968(II) p.475)

CRITERIA NOTIFIED UNDER THE TRANSPARENCY DIRECTIVE

Criteria notified to the European Commission under Article 7 of the Council Directive relating to the transparency of measures regulating the pricing of medicinal products for human use and their inclusion in the scope of national health insurance schemes (89/105/EEC)

The following six criteria have been separately notified by the UK Government to the European Commission since 1989 to comply with Article 7 of the Transparency Directive.

First, under the Selected List Scheme, medicinal products in seventeen therapeutic categories which are excluded from prescription on the grounds that, on expert advice, they had no clinical or therapeutic advantage over other, cheaper, drugs in the following categories:-

mild to moderate painkillers
indigestion remedies
laxatives
cough and cold remedies
vitamins
tonics
benzodiazepine sedatives and tranquillisers
anti-diarrhoeal drugs
drugs for allergic disorders
hypnotics and anxiolytics
appetite suppressants
drugs for vaginal and vulval conditions
contraceptives
drugs used in anaemia
topical anti-rheumatics
drugs acting on the ear and nose
drugs acting on the skin

Second, products may be considered as "borderline substances" which are not truly medicinal products with clinical or therapeutic value and are excluded from NHS prescription on that ground.

Third, as well as being freely available on sale over the counter to the general public the cost to the NHS if the product(s) were to be supplied on prescription could not be justified at any price likely to be economic to the manufacturer and that the supply of the product is not considered a priority for the use of the limited resources available to the NHS.

Fourth, that products which nonetheless may meet a legitimate clinical or therapeutic need when properly prescribed, are subject to misuse by drug misusers, and such misuse, or the manner in which the product is administered by drug misusers, gives rise to the risk of physical or mental morbidity and alternative products are available to meet all legitimate clinical or therapeutic needs.

Fifth, a medicinal product or a category of medicinal products may be excluded entirely from supply on NHS prescription. It may alternatively be excluded except in specified circumstances, or except in relation to specified conditions or categories of condition, or specified categories of patient. A medicinal product or a category of them may be so excluded where the forecast aggregate cost to the NHS of allowing the product (or category of products) to be supplied on NHS prescription, or to be supplied more widely than the permitted exceptions, could not be justified having regard to all the relevant circumstances including in particular: the Secretary of State's duties pursuant to the NHS Act 1977 and the priorities for expenditure of NHS resources.

Sixth, products which comprise an injection device prefilled with a drug may be excluded from supply on NHS prescription if the same drug is available and can be used more economically in a container which may be used in conjunction with a refillable injection device.

XVIIIC

CRITERIA NOTIFIED UNDER THE TRANSPARENCY DIRECTIVE

This Page is Intentionally Blank

PAYMENTS TO CHEMISTS SUSPENDED BY A PRIMARY CARE TRUST OR BY DIRECTION OF THE FHSAA

This Determination is made by the Secretary of State under regulation 58 of the National Health Service (Pharmaceutical Services) Regulations 2005[1] and regulation 18A of the National Health Service (Pharmaceutical Services) Regulations 1992.

1.   **Interpretation**

      1.1   Unless the context otherwise requires, words and phrases used in this Determination have the same meaning as they have in the National Health Service (Pharmaceutical Services) Regulations 2005 ("the 2005 Regulations") in relation to England, and the same meaning as they have in the National Health Service (Pharmaceutical Services) Regulations 1992 ("the 1992 Regulations") in relation to Wales.

2.   **Calculation of payments to be made to suspended chemists**

      2.1   Where a chemist is suspended by direction of the FHSAA, or by a Primary Care Trust (PCT) in England or a Local Health Board (LHB) in Wales as the case may be, a PCT in England or a Local Health Board shall make payments to him, calculated in accordance with this Determination.

      2.2   Where the suspended chemist has undertaken to provide pharmaceutical services from two or more premises in the area of a PCT or the area of a LHB, payments shall be calculated separately in respect of each of those premises.

      2.3   Upon receipt of a claim from the chemist, the PCT or LHB shall pay to the suspended chemist in respect of each complete calendar month during which he is suspended an amount equal to his reference remuneration, calculated in accordance with paragraph 3.

      2.4   For any calendar month during which the chemist was suspended for less than the whole month, payment shall be reduced pro rata to the number of days (including weekends and Bank Holidays) during which the chemist was suspended.

      2.5   If when the chemist is first suspended, the PCT or LHB does not have available to it all the details of the fees and allowances which it needs in order to calculate reference remuneration in accordance with paragraph 3, it shall estimate the reference remuneration on the basis of the information which is available to it, and make payments accordingly. When the full information becomes available, it shall recalculate the reference remuneration, and adjust its payments accordingly.

      2.6   The PCT or LHB shall also recalculate the reference remuneration (and, where appropriate, any additional payment or deduction under paragraphs 6 to 9 below) if the chemist ceases to be included in the pharmaceutical list in respect of any premises, or if the PCTs for England or LHBs for Wales receive new information about the fees and allowances to which he was entitled. The PCT or LHB shall adjust its monthly payments accordingly.

3.   **Reference Remuneration**

      3.1   A chemist's 'reference remuneration' is the total of the relevant fees and allowances (as defined in paragraph 4 below) to which he was entitled in respect of the relevant period (as defined in paragraph 5 below) in relation to the premises in question, divided by the number of months in the relevant period.

      3.2   For example, if the relevant fees and allowances for a given set of premises come to £12,000, and the relevant period for those premises is ten months, the reference remuneration will be £12,000/10 = £1200.   If the relevant period is the full twelve months, the reference remuneration would be £12,000/12 = £1000.

      3.3   Where a chemist is included in the pharmaceutical list of a PCT or a pharmaceutical list of a LHB both as a person who has undertaken to provide pharmaceutical services by way of the provision of drugs and by way of the provision of appliances in respect of the same premises, and the relevant period for the two types of service differ, the two sets of relevant fees and allowances shall be calculated separately for the purposes of determining reference remuneration.

XIX

[1] S.I.2005/641

PAYMENTS TO CHEMISTS SUSPENDED BY A PRIMARY CARE TRUST OR BY DIRECTION OF THE FHSAA

4. **Relevant Fees and Allowances**

    4.1   Relevant Fees and allowances means:

        (a) Professional Fees payable under clause 1 of Part IIIA of the Drug Tariff;

        (b) Additional or Special Fees payable under clause 2 of Part IIIA;

        (c) Fees for dispensing appliances, payable under Part IIIB;

        (d) Payment for Essential Services (Pharmacy Contractors) payable under Part VIA;

        (e) On-Cost Allowance for Appliance Contractors payable under Part VIB;

        (f) Payment for advanced services (pharmacy contractors) payable under Part VIC;

        (g) Payments for any enhanced services (pharmacy contractors) payable under Part VID;

        (h) Payments under the Essential Small Pharmacies Scheme payable under Part XII;

        (i) Payments in respect of Pre-Registration Trainees under Part XIII;

        (j) Payments for Oxygen Therapy Services (including service element and hardware, but excluding compensation for financial loss in respect of oxygen equipment paid under regulation 56(1)(j) of the 2005 Regulations as determined by the PCT or paid under regulation 18(1)(i) of the 1992 Regulations as determined by the LHB).

    4.2   For the purposes of calculating reference remuneration, relevant fees and allowances to which the chemist was entitled in respect of any part of the relevant period (as defined in paragraph 5) prior to 1 April 2005, other than those listed at (c) and (e) in paragraph 4.1, shall be increased by 3.225%.

    4.3   For example, if the relevant period were to be July 2004 to June 2005, reference remuneration would be calculated by reference to

        the relevant fees and allowances for July 2004 to March 2005, increased by 3.225%; and

        the relevant fees and allowances for April to June 2005, without any increase.

5. **Relevant Period**

    5.1   Where, prior to the suspension, the chemist has been included in the pharmaceutical list in respect of premises for less than 12 complete calendar months, the relevant period for those premises is the number of complete calendar months during which the chemist was so included in the pharmaceutical list.

    5.2   In all other cases, the relevant period is the last twelve complete calendar months immediately prior to the suspension.

    5.3   For example, if a chemist is suspended on 12 November 2005, the relevant period for each set of premises would normally be 1 November 2004 to 31 October 2005 (i.e. 12 months). But if the chemist was first included in the pharmaceutical list on 3 April 2005, the relevant period will be 1 May 2005 to 31 October 2005 (i.e. 6 months).

    5.4   Where a chemist has, under regulation 5 (1) (b) (ii) or 5 (1) (c) of the 2005 Regulations (where the premises are in England) or 4 (3) (a) of the 1992 Regulations (where the premises are in Wales), relocated the premises from which he provides pharmaceutical services, only the period after that relocation (or the last such relocation) is to form part of the relevant period.

    5.5   The provisions in paragraph 5.4 do not apply where a chemist has already been suspended and a relocation of the premises from which he provides pharmaceutical services takes place subsequent to that suspension (for example by virtue of a temporary chemist applying to change premises on behalf of the suspended chemist under regulation 9 (3)).

    5.6   Where a chemist began to provide pharmaceutical services from premises in place of another chemist under regulation 8 (1) of the 2005 Regulations (if the premises are in England) or 4 (3) (b) of the 1992 Regulations (if the premises are in Wales) and is then suspended, only the period after that change of ownership is to form part of the relevant period.

PAYMENTS TO CHEMISTS SUSPENDED BY A PRIMARY CARE TRUST OR BY DIRECTION OF THE FHSAA

6.   Additional Payments

6.1   Where the PCT or LHB is satisfied that, but for suspension, a pharmacy contractor would have been entitled to a higher rate of payment for Essential Services in Part VIA in respect of the month in which he was suspended than he in fact received, the PCT for England and LHB for Wales shall make an additional payment to him.

6.2   That payment shall be the difference between the amount the contractor received in respect of that month and the amount to which, by reference to payments in previous months, the PCT or LHB believes he would have been entitled but for the suspension.

6.3   Payment shall be made as soon as practicable after the PCT or LHB has available to it final details of the amount of Payment for Essential Services that was actually made to the contractor in respect of the month in question.

Payments for temporary chemists

6.4   Where the PCT for England has granted, under the provisions of regulation 54 of the 2005 Regulations, approval to a temporary chemist to provide pharmaceutical services at the relevant premises in place of the suspended chemist, and is further satisfied that the suspended chemist is paying to the temporary chemist a payment whether by way of fee, salary or other emolument, additional to any agreed share of payments made under paragraph 4 above, in respect of the month in which he was suspended, the PCT for England shall reimburse the suspended chemist the fee, salary or other emolument, up to a maximum of £150 per day.

7.   Deductions from Payments

7.1   *Essential Small Pharmacies Scheme*

7.1.1   Where the PCT or LHB is satisfied that, but for suspension, a pharmacy contractor would have been entitled under Part XII of the Drug Tariff to lower payments under the Essential Small Pharmacies Scheme in respect of the month during which he was suspended than he in fact received, the PCT or LHB shall make a deduction from its monthly payment to him.

7.1.2   That deduction shall be the difference between the amount the contractor received in respect of that month and the amount to which, by reference to payments in previous months, the PCT or LHB believes he would have been entitled but for the suspension.

7.1.3   Such deduction shall be made as soon as practicable after the PCT or LHB has available to it final details of the amount of payments under the Essential Small Pharmacies Scheme that was actually made to the contractor in respect of the month in question.

7.2   *On-cost allowance for Appliance Contractors*

7.2.1   Where the PCT or LHB is satisfied that, but for suspension, a supplier of appliances would have been entitled under Part VIB of the Drug Tariff to a lower level of on-cost allowance in respect of the month during which he was suspended than he in fact received, the PCT or LHB shall made a deduction from its monthly payment to him.

7.2.2   That deduction shall be the difference between the amount the supplier of appliances received in respect of that month and the amount to which, by reference to payments in previous months, the PCT or LHB believes he would have been entitled but for the suspension.

7.2.3   Such deduction shall be made as soon as practicable once the PCT or LHB has available to it final details of the level of on-cost that was actually paid to the supplier of appliances in respect of the month in question.

XIX

PAYMENTS TO CHEMISTS SUSPENDED BY A PRIMARY CARE TRUST OR BY DIRECTION OF THE FHSAA

8.   Claims for payment

8.1   The suspended chemist shall claim payments under this determination, by notifying the PCT or LHB in writing. When first making the claim, and subsequently as necessary, the suspended chemist shall provide such information as the PCT or LHB may reasonably require for the purposes of establishing the chemist's entitlement to, or the level of, payments.

9.   Arrangements for payment

9.1   Upon receipt of a claim from the suspended chemist, payments shall be made in arrears as soon as practicable following the end of each calendar month, starting at the end of the month following that in which the chemist was suspended. For example, if the chemist is suspended on 27 August, the first payment will be due as soon as practical after 30 September.

10.   Termination of payment

10.1   No claim for payment may be made in respect of any period after which the suspended chemist has, under regulation 9 (1) of the 2005 Regulations, disposed of the premises from which he was providing pharmaceutical services prior to his suspension.

Signed and dated by Jeanette Howe, Head of Pharmacy, Dept of Health, 1 April 2005

PRIVATE PRESCRIPTIONS FOR CONTROLLED DRUGS

For England only, following the Government's response to the Fourth Report of the Shipman Inquiry (Safer Management of Controlled Drugs), the requirements for private prescriptions for controlled drugs have changed.

From 1 April 2006 all private prescriptions issued for controlled drugs in Schedule 2 or 3 to the Misuse of Drugs Regulations 2001 must be ordered using the prescription form designed specially for this purpose (FP10PCD). Following dispensing, photocopy FP10PCD prescription forms must be submitted to the NHS Business Services Authority (NHSBSA) for audit purposes.

Submission of Forms

One FP34PCD submission document must be completed and submitted with each monthly submission of photocopy FP10PCD prescription forms. The submission document is available at www.ppa.org.uk along with guidance on how to complete the document.

The photocopy prescriptions must be packed securely and dispatched to the NHS Business Services Authority by no later than the fifth day of the month following that in which they were supplied.

The FP34PCD submission document and photocopy FP10PCD prescription forms must be submitted to the following address:

NHSBSA, Prescription Pricing Division
Division 3 Newcastle
Goods Entrance (off Dean Street)
Bridge House
152 Pilgrim Street
Newcastle upon Tyne
NE1 6SN

Please ensure that photocopy FP10PCD prescription forms are only sent with the relevant FP34PCD submission document and are not included in the monthly submission of NHS prescription forms.

XX

PRIVATE PRESCRIPTIONS FOR CONTROLLED DRUGS

This Page is Intentionally Blank

INDEX

INDEX

INDEX

INDEX

NOTES

Printed in the United Kingdom for The Stationery Office
978-0-11-783162-9 C255 02/07